XXV International Conference on Sports Rehabilitation and Traumatology

FOOTBALL MEDICINE STRATEGIES RETURN TO PLAY

In partnership with
FIFA Football for Health F-Marc

Abstract book

Editors
Giulio Sergio Roi
Stefano Della Villa

SALUS SCIENTIA SPORT
EDUCATION RESEARCH DEPARTMENT
ISOKINETIC

CALZETTI MARIUCCI
e d i t o r i

Football Medicine Strategies - Return to play

ISBN 978-88-6028-466-2

Roberto Calzetti Editore srl
Via del Sottopasso, 7 – Loc. Ferriera
06089 Torgiano PG
www.calzetti-mariucci.it
e-mail: sport@calzetti-mariucci.it
Tel./Fax 075 5997310

Graphic designers and proofreaders: Dino Festa, Daniele Calzoni
Cover designer: Massimiliano Baccanti

ABSTRACT BOOK

FOREWORD

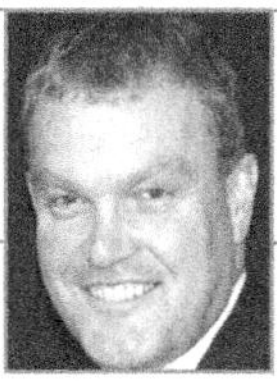
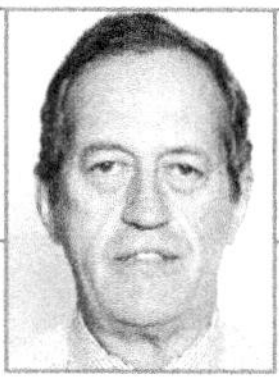
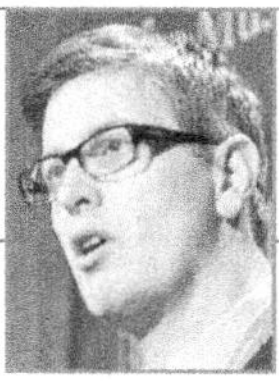
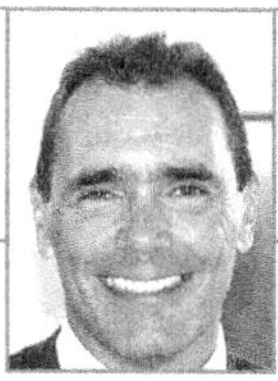
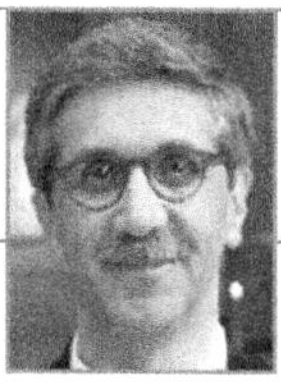

A recent study showed that only 55% of players return to competitive sport following an Anterior Cruciate Ligament (ACL) reconstruction (1). Furthermore, it is also demonstrated that the risk of sustaining a subsequent new ACL injury is 5.8% for the ipsilateral and 11.8% for the contralateral limb at a minimum of five years follow up (2).
At the fundamental base, it is all about Return To Play (RTP), and the only question doctors, players and teams seem to care about is: "When will the player be back on the field, safely?"

RTP is a broad subject, and this abstract book of the XXV International Conference on Sports Rehabilitation and Traumatology is dedicated to the topic of Football Medicine Strategies for Player Care. The aim is to give to the reader a wider vision; one which can help to be successful in her/his career. We try to do this by sharing the expertise and knowledge that has taken those individual practitioners and professionals to the top of Football Medicine and Science.

Indeed, the Conference is, above all, an opportunity for discussion and represents an opportunity for the exchange of ideas and experiences. Therefore in this book, in addition to the abstracts the invited speakers sent to us before the conference, we have inserted all of the abstracts that have been accepted for free oral communication, poster presentation and workshops.
More specifically, Return to Play is analysed through sharing different points of view and disciplines: sports science, sports medicine, orthopaedics, physical therapy, psychology, general medicine, radiology, chiropractic and osteopathy, podiatrists, athletic training and team coaching. Through this multidisciplinary approach the reader can gain a deeper understanding of the whole sports medicine and rehabilitation process, and not only the techniques themselves.

Our overall purpose is to bring health in the world of Football. There are nearly 300 million football players in the world and we want to help, so that when you are part of the team caring for player health, you will have the skills to be at the top of the world's Football Medicine Community.
We are confident from previous experience of editions of the International Conference on Sports Rehabilitation and Traumatology that this volume will further feed the debate on the Football Medicine Strategies for Player Care, and we thank all of the Authors who contributed to the realisation of this book.

Phil Batty
Peter Brukner
Mike Davison
Stefano Della Villa
Giulio Sergio Roi

London, March 2016

References

1. Ardern CL, Taylor NF, Feller JA, Webster KE. Fifty-five per cent return to competitive sport following anterior cruciate ligament reconstruction surgery: an updated systematic review and meta-analysis including aspects of physical functioning and contextual factors. Br J Sports Med 2014; 48: 1543-1552
2. Wright RW, Magnussen RA, Dunn WR, Spindler KP. Ipsilateral graft and contralateral ACL rupture at five years or more following ACL reconstruction: a systematic review. J Bone Joint Surg Am 2011; 93: 1159-1165

CONTENTS

Saturday 9th April, 2016 (morning)
FLEMING ROOM

INVITED SPEAKERS

THE INTERNATIONAL LANDSCAPE OF RETURN TO PLAY

Chairs

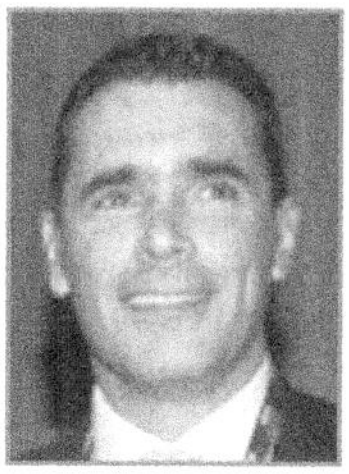

Stefano Della Villa
(Bologna, Italy)

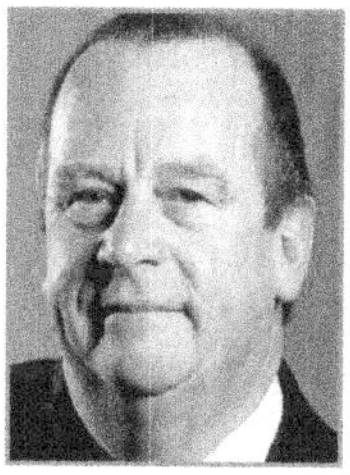

Michael D'Hooghe
(Bruges, Belgium)

9:15 Scientific review on return to play
Roald Bahr (Oslo, Norway)

9:30 Surgical implications for return to play in the elite athlete
Riley Williams III (New York, USA)

9:45 Role of clinical judgement in return to play decisions
Phil Batty (London, United Kingdom)

10:00 The historical battle in return to play decisions: criteria vs time
Lynn Snyder-Mackler (Newark, USA)

10:15 Return to play: the role of the team doctor
Jiri Dvorak (Zürich, Switzerland)

10:30 Diploma in Football Medicine
Mark Fulcher (Aukland, New Zeland)

10:45 Discussion

11:00 End of the Session

SURGEON PERSPECTIVES ON RETURN TO PLAY IN THE ELITE ATHLETE

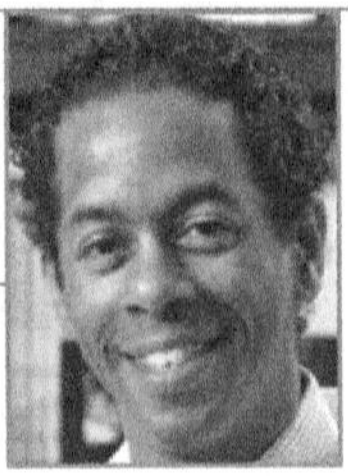

Williams RJ III

New York Red Bulls and Hospital for Special Surgery, FIFA Medical Centre of Excellence, New York, USA

Return To Play (RTP) decisions require judgement under pressure. This presentation aims to offer an insight from a surgeon's perspective on how to deal with this.

Sporting Environment

Elite athletes inhabit a unique environment. It is inappropriate to treat them in the same way as a non-sporting patient. Conditions may be the same, but their implications are very different. Understanding the environment in which a player has to be involved makes it easier for a surgeon to accept RTP that is as soon as feasible. Never forget that a RTP time must not put a player at risk.

'It's a Team Game'

At the beginning of my work with athletes in '99, I would be sent a player by a Club for surgery and I would set a RTP date, which would be adhered to without question. Whilst my life was easier then, it was not necessarily the best way to treat many athletes! Now at times I am challenged to justify my RTP plan. If I cannot I must acknowledge the expertise of others in the medical team and I will alter my RTP regime. Quite rightly RTP planning involves discussion between the surgeon and Club medical staff as well as the player.

The team I refer to is a multidisciplinary one. Since a surgeon is the only member of this team practising outside the club environment, it is easier to notice differences in progress as assessment is made at intervals in clinic, and surgeons' pronouncements can help take pressure off the medical team and player back at the Club. Within the decision making group the surgeon is the one with the largest experience of recoveries following surgery. To help gain most from this experience surgeons must record data and be committed to investigating apparent differences in recovery between certain cases. E.g., the fact that in footballers the outcome after meniscectomy is much worse in the lateral rather than medial meniscus (3).

The surgeon must resist the temptation to use a 'cookbook' approach to rehabilitation. Not all cases are the same in terms of the pathology and therefore surgical detail, nor the individual's physiological response. Because of this it is essential that there is an appreciation that therefore progression in rehabilitation has to be according to achievement of certain milestones (the 'traffic light philosophy' - see below).

It is easy to forget we cannot beat Nature! The time to return to play is usually either specific to the tissue damaged and operated upon, e.g. chondral damage versus meniscal versus ligamentous surgery, or related to the time required to restore adequate neuromuscular control to make it safe to return to play.

Surgeons Role in Quality Control

Whilst respecting all team-members involved in deciding on RTP, if clearly what is planned for a player is wrong in my opinion, then I must tactfully state my view.
One of the privileges of working with professional athletes is the opportunity for clinical research, which can lead to improvements in the medical care of not only athletes but all patients. E.g., my data shows the re-rupture rate following Anterior Cruciate Ligament (ACL) reconstruction in professional footballers is around double when hamstring tendons are used compared with patellar tendon graft- in my hands (2).
Basic science study is valuable. At Imperial College we described the anterolateral ligament (1). Whilst this caused considerable interest, further study showed it is not very important but connections of the iliotibial band to the femur provide very powerful control of internal rotation (Kittl C, El Daou H, Athwal KK, Gupte CM, Weiler A, Williams A, Amis AA. The role of the anterolateral structures and the ACL in controlling laxity of the intact and ACL-deficient knee. Am J Sports Med Dec 10. pii: 0363546515614312. [Epub ahead of print]). This work may lead to refining of ACL reconstruction techniques.

'Naming the Day'

After surgery an estimate of time to RTP is made. My personal approach is described as follows:
1. The 'traffic light' approach to rehabilitation, as popularised by the Isokinetic group, is employed so that the player has passed every landmark appropriately during recovery.
2. Aerobic fitness: the player must be fit or they will fatigue and their neuromuscular control will be compromised.
3. No swelling.
4. The player must be confident.
5. Symmetry – in many ways this is the most important factor. The closer the operated limb muscle function limb is to normal the better. My preference is for a deficit on functional testing or isokinetic testing to be within 10% of the other side. This is a worse scenario and of course I like it to be better.

Conclusions

Decision making to guide RTP after surgery for an athlete is not easy. There is objective evidence to help, but experience and a team approach is invaluable.

References

1. Clatworthy M, Pearle A, Williams A, Lind M. Current concepts: femoral tunnel placement in ACL-reconstruction: central footprint versus AM Bundle. ISAKOS Newsletter 2015; 2: 24-31
2. Dodds AL, Halewood C, Gupte MC, Williams A, Amis AA. The anterolateral ligament: anatomy, length changes and association with the Segond fracture. Bone Joint J 2014; 96-B: 325-331
3. Nawabi NH, Cro S, Hamid IP, Williams A. Return to play after lateral meniscectomy compared with medial meniscectomy in elite professional soccer players. Am J Sports Med 2014; 42: 2193-2198

ROLE OF CLINICAL JUDGEMENT IN RETURN TO PLAY DECISIONS

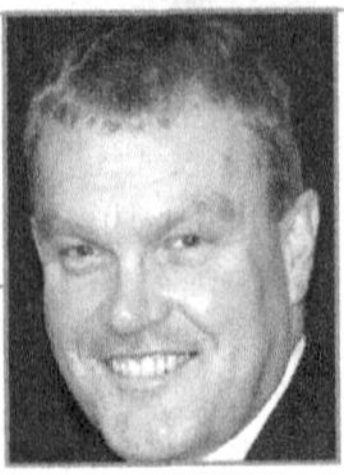

Batty P

Isokinetic Medical Group, FIFA Medical Centre of Excellence, London, United Kingdom

Professional football is well resourced to provide state of the art rehabilitation facilities and to be at the cutting edge of rehabilitation from injury. There has been an increase in investment as revenue has increased, and this includes the medical and rehabilitation teams. Studies identified methods to quantify functional rehabilitation in football (Fuller CW, Walker J. Quantifying the functional rehabilitation of injured football players. Br J Sports Med 2006; 40: 151-157; discussion 151-157), however there remains a paucity of high quality evidence to show the effectiveness of football rehabilitation interventions and particular transference of these methods to the exercising population at large (Lohmander LS, Roos EM. The evidence base for orthopaedics and sports medicine. BMJ. 2015 Jan 2;350:g7835. doi: 10.1136/bmj.g7835.).

The lack of good evidence creates an environment of uncertainty in professional sport, with conflicting pressures for an athlete to Return To Play (RTP). Medical teams will vary in their perception of risk, and this can also influenced by the patient, coach and fixture list.

Risk is mitigated through informed consent, patient autonomy, continuous close monitoring, open communication and the application of common sense despite a limited evidence base (3).

Concussion is possibly the only area where there is consensus regarding diagnosis and clear RTP criteria (2). This protocol involves limited use of diagnostic investigations, with tools to support RTP based on clinical criteria and assessment. There is very little consensus regarding RTP criteria for hamstring injury (Van der Hortst N, van de Hoef S, Reurink G, Huisstede B, Backx F. Return to play after hamstring injuries: a qualitative systematic review of definitions and criteria. Sports Med 2016 Jan 14. [Epub ahead of print]), of which there has been an increase since 2001 (1).

Clinical judgment is increasingly undervalued with the technological advances in diagnostics (Kienle GS, Kiene H. Clinical judgement and the medical profession. J Eval Clin Pract 2011; 17: 621-627). Are we becoming more interested in what the scan or test shows rather than what the patient informs us by way of history and examination?

RTP criteria needs to be based on clinical and functional information. Consensus is not possible in elite football where there are competing interests and a lack of evidence.

References

1. Ekstrand J, Waldén M, Hägglund M. Hamstring injuries have increased by 4% annually in men's professional football, since 2001: a 13-year longitudinal analysis of the UEFA Elite Club injury study. Br J Sports Med. 2016 Jan 8. pii: bjsports-2015-095359. doi: 10.1136/bjsports-2015-095359. [Epub ahead of print]
2. McCrory P, Meeuwisse WH, Aubry M, Cantu B, Dvorák J, Echemendia RJ, Engebretsen L, Johnston K, Kutcher JS, Raftery M, Sills A, Benson BW, Davis GA, Ellenbogen RG, Guskiewicz K, Herring SA, Iverson GL, Jordan BD, Kissick J, McCrea M, McIntosh AS, Maddocks D, Makdissi M, Purcell L, Putukian M, Schneider K, Tator CH, Turner M. Consensus statement on concussion in sport: the 4th International Conference on Concussion in Sport held in Zurich, November 2012. Br J Sports Med. 2013; 47: 250-258
3. Weiler R, Monte-Colombo M, Mitchell A, Haddad F. Non-operative management of a complete anterior cruciate ligament injury in an English Premier League football player with return to play in less than 8 weeks: applying common sense in the absence of evidence. BMJ Case Rep. 2015 Apr 26;2015. pii: bcr2014208012. doi: 10.1136/bcr-2014-208012

THE HISTORICAL BATTLE IN RETURN TO PLAY DECISIONS: CRITERIA VS TIME

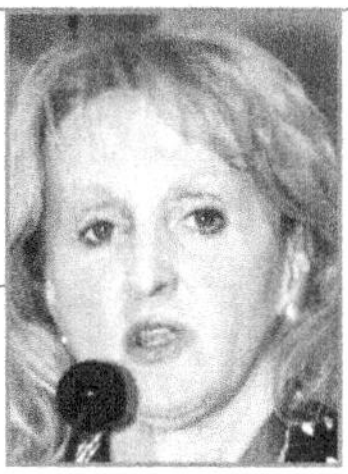

Snyder-Mackler L

University of Delaware, Newark, USA

The question of how quickly to allow patients to safely return to sport after injury has driven clinical practice and research for years. The ultimate battle is painted as timed based (based on healing) versus criterion-based. The answer is we must use both!

Ultimately, surgical success is a race between biologic healing and failure of fixation. In our football players, pathology involves healing of soft tissue, bone, and articular cartilage. All soft tissue healing is not equal. Both the quality of the injured tissue and its intrinsic healing potential determine the timing and magnitude of the stress we can apply to the healing structures (e.g., functional activities, exercises, mobilization).

Surgical repair is restricted to structures with healing potential. Repair restores normal anatomy (e.g., suturing an injured structure back together). When healing potential is limited, either because of the inherent properties of the tissues involved (e.g., Anterior Cruciate Ligament) or because the extent of the injury is too great (e.g., complex tear of the meniscus), repair is unlikely to be successful even with significantly modified rehabilitation. Repair in this instance would be a failure for the surgeon, the rehabilitation specialist, and most importantly, the patient; therefore, the structure must be resected (removed) or preferably, reconstructed (replaced).

Rehabilitation specialists strive to resolve impairments (e.g., range of motion, weakness, inflammation) as quickly as safely possible. Not all tissue is of good quality, and not all fixation is rigid. Therefore, adjustments in protocol are necessary to protect the surgical site until biologic healing has progressed to permit the demands of a rehabilitation program. Primary and associated pathologies, the primary surgical procedure, and the associated, intraoperative measures taken to allow accelerated rehabilitation (i.e., rehabilitation-modified surgery), and intraoperative and postoperative surgical concerns are discussed. All must be considered by the clinician to create and modify the rehabilitation pathways.

The sports medicine team needs to consider player age, experience, talent, importance of the competition, time left in the competitive season, in the return to play decision, but only after the tissue is deemed healed enough to safely return.

When the athlete has progressed through a criterion based rehab progression and achieved all the milestones necessary, return-to-play progression may begin. The basic return-to-play lower extremity progression incorporates the following: straight-plane movements, lateral movements, cutting at progressive angles, sport-specific agility, mirroring practice, return to practice, and return to play. When to advance athletes along this continuum is based on clinical decision making involving all the aforementioned aspects mentioned in this chapter. The basis behind this is to slowly introduce these complex movements in a controlled environment before returning to play. The intensity and difficulty can be altered as progression continues. The athlete must be able to complete each progression at 100% intensity before moving to the next level. An often forgotten aspect of the return-to play-progression is psychologic readiness to return to play. One way to objectively assess this factor is through the use of outcome measures. When the time comes for return to sport, the athlete may be permitted either full return or a graded return. A graded return to sport occurs when the athlete is limited to a certain amount of playing time, which is then progressed until unlimited play occurs. The last step in formulating treatment pathways is to develop a way to help prevent the athlete from becoming reinjured. The biggest predictors of risk for injury is previous injury. The athlete must have a plan in place to minimize this risk.

RETURN TO PLAY: THE ROLE OF THE TEAM DOCTOR

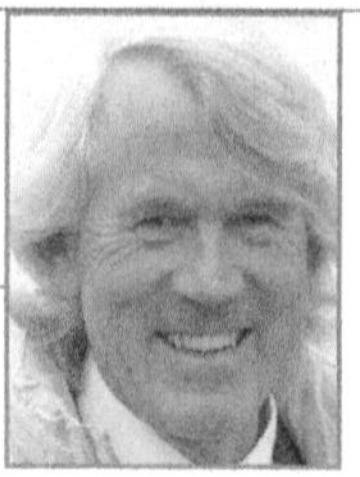

Dvorak J

FIFA Medical Assessment & Research Centre (F-MARC),
Schulthess Clinic, Zürich, Switzerland

Maintaining the player's health is the primary objective of team doctors - the prevention of injuries and the appropriate management in the event of an injury on the pitch and/or at the sideline.
The team doctor also determines the decision whether the player returns to the pitch or how long he/she should be absent from training and matches.
The primary duty of a doctor is to act in the best interest of the patient, which in our case, is the player.
We follow the Hippocratic Oath including our professional medical ethical principles.
The Team Physician is quite often under pressure by the manager, the coach and even by the player himself/herself to return quickly to the field of play.
There are two emergency situations that require immediate action and the team doctor's decision, unrelated to the constraints, the coach or even the referee's opinion and these are, the suspicion of a sudden cardiac arrest and a head injury with suspected concussion.
In order to prevent potential conflicts between the doctor's opinion/decision, and the coach, education on team spirit is necessary.

"11 for coaches" – Recommendations for health within football teams

1. Respect your medical team, understand each other and communicate consistently.
2. Organise at the beginning of the season: prevention, first-aid, treatment & rehab management in your team.
3. Customise your training sessions & consider environmental factors (heat/cold).
4. Allow player's time to recover (consider different age group regeneration!).
5. Implement prevention programmes like the 11+.
6. Offer education in active ways on how to avoid injuries.
7. Encourage a balanced nutrition and avoid supplements and drugs (consider the 2015 World Anti-Doping Code).
8. Respect mental and psychological status of the players.
9. Help build a consensus within the players, coaches, medical staff and athletic trainers.
10. Promote safe and effective return to play after injuries and illness.
11. Be fair and open for changes and improvement in football medicine and science.

From the medical viewpoint, following and understanding the recommendations will no doubt reduce potential conflicts of interest, ensuring that the health of the player is the main objective.

Saturday 9th April, 2016 (morning)
FLEMING ROOM

INVITED SPEAKERS

BASIC SCIENCE AND RETURN TO PLAY

Chairs

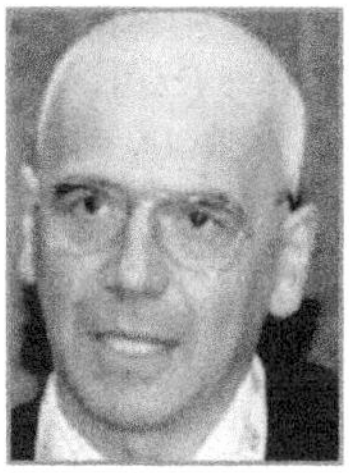

Alberto Gobbi
(Milan, Italy)

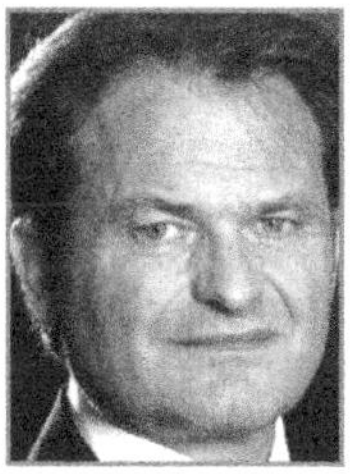

Bertrand Sonnery-Cottet
(Lyon, France)

11:30 Injury pattern and return to play principles
Ian Shirer (Montreal, Canada)

11:45 Overview of biomechanics, orthobiologics and return to play issues
Bert Mandelbaum (Santa Monica, United States)

12:00 Surgical advances for earlier return to play
Christoph Erggelert (Zürich, Switzerland)

12:15 Progressive mechanical stimuli in the recovery process
Jill Cook (Melbourne, Australia)

12:30 Neuroscience: "brain pain" and sport recovery
Mark Lindsay (Toronto, Canada)

12:45 Discussion

13:00 End of the Session

1

INJURY PATTERNS AND RETURN TO PLAY PRINCIPLES

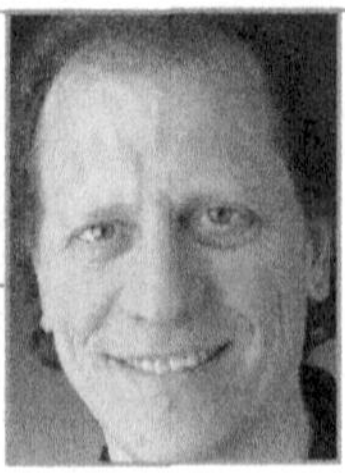

Shrier I

Centre for Clinical Epidemiology, Lady Davis Institute, Jewish General Hospital, McGill University, Montreal, Canada

Every patient visiting a clinician with an injury wants to know when it is safe to Return To Play (RTP). Recommendations for RTP are based on a large number of factors including the history of the injury, physical examination, type of injury, rehabilitation, type of activity, psychological state, competitive level and ability to protect the injury. In addition, the clinician must weigh the risk of reinjury in the short term as well as long term consequences and other issues. The different combinations of these factors sometimes make it difficult for the clinician to navigate through the decision-making process. In addition, the athlete may receive conflicting opinions from other clinicians, family, friends, coaches and agents. Such conflicts can lead to negative consequences including loss of trust, unnecessary fear of reinjury when risk is low, and serious medical complications when athletes return to activity while still at unacceptable levels of risk for subsequent sport-related injury.

One factor that may minimize such conflict is to have a formal structure that makes the RTP decision reasoning more transparent. The Strategic Assessment of Risk and Risk Tolerance (StARRT) framework is an updated version of a decision theoretic model for RTP decision-making originally published in 2010, in which the decision-making process is divided into three steps (1).

The first two steps, Tissue Health (stress the tissue can withstand) and Tissue Stresses (stress applied to the tissue) assess risk, and the third step evaluates the effect of factors that modify the clinician's tolerance to risk (Risk Tolerance modifiers).

The model has been shown to be consistent with clinician RTP decision making based on simulated clinical vignettes.

Recent pilot work on actual case studies suggests risk estimates from different clinicians evaluating the same case can be considerably different, and that risk tolerance modifiers are considered during routine clinical care.

References

1. Shrier I. Strategic Assessment of Risk and Risk Tolerance (StARRT) framework for return-to-play decision-making. Br J Sports Med 2015; 49: 1311-1315

OVERVIEW OF ORTHOBIOLOGICAL AND BIOMECHANICAL AND RETURN TO PLAY ISSUES

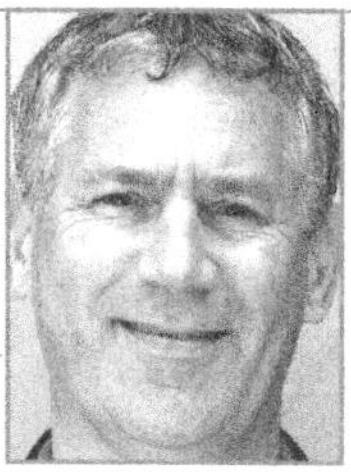

Mandelbaum BR

Clinical Affairs Kerlan Jobe Institute and Cedars Sinai, FIFA Medical Center of Excellence, Santa Monica; LA Galaxy, Los Angeles; Pepperdine University, Malibu, USA

Return To Play (RTP) is a multilevel, multidisciplinary and multimodal process that requires harmonious and synergized and specific approaches to athletes with Knee issues. At this time we must consider the fundamental aspects of the 15 elements that must be considered in today's athlete.

1. The history and sport and the demands, loads of the commitment to training and competition. Time of year and season. Number of games played Age of athlete? Is this a 16 years old or a previous injury was 16 years ago. Previous treatment including articular cartilage, bone, ligament or meniscus.
2. The player's athlete details of contract, commitment, scholarship and investment in sport. Success in the sport, the stage of career? Development or preparing for retirement. The contralateral extremity. Motivated and inspired to continue competition and training.
3. The mechanism of injury overuse vs. traumatic. Contact vs. noncontact, vs. mild perturbation. The energy of injury. Time of the injury the role of fatigue. The position of the lower extremity, dynamic valgus vs. varus in the coronal and sagittal planes. Positioned played defending or offending. Dominant vs. non-dominant leg. Study the video in the non-contact mechanisms so it doesn't reoccur in the future.
4. The Spectrum of injury. Stratifiable. Multi ligamentous vs. isolated Anterior Cruciate Ligament (ACL). Articular the size and dimensions the location, osteochondral, or bone marrow lesion. The location, the magnitude all should be considered.
5. The interventions required to regenerate, repair, reconstruct and restore full function. Non-surgical vs. surgical. Timing, staging in relationship procedures and postoperative protocols.
6. The orthobiological status of the knee joint. Catabolic or anabolic previous presence of chondropenia or osteoarthritis (OA) must be considered. The use of orthobiological Performance Enhancing Adjuncts (PEA) including glucosamine, hyaluronic acid, Platelet Rich Plasma (PRP) and type in relationship to high or low White Blood Cells (WBC), stem cells adipose derived, lipo-aspirate, manipulated or not, Bone Marrow Aspirate Concentrate (BMAC), induced pluripotential stem cells, amniotic fluid, or hormonal deficiency. Each of these adjuncts perhaps were used previously in today's world or may be considered after injury as non-operative treatment, in preparation for surgery , during surgery or as a postoperative adjunct at different time intervals.
7. Postoperative protocol. Weight bearing progressions, mobilization. Neuro-muscular stimulation. Focus and functional performance at every step.
8. The Rehabilitation progression. Exercises. Cross training, the pool, the ALTER G.
9. Use of Prevention programs such as Prevent injury Enhance Performance (PEP) or FIFA 11+ should be utilized in all.
10. Biomechanical and neuromuscular control readiness and testing threshold.
11. On field and court sport's specific finite progressions.
12. Fatigue in relation to demand issues and loss of neuromuscular control.
13. Release to team practice and training, contact vs. non-contact progressions and game progressions.
14. Full unrestricted participation. Training for the athlete same or different than normal others.
15. Chondro-protection and chondro-facilitation, and periodicity with also the goal of disease modification and preventing OA and the decline slope!

SURGICAL ADVANCES FOR EARLIER RETURN TO PLAY

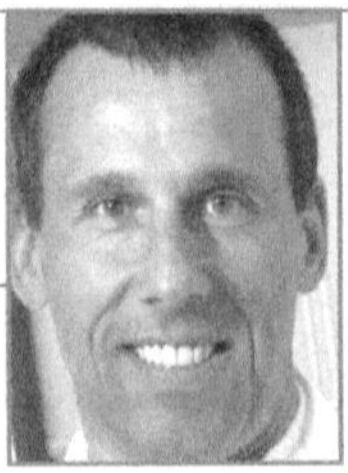

Erggelet C

University of Freiburg Medical Centre, Centre of Biologic Joint Surgery, Zürich, Switzerland

To discuss this topic two question have to be addressed: 1) Can advanced surgical techniques enable an earlier return to play? 2) Does a modern surgical intervention provide a faster rehabilitation and return to sport than a non-operative treatment ?
For the most common sport injuries there is no significant benefit for a surgical intervention regarding Return To Play (RTP). However, surgical procedures might be necessary to Stay In Play (SIP) over the years.

Tendons

Tendons do not heal and are usually under tension. Non-operative self-healing will result in the formation of bridging scar tissue and of loss of function due to reduced stability of the tissue and lengthening of the tendon. Partial compensation is possible with muscle strengthening. Usually the non-operative approach allows for a faster RTP compared to surgical reconstruction at the price of a reduced SIP period due to failing compensation mechanisms when getting older.
An unstable knee after Anterior Cruciate Ligament (ACL) Rupture will lead to an early career ending osteoarthritis without surgery. After surgical ACL reconstruction a RTP after 6-12 months are most common and enables SIP with a high probability. Modern surgical developments like double bundle reconstruction, anatomic single bundle or graft choice/allograft treatment show no conclusive benefits for an earlier RTP. For stable knees a non-operative treatment might allow for a RTP after 3-4 months. The same applies to Medial Collateral Ligament (MCL) or Lateral Collateral Ligament (LCL) lesions Advanced techniques for surgical reconstruction of e.g. acute lesions of the Achilles tendon allow for early rehabilitation and loading, preventing muscle loss and stiffness of the ankle.

Meniscus and Labrum

Like tendons this cartilaginous tissue only heals with scarring. When protected in a physiological position self-healing without elongation or dislocation can occur. In that case, an early RTP is possible after regaining muscle strength and full Range Of Motion (ROM) of the joint. If healing does not occur, a secondary reconstruction or partial resection becomes necessary with reduced chances of success. With more advanced techniques and instruments primary surgical interventions seem to be advisable to prevent pain and instability e.g. in knee, shoulder or hip. This will lead not necessarily to an earlier RTP but to a higher chance to SIP.

Cartilage

For the repair of cartilage lesions surgical interventions, not even the most advanced ones, do not offer any benefit regarding RTP. Long-term outcome e.g. for autologous chondrocyte transplantation seem to indicate a higher chance of SIP.

Fractures

Fractures need a certain time to heal, depending on the location/bone, with or without surgical intervention. But a surgical stabilization promotes faster rehabilitation, a decreased loss of joint function and in consequence a faster RTP. Advanced implants and operation techniques reduce the morbidity of a surgical intervention.

Conclusion

To date surgical interventions cannot beat the natural healing process but the combination of advanced techniques and a progressive and well balanced rehabilitation will lead to an safer return to play and a higher chance to stay in play.

PROGRESSIVE MECHANICAL STIMULI IN THE RECOVERY PROCESS

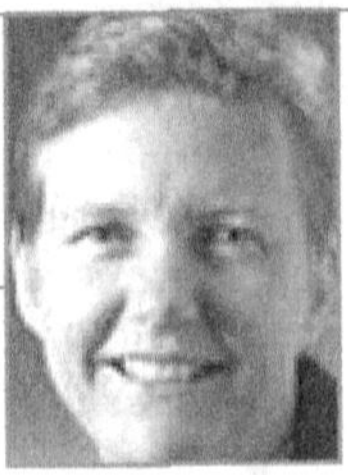

Cook J

La Trobe University, Melbourne, Australia

Tissue capacity must exceed or at least be equal to the amount of load placed on it. The loading placed on musculoskeletal tissue can be short and extreme in nature, or prolonged at a lower level of tissue stress. Both these types of loads have the potential to exceed the tissue capacity and training the tissue to be tolerant to the athlete's load is a central part of rehabilitation and treatment of injury. Individual factors such as age and gender can affect this sensitivity to injury and identifying tissues under stress must account for these intrinsic factors. Systemic factors and genetics also can alter tissue capacity and ability to recover, as can previous injury history, and pain processing of the individual.

Unfortunately, tissue capacity is slow to adapt, meaning that measures to increase the capacity must be placed over some time. Each tissue has its own adaptation periods, overall collagen-based tissues are notoriously slow to respond to loading and the lecture will consider these tissues only, as muscle tissue has completely different adaptation responses. It is also evident that progressive loads are critical, and although there are standard protocols for tendon loading programs, ligament and bone adaptation are usually only considered as part of overall musculoskeletal reloading.

Progressive laoding must begin where the tissue capacity is, and this depends on previous unloading and tissue injury or pathology. Clearly it must end at the level of loading that the athlete requires. Over-adaptation, i.e. taking the tissue beyond the sporting demands of the athlete is not beneficial as the tissue capacity will always only maintained at the level of loading placed on it.

Clinicians must be receptive to the loading adaptation of tissues as it is evident that there are few treatment strategies that can hasten the tissue response. This raise issues of extended time frames for recovery that are not acceptable in elite sport and the expert clinician can recognise tissues and individuals that can be pushed to and beyond the tissue capacity and those who will respond negatively to this.

Saturday 9th April, 2016 (morning)
CHURCHILL AUDITORIUM

INVITED SPEAKERS

RETURN TO PLAY IN SHOULDER AND SPINAL PATHOLOGIES

Chairs

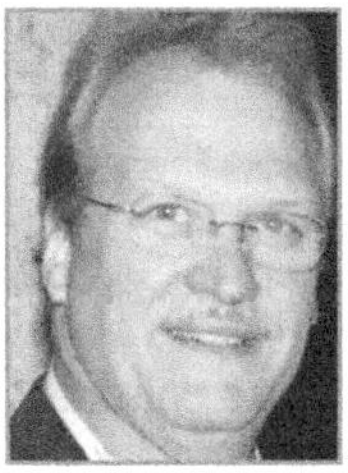

Michael Axe
(Newark, United States)

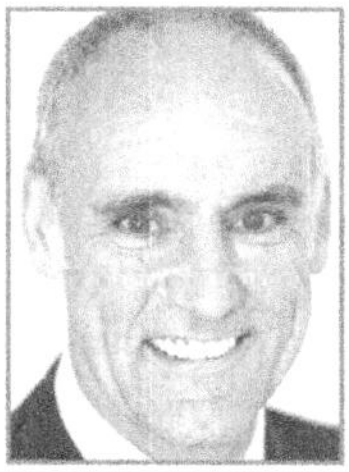

Michael Mayer
(Münich, Germany)

11:30	Return to play after shoulder surgical stabilisation **Philippe Landreau (Doha, Qatar)**
11:45	Return to play after rotator cuff injuries **Pietro Randelli (Milan, Italy)**
12:00	Return to play in spondylolysis and vertebral pedicle fracture **Damian Fahy (London, United Kingdom)**
12:15	Return to play for conservatively managed low back pain **Carl Todd (Bath, United Kingdom)**
12:30	Return to play after herniated disc surgery **Fabrizio Tencone (Turin, Italy)**
12:45	Discussion
13:00	End of the session

1

RETURN TO PLAY AFTER SHOULDER SURGICAL STABILIZATION

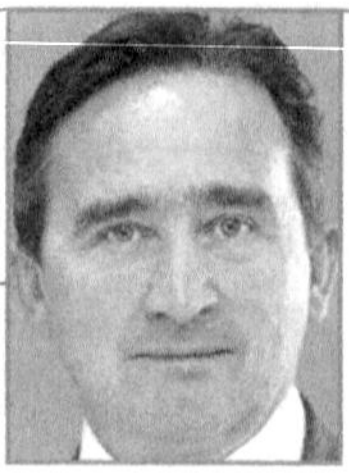

Landreau P

Aspetar, Orthopaedic and Sports Medicine Hospital, Doha, Qatar

The impact of shoulder instability is probably underestimated in the football population. The acute, primary dislocations of the gleno-humeral joint occurred in 8 to 25 per 100,000 person years. The dislocation rate among athletes is higher than the general population: 0.12 episodes of gleno-humeral instability occurring per 1,000 sporting exposures (defined as a practice session or competition session without reference to duration). Men are 2.5 times more involved than women. Contact sports, like football, are the most injurious, with the majority of dislocations occurring during contact with other athletes during competition.

After a first episode of anterior shoulder dislocation, 75% of male athletes under 25 years will develop recurrent instability by 2 years, rising to 85% at 5 years. The risk of recurrence is correlated with the young age and the bony lesions. In comparative studies, there is a sevenfold reduction in the risk of recurrent instability after arthroscopic stabilization, when compared with non-operative treatment for the first-time dislocation. Therefore, it has been advocated to do a Bankart repair after a first episode of dislocation to reduce the risk of recurrence.

In case of chronic shoulder instability, either an arthroscopic Bankart repair or a Latarjet procedure can be performed. Overall, the incidence of recurrence appears to be higher for arthroscopic surgery than for open surgery. Failure to address significant glenoid and humeral head bone loss are an increasingly recognized cause of failed shoulder stabilization. Patient factors specifically associated with recurrent instability following arthroscopic stabilization include: multiple episodes of instability before stabilization, younger age at the time of surgery, hyperlaxity, noncompliance with post-operative immobilization, involvement in competitive football, and an early return to play.

After surgical stabilization, the time to return to sport is a minimum of four months, but it seems to be faster for goalkeepers. Between 70 to 75% of patients return to the same level and only 3 to 4% have to quit football activity completely. In addition to the difference in recurrent rate between the two main techniques of shoulder stabilization, it has been shown that after a Latarjet procedure, the shoulders remained stable over time, whereas stability declined after an arthroscopic Bankart repair.

In the football population, in case of a first episode of shoulder dislocation, we suggest that an early Bankart repair should be proposed to the patient according to his age, position in the team and gleno-humeral bone lesions. If the patient is complaining of a recurrent shoulder dislocation, the choice between an arthroscopic Bankart repair and a Latarjet procedure should be mainly dictated by the Instability Severity Index Score.

RETURN TO PLAY AFTER ROTATOR CUFF INJURIES

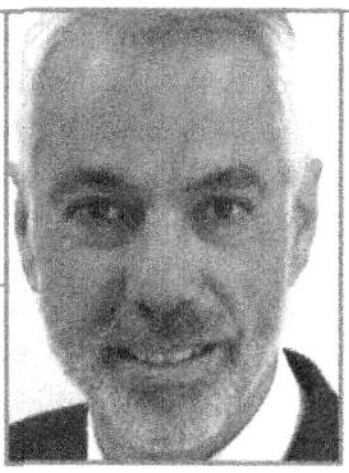

Randelli P, Pulici L

Orthopedics and Traumatology, Biomedical Science for Health Department, Università degli Studi di Milano, and 2nd Orthopaedics Department, IRCCS Policlinico San Donato, Milan, Italy

Rotator Cuff Tear (RCT) is a common pathology, which prevalence increases with aging, from a 2.5% in 30s to a 50% in 80s (3).

In elderly patients RCT is usually degenerative while in young patients is traumatic, especially in athletes who practice overhead (baseball, tennis, baskeball) or contact sport (rugby, american football, ice hockey, soccer).

Surgical approach is often used in athletes to treat RCT. Nowadays arthroscopic repair is the gold standard to treat RCT. There is no evidence for better outcome using suture anchor technique or trans-osseous technique for RCT.

An accelerated rehabilitation protocol, especially in professional athletes, is used after RCT repair and it consists of the following phases:

- Phase 1 (Immobilization and ROM recovery): brace immobilization for two/four weeks and passive mobilization to achive full ROM starting at two weeks post-op.
- Phase2 (active mobilization): at five weeks post-op using active and isometric exercises.
- Phase 3 (basic strenghtening and proprioceptive exercises): at minimum two months post-op with elastic band and basic proprioception exercises.
- Phase 4 (advanced strenghtening and proprioceptive exercises): at minimum three months post-op with isotonic and isokinetic exercises, advanced proprioception exercises.
- Phase 5 (sport specific exercises): from basic exercise to full sport practice.

The progression from one phase to the other one is clinically based.

Return To Play (RTP) after RCT repair should be at least five months after surgery using the decision-based RTP model, proposed by Creightow et al. (1), consisting in three steps:

- Step 1: evaluation of health status (medical factors, e.g. sign and symptoms, laboratory tests).
- Step 2: evaluation of participation risk (sport risk modifiers, e.g. type of sport, position played).
- Step 3: decision modification (decision modifier, e.g. timing of season, external pressure).

RTP after RCT repair, according with the meta-analysis of Klouche et al. (2), is 84.7%, with a delay ranging from 4.1 to 17.0 months, but the RTP at the same level of professional athletes in significantly lower than recreational ones (49.9% vs 81.4%).

References

1. Creightow DW, Shrier I, Shultz R, Meeuwisse WH, Matheson GO. Return-to-play in sport: a decision-based model. Clin J Sport Med 2010; 20: 379-85
2. Klouche S, Lefevre N, Herman S, Gerometta A, Bohu Y. Return to sport after rotator cuff tear repair. A systematic review and meta-analysis. Am J Sport Med 2015 Aug 27. pii: 0363546515598995. [Epub ahead of print]
3. Yamamoto A, Takagishi K, Osawa T , Yanagawa T, Nakajima D, Shitara H, Kobayashi T. Prevalence and risk factors of a rotator cuff tear in the general population. J Shoulder Elbow Surg. 2010; 19(1): 116-120

4

RETURN TO PLAY CONSIDERATIONS AND APPROACHES FOR CONSERVATIVELY MANAGED LOWER BACK PAIN

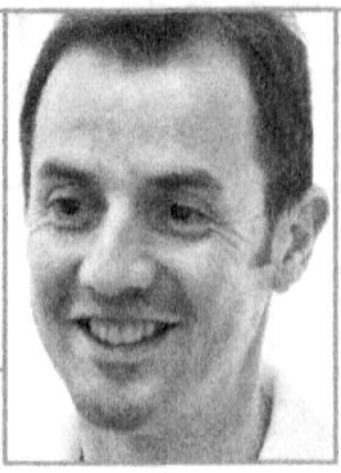

Todd C

The Football Association, London; England Men's Senior Team; Chelsea FC; The Carl Todd Clinic Bath, United Kingdom

Introduction and Purpose

The return to play considerations and approaches for conservatively managed low back pain in elite football appears, to lack structured clinical guidelines with limited levels of published evidence available. To date, there are no standardised criteria utilising the conservative approaches to manage spinal pathologies in athletes for returning to play (2). Moreover, a literature search from PubMed shows no current published studies for the conservative management on the return to play for low back pain in footballers. The majority of decisions on return to play appear to be based upon expert opinion and clinical experience (1). Therefore, the purpose of this presentation to provide a review of a clinical case report highlighting the return to play conservative management strategy for a football player presenting with chronic low back, hip and groin pain.

Methods

Player was a male, right-footed central defender, (22 years) in age, stature (190 cm), and body mass (82 kg) and had been privately referred by an orthopaedic surgeon. Presenting complaint was long-term low back, hip and groin pain (Vas 8/10), duration 8/12 pre/post surgery, current symptoms increased with physical activity, unable to jog, strike a ball or sit for prolonged periods. Previous medical history with Magnetic resonance Imaging (MRI) highlighted L4-5 spondylolysis, player had undergone bilateral hip arthroscopy for Cam Femoro-Acetabular Impingement (FAI) repair combined with labral reconstruction and subsequent right-sided psoas release. Quantitative measurements were recorded and included the use of: 1) Visual Analogue Scale (VAS); 2) MicroFET 2 Wireless Digital Handheld Dynamometer (HHD; Hogan Scientific LLC, Salt Lake City, USA); 3) 66fit Pressure Bio Feedback Unit (PBU), Taiwan (Republic of China).
Standing active spinal and pelvic examination revealed pain at end of Range of Motion (ROM) in flexion and extension. Hypermobility was noted on active flexion at the L4-5, L5-S1 segments and on active extension 'hinging' was noted at the L4-5 segment. Right-sided load/unload Trendelenburg test was positive. Passive evaluation highlighted segmental facet joint restrictions T12-L1 and T7-9 and increased palpatory spinal hypermobility over right-sided lower lumbar segments and Sacro-Iliac Joint (SIJ). Hip examination highlighted pain and restriction in motion with standing and sitting active Hip Flexion (HF) and tested positive for hip joint Flexion, Adduction and Internal Rotation (FAIR). Active Straight Leg Raise (ASLR) was 'laboured' but improved with pelvic force closure. HHD testing for inner range Hip Flexion (HF) and Hip Abduction (ABD) was not recorded on initial consultation due to pain but was measured during the second and final consultations. PBU squeeze test on first consultation; Straight Leg (SL) 150 mmHg and Bent Knee (BK) 60° 120mmHg. Working Hypothesis was a triad of multifaceted related issues; reduced hip joint motor control and intolerance to work capacity load resulting in a breakdown of spinal and pelvic compensatory mechanisms.

Management was 4 treatment sessions throughout a 5/52 period involving patient education, correction of spinal somatic dysfunctions at T12-L1, T7-9, soft tissue mobilisation for overactive muscles. Neuromuscular facilitation techniques to improve inhibited muscles, progressing to work capacity tolerance and spinal conditioning programme encompassing segmental motor control, dissociation and work capacity. Player used a serloa SIJ belt for initial 2/52 to help reinforce pelvic closure and performed daily water based recovery sessions. The player was able to resume modified training at 10/7, played 45 minutes at 3/52 and 90 minutes 5/52 with no reaction.

Results

Follow up at 1/52 the VAS 4/10, with pain free spinal ROM, negative load/unload, Sorensen test 170 seconds, HHD inner range HF 5.03 kg, ABD 5.5 kg, PBU squeeze test SL 150 mmHg, BK 60° 120 mmHg.
Follow up at 3/52, VAS 1/10, pain free spinal ROM, negative load/unload, Sorensen test 220 seconds, HHD inner range HF pain free, 7.12 kg, ABD 13.3 kg, PBU squeeze test SL 240 mmHg, BK 60° 280 mmHg.
Follow up at 5/52 VAS 0/10, Sorensen test 240+ seconds, HHD HF 8.7 kg, ABD 14.2 kg, PBU squeeze test SL 280 mmHg, BK 60° 300+mmHg.
Follow up at 1 year; participant had played over 40 games and remained injury free.

Conclusions

This case reports on the conservative approach for return to play, in a footballer with chronic, low back, hip and groin pain. In spite of a lack of specific guidelines regarding the return to play criteria for the conservative management of low back pain in footballers, the general consensus are, that players should be symptom free, absent of neurological deficits, have full range of motion and developed a work capacity tolerance to load and strength (1). Moreover, some studies have shown the time scale for the return to play with conservative management to appear similar compared with surgical intervention (3). However, a shorter duration for return to play has been shown for the conservative management of specific spinal pathologies (2). It is suggested that for the conservative management of a footballer with chronic low back, hip and groin pain, the spino-pelvic-hip complex should be viewed as a functional integrated unit and therefore, should be treated as such.

References

1. Huang P, Anissipour A, McGee W, Lemak L. Return to play recommendations after cervical, thoracic and lumbar spine injuries: A comprehensive review. Sports Health. 2015 Oct 14. pii: 1941738115610753. [Epub ahead of print]
2. Iwamoto J, Sato Y, Takeda T, Matsumoto H. The return to sports activity after conservative or surgical treatment in athletes with lumbar disc herniation. Am J Phys Med Rehabil 2010; 89: 1030-1035
3. Mortazavi J, Zebardast, J, Mirzashahi B. Low back pain in athletes. Asian J Sports Med 2015 June: 692):e24718

RETURN TO PLAY AFTER HERNIATED DISC SURGERY

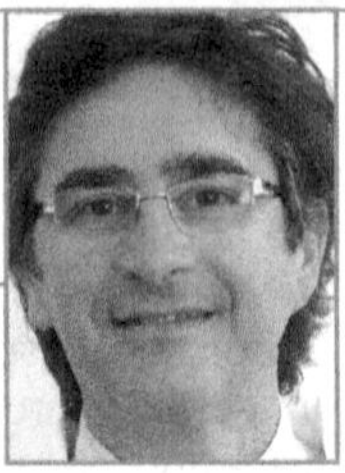

Tencone F

Isokinetic Medical Group, FIFA Medical Centre of Excellence Torino, Italy

Introduction

Up to today there is still no ideal rehabilitation protocol and the topic is still researched; our experience leads us to think that in the management of a professional football player it is crucial to build a personalized protocol considering five factors:

1. Morphological characteristics of the player.
2. Pre-operative clinical and metabolic conditions.
3. Role of the player.
4. Eventual residual neurological deficit.
5. Psychological and motivational characteristics of the player.

During the entire rehabilitation process it is necessary:

I) to measure the results obtained;
II) to constantly monitor the clinical and functional progress of the player;
III) to critically analyze the results obtained so that is possible to properly modify the therapeutic planning.

The aim of the rehabilitation program is to protect the surgery site by avoiding biomechanical stress and respecting the biological healing times (3).

Epidemiology

Although lumbar discectomy for treatment of lumbar disc herniation (1) in the general population generally improves patients' pain, function, and validated outcomes scores, results of treatment in elite athletes may differ because of the unique performance demands required of competitive athletes (2).

Rehabilitation protocol

Schematically the rehabilitation protocol is divided into 5 phases:

Phase I (Control of pain). Generally pain is quickly resolved by the surgery, but in some athletes can persist: in this case instrumental therapies such as the Transcutaneous Electrical Nerve Stimulation (TENS), antalgic postures, massage and if necessary NSAID can be used.

Phase II (Recovery of range of motion). The selective stretching (Gluteus, Ileopsoas, Piriformis, knee flexors muscles) and the mobilization of soft tissues are fundamental moments for the recovery of a correct mobility of the spine.

Phase III (Recovery of strength). Exercises to improve the isometric strength of stabilising muscles of the spine and erectors muscles (Multifidus, Quadratus Lumborum, Transversus Abdominis and Obliques) indispensable for reducing the discal and articular stresses. Exercises to improve the concentric and eccentric strength of the thoraco-lumbar muscles have been introduced subsequently.

Phase IV (Recovery of coordination). There is evidence that an optimal neuro-muscular control of the trunk allows to protect the site of surgery from sudden and unexpected loads. This is a very important rehabilitation phase, strictly interwoven to phase III and based on coordination exercises.

Phase V (Recovery of the technical gesture). It is the phase that leads to the return to team activities. It includes exercises that will complete the specific physical fitness for the soccer player, and the achievement of a psychological security in the execution of different sport specific gestures. The activities have been performed constantly monitoring the metabolic intensity through the heart rate corresponding to aerobic and anaerobic thresholds.

Conclusions

The rehabilitation project is based on the achievement of specific functional and clinical objectives monitoring the patient responses to stimuli.

The collected data are a valid motivational instrument for the athlete since, if shared, they are a feedback that proves the results achieved and stimulates the patient toward the maximum possible functional recovery.

References

1. Kamper SJ, Ostelo RW, Rubinstein SM, Nellensteijn JM, Peul WC, Arts MP, van Tulder MW. Minimally invasive surgery for lumbar disc herniation: a systematic review and meta-analysis. Eur Spine J 2014; 23: 1021-1043
2. Nair R, Kahlenberg CA, Hsu WK. Outcomes of lumbar discectomy in elite athletes: the need for high-level evidence. Clin Orthop Relat Res 2015; 473: 1971-1977
3. Watkins RG 4th, Hanna R, Chang D, Watkins RG 3rd. Return-to-play outcomes after microscopic lumbar discectomy in professional athletes. Am J Sports Med 2012; 40: 2530-2535

Saturday 9th April, 2016 (morning)
PICKWICK ROOM

FREE ORAL PRESENTATIONS

BASIC SCIENCE AND REGENERATIVE MEDICINE

Chairs

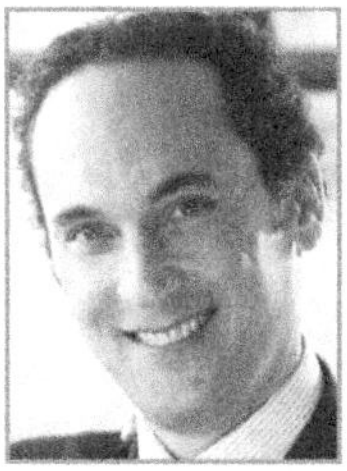
Vincenzo Madonna
(Verona, Italy)

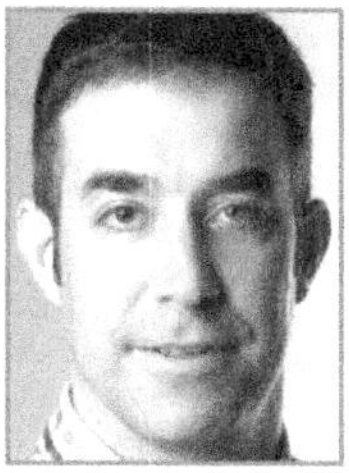
Gérgely Panics
(Budapest, Hungary)

11:30 Anterolateral ligament, fact or fiction?
Musahl V, Soni A, Rahnemai-Azar A, vanEck C, Guenther D, Shaikh H, Albers M, Fu FH (Pittsburgh, USA)

11:40 Moving research findings into action: the science of tendon/ligament repair in sports medicine
Zheng MH (Perth, Australia)

11:50 Can growth factors concentration modify timing of healing process after muscle injuries?
Cianforlini M, Gigante AP (Ancona, Italy)

12:00 Stem cell therapy for sport injuries and arthritis
Michalek J (Brno, Czech Republic)

12:10 Platelet-rich plasma for the treatment of musculoskeletal soft tissue injuriess
Chow G, Owusu D, Malik Q, Khan S (Essex, United Kingdom)

12:20 Eccentric exercise and platelet-rich plasma injection for hamstring injury
Saita Y, Kobayashi Y, Ikeda H (Tokyo, Japan)

12:30 Platelet rich plasma enhances neovascularisation after anterior cruciate ligament reconstruction
Vogrin M, Kelc R (Maribor, Slovenia)

12:40 Autologous tenocyte injection for chronic refractory tendinopathy: from cell biology to clinical trials
Rao KA, Zheng MH, Wang A, Bucher T, Wang T, Ebert J, Breidahl W (Perth, Australia)

12:50 Discussion

13:10 End of the session

ANTEROLATERAL LIGAMENT, FACT OR FICTION?

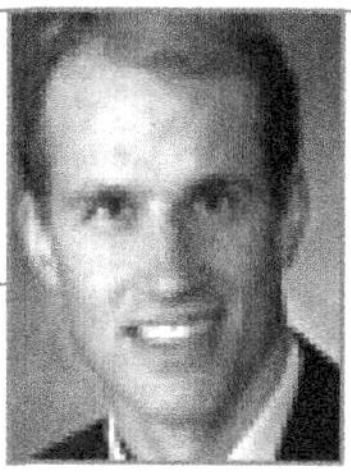

Musahl V, Soni A, Rahnemai-Azar A, vanEck C, Guenther D, Shaikh H, Albers M, Fu FH

University of Pittsburgh Medical Center, Department of Orthopaedic Surgery, UPMC Rooney Sports Complex, Pittsburgh, USA

Current literature provides a multitude of descriptions regarding the anatomy of the anterolateral capsule of the knee. Researchers have argued that the capsule contains a true ligament, while others suggest it merely displays a thickening. Therefore, the objective of this study is to meticulously evaluate the anatomy, histology, biomechanics, kinematics and clinical implication of the anterolateral capsule.

While performing anatomic dissections on 24 different animal species, we have consistently found a double Lateral Collateral Ligament (LCL) in three types of primates; however, not an Antero Lateral Ligament (ALL).

In fetus dissections aged 18-22 weeks, no distinguishable ALL was identified within the capsule.

When evaluating the macroscopic anatomy, histology and radiology of the anterolateral capsule in adult human cadaveric specimens, only 30% of the specimens showed a discrete capsular thickening of 2-4 mm on Magnetic Resonance Imaging (MRI). Histology of this capsular thickening showed some collagen alignment but not pronounced enough and less cellular then a true ligament.

Tensile testing of the anterolateral capsule of the knee showed that the anterolateral capsule has four times less stiffness, five times less load to failure and twice the ultimate elongation compared to other knee ligaments, which fails to support a ligamentous function of this structure.

During a simulated pivot shift test using a robotic testing system, the contribution of this section of the capsule to the knee stability was negligible.

In our experience of evaluating the anatomy of the anterolateral capsule in more than 150 patients with an Anterior Cruciate Ligament (ACL) injury during arthroscopy, no overt pathology of the anterolateral capsule was observed, nor was any thickening appreciated.

It appears that many questions regarding the anterolateral capsule of the knee remain.

Future studies are needed to better evaluate the role of anterolateral capsular injuries on knee stability, how to best restore the function of the anterolateral capsule, and the effect of extra-articular repairs or reconstruction on the outcome after ACL surgery.

Until these questions are answered, the focus should remain on restoring the native anatomy. If an anatomic structure is torn, the goal should be to reconstruct its anatomy to as close to native as possible. If an ACL reconstruction fails, we should first determine why it has failed, focusing on graft choice, size, bony morphology, reconstruction method and tunnel placement before looking for the cause in the anterolateral capsule structures.

Providing individualized care to ensure the best potential for a successful outcome for our patients should be our main goal.

2

MOVING RESEARCH FINDINGS INTO ACTION: THE SCIENCE OF TENDON/LIGAMENT REPAIR IN SPORTS MEDICINE

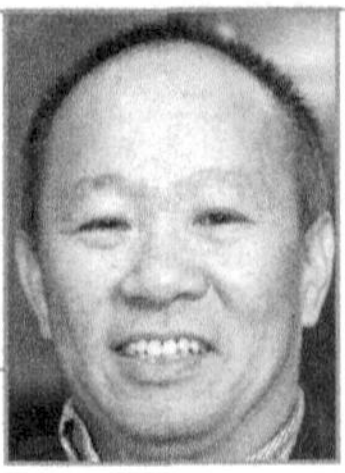

Zheng MH

Centre for Orthopaedic Research, School of Surgery, University of Western Australia, Perth, Australia

Ligaments and tendons are the fibrous tissues that facilitate joint stability by connecting bone to bone or muscle to bone. Tendons and ligaments are frequently damaged during rigorous activities such as sport or the process of aging. Despite their relatively high prevalence and morbidity of tendon and ligament injury in sport, most treatments have been proven to provide no, or only modest short-term benefits. Traditional first-line treatments might include rest and activity modification, exercises such as eccentric strengthening and bracing Topical or oral Non-Steroidal Anti-Inflammatory Drugs (NSAIDs) and local glucocorticoid injections may provide modest short-term benefits for pain. More recently, novel treatments including extracorporeal shock wave therapy, and injectable autologous blood products and botulinum have been studied but have either been proven to be ineffective or remain unproven. Current surgical and therapeutic treatment options include prosthetic devices, autografts, allografts, or xenografts, however these exhibit only limited success. Over the past 15 years, we focus exclusively on the translational medicine program of tendon repair and regeneration. We have identified key extracellular matrix molecules that involve in collagen assembly of tendon collagen fibers and tendon cell fate. We have also observed that depletion of the functional tenocyte pool in the region of the tear may account for fatigue of the normal healing response. On the basis of the pathology studies, we have developed numbers of novel therapeutic strategies for tendon and ligament repair in human. These include the development of ultrasound guided Autologous Tendon cell Injection (ATI) for tendon tear and the Matrix Argument autologous Tendon cell implantation (MATT) for surgical repair of tendon and ligament and human neo-tendon implant. We have showed that ATI, the first homologous cell therapy technique developed for the treatment of tendinopathy, has the potential to address this unmet clinical need by replenishing the pool of functional tenocytes in the site of tendinopathy. Clinical study of ATI in a pilot of 17 patients with chronic resistant lateral epicondylitis revealed significant improvement in mean Visual Analogue Scale (VAS) pain score from 5.73 at initial assessment to 1.21 (78% improvement) at final follow-up of 4.5 year (1). To date, over 250 patients with tendinopathy were treated with ATI and we are currently conducting double blind randomised control study of ATI. MATT technique by direct inoculating autologous tendon cells on the collagen matrix has been validated in the pre-clinical model of rabbit (2). Human clinical trial is on the way with the completion of two cases for the rotator cuff tendon tear. Finally, we have developed senor controlled bioreactor for the generation of neo-tendon tissue using autologous tendon cells from a needle biopsy. Histology and immunohistochemistry showed that the neo-tendon tissue mimics human tendon structure and express tendon cell markers including scleraxis, tenomodulin and type I collagen. It is anticipate that the first case of the human neo-tendon implant may occur in 2017 if the regulatory agency and ethic committee approve the study.

References

1. Wang A, Mackie K, Breidahl W, Wang T, Zheng MH. Evidence for the Durability of Autologous Tenocyte Injection for Treatment of Chronic Resistant Lateral Epicondylitis: Mean 4.5-Year Clinical Follow-up. Am J Sports Med 2015; 43: 1775-1783
2. Willers C, Chen J, Wood D, Xu J, Zheng MH. Autologous chondrocyte implantation with collagen bioscaffold for the treatment of osteochondral defects in rabbits. Tissue Eng 2005; 11: 1065-1076

CAN GROWTH FACTORS CONCENTRATION MODIFY TIMING OF HEALING PROCESS AFTER MUSCLE INJURIES?

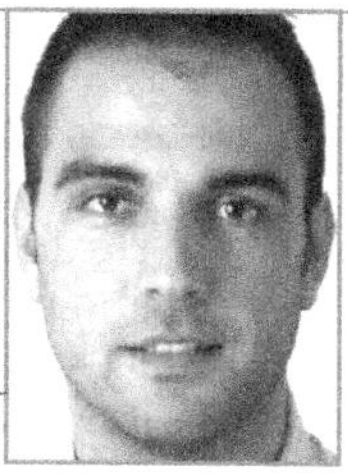

Cianforlini M, Gigante AP

Department of Clinical and Molecular Sciences, School of Medicine,
Università Politecnica delle Marche, Ancona, Italy

Introduction

Skeletal muscle injuries, mainly contusions and strains, are common causes of severe long-term pain and physical disability. They account for up to 55% of all sports injuries and for 31% of all damages in élite football (soccer) players. Muscle injury is a challenging problem in traumatology, as injured muscles heal very slowly and often with incomplete functional recovery; hence the critical importance of a correct evaluation, diagnosis and therapy of these disorders.
In sport, muscle lesion treatment is aimed to re-enable the athlete training and competing as soon as possible and without complications. Most current muscle injury treatments are based on limited experimental and clinical data and/or were only empirically tested. (2)
The role of Growth Factors (GFs) in the process of muscle regeneration and satellite cell activation is of outmost importance. Since scarring and fibrosis are both obstacles to a complete muscle recovery a correct management of GFs use in imperative to avoid an excessive fibrosis in the treatment of muscle lesions.
Platelet Rich Plasma (PRP) is commonly used in orthopaedic practice to enhance healing in sports-related skeletal muscle, tendon, and ligament injuries (1). However, the use of PRP in the treatment of skeletal muscle lesions is based on limited experimental data, and no meta-analysis studies or randomized controlled trials have been conducted to allow their safe and effective use. Only a few in vivo studies have shown that GFs are able to improve muscle regeneration and increase muscle strength after a trauma (3).
Due to the short half-life and rapid clearance of GFs injured muscles need to be treated with high concentrations of these molecules. The present study is therefore focused on the use of different concentrations of PRP in an experimental animal model.
The principal aim of the present experimental in vivo study is a morphological and morphometrical evaluation of the PRP effects on full thickness muscle lesions in an animal model to verify a relationship between concentrations of GFs, muscle regeneration and fibrosis and functional recovery.

Methods

Briefly, blood necessary for PRP preparation was obtained by intracardiac puncture from 14 rats using a 10 mL syringe containing Citrate Phosphonate Dextrose (CPD) in ratio 5:1. Three different concentrations of platelets were achieved (1.200x106 platelets/mmc, 1.700x10^6 platelets/mmc, 2.500x10^6 platelets/mmc).
Unilateral cutaneous incisions (3 cm in length) were performed in the paravertebral region, then, using a standard pincer technique, muscular tear lesions (0.7x0.3 cm) were executed on the Longissimus Dorsi muscle of 36 male Wistar rats (340±60 g of body weight).
PRP intramuscular injection (2 mL) in the lesion sites were performed 24 h after the surgical trauma: nine rats received the lowest PRP concentration (group A), nine rats received the second PRP concentration (group B), nine rats received the highest PRP concentration (group C) and nine rats were left untreated and used as Controls (CTRL).

This location was chosen since the presence of the supraspinatus ligament and fascia allow to carry out the wounds and, moreover, prevents rats from interfering (i.e. biting or scratching) with the surgical treatment. In all cases muscle was left unsutured, the fascia and skin were closed with a standard approach with a non-absorbable suture wire in order to identify the repair site at the time of necropsy. Animals were maintained with a normal diet and no forced exercise was induced. Histological, immunohistochemical (M-caderina, CD-34, V-CAM-1, Myo-D and myogenin) and histomorphometric analyses were performed to evaluate muscle regeneration, neovascularization, fibrosis and inflammation and the presence of metaplasic zones, calcifications and heterotopic ossification.
The policies and procedures of their use and maintenance were in accordance with those detailed by the directive n. 86/609/CEE regarding animal care and experimental usage.

Results

Gross examination did not show differences between PRP treated or untreated muscle lesions.
Histological score evaluation evidenced that muscular regeneration was greater in PRP treated samples in comparison with controls at the earlier time points (i.e. 3 and 15 days), whilst it was comparable at 60 days after surgery.
Comparison of the three PRP treated groups by histo-morphometric analysis showed that in the animals treated with PRP at a higher concentration of growth factors (group C), muscular regeneration was higher both at 3 and at 15 days after surgery, while no differences were detected 60 days after surgery.
This observations was corroborated by immunohistochemical analyses performed at 3 days after surgery. In PRP treated lesions, the higher Myogenin positivity and MyoD immune-staining were directly proportional to the concentration of GFs.
Data on muscle regeneration go hand in hand with those of neovascularization. This feature was greater in PRP treated samples in comparison with controls at the earlier time points of 3 and 15 days, but it was comparable 60 days after surgery. Also in this case the use of a higher concentration of GFs significantly affect neovascularization at 3 and 15 days after surgery, but it seems ineffective after 60 days.
As far as inflammation is concerned, no differences were detected between all the groups throughout the follow-up, even though a significant reduction of inflammatory cells was observed at 60 days from surgery.
At last a reduction in fibrosis was observed at 15 days after surgery, with no significant among the groups, even though faint differences in Sirius Red staining were detected at 60 days after surgery.

Conclusions

The present study confirmed previous data about the usefulness of PRP in the treatment of muscle injury and demonstrated that this process is dependent on the concentration of administered GFs. Even though these experimental results are lacking in data on pain and functional recovery, they open a clinical debate on the appropriate dose of PRP for sportsmen muscle lesion treatment.

References

1. Anitua E, Andia I, Ardanza B, Nurden P, Nurden AT. Autologous platelets as a source of proteins for healing and tissue regeneration. Thromb Haemost 2004; 91: 4-15
2. Gharaibeh B, Chun-Lansinger Y, Hagen T, Ingham SJ, Wright V, Fu F, Huard J. Biological approaches to improve skeletal muscle healing after injury and disease. Birth Defects Res C Embryo Today 2012; 96: 82-94
3. Gigante A, Del Torto M, Manzotti S, Cianforlini M, Busilacchi A, Davidson PA, Greco F, Mattioli-Belmonte M. Platelet rich fibrin matrix effects on skeletal muscle lesions: an experimental study. J Biol Regul Homeost Agents 2012; 26: 475-84

STEM CELL THERAPY FOR SPORT INJURIES AND ARTHRITIS

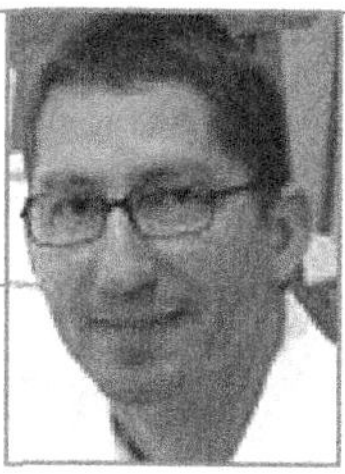

Michalek J

International Consortium for Cell Therapy and Immunotherapy, Brno, Czech Republic

Therapy of sport injuries and arthritis relies on non-steroid analgesics, chondroprotectives and in late stages total joint replacement is considered as a standard of care.
We performed a case-control study using novel stem cell therapy approach that optimizes healing process for active football players suffering from sport injuries as well as patients suffering from osteoarthritis or degenerative arthritis.
Stem cell therapy relies on one surgical procedure which consists of abdominal lipo-aspiration of 50-200 mL of fat, processing of adipose and connective tissue to Stromal Vascular Fraction (SVF) cells that typically contain large amounts of mesenchymal stromal and stem cells. SVF cells were prepared by patented technology to obtain high yields of viable cells and at least 20 million of nucleated cells were injected immediately as a single injection to the target joint or to the connective tissue of the target joint. Up to 4 joints were injected at the same occasion. After one week a rest patients started physiotherapy to get to normal physical activities within 6 weeks after the SVF cell application.
Since 2011, total of 1,128 patients have been recruited and followed for up to 60 months to demonstrate the therapeutic potential of freshly isolated SVF cells. At the same time, one to four joints (knees and hips) were injected with SVF cells per patient.
A total number of 1,856 joints were treated. Clinical scale evaluation including pain, non-steroid analgesic usage, limping at walk, extent of joint movement and stiffness was used as measurement of the clinical effect.
All patients were diagnosed with sport injury including chondropathy or with stage II-IV osteoarthritis using clinical examination and X-ray, in some cases Magnetic Resonance Imaging (MRI) was also performed to monitor the changes before and after stem cell therapy.
After 12 months from SVF therapy, at least 50% clinical improvement was recognized in 91%, and at least 75% clinical improvement in 63% of patients, respectively.
Within 1-2 weeks from SVF therapy 72% of patients were off the non-steroid analgesics, active in sports and most of them remain such for 12-60 months.
No serious side effects, infection or cancer was associated with SVF cell therapy at 12-60 months follow-up.

Conclusions

Autologous stem cells from adipose and connective tissue can contribute significantly to healing process of sport injuries and arthritis.
Time to return to play was decreased to 1-2 weeks in case of sport injuries.
Autologous stem cell therapy represents novel, safe, minimally invasive and highly effective treatment strategy for sport injuries as well as degenerative arthritis.
There is no age limitation for cell therapy and no serious side effects were present in association with SVF cell therapy.

This work was supported in part by the International Consortium for Cell Therapy and Immunotherapy (www.iccti.eu) and Czech Ministry of Education Grant No. CZ.1.07/2.3.00/20.0012.

5

PLATELET-RICH PLASMA FOR THE TREATMENT OF MUSCULOSKELETAL SOFT TISSUE INJURIES

Chow G, Owusu D, Malik Q, Khan S

Basildon Hospital, Essex, United Kingdom

Introduction

Platelet-Rich Plasma (PRP) is a fragment of whole blood that contains a much higher concentration of platelets compared to whole blood itself. Its predicted benefit is enhanced healing of soft tissues through improved clotting and delivery of growth factors (1, 2).

PRP's popularity in professional sports, such as football, has grown in recent years due to well-publicised success stories. An example is that of Xavi, Barcelona and Spanish International footballer who, initially sidelined with a season-ending grade two Achilles tendon tear, returned in two months following treatment with PRP.

High-profile cases like this have resulted in PRP moving from the spotlight of professional sports to that of the amateur sportsman and those simply aiming to return to their pre-injury functional state, whether that is sport related or not.

Unfortunately the literature is currently inconclusive and difficult to interpret due to varying techniques in preparation of PRP, each leading to different final products; lack of a universally agreed classification and poor descriptions of techniques and types of PRP used in current studies (1). Varying PRP products could potentially have a wide range of effects on healing and patient outcomes. In addition, this disparity restricts our ability to make useful comparisons between studies.

Our aim was to assess the use of ultrasound-guided PRP injections for the treatment of musculoskeletal soft tissue injuries at Basildon Hospital, including those commonly experienced by football players, such as patella and Achilles tendonitis.

Methods

This was a retrospective review of 18 patients affected by tendonitis of the patella (n=7), Achilles (n=3), quadriceps (n=1), bicipital (n=1), peroneus brevis (n=1), pes anserinus (n=2) and plantar fascia (N=3). The sample group included patients playing sport at a recreational level as well as those not participating in sport but simply aiming to return to their pre-injury functional state. The mean age of our sample group was 38±19 with 43% male, 57% female.

Diagnosis was confirmed using ultrasound or Magnetic Resonance Imaging. Average duration of symptoms was 22 months (range 3 months – 4 years). All patients had previously failed conservative therapy including physiotherapy or steroid injections but had no previous surgical treatment.

PRP used was the Tropocells Basic preparation provided by Lavender Medical (Stevenage, United Kingdom) in which the platelet concentration is 4-5 x that of whole blood. Growth factor concentrations were as follows: Platelet-Derived Growth Factor (PDGF) 2048 pg/mL; Vascular Endothelial Growth Factor (VEGF) 220 pg/mL, and Epidermal Growth Factor (EGF) 269 pg/mL.

The six step preparation process involved centrifugation of a whole blood and anticoagulant mix for 10 minutes at 1,500 g. The gel within the vacuum tube allowed separation of the whole blood into Platelet Poor Plasma (PPP), a platelet layer and red blood cell layer. PPP was then mixed with the platelet layer to produce PRP. Each patient received a single 2 mL injection followed by a 2-week rest period. No specific rehabilitation protocol was followed.

Patients were evaluated using subjective impression of their pain severity expressed on a Visual Analogue Scale (VAS) and their functional state. The VAS was scored out of 10, with 10 representing the most severe pain. Follow up was at 1 and 3-4 months.

Results

To investigate the incidence and nature of knee injuries in professional footballers.

	Pre-PRP	1 month	3-4 months
VAS	6.9±2.3	6.6±1.4	6.8±2.3

Table 1. Visual Analogue Scale (VAS) before and after Platelet-Rich Plasma (PRP) treatment.

At one month, 8 patients reported improvement in symptoms, with 1 patient's symptoms completely resolving resulting in a return to sports by month 3.
At 3 months, 11 patients reported improvement in symptoms, with complete resolution in 2 cases.
There was sustained improvement throughout the follow up period for 5 patients, with 3 patients discharged due to resolution of their presenting complaint.
There were no documented complications.
Three patients reported worsening symptoms and 5 patients went on to receive other treatment methods, such as surgery.

Conclusions

Our data demonstrated modest symptomatic improvement at short term (1 month: 44%), at medium term (3-4 months: 61%), with only 17% formally discharged from orthopaedic care at 3-4 months. Mean VAS remained relatively consistent throughout the follow up period.
The benefits of PRP may take longer than one month to truly materialise.
In addition, 28% of patients required further treatment, either repeat PRP injections or surgical treatment.
Despite these mixed experiences there were no reported complications up to 3-4 months.
Further work is required to consolidate PRP's role within this field, particularly with respect to long term outcomes and sustained return to sports. This should be in the form of a controlled study, with carefully chosen outcome measures and a single of type of PRP.

References

1. Dohan Ehrenfest DM, Rasmusson L, Albrektsson T. Classification of platelet concentrates: from pure plateletrich plasma (P-PRP) to leucocyte- and platelet-rich fibrin (L-PRF). Trends in Biotechnology 2009; 27(3): 158-167
2. Foster TE, Puskas BL, Mandelbaum BL, Gerhardt MB, Rodeo SA. Platelet-rich plasma: from basic science to clinical applications. American Journal of Sports Medicine 2009; 37: 2259-2272

ECCENTRIC EXERCISE AND PLATELET-RICH PLASMA INJECTION FOR HAMSTRING INJURY

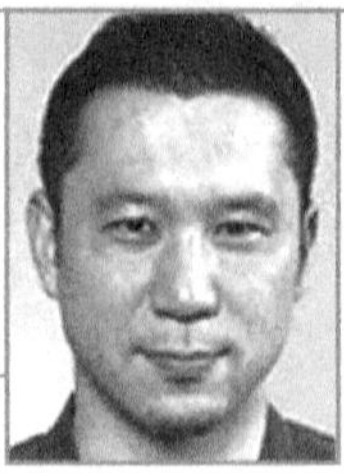

Saita Y, Kobayashi Y, Ikeda H

Orthopedics and Sports Medicine, Juntendo University,
FIFA Medical Centre of Excellence, Tokyo, Japan

Introduction

Hamstring injury is the most common muscle injury in football players and its treatment remains major concern in the area of football medicine. Recent works confirmed the Eccentric exercise (EC-Cex) successfully shortened the time to Return To Play (RTP), whereas the effect of Platelet-Rich Plasma (PRP) injection for muscle injuries is still controversial.
The purpose of this study is to reveal the efficacy of ECCex and PRP therapy for the treatment of hamstring injuries.

Methods

Twenty three muscle-tendon junction injuries combined with partial tear of central tendon of biceps femoris occurred in the male professional football players in Japan from 2010 to 2015.
The age of players was 25.6 4.6 years old, the height was 18 ±8 cm, and the body weight was 72.96.5 kg on average ±SD. The 3 Tesla Magnetic Resonance Imaging (3T-MRI) performed within 48 hours post-injury and at least two team physicians as well as one radiologist confirmed the diagnosis of muscle strain.
The treatments of these players were changed by two seasons:
- 2010-11: conventional physiotherapy mainly consisted with concentric exercises (group A, n=7);
- 2012-13: conventional physiotherapy plus PRP therapy (group B, n=8);
- 2014-15: early progressive ECCex plus PRP therapy (group C, n=8).

There were not significant differences in age, height, body weight, and body-mass-index among these three groups. With regard to the PRP therapy, we prepared three mL of PRP from 30 mL of peripheral blood using commercially available PRP kit (MyCells-PRP kit, Kaylight Technologies Ltd, Holon, Israel).
PRP typically contains 2-4 times the concentration of normal platelet levels, while white blood cells were below the base line (Leukocyte-poor PRP). PRP was percutaneously injected with 23G Cattelan needle under the Ultrasound (US) guide at the partial tendon rupture site confirmed with Magnetic Resonance Imaging (MRI) and US.
The initiation of PRP therapy was 7±2 days post injury. PRP therapy performed from one to two times in every week or every another week depends on the severity of injury and clinical course. The progressive ECCex was a accelerate rehabilitation protocol emphasizing lengthening exercises similar to Askling's L-protocol (1). The outcome measure was the days to return to full team training and availability for match selection. Reinjury was defined as re-rupture of biceps femoris intramuscular tendon during a period of six months after return to play.
RTP permission criteria was as follows: i) All of the physical findings are negative including the discomfort during concentric and eccentric muscle contractions; ii) Athletes feels nothing during football specific motions on the pitch; iii) More than 90% of recovery of peak isokinetic torque (60 degree/s) both in knee extension and flexion compared to unaffected leg and/or pre-injured muscle strength.

Results

The time to RTP in group A, B, and C were 38.9±15.2, 30.4±2.3, and 17.8±9.2 days respectively (Figure 1), and the incidences of recurrence were 2/7 (28.6%), 1/8 (12.5%), and 0/8 respectively. The time to RTP was statistically significantly shortened in group C compared to group A ($p<0.01$, one-way ANOVA with post-hoc tests), while there were no significant differences between group A and B ($p=0.40$), and B and C ($p=0.13$) (Figure 1).

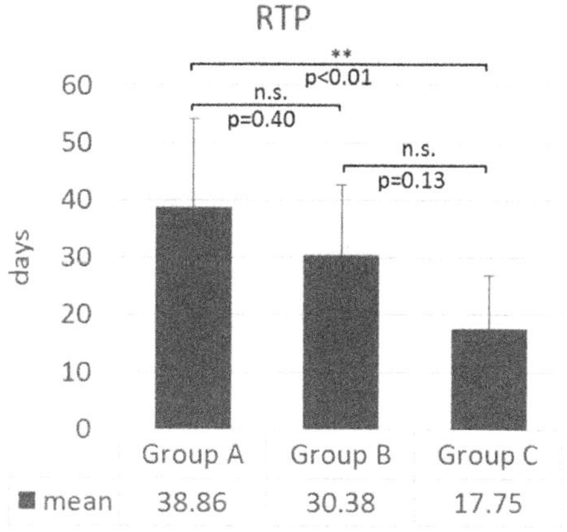

Figure 1. Time to RTP in the three groups.

Conclusions

ECCex plus PRP injection for hamstring injury shortened the time to RTP and it may decrease the re-injury rate as well. ECCex is the most effective treatment for hamstring injuries and PRP might be one of the optional tools to assist the repair process of injured intramuscular tendon.

References

1. Askling CM, Tengvar M, Thorstensson A. Acute hamstring injuries in Swedish elite football: a prospective randomised controlled clinical trial comparing two rehabilitation protocols. Br J Sports Med 2013; 47: 953-959

PLATELET RICH PLASMA ENHANCES NEO-VASCULARISATION AFTER ANTERIOR CRUCIATE LIGAMENT RECONSTRUCTION

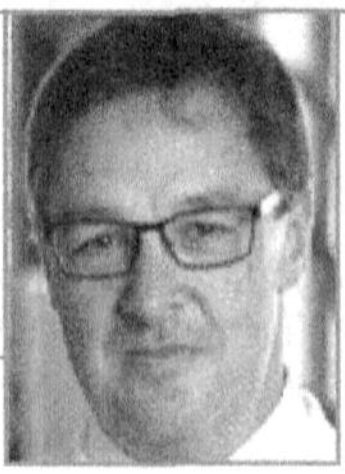

Vogrin M, Kelc R

Department of Orthopaedic Surgery, University Medical Center, Maribor, Slovenia
Institute of Sports Medicine, Faculty of Medicine, University of Maribor, Slovenia

Introduction

Long rehabilitation after arthroscopic Anterior Cruciate Ligament (ACL) reconstruction represents big problem for mainly due to a slow process of ligamentization.
The purpose of the study was to determine if the use of Platelet Gel (PG) accelerates graft revascularisation after ACL reconstruction, and whether it has any morphological and clinical relevance for the operation outcome.

Methods

Fifty patients were included, 25 treated with Platelet Riche Plasma (PRP; PG group) and 25 in a Control group, all aged between 18 and 50 years. During the procedures Gracilis and Semitendinosus tendons were used as grafts.
Platelet gel was produced from PRP in a standard procedure using Magellan autologous platelet separator. Six mL of platelet- and leukocyte-rich plasma were injected in the knee joint as a single injection into the femoral and tibial tunnels intraoperatively.
All patient followed the same rehabilitation protocol, with permission for immediate weight bearing and full range of motion. Closed kinetic chain exercises were permitted immediately after the surgical procedure. Running was allowed at 12 weeks and contact sports at 6 months in cases with no-knee joint effusions, full range of motion and obtained muscle strength of 90% compared with the contralateral leg.
We quantitatively evaluated the process of revascularization. Contrast enhanced Magnetic Resonance Imaging (MRI) studies were carried out at 4-6, 10-12 and 25-27 weeks post-surgery. The vascularization rate was defined as the MRI signal enhancement of the osteo-ligamentous interface between the wall of the tibial tunnel and the graft and in the intra-articular part of the graft itself after paramagnetic contrast medium administration.
Differences in characteristics between the two therapeutic methods were compared by chi-square tests for categorical variables and by Mann-Whitney rank test for continuous variables. Linear regression was used to adjust the effect of age and body mass index on the two therapeutic methods.

Results

Patients treated with PG demonstrated a significantly higher level of vascularization in the osteo-ligamentous interface at the first control.
At the second control, the level of vascularisation decreased in the PG group and increased in the control group. In the intra-articular part of the graft we found minimal levels of revascularization but no differences among the groups.
At third control the level of vascularisation decreased in both groups. The amount of new sclerotic bone formation was significantly higher in group treated with PRP, as well as the antero-posterior knee stability.

Groups	S (tib) K1	S (art) K1	S (noise) K1	S (tib) K2	S (art) K2	S (noise) K2
PG group Before CM	290.9	94.8	1,029.8	283.9	108.2	1,098.2
PG group After CM	657.7	91.9	1,074.6	527.7	132.1	1,198.9
Control group Before CM	311.3	66.7	1,141.1	270.4	79.4	1,167.8
Control group After CM	509.6	77.8	1,177.8	494.6	102.5	1,201.9

Table 1. MRI signal intensity (S) in the PG group and the Control group before (K1) and after (K2) the application of the Contrast-enhanced Medium (CM).

Vascularization rate	Control (n=20)	PG (n=21)	P value
V(tib)K1 (4-6 weeks)	0.16±0.09	0.33±0.09	<0.001
V(tib)K2 (10-12 weeks)	0.17±0.10	0.20±0.13	0.404
V(art)K1 (4-6 weeks)	0.01±0.02	-0.01±0.08	0.262
V(art)K1 (10-12 weeks)	0.02±0.04	0.01±0.06	0.404

Table 2. Vascularization rate in the interface zone between the graft and bone tunnels, V(tib), and the intra-articular part of the graft, V(art), at the first (K1) and second (K2) control follow-ups.

Conclusions

The PG enhances early revascularization of the graft in the zone of the osteo-ligamentous interface after ACL reconstruction.

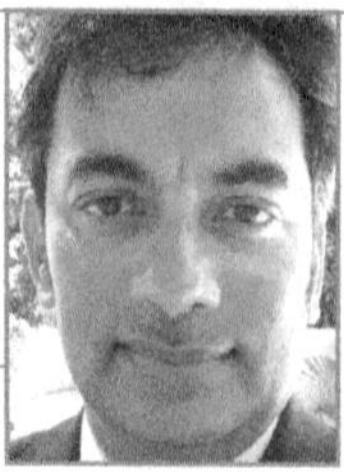

AUTOLOGOUS TENOCYTE INJECTION FOR CHRONIC REFRACTORY TENDINOPATHY: FROM CELL BIOLOGY TO CLINICAL TRIALS

Rao KA[1], Zheng MH[2], Wang A[2], Bucher T[3], Wang T[2], Ebert J[4], Breidahl W[5]

[1]Specilaist Sportscare WA, Inglewood, Perth; [2]Centre for Orthopaedic Research, School of Surgery, University of Western Australia, Perth; [3]Department of Orthopaedics, Fremantle Hospital, Fremantle; [4]School of Sport Science, Exercise and Health, University of Western Australia, Crawley, Perth; [5]Perth Radiological Clinic, Subiaco, Perth, Australia

Introduction

Histological studies of tendinopathy show that the functional tenocyte population is significantly decreased in areas of severest damage. We hypothesized that restoration of the functional tenocyte pool using our Autologous Tenocyte Injection (ATI) technique might be an effective therapeutic strategy. The autologous cells displayed tendon characteristics including expression of tendon transcription factors, type I collagen, tenomodulin and tendon related growth factors. Additionally, they were able to form neotendon tissue when cultured in a bioreactor system with cyclic mechanical stimulation.

After completing successful animal studies, we commenced clinical studies of ATI in patients with chronic tendinopathy.

Methods

A total of 57 patients with chronic, refractory tendinopathy with age ranged from 25 to 60 with M:F 1:1.5, most are weekend warriors and work-related injury. Most of them had failed to respond to more than one previous injection therapies (PRP or Steroid) and eccentric exercises.

Average symptom duration was 18 months with ranged from 8 month to 240 months, and they were affected by lateral epicondylitis (n=37), gluteal tendinopathy (n=12), rotator cuff tear (n=5), Achilles tendinopathy (n=3).

Autologous tendon cells were sourced from a needle biopsy of healthy tendon (usually the patellar tendon). The cells were isolated by enzymatic digestion and expanded in a Good Manufacturing Practices (GMP) certified laboratory. Characterization studies were conducted to examine purity, potency, identity and viability.

Approximately three weeks after patellar tendon biopsy, cells were implanted in the site of tendinopathy by ultrasound-guided injection. Up to 2 mL of autologous tenocytes (2-5 3 106 cells/mL) suspended with 10% autologous human serum were injected using an 18-gauge needle into the tendinosis or tear as identified. After the injection, there is no specific rehabilitation required except normal daily activity. Clinical assessments on VISA pain score, functional assessment and Magnetic Resonance Imaging (MRI) were performed at baseline (before biopsy) and up to 5 years post-treatment.

Results

As this is a collective cases study from different anatomical site of tendinopathy, representative data on the assessment for lateral epicondylitis are presented. The result showed that clinical evaluation revealed significant improvement (35; $p<0.001$) in mean VAS pain score from 5.73 at initial assessment to 1.21 (78% improvement) at final follow-up.

Mean QuickDASH, UEFS and grip strength scores also significantly improved ($p<0.001$) from initial assessment to final follow-up (45.88 to 6.61, 84%; 31.73 to 9.20, 64%; 19.85 to 46.60, 208%, respectively). There was no difference in mean QuickDASH and UEFS scores at one year and final follow-up ($p>0.05$), however grip strength continued to improve ($p<0.001$). At final follow up, 93% of patients were either highly satisfied or satisfied with their ATI treatment.

Using a validated MRI scoring system, the mean grade of tendinopathy at the common extensor origin improved significantly ($p<0.001$) from initial assessment (4.31) to one year (2.88) and was maintained ($p>0.05$) at final follow-up (2.87).

Over all, patients experienced significant improvements in pain and function starting from one month post-treatment, and the improvements were maintained for up to 5 years.

Conclusions

These studies show that ATI facilitates structural repair and improves pain and function in patients with tendinopathy. Further study using randomized control study protocol is needed to confirm the efficacy.

References

1. Wang A, Mackie K, Breidahl W, Wang T, Zheng MH. Evidence for the durability of autologous tenocyte injection for treatment of chronic resistant lateral epicondylitis: mean 4.5-year clinical follow-up. Am J Sports Med 2015; 43: 1775-1783
2. Wang A, Breidahl W, Mackie KE, Lin Z, Qin A, Chen J, Zheng MH. Autologous tenocyte injection for the treatment of severe, chronic resistant lateral epicondylitis: a pilot study. Am J Sports Med 2013; 41: 2925 2932
3. Wang AW, Bauer S, Goonatillake M, Breidahl W, Zheng MH. Autologous tenocyte implantation, a novel treatment for partial-thickness rotator cuff tear and tendinopathy in an elite athlete. BMJ Case Rep 2013 Jan 11;2013. pii: bcr2012007899. doi: 10.1136/bcr-2012-007899.

Saturday, 9th April, 2016
POSTER AREA

FREE POSTER PRESENTATIONS

REHABILITATION AND RETURN TO PLAY

Chairs

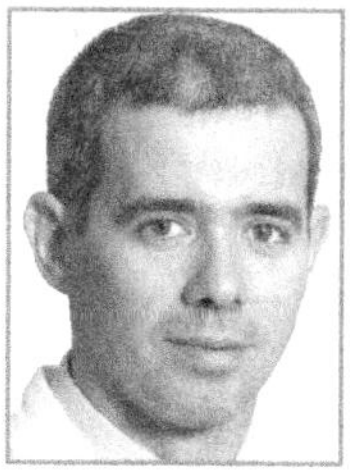

Lorenzo Boldrini
(Milan, Italy)

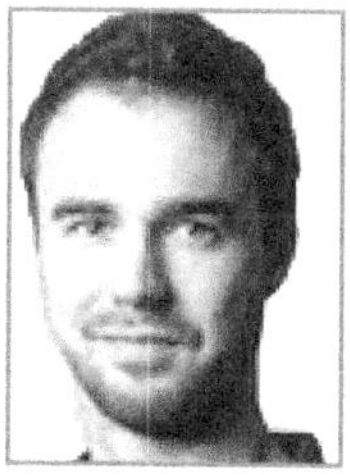

Alessandro Marconato
(London, United Kingdom)

PC01 Return to play training after a fifth metatarsal stress fracture in a professional football player: a case report
Cavaggioni L, Ongaro L, Alberti G (Milan, Italy)

PC02 Return-to-play criteria after anterior cruciate ligament reconstruction: actual medicine practice in professional soccer teams
Delvaux F, Rochcongar P, Bruyère O, Bourlet G, Daniel C, Diverse P, Reginster JY, Croisier JL (Liege and Verviers Belgium; Rennes, France)

PC03 Bridging the gap: an exercise intervention to return to play after hip arthroplasty **Pozzi F, Zaffagnini S, Snyder-Mackler L (Los Angeles and Newark, USA; Bologna, Italy)**

PC04 Return to play after minimal muscular injury in La Liga football club
Jablonski J, Turmo-Garuz A, Garcia-Diaz M, Gasol X, Lupon G, Til L (Barcelona and Sant Cugat del Valles, Spain; Lodz, Poland)

PC05 Injury rates and return to play times in under 16-18 academy footballerst
Davies GP (Sheffield, United Kingdom)

PC06 The functional movement screen and prediction of time to return to play
Nagao M, Okazaki T, Miyamori T, Yoshimura M (Tokyo, Japan)

PC07 Comparison of time to return to play between elite Spanish football and futsal **Vivo-Fernández I, Lopez-Segovia M, Salinas-Palacios V, Herrero-Carrasco R, Pareja-Blanco F (Murcia and Seville, Spain)**

PC08 Is single leg hop test at the end of the assisted rehabilitation predictive of full RTP in football players after ACL reconstruction?
Danelon F, Pisoni D, Caminati D, Gamberini J, Della Villa F (Milan and Bologna, Italy)

PC09 Physiotherapy in revision reconstruction of ACL of football players
Kępczyński A, Krzyżak Ł, Luboiński Ł (Warsaw, Poland)

PC10 Return to play after functional movement analysis in soccer players with long-standing muscle-related pain
Dewitz H, Yildirim B, Stock Th, Klein P (Cologne, Germany)

PC11 Fast bleeding recovery with whole body cryo-therapy after muscular injury
Freschi M, Genovese E, Tavana R (Milan and Cagliari, Italy)

RETURN TO PLAY TRAINING AFTER A FIFTH METATARSAL STRESS FRACTURE IN A PROFESSIONAL FOOTBALL PLAYER: A CASE REPORT

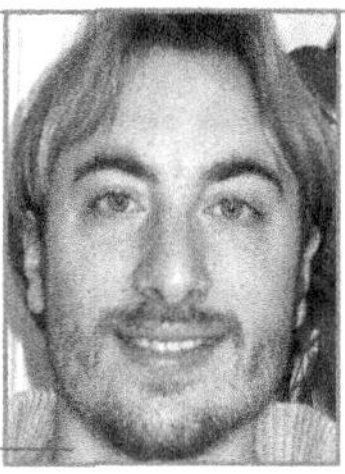

Cavaggioni L, Ongaro L, Alberti G

School of Exercise Science, Department of Biomedical Sciences for Health, Università degli Studi di Milano, Italy

Introduction

In professional football players, of 1.3754 injuries, 0.5% derived to be fifth metatarsal fractures (2). Ekstrand & Torstveit (2012) found that the distribution of stress fractures in 2.379 football players affected the lower extremities and 58% of them affected the fifth metatarsal bone.
A stress fracture is a partial or complete bone fracture that results from repeated application of stress lower than the stress required to fracture the bone in a single loading. Many factors may be involved, such as biomechanical predisposition in running or jumping patterns, feet postural disorders, training methods, gender differences and other factors such as diet, muscle strength or flexibility. For this type of injury, surgery provided to be the best result with a period of non-weight-bearing, mobilization and follow-up X-rays to assesses the fracture healing.
The purpose of this case report is to describe the post-surgery reconditioning training routine with a professional football player affected by a fifth metatarsal stress fracture which allowed him returning to prior level of sport participation.

Methods

The subject is a professional male football player (36 years old; 1.80 m; 75 kg; 23.1 kg/m^2) who stopped playing on 13th of February because of a fifth metatarsal stress fracture on the left foot during an official game. After surgery (on the 3rd of March it was made a stab incision with an intramedullary screw) the athlete could not bear any weight for 13 days. He started immediately physical therapy treatments (weight-bearing walking exercises in the pool and in the gym on bicycle, elliptical machines and treadmill).
On the 5th of April he started the conditioning programme, which finished on 25th April.
The return to play routine was based on different levels: the first step (6 session/week, 90 minutes each) included a core muscles programme through a progression of neuro-developmental exercises using a diaphragmatic breath, motor patterns like rolling, chopping, lifting or rotational movements, strengthening with slow speed of muscular action (1), mobility through global stretching Mézières method, kinaesthetic feet awareness on sand (3) and cardio-respiratory development on treadmill. The second step was always based on motor patterns and conditioning drills on court, more focused on sport-specific demands in order to achieve the adequate flexibility, motor control and balance required for return to play (5 session/week, 60 minutes each).
To evaluate the postural, functional and strength parameters a photographic Morphological Mapping, Functional Movement Screen (FMS), and a Counter Movement Jump (CMJ) with an infrared validated device (Optojump system) were used. All these measurements were taken on three different occasions: during training before the injury, at the end of the retraining period after injury, and two months after the return to play for a follow-up.

Results

Results of FMS and CMJ are shown in Table 1. Observing photographs we can appreciate a reduced pelvic inclination on the right side, a lower left knee intra-rotation and feet supination (Figure 1).

	DS	HS R	HS L	ILL R	ILL L	SM R	SM L	ASLR R	ASLR L	TSPU	RS R	RS L	COM-POSI-TE	CMJ	CMJ R	CMJ L
Before injury	2	2	1	2	1	2	2	1	1	2	2	2	11	35.2	22.1	23.5
End of retraining	2	2	2	2	2	3	2	2	2	3	2	3	15	41.8	24.7	26.1
Follow-Up	2	2	2	2	2	3	2	2	2	2	2	2	14	40.1	23.5	25.4

Table 1. Results of Functional Movement Screen (arbitrary units) and Counter Movement Jump (CMJ) test (cm) also for Right (R) and Left (L) limbs. DS=Deep Squat, HS=Hurdle Step, ILL=In Line Lunge, SM=Shoulder Mobility, ASLR=Active Straight Leg Raise, TSPU=Trunk Stability Push Up, RS=Rotary Stability.

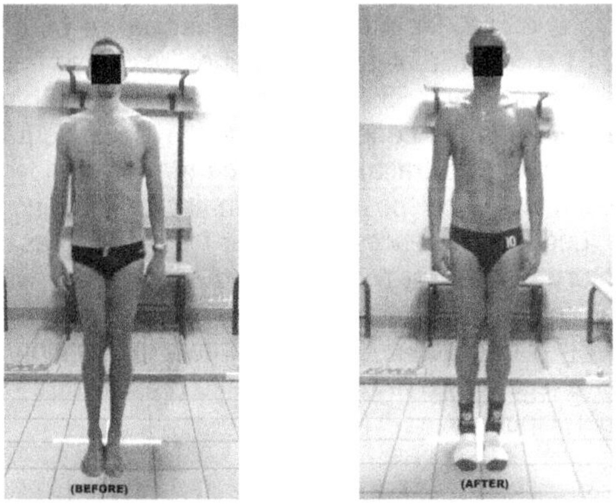

Figure 1. Photographic Morphological Mapping before and at the end of the conditioning

Conclusions

The conditioning program based on a movement-guided routine in order to improve mobility, stability, strength on the injured foot, and to reduce the regional impairments allowed the player to improve motor control, flexibility and strength from the baseline compared to end of the conditioning period. These improvements were maintained at two months follow-up.

The FMS scores showed a decrease in asymmetries from the beginning until the end especially on the left (injured) side (Hurdle Step, In Line Lunge), and an increase in posterior chain mobility and pelvic stability (Active Straight Leg Raise). A structured training routine addressed essentially postural alignment, proper breathing pattern and functional movement, potentially allows athletes to return to sport with this type of injury.

References

1. Alberti G, Cavaggioni L, Silvaggi N, Caumo A, Garufi M. Resistance training with blood flow restriction using the modulation of the muscle's contraction velocity. Strength Cond J 2013; 35: 42-47
2. Ekstrand J, van Dijk CN. Fifth metatarsal fractures among male professional footballers: a potential career-ending disease. http://www.ncbi.nlm.nih.gov/pubmed/23467966 Br J Sports Med 2013; 47: 754-758
3. Gaudino P, Gaudino C, Alberti G, Minetti AE. Biomechanics and predicted energetics of sprinting on sand: hints for soccer training. J Sci Med Sport 2013; 16: 271-275

RETURN-TO-PLAY CRITERIA AFTER ANTERIOR CRUCIATE LIGAMENT RECONSTRUCTION: ACTUAL MEDICINE PRACTICE IN PROFESSIONAL SOCCER TEAMS

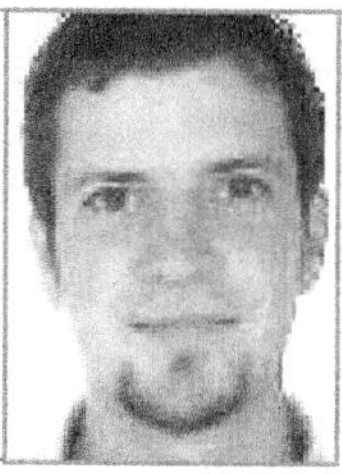

Delvaux F[1], Rochcongar P[2], Bruyère O[3], Bourlet G[1], Daniel C[4], Diverse P[5], Reginster JY[3], Croisier JL[1]

[1]Department of Sport and Rehabilitation Sciences, University and CHU of Liege, Belgium; [2]Department of Biology and Sports Medicine, CHU Pontchaillou, Rennes, France; French Federation of Soccer, Professional Football League; [3]Department of Public Health, Epidemiology and Health Economics, University and CHU of Liege, Belgium; [4]Department of Orthopaedic Surgery, CHU of Liege, Belgium; [5]Department of Orthopaedic Surgery, Saint-Elisabeth Hospital, Verviers, Belgium

Introduction

Return To Play (RTP) decisions are a crucial component in sports medicine, but they may vary according to differences of scientific knowledge, personal experience or personal values of physicians (1). The purpose of this study was to analyze how sport physicians decide, in their daily practice, when an Anterior Cruciate Ligament (ACL) reconstructed professional soccer player is able to get back to competitive activities.

Methods

Thirty-seven physicians (age: 46.3±7.1 years; experience in professional soccer: 12.3±6.4 years) for professional French and Belgian soccer teams filled in a specific questionnaire dedicated to: i) return-to-play criteria after ACL reconstruction; ii) the importance they assigned to each of these criteria in the return-to-play decision; iii) the potential role of professionals such as physiotherapists, physical coaches or soccer coaches in this decision.

Results

Eighty per cent of the responders declared to use at least eight criteria in order to assess player's ability to return to competitive soccer after ACL reconstruction. The most important ones were (in order of importance): dynamic knee stability during a specific soccer exercise, muscle strength performance, normalization of knee flexion and extension ranges of motion, and subjective feeling reported by the player (Table 1).

1	Dynamic knee stability during a specific soccer exercise
2	Muscle strength performance
3	Normalization of knee flexion and extension ranges of motion
4	Subjective feeling reported by the player
5	Complete pain relief

Table 1. Return-to-play criteria ranking in order of importance

For most of these criteria, there was a lack of consensus about the choice of assessment parameters and the limit values allowing physicians to authorize or forbid the return-to-competition. For example, a bilateral balance of isokinetic strength performance represents an essential RTP criterion for all the physicians. However, 24% of the responders tolerate less than 5% of bilateral deficit, 36% tolerate up to 10% of deficit and 31% declared to allow RTP in spite of bilateral differences of 15%.
A very large majority of participants stated to take into consideration advices from physiotherapists (97%) or physical coaches (91%) in the RTP decision, while only 40% of physicians take the opinion of the soccer coach for the RTP decision.

Conclusions

Sport physicians for professional soccer teams use relevant criteria to assess player's ability to return to full sport after anterior cruciate ligament reconstruction. Nevertheless, it appears that there is a lack of consensus about the choice of the assessment parameters and the limit values allowing doctors to authorize or forbid RTP. Even if the scientific evidence about this topic is not sufficient at the moment, some objective criteria have been scientifically demonstrated to lower re-injury rate and their implementations are now possible.

References

1. Delvaux F, Rochcongar P, Bruyère O, Bourlet G, Daniel C, Diverse P, Reginster JY, Croisier JL. Return-to-play criteria after hamstring injury: actual medicine practice in professional soccer teams. J Sports Sci Med 2014; 13: 721-723

BRIDGING THE GAP: AN EXERCISE INTERVENTION TO RETURN TO PLAY AFTER HIP ARTHROPLASTY

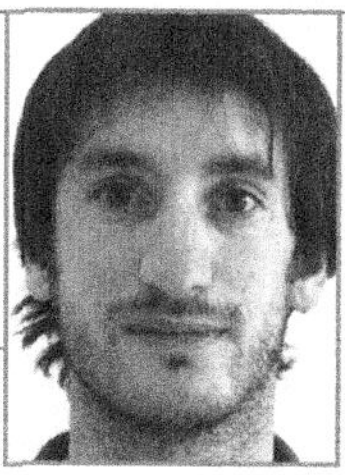

Pozzi F[1], Zaffagnini S[2], Snyder-Mackler L[3]

[1]University of Southern California, Los Angeles, USA;
[2]Rizzoli orthopaedic Institute, Bologna, Italy; [3]University of Delaware, Newark, USA

Introduction

Many patients stop participating in recreational activities after Total Hip Replacement (THA) (1). Current rehabilitation protocols following THA do not typically address factors that could promote exercise participation (2). An exercise intervention is needed to target persistent deficits and promote return to play. This type of intervention may be extremely beneficial after surgery as pain, the major barrier to exercise (3), is often resolved. The purpose of this study was to assess the feasibility and the preliminary effectiveness of a transitional exercise program on patients' outcome and sport participation following THA.

Methods

One male patient (62 years old, 31.5 kg/m^2 of Body Mass Index) who underwent unilateral THA with an anterolateral approach participated in this intervention. He previously completed 5 home and 12 outpatient physical therapy sessions. Seven-months after THA, he participated in 18 one-to-one, hour long exercise sessions over 6 weeks. Each session included two 15-minutes aerobic exercise components, one 20 minute strengthening component, and 10 total minutes of recovery between exercises. Methods of aerobic and resistive weight training were tailored to his baseline status and goals, according to his Patient Specific Functional Scale (PSFS). Aerobic exercises were progressed to maintain an intensity level of 65% of the maximal predicted heart rate. The strengthening component targeted muscle groups in the lower leg. Resistance was adjusted to maintain the appropriate exercise intensity (3 sets of 10 repetitions). Adverse effects, such as joint pain, swelling, and excessive soreness, were monitored at the end and before the start of each session. The patient underwent a functional evaluation before and at the end of the exercise intervention. Functional outcomes included the PSFS, the Fatigue Severity Scale (FSS), the International Physical Activity Questionnaire short form (IPAQ), hip range of motion, and hip abductor and quadriceps strength test. For all these variables, percentage change between baseline and at the end of the intervention time points was calculated.

Results

The patient completed all 18 sessions without reporting adverse outcomes. He did report hip pain after the first and second session (1 and 2 out of 10, respectively), which may be related to the beginning of an exercise routine. At final follow-up, his body weight decreased 5%; hip abduction and adduction range of motion increased 67 and 36%, respectively; hip abductor and quadriceps strength on the surgical side increased 22 and 31%, respectively; FSS score decreased 47%; and weekly metabolic equivalent (derived from the IPAQ scale) increased from 891 MET/week to 4760 MET/week (Table 1). At the end of the intervention, his perceived ability to run and play golf, as measured with the PSFS, increased 50 and 75%, respectively (Table 1).

		Baseline	End	Diff. %
Demographic	Weight (kg)	108	103	-5
	BMI (kg/m^2)	31.5	29.8	-5
Surgical leg, average joint pain	Hip (0-10)	0	0	0
	Knee (0-10)	2	0	-100
Surgical leg, strength	Hip abductors (% Body mass)	0.09	0.11	22
	Knee extensors (Nm/kg)	1.67	2.19	31
Surgical hip, range of motion	Flexion (°)	120	110	-8
	Abduction (°)	15	25	67
	Adduction (°)	11	15	36
	External rotation (°)	43	43	0
	Internal rotation (°)	33	32	-3
Activity level	IPAQ (METs/week)	891	4760	434
	FFS (0-63)	43	23	-47
Ability to participate in sports	Golf (PSFS 0-10)	6	9	50
	Running (PSFS 0-10)	4	7	75

Table 1. Clinical measures before (Baseline) and at the end of the exercise intervention (End) for the patient, and change from baseline (Diff. %).

Conclusions

This case study suggests that an exercise intervention that includes aerobic and strengthening exercises is feasible in patients after THA. The intervention successfully increased hip range of motion and leg strength. Greater activity level was measured with decreased level of perceived fatigue. The higher level of activity may have promoted clinically significant weight loss. The increased ability to perform high level of recreational activity may suggest that this type of intervention may also foster return to play in this population.

References

1. Delasotta LA, Rangavajjula A V, Porat MD, Frank ML, Orozco FR, Ong AC. What are young patients doing after hip reconstruction? J Arthroplasty 2012; 27: 1518-1525.
2. Minns Lowe CJ, Barker KL, Dewey ME, Sackley CM. Effectiveness of physiotherapy exercise following hip arthroplasty for osteoarthritis: a systematic review of clinical trials. BMC Musculoskelet Disord 2009 Aug 4; 10:98. doi: 10.1186/1471-2474-10-98
3. Wilcox S, Der Ananian C, Abbott J, Vrazel J, Ramsey C, Sharpe PA, Brady T. Perceived exercise barriers, enablers, and benefits among exercising and nonexercising adults with arthritis: results from a qualitative study. Arthritis Rheum 2006; 55: 616-627

RETURN TO PLAY AFTER MINIMAL MUSCULAR INJURY IN LA LIGA FOOTBAL CLUB

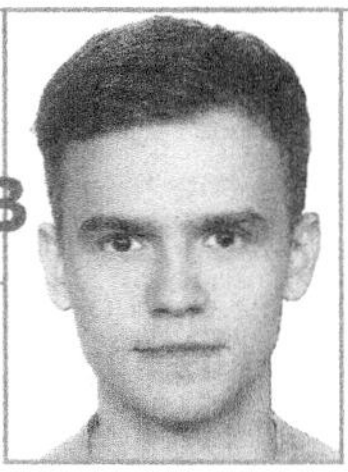

Jablonski J[1,4], Turmo-Garuz A[2,3], Garcia-Diaz M[3], Gasol X[3], Lupon G[2,3], Til L[2]

[1]Sport Medicine School - Univesity of Barcelona, Barcelona, Spain; [2]High Performance Center (CAR), Sant Cugat del Valles, Spain; [3]Reial Club Deportiu Espanyol Barcelona, Barcelona, Spain; [4]Orto Med Sport, Lodz, Poland

Introduction

Muscle injuries constitute a high percentage of all injuries in football causing a significant amount of missed game time. Minimal muscle injury, as defined by the Munich consensus statement (1, 3), encompasses all functional muscle disorders without macroscopic evidence of fibre tear (examined with expert ultrasound or Magnetic Resonance Imaging) including fatigue induced muscle disorders, Delayed Onset Muscle Soreness (DOMS), as well as muscle and spine related neuro muscular muscle disorders. Management of minimal muscle injury is now being recognized as an important area of focus due to its diagnostic difficulties as well as associated time-loss.
The purpose of this study was to determine if a correlation exists between return to play time and this type of muscle injury.

Methods

This was a retrospective study of male elite football players from the first and second teams of Reial Club Deportiu (RCD) Espanyol Barcelona during four regular seasons of La Liga from 2011 to 2015. Injury data was collected by team doctors.
The Orchard Sports Injury Classification System (OSICS-10.1) was used for coding the injuries (2). Muscular injury rates and time-loss were calculated using previously reported team rates.
Injuries were separated into two groups of structural and functional muscle injuries using the Munich classification of muscle injuries.

Results

During the four year study period a group 121 players were injured with a total of 564 of injuries and time-loss of 5,427 days.
189 (33.5%) of the injuries were muscle injuries, accounting for 1,233 missed days (22.7%).
Most of the muscle injuries 81 (42.9%) were fatigue induced muscle disorders with no or minimal (1-2 days) time missed total of 66 days (5.4%) of time-loss, 61 (32.3%) were structural muscle injuries with a total of 852 days (69.1%) of time-loss, 47 (24.8%) were functional muscular disorders (excluding fatigue induced disorders) resulting in a total 315 days (25.6%) of time-loss (Table 1).

Minimal Muscle Injury	**Number**	**Days of Time-loss**
Rectus Femoris	13	93
Semitendinosus	10	96
Biceps Femoris	8	46
Adductor Longus	4	14
Gastrocnemius	4	11
Peroneal	3	2
Soleus	2	42
Semimembranosus	2	7
Psoas	1	4
Totals	47	315

Table 1. Minimal Muscle Injury per muscle.

Conclusions

Both structural muscle disorders and functional muscle disorders have significant impact on return to play. The diagnosis of Minimal Muscle Injuries is mainly clinical examination due to lack of specific diagnostic support.
Medical staff should pay more attention to Minimal Muscular Injuries considering high possibility of long return to play.
Further studies are required to determine proper diagnostic base for therapeutic decision-making and prognostication to support return to play.

References

1. Ekstrand J, Askling C, Magnusson H, Mithoefer K. Return to play after thigh muscle injury in elite football players: implementation and validation of the Munich muscle injury classification. Br J Sports Med 2013; 47: 769-774
2. Pollock N, James SL, Lee JC, Chakraverty R. British athletic muscle injury classification: a new grading system. BR J Sports Med 2014; 48: 1347-1351
3. Mueller-Wohlfahrt HW, Haensel L, Mithoefer K, Ekstrand J, English B, McNally S, Orchard J, van Dijk CN, Kerkhoffs GM, Schamasch P, Blottner D, Swaerd L, Goedhart E, Ueblacker P. Terminology and classification of muscle injuries in sport: The Munich consensus statement. Br J Sports Med 2013; 47: 342-350

INJURY RATES AND RETURN TO PLAY TIMES IN UNDER 16 -18 ACADEMY FOOTBALLERS

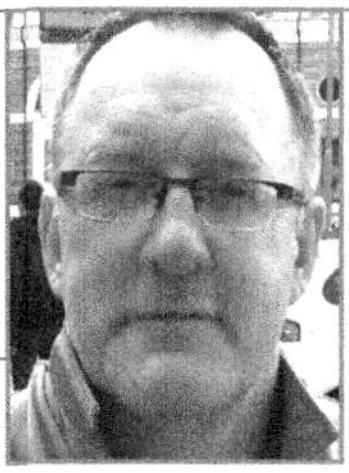

Davies GP

Sheffield Wednesday Football Club, Sheffield, United Kingdom

Introduction

The Injury rate in under-18 (U18) footballers has impact on their availability for training and match play during their two year scholarship. The time lost due to injury may have impact on player development and progression to full time adult football. There have been few recent studies of injury rates in U18 footballers in English Professional Academies.

This poster reviews the date in the season, the rate and site of injury, and the time to return to play of academy players over nine seasons at U18 level at single club in the English football league.

Methods

A review was made of nine seasons of player injury records and club audit for the seasons 2006-07 to 2015-16.

A total of 184 individual players were studied and a total of 297 injuries leading to a total time loss of 7407 days recorded.

Annual audits were compiled at the close of each season from the player records. The definition of an injury and data were recorded according to the consensus statement on injury definitions and data collection procedures in studies of football injuries (1).

Results

The time loss from injury per player a season was an average of 39.6 days (13.7% of playing season).

The season total time loss was an average of 823 days with an average squad size of 20.4 players during the study period. The commonest sites of injury were ankle (7.9 injuries/season, average time to Return To Play (RTP) 20 days), knee (5.44 injuries/season; RTP: 45 days), groin (3.77 injuries/season; RTP: 42 days) and back (3.11 injuries/season; RTP: 29 days).

Injury rates peaked in the pre- season and early playing season from July to September then a second smaller peak occurred late in the playing season in March.

Conclusions

The two year period spent between 16 and 18 years on the academy programme is regarded as a vital stage in the development of a professional footballer.

The loss of a significant amount of the player's two year academy programme may be a factor in the failure of players to progress to professional football.

References

1. Fuller CW, Ekstrand J, Junge A, Andersen TE, Bahr R, Dvorak J, Hägglund M, McCrory P, Meeuwisse WH. Consensus statement on injury definitions and data collection procedures in football (soccer) injuries. Br J Sports Med 2006; 40: 193-201

6

THE FUNCTIONAL MOVEMENT SCREEN AND PREDICTION OF TIME TO RETURN TO PLAY

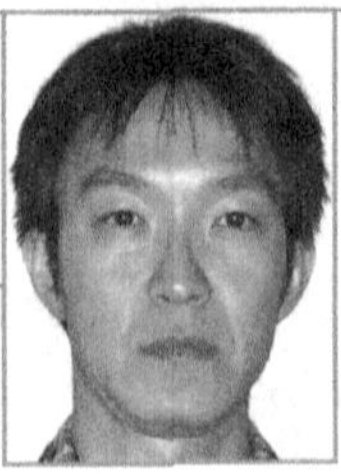

Nagao M, Okazaki T, Miyamori T, Yoshimura M

Orthopedics and Sports Medicine, Juntendo University, Tokyo; FIFA Medical Centre of Excellence Tokyo, Japan

Introduction

Football is the most popular sports in the world and the popularity and participation rates are continuously growing. Most of the football athletes experience injuries occur mainly at the lower extremities and the short- to long-term deficit from games could potentially affect their career.
Numerous individual factors have been proposed as risk factors for overall injuries related to fo-otball. Recently, the attention has been directed to the multifactorial influence of risk factors.
The Functional Movement Screen (FMS) is an evaluation tool that attempts to assess fundamental movement patterns of an individual. Recent cohort studies demonstrated that low FMS score is associated with serious injuries (1, 2). However, FMS appears to be not a suitable screening tool for identifying risk for injuries because of low predictive value. Also whether it can be applied for Asian soccer athletes has not been examined. The purpose of this study is to explore whether the FMS score predict the overall incidence of injury or time to return to play on Japanese college football athletes

Methods

One-year prospective cohort study from March 2014 was performed. All subjects were members of collage soccer team, which is classified as division 1 according to the Kanto University Football Association in Japan. Athletes who had recent musculoskeletal and head injuries within the past six weeks or had used mobility aid or a prophylactic device were excluded.
A total of 75 (men 48 and women 27) athletes were enrolled in the study.
Mean±SD age and BMI were 19.9±1.4 yrs and 22.0±1.4 kg/m^2, respectively.
Injury and time to Return To Play (RTP) were monitored.
The FMS was evaluated by experienced two physiotherapists before the study.
Inter-rater reliability was evaluated by Kappa. Associations between FMS score and the incidence of injury or time to return to play were analyzed in two different ways. First, Receiver Operating Characteristic (ROC) curve was determined including the Area Under the Curve (AUC) to set an optimal cut-off point. Second, FMS score of ≤14, ≤15, ≤16, ≤17, ≤18 or ≤19 was used as cut-off points and the associations between FMS score and the incidence of injury or time to return to play were evaluated by logistic regression analysis controlling for age, BMI and sex.

Results

A total of 82 injuries were reported and 88% were at lower extremities. 34% were non-contact injuries.
Mean FMS scores for male and female were 16.0±1.4 and 16.3±1.5 respectively, and has no statistical difference.
FMS inter-rater reliability was 0.92, indicating excellent reliability.
There are no significant associations between BMI or age with total FMS score (p=0.8 and p=0.14 respectively), while Active Straight Leg Rise (ASLR) score in women were higher than in men (P=0.04).
Cut-off points determined to be optimal for injury screening and time to return to play by ROC analysis was FMS scores of ≤16, and the AUCs were 54.6% and 53.4%, respectively.
Table 1 demonstrates the association of the FMS score with the injury risk or time to return to play. Multivariate logistic regression analysis shows that each cut-off point was not a significant risk factor for overall injury or time to return to play.

FMS score	N	%	Overall injury		Time to Return To Play	
			Odds ratio (95%CI)	p	Odds ratio (95%CI)	p
≤14	10	2.6	1.70 (0.42-6.92)	0.75	1.15 (0.63-2.10)	0.45
≤15	20	26.7	1.55 (0.51-4.74)	0.44	1.12 (0.73-1.72)	0.53
≤16	47	62.7	1.31 (0.44-3.96)	0.49	0.76 (0.49-1.18)	0.23
≤17	62	82.7	0.88 (0.22-3.60)	0.87	0.98 (0.58-1.65)	0.95
≤18	70	93.3	2.45 (0.16-38.17)	0.52	1.21 (0.62-2.39)	0.58

Table 1. Functional Movement Screen (FMS) scores and one-year injury risk or time to return to play.

Conclusions

Although a FMS score of ≤16 indicates a higher injury risk or longer time to RTP by ROC analysis, FMS is not a suitable screening tool for identifying those in this population.

References

1. Bushman TT, Grier TL, Canham-Chervak M, Anderson MK, North WJ, Jones BH. The Functional Movement Screen and injury risk association and predictive value in active men. Am J Sports Med 2015 Dec 10. pii: 0363546515614815. [Epub ahead of print]
2. Kiesel K, Plisky PJ, Voight ML. Can serious injury in professional football be predicted by a preseason functional movement screen? N Am J Sports Phys Ther 2007; 2: 147-158

COMPARISON OF TIME TO RETURN TO PLAY BETWEEN ELITE SPANISH FOOTBALL AND FUTSAL

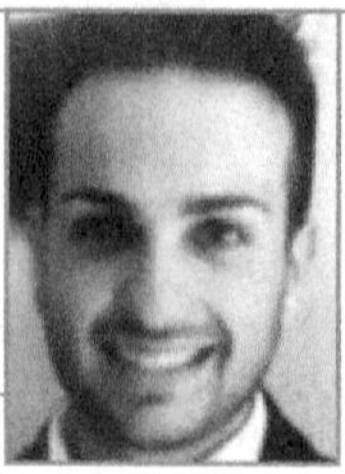

Vivo-Fernández I[1,2,3], Lopez-Segovia M[1,3], Salinas-Palacios V[1], Herrero-Carrasco R[3], Pareja-Blanco F[4]

[1]Innova, Health and Sport Institute, Murcia; [2]Department of physiotherapy, University of Murcia, Murcia; [3]Research Centre of Murcia Soccer Federation; [4]Sports and Athletic Performance Research Centre, Faculty of Sport, Pablo de Olavide University, Seville, Spain

Introduction

One of the main objectives of the medical staff of sports teams is to maintain the availability of the players in the pitch. Injuries had a negative influence on the performance (2) and the cost of an injury per month in elite player is very high, therefore professional teams can expect to reduce the time-loss in each injury. Lots of studies describe epidemiology, injury incidence and time to Return To Play (RTP) in professional and elite football, however, although futsal is a sport also registered by International Federation of Association Football (FIFA) that has in common with soccer the high risk of injury as a result of continuing sprints, changes of direction, accelerations and decelerations that occur during the game, we didn't find in the literature any study that contrast the injury patterns and time to RTP between both sports. As consequence, the aim of this study is to compare the time to RTP between Football and Futsal Elite Players.

Methods

A prospective cohort study was carried out during one season. Injuries of 24 elite football players (Spanish LaLiga, UEFA Europe League), and 24 elite futsal players (First Division of Spanish Futsal League, LNFS) were registered. The medical staff of the teams recorded injuries and time-loss. Injury definitions and data collection procedures were in accordance with the respective consensus statement for football (1). Statistical analyses were completed with IBM SPSS Statistics V.2.1.0 (IBM, Armonk, New York). Independent t-tests were used to determine whether it was significance difference in time to RTP between elite football and elite futsal groups.

Results

Injuries of 24 elite football players (26.5±4.1 years) and 24 elite futsal players (28.1±4.6 years) were registered during an entire season (Table 1).

Injury		Football		Futsal	
Location	Type	N	Days of absence	N	Days of absence
Head-neck	Muscle rupture, strain, cramps	0	0	1	1
	Haematoma, contusion	1	1	0	0
Sternum, ribs, upper back	Meniscus, cartilage	0	0	1	15
Shoulder, clavicula	Sprain, ligament	0	0	1	10
Wrist	Sprain, ligament	1	94	0	0
Abdomen	Tendon	0	0	2	2
Lower back, pelvis, sacrum	Other bone injuries	1	9	0	0
Hip, groin	Muscle rupture, strain, cramps	14	50	12	55
Thigh	Muscle rupture, strain, cramps	18	204	10	76
	Tendon injury	1	14	1	8
Knee	Haematoma, contusion	2	3	2	9
	Lesion meniscus	6	32	1	16
	Sprain, ligament	2	171	4	195
	Tendon injury	1	6	4	38
Lower leg	Muscle rupture, strain, cramps	2	2	3	3
	Haematoma, contusion	4	35	1	7
	Fracture	1	45	0	0
	Tendon injury	0	0	1	12
Ankle	Sprain, ligament	3	24	14	76
	Haematoma, contusion	1	1	2	2
Foot, toe	Haematoma, contusion	1	4	6	36

Table 1. Injury distribution by location and type and days of absence type in both groups.

	Football			Futsal		
Location	N	Days of absence	%	N	Days of absence	%
Head-neck	1	1	0.1	1	1	0.2
Sternum, ribs, upper back	0	0	0.0	1	15	2.7
Shoulder, clavicula	0	0	0.0	1	10	1.8
Wrist	1	94	13.5	0	0	0.0
Abdomen	0	0	0.0	2	2	0.4
Lower back, pelvis, sacrum	1	9	1.3	0	0	0.0
Hip, groin	14	50	7.2	12	55	9.8
Thigh	20	220	31.6	12	87	15.4
Knee	11	212	30.4	11	258	45.6
Lower leg	7	82	11.8	5	22	3.8
Ankle	4	25	3.5	16	78	13.9
Foot, toe	1	4	0.6	6	36	6.4
TOTALS	**60**	**697**	**100**	**67**	**564**	**100**

Table 2. Injury distribution by location and days of absence (total and %) in both groups.

Total number of injuries was 61 in football, while in futsal 67 injuries were registered (Table 2). In average, each football player sustained 2.54 injuries, and 29.0 days loss. In futsal, each player sustained 2.79 injuries, with 23.5 days off because of injuries.
Differences in mean time to RTP for injury were not statistically significant between football and futsal group, with 11.4±23.5 days in football and 8.4±16.6 days for futsal group ($p=0.046$). Injury patterns by location and type are shown in next table.

Conclusions

Despite there are some differences in injury distribution (for example, four more times ankle sprains in futsal or almost two more times muscle thigh injuries in football), there are not significant differences between injury incidence and time to RTP between Spanish elite football and futsal players during a season.

References

1. Fuller CW, Ekstrand J, Junge A, Andersen TE, Bahr R, Dvorak J. Consensus statement on injury definitions and data collection procedures in studies of football (soccer) injuries. Br J Sports Med 2006; 40: 193-201
2. Hägglund M, Waldén M, Magnusson H, Kristenson K, Bengtsson H, Ekstrand J. Injuries affect team performance negatively in professional football: an 11-year follow-up of the UEFA Champions League injury study. Br J Sports Med 2013; 47: 738-742

IS SINGLE LEG HOP TEST AT THE END OF THE ASSISTED REHABILITATION PREDICTIVE OF FULL RTP IN FOOTBALL PLAYERS AFTER ACL RECONSTRUCTION?

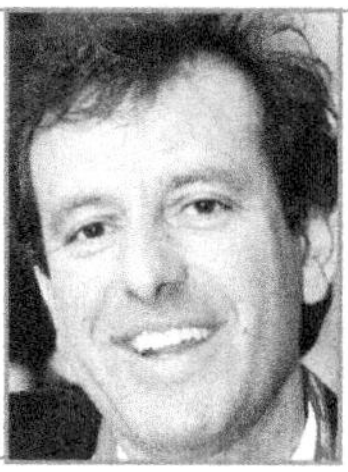

Danelon F[1], Pisoni D[1], Caminati D[2], Gamberini J[2], Della Villa F[2]

Isokinetic Medical Group, FIFA Medical Centre of Excellence, [1]Milan and [2]Bologna, Italy

Introduction

Testing functional skills at the end of rehabilitation is part of the strategy suggested to give consensus for a safe Return To Play (RTP) after Anterior Cruciate Ligament (ACL) surgery (1). According with this statement we usually evaluate patients with some tests, exploring recovery of hopping skills and speed and verifying if the players got the desired level of performance. Hop tests should help to ensure that players recovered ability to jump with the injured or operated limb the same distance than they do with the healthy one. The most popular and simple test are the Single leg Hop Test for distance (SHT) and the Triple leg Hop Test for distance (THT). For this reason we adopt them and calculate the Limb Symmetry Index (LSI), consisting in the percent ratio between distances jumped with the operated limb and with the healthy one. From the literature a cut off of 90% in the LSI is used to give the patient the consensus to return to play.
Aim of our study is to verify if the 90% cut-off in the single leg hop test can predict the self-reported functional level and the feeling to be returned to play at the same level of pre-injury in football players at the follow-up one year after ACL reconstruction.

Methods

We evaluated 31 consecutive Italian male non-professional football players aged 23±7 (mean±SD) years, submitted to ACL reconstruction with different techniques and rehabilitated between 2009 and 2014. We divided them into three groups based on the LSI obtained at the last SHT of the assisted rehabilitation done under our care, in our Clinic. The first group is made by 8 players that obtained a LSI higher than 100%, because they jumped longer distance with the operated leg (>100 group), the second group includes 19 players that obtained a LSI from 90 to 100 % (>90 group) and a third group which includes, for different reasons, mainly social and economic, 4 patients released with a LSI lower than 90 (<90 group). In each of the three group we verify the self reported functional level with the International Knee Documentation Committee (IKDC) subjective knee evaluation form and the ratio of players that feels to be fully returned to play at the same level of pre-injury through an individual phone call interview at 12 months after surgery. The question we asked patients during the interview was: "Do you really feel to be returned to the same sport at the same level of pre-injury?"

Results

Results are shown in table 1.

N°	SLH operated	SLH non-operated	LSI	IKDC	RTP at the same level
8	1.77±0.15	1.70±0.16	≥100	95.9±3.0	100%
19	1.68±0.24	1.74±0.25	>90	94.8±6.6	69%
4	1.52±0.15	1.78±0.12	<90	94.4±2.5	25%
31	1.68±0.21	1.74±0.21	All	95.0±5.3	--

Table 1. Functional self-reported outcome (IKDC) and % of full RTP (Return To Play) at one year assessed by phone call. LSI: Limb Symmetry Index (%); SLH: Single leg Hop Test (m) in operated and non-operated limb.

Conclusions

Considering the limitations related to the low number of patients studied, and the inconsistence of the difference among group in functional outcome (IKDC) we can observe that: i) at the end of assisted rehab jumping test for distance longer with the operated leg than with the non- injured one seems to be very positively related with a full RTP at the same level of pre-injury after one year. ii) a LSI higher than 90 % is not a guarantee of a full RTP at same level injury after one year. This indicates that jumping power is just one of the important aspect of the rehab for football players that need to be recovered; iii) a LSI lower than 90 % seems to be a bad prognostic factor for RTP at same level at one year after surgery.
Evaluating SHT at end-rehab and taking LSI index as a tool to predict RTP is a useful strategy but it must be evaluate together with other more complex evaluation, as biomechanical and psychological measures.

References

1. Logerstedt D, Grindem H, Lynch A, Eitzen I, Engebretsen L, Risberg MA, Axe MJ, Snyder-Mackler L. Single-legged hop tests as predictors of self-reported knee function after anterior cruciate ligament reconstruction: the Delaware-Oslo ACL cohort study. Am J Sports Med 2012; 40: 2348-2356

PHYSIOTHERAPY IN REVISION RECONSTRUCTION OF ACL OF FOOTBALL PLAYERS

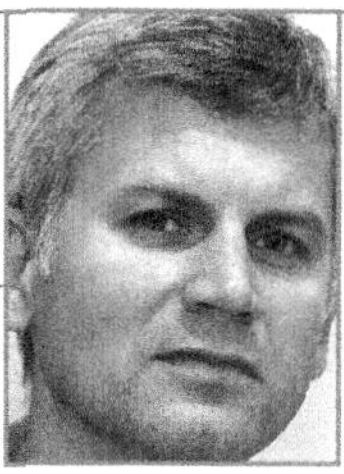

Kępczyński A[1], Krzyżak Ł[1], Luboiński Ł[1,2]

[1]Klinika Ruchu, Warsaw; [2]Warsaw Central Clinical Hospital of The Internal, Warsaw, Poland

Objectives

To determine the main goals of physiotherapy in athlets after Revision Reconstruction of Anterior Cruciate Ligament (RRACL). To prove importence of the prevention of Anterior Cruciate Ligament (ACL) injury taking into account football specific exercises. Recovery of the patient after RRACL regarding the accomplaying injuries.

Methods

Eleven football players (age range 22-54 years) after RRACL performed by only one surgeon, had a physiotherapy treatment in our Clinic in years 2012-2014. Three of them were profesional football players of Premiere League- Ekstraklasa-Legia Warszawa Sports Club. Eight of the patients were amateur. There were two woman and nine men in our sudy.
The time between first and second RRACL was 1-3 years and the time of RRACL was 6-12 weeks after injury.
Six patients had hamstrngs autografts; three patients autograft of patella tendon and two patients allograft of tibialis anterior muscle. Double boundle RACL as a first reconstruction were made in 4 cases. Single boundle RACL were performed in 7 cases. Menisectomy of the medial meniscus had 4 and lateral 3 of our patients with secondary rupture of the ACL. Microfracture treatment was nessesery in one patient.
The physiotherapy protocol was carried out according with this timing: 1) unloading or partial weightbearing with cruthes in average 3-4 weeks; 2) bracing the knee, specialy during night in 3 weeks; 3) Continuous Passive Motion (CPM) 4 hours /day in patient with microfractures; 4) full range of motion from the first day after surgery; 5) open and closed kinetic chain exercises of quadriceps and hamstring muscles- 2 weeks after surgery; 6) proprioception exercises started 2 days after surgery; 7) pool exercises 6 weeks after surgery; 8) runnig protocol started 14 weeks after surgery; 9) on the field exercises in cooperation with trainer in 3 cases started 7 months after RRACL; 10) physiotherapy protocols were completed within 6-8 months after RRACL; 11) players returned to play within 9-12 monts after RRACL.

Conclusions

All of the eleven patients return to football at the same level within 1 to 1.5 years after RRACL. At one year follow-up, only one patient, a profesional player, had a partial meniscectomy 9 months after RRACL.

10

RETURN TO PLAY AFTER FUNCTIONAL MOVEMENT ANALYSIS IN SOCCER PLAYERS WITH LONG-STANDING MUSCLE-RELATED PAIN

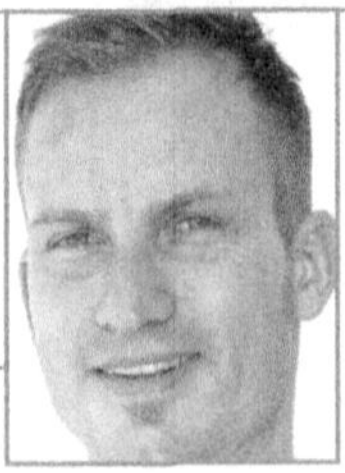

Dewitz H[1,2], Yildirim B1, Stock Th[1,2], Klein P[1,2]

[1]Mediapark Klinik, Department of Orthopaedic Surgery, Sports medicine, Cologne;
[2]Institute for Functional Diagnostics (IFD-Cologne), Cologne, Germany

Introduction

Muscle injuries are a substantial problem for athletes and their clubs. These injuries are one of the major problems in soccer players and are reported with up to 37% of time-loss injuries in literature. Usually Magnetic Resonance Imaging (MRI) scans are used to diagnose muscle injuries and to assess their healing process. The decision for the right time for a return to competition in professional sports often refers to MRI scans, clinical findings and the experience of the medical team.
After muscle injuries, other injuries or in preventive screenings it could be very helpful to detect deficits in the athlete movement based on functional movement analysis. In addition to kinematic and kinetic parameters you could also detect substantial deficits in the muscle activity using an Electromyographic (EMG) screen of sport-specific/important muscle groups. Whereas a Magnetic Resonance Imaging (MRI) can point out the injured structure, the high-precision motion analysis tries to detect the respective causes of an injured structure.

Methods

Three high level soccer players from the 1st German Bundesliga were screened in the IFD-Cologne, because of different reasons: 1) Player 1 got the first check-up after muscle tear of the Rectus Femoris (load/training regulation depending upon his movement biomechanics). 2) Player 2 with recurrent muscle discomforts of the Biceps Femoris over months got a motion analysis because MRI Scans were without explainable findings). 3) Player 3 got a preventive screen to detect possible deficits.
The three-dimensional motion analysis was performed using a 12 camera motion analysis system (250 Hz; Vicon Motion Systems, Oxford, UK) including two force plates (2500 Hz; AMTI, Watertown, USA). Standard kinematic and kinetic parameters were calculated using a five segment, rigid body inverse dynamics model of the lower extremity bilateral. The EMG data were collected with a sampling rate of 4000 Hz using a 16 channel wireless system (Myon 320, Myon AG, Switzerland). After shaving and cleaning the skin with alcohol, disposable surface electrodes (Ambu Blue Sensor N, Ambu A/S, Ballerup, Denmark) were placed over the selected muscles. The kinematic, kinetic and EMG data were recorded during different motions (gait, running, squatting, jumping, cutting). Detected deficits of muscle activation were trained in combination with biofeedback technique at the clubs (Myotrace 400, Noraxon USA Inc, Scottsdale, USA). In order to regulate the correct trainings load or to control successful / physiological muscle activation, re-tests for the players were realized after some weeks (time points for the controls by the Institute for Functional Diagnostics (IFD-Cologne) were definite from the medical team of the club).

Results

Player 1 shows non physiological EMG of his Rectus Femoris which was injured, but also of the Semitendinosus on both sides show non physiological muscle activation. In this case a part of the hamstring structure could be detected perhaps before an injury. At the re-test three weeks after training, including biofeedback, the EMG signals were physiological (Figure 1).

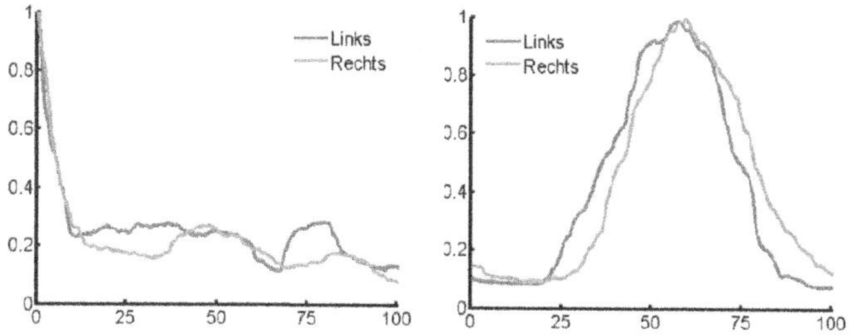

Figure 1. Non physiological activation of both (left+right) Semitendinosus (left), and physiological activation after biofeedback treatment a (right) during running. x-line: 0 (%)initial contact and 100 (%) toe off.

Player 2 had recurrent muscle discomforts of the Biceps Femoris (right) after a subtotal tendon rupture of the Semimembranosus (right). Repetitive MRI could not detect the reason for the recurrent problems. After the three-dimensional motion analysis with EMG a non physiological EMG activation of the right-continuous Semi-group and the Biceps Femoris was shown (Figure 2).

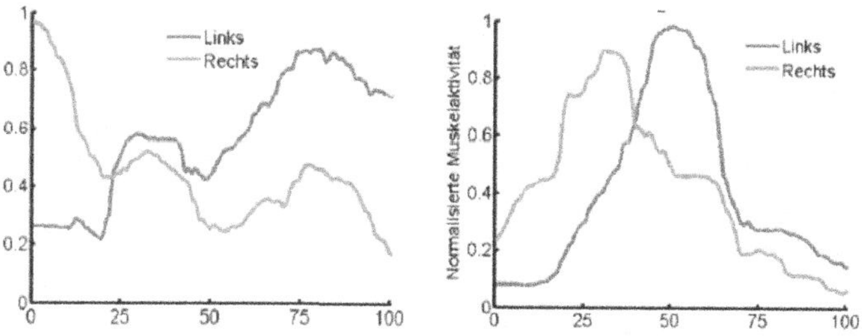

Figure 2. Non physiological activation peak of the right Semimembranosus (left panel) and a too early activation of the right Biceps Femoris (right panel). x-line: 0 (%)initial contact and 100 (%) toe off.

The reason was a disturbed activation of the Semi-group (right) after the injury. This led the Biceps Femoris trying to handle the less semi activity with earlier and more not physiological activity with the consequence of an excessive demand. After a consequent biofeedback training to activate the muscles of the semi-group, the player had not this discomfort until now and could play again at high level over 90 minutes for the whole season. Player 3 had a non physiological EMG activity of the Biceps Femoris (right-continuous) which was shown and documented after the screen in our motion laboratory. After this screen the player was involved in the pre-season training-camp where he injured his Biceps Femoris while training with the team. Afterwards the club and the player want the IFD to check the player himself during his rehabilitation time at different time points (depending on the questions from the medical team for the next and correct decrease of load). The follow-up of Biceps Femoris activation enabled to release demanding movements like running at more than 3 m/s, jumping or cutting. Since the player returns to competition he feels no discomfort and in some units/week he trains with the EMG biofeedback system at the club.

Conclusions

Longstanding muscle problems can be solved thanks to the professional implementation of the intervention. Also during the preventive diagnostic, some abnormalities of muscle activations could be detected, and for this reason a possible muscle injury could be avoided. In professional sports is mainly important not only to detect structural but also functional deficits in order to reduce these frequent injuries.

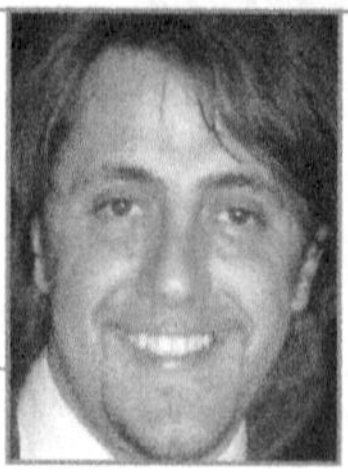

FAST BLEEDING RECOVERY WITH WHOLE BODY CRYOTHERAPY AFTER MUSCULAR INJURY

Freschi M[1,2], Genovese E[3], Tavana R[1]

[1]AC Milan Medical Staff; [2]Isokinetic medical Group, FIFA Medical Centre of Excellence, Milan; [3]Istituto di Radiologia, Università di Cagliari, Italy

Introduction

Ice and cold therapy is the most common therapy used in acute or overuse injuries to relieve pain symptoms, and also in inflammatory diseases. A form of cold therapy (or stimulation), called Whole-Body Cryotherapy (WBC) was proposed since eighties for the treatment of rheumatic diseases, and is now recommended for the treatment of arthritis, fibromyalgia and ankylosing spondylitis. The therapy consists of exposure to very cold air that is maintained at -110°C to -140°C in special temperature-controlled cryo-chambers, generally for 2 or 3 minutes.

In sports medicine WBC has gained wider acceptance as a method to improve recovery from hard training or muscle injury, because seems to be effective on these levels: 1) antioxidant capacity, 2) Creatine Kinase (CK) faster reduction, 3) anti-inflammatory effect.

1) Physical exercise leads to increased production and release of reactive oxygen species, which induce oxidative stress mainly as lipid peroxidation, and consequently membrane damage. The WBC effect on pro-oxidant-antioxidant balance was studied in 20 top-level kayakers from the Polish Olympic team and in 10 untrained men. WBC preceding kayakers' training induced positive adaptive changes in cells protecting organisms from pro-oxidative-antioxidative equilibrium disturbances (3). The lower activity of antioxidant enzymes during training accompanied by WBC, at the same time as a lower concentration of lipid peroxidation molecules, indicates a decrease in the generation of reactive oxygen species. Considering the antioxidant enzymes activity during training without WBC, the increase of superoxide dismutase and glutathione peroxidase activity was observed after the third day of training. The level of lipid peroxidation products also increased after the training without WBC. The use of WBC prior to training may reduce the risk of oxidative stress and the extent of muscle fiber injuries provoked by intense exercise (1).

2) The cold stimulation shows positive effects on CK and Lactate Dehydrogenase (LDH), and it should be considered a procedure that facilitates athletes' recovery as described in top-level rugby players after training, where WBC induced a clear and significant decrease in the mean values of CK and LDH after one week of treatment (1). It seems that short-time cold air exposure induces an enhancement of muscle fibre repair, reducing the breakdown of the cell membrane or reducing its increased permeability, which is generally caused by oxidant agents produced by physical exercise, the significant decrease of serum total CK and LDH concentrations resulted in proper and rapid recovery of muscular damage (1). The reduction of micro-injuries to muscle fibres caused by exercise (shown by a decrease in CK serum concentration) was confirmed in 21 kayakers performing two 10-day training cycles, one cycle without treatment and the other with WBC preceding each training session. The CK values in both groups were higher than those before training, as expected. The values during training with WBC were significantly lower than those observed during training without WBC (1).

3) An anti-inflammatory effect of WBC was found in rugby players who were treated for one week, where an increase in the anti-inflammatory cytokine IL-10, and a decrease in the proinflammatory cytokine IL-2 and chemokine IL-8 was seen. Moreover, the decrease in intercellular adhesion molecule-1 (ICAM-1) supported the anti-inflammatory response (1).

With this premises our hypothesis is WBC can works also when major muscular lesion happen.

Case report

This case report is aimed to present the effects of repeated session of WBC after a muscle injury. The player was 18 years old male of a top Italian football U19 team, midfielder, 173 cm, 68 kg. The injury happens at sixth minute of a match during a sprint. He was immediately substituted and Rest, Ice, Compression and Elevation (RICE) was applied. A Magnetic Resonance Imaging (MRI) performed 2 days after the injury showed a 3B lesion (München classification; 2) of the left Biceps Femoris, with proximal miotendineous lesion and a big interstitial, fascial bleeding that goes around Ischiatic Nerve as shown in the images on the left. After MRI, the player started physiotherapy that in the first five days consisted in electrotherapy and walking protected by crutches plus WBC. When pain disappeared he started isometric contractions under pain level at different knee and hip angles simulating knee flexion and hip extension without length muscle change, plus hydrokinesitherapy and WBC. At ten days he started concentric contraction, pulsed Ultrasounds and continued WBC till next MRI. Pain was very low and he come back to the pitch in 31 days. He had before other muscle lesion and his time for Return To Play (RTP) was 25 and 20 days for a 3A lesion of right Rectus Femoris and right Biceps Femoris respectively. During the rehabilitation period we applied eight sessions of cryotherapy done on days 3, 4, 5, 6, 9, 10, 11, and 12 after the injury, thanks to the availability of a mobile cryochamber (KR-2010 Sapio Life, Sapio, Monza, Italy). A session lasted three minutes at a temperature of -130°C after the rehabilitation session; in the last 3 sessions he can perform bike exercise at aerobic level after the WBC, in the previous session he can't for the pain.

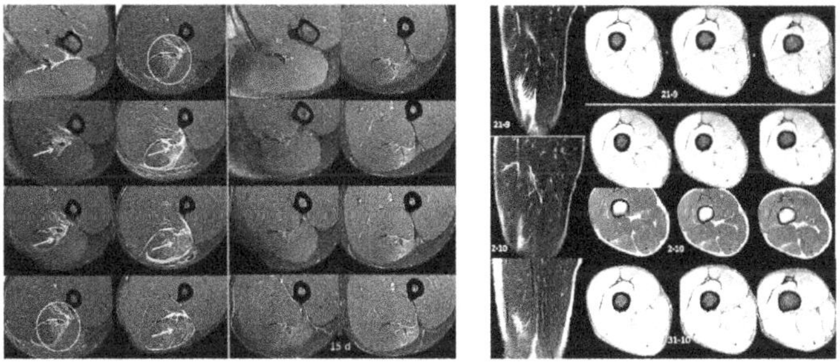

Figure 1. Left: progressive reduction of the fluid in the fascial bend and of the interstitial hemorrhage after 15 days after 8 session of cryochamber (3B lesion). Right: slower reduction of the interstitial fluid in control with 3A lesion (no cryochamber).

After 15 days the MRI showed a big reduction of the fluid in the fascial space and of the interstitial bleeding. As control we show another MRI with control after 12 days with similar images but with an injury less serious than case-report (3A lesion (2)).The player returned complete training after 31 days without match for other 20 days because the season ends during his rehabilitation, but he starts the new season with all the group with two session per days. At a 8 months follow-up he is still playing without relapses.

Conclusions

Whole-Body Cryotherapy can help the recovery process after muscle injury in professional football players.

References

1. Banfi G, Lombardi G, Colombini A, Melegati G. Whole-body cryotherapy in athletes. Sports Med 2010; 40: 509-517
2. Mueller-Wohlfahrt HW, Haensel L, Mithoefer K, Ekstrand J, English B, McNally S, Orchard J, van Dijk CN, Kerkhoffs GM, Schamasch P, Blottner D, Swaerd L, Goedhart E, Ueblacker P. Terminology and classification of muscle injuries in sport: a consensus statement. Br J Sports Med 2012; 47: 342-350
3. Wozniak A, Wozniak B, DrewaG, Mila-Kierzenkowska C, Rakowski A. The effect of whole body cryostimulation on the prooxidant-antioxidant balance in blood of elite kayakers during training. Eur J Appl Physiol 2007; 101: 533-7

Saturday, 9th April, 2016
POSTER AREA

FREE POSTER PRESENTATIONS

ORTHOPAEDIC SURGERY

Chairs

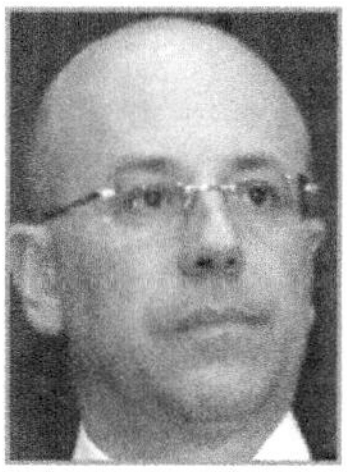

Stefano Respizzi
(Milan, Italy)

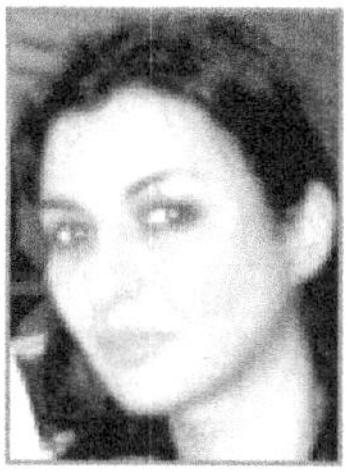

Francesca Vannini
(Bologna, Italy)

PE01 Evaluation of the development of jones fractures in terms of the dynamic factors **Murakami K, Nishio H, Kobayashi Y, Saita Y, Akiyoshi N (Miyagi, Tokyo and Chiba, Japan)**

PE02 Surgical treatment after rupture of rectus femoris direct head tendon in a professional soccer player
Papadimas D, Theos Ch (Athens, Greece)

PE03 Treatment of chronic lateral ankle instability using the Broström-Gould technique in athletes: long-term results
Russo A, Giacchè P, Marcantoni E, Arrighi A, Molfetta L (Firenze, Genova and La Spezia, Italy)

PE04 Clinical outcomes of meniscal repairs for isolated meniscal tears in soccer players **Matsushita T, Tanaka T, Nagai K, Araki D, Kuroda R, Kurosaka M (Kobe, Japan)**

PE05 Insertional Achilles tendinosis: surgical treatment with calcaneoplasty, reattachment of the Achilles tendon with Speedbridge Arthrex technique
Risi M, Miceli M, Carboni L, Molinari M, Zunarelli P (Bologna, Italy)

PE06 Muscle injuries: antifibrotic therapy, effective healing, faster return to play?
Kelc R, Vogrin M (Maribor, Slovenia)

PE07 Revision of anterior cruciate ligament with ligament advanced reinforcement system
Picchetti F, Giannini E, Michelotti M (Pisa and Firenze, Italy)

PE08 Lateral compartment osteoarthritis in a soccer player with varus knee: a case report
Cohen M, Debieux P, Gomes T (São Paulo, Brazil)

PE09 Serious shoulder injury in a high level soccer player. Return to participation after surgery
Theos Ch, Kostas N, Koinis A (Athens, Greece)

EVALUATION OF THE DEVELOPMENT OF JONES FRACTURES IN TERMS OF THE DYNAMIC FACTORS

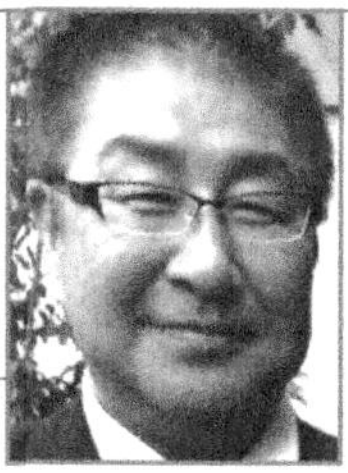

Murakami K[1], Nishio H[2], Kobayashi Y[2], Saita Y[2,3], Akiyoshi N[4]

[1]Sendai University Graduate School of Sports Science, Miyagi; [2]Department of Orthopaedics and Sports Medicine, Juntendo University, Tokyo; [3]FIFA Medical Centre of Excellence, Tokyo; [4]Oyumino Central Hospital Department of Rehabilitation, Chiba, Japan

Introduction

A Jones fracture (2) is defined as a stress fracture of the proximal metaphyseal and diaphyseal part of fifth metatarsal bone caused by sports activities (broad definition). However, in general, fractures which develop specifically at the proximal metaphyseal-diaphyseal junction of the fifth metatarsal bone are referred to as Jones fracture (narrow definition).

Especially it occurs more frequently in sports requiring more cutting motions, stepping motion, stopping motion, such as football and basketball and kicking motion for football.

In the past, the factors leading to the development of Jones fractures (narrow definition) have been evaluated by dividing them into individual factors (poor body alignment), surface factors, and shoe factors. At the same time, no detailed evaluations in terms of sports movement have been carried out. Therefore, the objective of this study was to simulate the development of Jones fractures (narrow definition) based on the dynamic factors acting on the fifth metatarsal bone when moving and prevent recurrence.

Methods

A total of four healthy adult male amateur football players (mean age 24.4±2.3 yrs) were measured for football kicking movement (instep kicking) using a three dimensional movement analyzing device (Vicon N10, Oxford Metrix, Oxford, United Kingdom) synchronized with a Ground Reaction Force (GRF) measuring device (9281-1, Kistler, New York, USA), after which the results were analyzed by musculoskeletal modeling and analysis system SIMM 6.0 (Musculo Graphic, Santa Rosa, USA), calculating the GRF z component for each movement and the Muscular Tension Force (MTF) of the pivoting leg (peroneus brevis, third peroneal muscle) at the time of kicking.

In addition, foot finite element models were created based on the Computed Tomography (CT) data of an identical subject whose movement was measured. The loading conditions were as follows: the maximum GRF value (the value for the z component alone) right after the Foot Contact the ground (FC) for each movement was provided as the fifth metatarsal distal head arbitrary point, and the MTF (peroneus brevis/third peroneal muscle) at the time maximum GRF was generated was provided as the muscular action. Regarding the constraint conditions, the fifth metatarsal surface of the cuboid and the fifth metatarsal proximal fourth metatarsal surface were fully restrained. The load position was set with reference to the coordinate system of the finite element model: the same direction as the z axis; an inclined direction of 30° to the z axis; and an inclined direction of 45° to the z axis. These angles were based on the assumption of the foot position at the time the foot touches the ground.

The Finite Element Method was used for analysis (1), and a bone fracture analysis, which divides each value into 40 steps with the maximum GRF value of each movement as the load, was conducted by Finite Element Analysis software Mechanical Finder 7.0 (Research Center of Computational Mechanics, Tokio, Japan).

Results

While the fracture lines were mainly observed in more distal part of the fifth metatarsal bone for loads in the same direction as the z axis, for loads at an inclined direction of 30° to the z axis, and an inclined direction of 45° to the z axis, the fracture lines were observed in the proximal metaphyseal-diaphyseal junction of the fifth metatarsal bone (Figure 1). Further, more fracture lines observed in models without taking MTF into account.

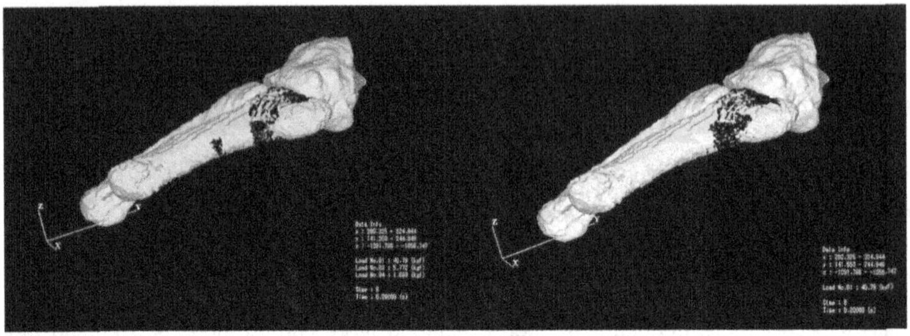

Figure 1. Left: fracture lines of 30°; right: fracture lines of 45°.

Conclusions

Based on the present results, in the pivoting leg when kicking, results without MTF acting demonstrated more fracture lines than the results taking the inclined direction of 30° and 45° to the z axis and MTF into consideration. This was probably because each muscle was acting on the fifth metatarsal to reduce the stress after the foot touched the ground.

In order to prevent Jones fractures from occurring in the pivoting leg during kicking movement in football, it was revealed that the most important factor is to make the player to acquire the movements that will not place an outer load on the foot. Should a fracture occur, to prevent recurrence, careful consideration should be taken regarding outer loading during movement at the time of rehabilitation.

References

1. Arangio GA, Xiao D, Salathe EP. Biomechanical study of stress in the fifth metatarsal. Clin Biomech 1997; 12: 160-164
2. Jones R. Fracture of the base of the fifth metatarsal bone by indirect violence. Ann Surg 1902; 35: 697-670

2

SURGICAL TREATMENT AFTER RUPTURE OF RECTUS FEMORIS DIRECT HEAD TENDON IN A PROFESSIONAL SOCCER PLAYER

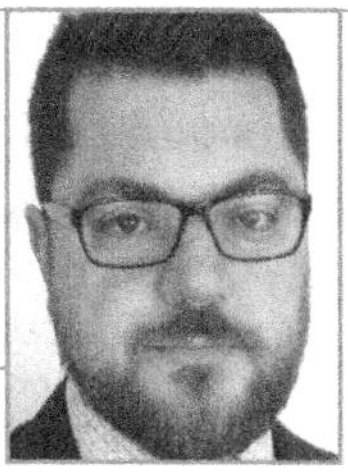

Papadimas D, Theos C

Metropolitan Hospital, N Faliro, Greece

Introduction

Muscle injuries in sport activities are quite common. Most of the injuries regarding muscles are typically treated conservatively. The most common muscle injuries in football players are those regarding the hamstrings, while quadriceps injuries are not frequently encountered, with the latter when present usually located in the Rectus Femoris muscle. Most injuries of the Rectus Femoris most commonly are located at the level of the musculotendinous junction or the quadriceps tendon. Proximal ruptures of the Rectus Femoris are considered rather uncommon, as they are estimated less than 1% of the quadriceps injuries. These injuries are very important in sports such as soccer, which require repetitive and at the maximum level running, sprinting and kicking. Thus the need for proper treatment and rehabilitation is highlighted in professional athletes, whose performance is severely affected and the need for fast and safe return to play, with minimal risk of recurrence is of primary concern. In the literature there are not many case reports and studies regarding such injuries and with on consensus of the optimal treatment.

Case report

A case of a 29-year old, 197 cm height and 93 kg of weight, male professional soccer player with rupture of the tendon of the direct head of the right Rectus Femoris muscle is presented. The player (goalkeeper) was injured at the time of kicking the ball in motion during training of his club, which participates in the Greek Super League.

The clinical examination revealed pain during muscle contracture, in active and active-resisted hip flexion and knee extension. Local tenderness in the proximal anterior thigh in line with the proximal Rectus Femoris. A palpable gap was evident in the site of rupture, which became even more evident during the muscle contraction, as the muscle belly was retracted distally. The Magnetic Resonance Imaging (MRI) scan showed rupture of the tendon of the direct head of Rectus Femoris. The patient was informed of the non-operative and the operative (1, 2) options of treatment, the patient decided to proceed with the surgical repair of the tendon. Under general anesthesia, a modified Smith-Petersen approach was used; anterior approach, starting 2 cm below the anterior inferior iliac spine, extending 5 cm distally, dissection in the plane between Sartorius and Quadriceps muscles. The tear of the tendon was identified at the level just distal to its bony origin. The tendon was repaired using two metal anchors (5.0 Wedge Anchor II, Stryker, Kalamazoo, USA), with two non-absorbable sutures each (Force Fiber, Stryker, Kalamazoo, USA). Each anchoring suture was used in Krackow technique manner. The stability of the construct was assessed with intraoperative forced knee flexion. Postoperatively, the patient had his knee immobilized in a knee brace locked in extension for four weeks. Passive hip range of motion was initiated immediately postoperatively. The patient postoperatively walked with the aid of crutches, weight bearing as tolerated, at first touchdown, proceeding to partial weight-bearing. Full weight bearing was allowed after four weeks postoperatively. Ergometer training was started at six weeks postoperatively, with mild resistance. Running was started at 8 weeks and training with the ball at 10 weeks postoperatively. Return to training with the team was allowed at 12 weeks postoperatively and return to play was allowed at 6 months postoperatively. 14 months after his surgery he participates in full squad's program without any problems.

Conclusions

Although non-operative treatment of a proximal rupture of Rectus Femoris may be a realistic option for the low-demand patient, it would most likely be unacceptable for the high-demand professional athlete. The surgical repair has shown good outcomes and therefore should be considered as the treatment of choice in high-demand patients, such as professional soccer player.

References

1. Bottoni CR, D'Alleyrand JC. Operative treatment of a complete rupture of the origination of the Rectus Femoris. Sports Health 2009; 1: 478-480
2. García VV, Duhrkop DC, Seijas R, Ares O, Cugat R. Surgical treatment of proximal ruptures of the Rectus Femoris in professional soccer players. Arch Orthop Trauma Surg 2012; 132: 329-333

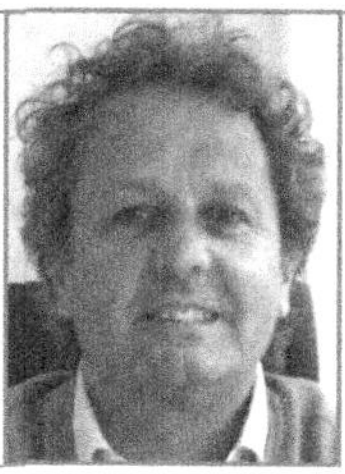

TREATMENT OF CHRONIC LATERAL ANKLE INSTABILITY USING THE BROSTRÖM-GOULD TECHNIQUE IN ATHLETES: LONG-TERM RESULTS

Russo A[1], Giacchè P[1], Marcantoni E[1], Arrighi A[2,3], Molfetta L[2]

[1]Istituto Ortopedico Fiorentino (IFCA), Villa Ulivella e Glicini, Firenze; [2]Università di Genova, Facoltà di Scienze Mediche e Farmaceutiche, Genova; [3]AD Motum, La Spezia Italy

Introduction

Conservative treatment of ankle ligament injuries does not always result in anatomical and functional healing of the injury itself and resolution of the instability. There exist numerous surgical techniques for treating chronic instability due external ankle ligament injury (1). Cadaveric studies have shown greater mechanical stability obtained with the modified Broström technique as opposed to Watson-Jones, which encourages to apply this method in athletes and football players (3). The aim of this study was to understand if the Broström-Gould technique can be considered as an effective technique for the treatment of chronic lateral ankle instability in athletes practicing high demanding sport activities.

Methods

Our sample comprised 18 athletes (7 females, 11 males), aged between 17 and 32 years at the time of surgery. The right side was affected in 12 patients and the left side in six. The duration of instability ranged from one to four years. All the subjects practiced sports at football competitive level.

Criteria of inclusion were: 1) failure of previous conservative treatment; 2) clinically evident anterior drawer sign, when compared with the healthy contralateral side, at 20° of plantar flexion and a positive talar tilt test; 3) complete rupture of the anterior talo-fibular ligament with intact calcaneo-fibular ligament and posterior talo-fibular ligament documented by MRI; 4) subjective feeling of instability associated with pain during normal walking.

The surgical procedure was performed using standard arthroscopy instruments. We begin reconstructing the ligament using the Broström-Gould technique which proved to be simple and rapid, and free from intra- or post-operative complications (2).

A group of five athletes with associated osteochondral lesions and/or lesions of the tibiofibular syndesmosis were excluded from the study.

The day after surgery all patients were fitted with a protective ankle brace with two valves and permitted to load the joint very lightly (i.e. to graze the floor) using two crutches.

From the fifteenth day post-surgery, walking was allowed with partial loading (progressively increasing), and a rehabilitation programme started with flexion-extension exercises of the ankle and knee followed by exercises to strengthen the peroneal tendons and proprioception exercises. Running was resumed from the third month post-surgery and the patients gradually returned to their sporting activities as from the fourth month post-surgery, with protective taping used for a further two months.

All the patients were reassessed after a minimum of 10 years to a maximum of 15 years after surgery using the American Orthopaedic Foot and Ankle Society (AOFAS) scoring system.

Results

After surgery, the patients return to play at the same level of pre-injuries within 120 days. We observed a presence of a moderate anterior drawer sign in only one patient, while the varus-valgus stability was good in all the operated athletes, with subjective feeling of good stability.
The AOFAS score rose from a mean of 67.6±3.9 before surgery to a mean of 98.8±1.4 at final follow-up, which corresponded to a mean increase of 31.2 points.
The long-term results were excellent in 94.5% of the cases and good in the remaining 5.5% (comparison with Ankle-Hindfoot Scale). There were no unsatisfactory results in this series of patients.

Conclusions

These results indicate that the Broström-Gould method can be considered as a successful surgical technique for the treatment of ankle instability due to isolated rupture of the anterior talo-fibilar ligament in athletes practicing high demanding sport activities.

References

1. Bordmann DL, Liu SH. Contribution of the anterolateral joint capsule to the mechanical stability of the ankle. Clin Orthop Relat Res 1997; 341: 224-232
2. Giannini S, Ceccarelli F, De Benedictis M, Perna L, Faldini C. Lesioni capsulo legamentose croniche della tibiotarsica. In: Progressi in chirurgia del piede [Congress Proceedings]. Il piede nello sport 1997; 7-139
3. Liu SH, Baker CL. Comparison of lateral ankle ligamentous reconstruction procedures Am J Sports Med 1994; 22: 313-317

4

CLINICAL OUTCOMES OF MENISCAL REPAIRS FOR ISOLATED MENISCAL TEARS IN SOCCER PLAYERS

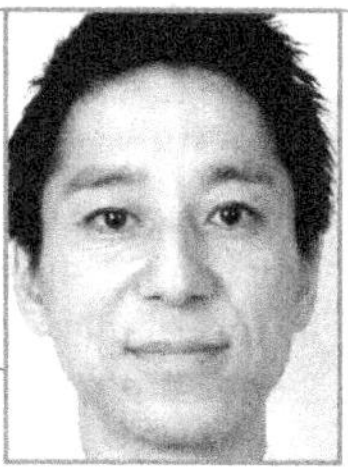

Matsushita T, Tanaka T, Nagai K, Araki D, Kuroda R, Kurosaka M

Department of Orthopaedic Surgery, Kobe University Graduate School of Medicine, Kobe, Japan

Introduction

Meniscal tears are one of the common injuries in soccer players (2). Menisectomy has been performed to allow patients an early return-to-play. However menisectomy often causes progression of osteoarthritis and it also can lead to early termination of the career. Therefore preservation of the torn meniscus by meniscal repair is an important step to provide players better treatments. However outcomes of meniscal repairs in soccer players are not fully examined. In the present study, clinical outcomes of isolated meniscal repair were examined.

Methods

Eighteen meniscal tears in 18 patients (15 males, 2 females) who received a meniscal repair in our hospital were examined. All the players were competitive players (Tegner >7) including two professional and 14 amateur players.
The mean preoperative Tegner activity scale was 8.6±1.0 (range 7-10). The mean follow-up was 24.7±19 months with a minimum of 1 year (1-3 years) and the mean age at the time of the surgery was 18.8±4.9 years old.
The mean time from injury to surgery was 4.9±5.1 months.
Meniscal tears includes 7 medial and 11 lateral meniscal tears.
The type of the tears were 14 longitudinal tears and 4 radial tears.
An all-inside technique was used in 3 knees and an inside-out technique was used in 15 knees. Complete return-to-play was allowed 6 months after surgery. Clinical outcomes were evaluated by retear rate, Lysholm score, and return-to-play. In addition, factors affecting the retear were evaluated.

Results

Sixteen patients (88.9%) returned to the original activity level.
The mean Lysholm score improved from preoperatively 62.3±7.4 to postoperatively 95.7±3.4.
Re-tear was observed in 6 knees (33.3%) after the return-to-play.
The average timing of the re-tear was 12.4±6.7 months.
Of the 6 torn menisci, 3 knees were medial (43%) and 3 knees (27%) were lateral menisci.
One player received meniscal re-repair and rest of the 5 players received meniscectomy. The re-repaired meniscus re-teared 3 years after the re-repair. All the 6 players returned to the original activity level.
There was no statistically significant difference in the age, time since injury to operation, side of the meniscus (medial or lateral), the length of the tear and the Tegner activity scale between the re-tear group and the non-re-tear group.
Higher re-tear rate was observed in the menisci repaired by the all-inside out technique (67%), but it did not reach significant difference compared with menisci repaired by the inside-out technique (27%).

Conclusions

Most of the soccer players who received a meniscal repair successfully returned to the original activity level. However re-tear was observed in not a few players and a high failure rate was observed in the menisci repaired by the all inside-out technique contradicting to a previous report (1). No significant cause of the failure was confirmed.
Surgeons should carefully discuss with players about the treatment plan and an improvement of outcomes of meniscal repair are required.

References

1. Avarez-Diaz P, Alentorn-Geli E, Llobet F, Granados N, Steinbacher G, Cugat R. Return to play after all-inside meniscal repair in competitive football players: a minimum 5-year follow-up. Knee Surg Sports Traumatol Arthrosc 2014 Sep 27. [Epub ahead of print]
2. Logan M, Watts M, Owen J, Myers P. Meniscal repair in the elite athlete: results of 45 repairs with a minimum 5-year follow-up. Am J Sports Med 2009; 37: 1131-1134

INSERTIONAL ACHILLES TENDINOSIS: SURGICAL TREATMENT WITH CALCANEOPLASTY, REATTACHMENT OF THE ACHILLES TENDON WITH SPEEDBRIDGE ARTHREX TECHNIQUE

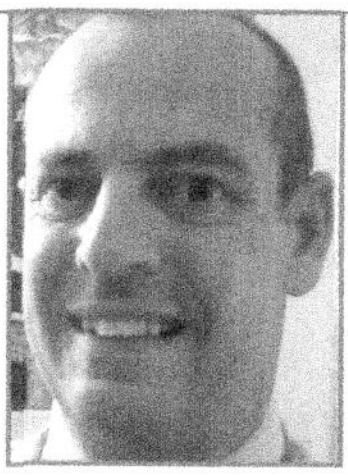

Risi M[1], Miceli M[2,3], Carboni L, Molinari M[1], Zunarelli P[3]

[1]Orthopedic and Traumatology Department and [2]Radiology Department, Maggiore and S. Giovanni Hospital, Bologna; [3]Isokinetic Medical Group, FIFA Medical Centre of Excellence, Bologna, Italy

Four heels in six patients (4 soccer an 2 basketball players) treated surgically for a primary diagnosis of insertional Achilles tendinosis (2) were reviewed on the basis of preoperative and postoperative examinations, office records, and a comprehensive questionnaire administered to each subject. Each patient had an associated prominent calcaneal bursal projection with lateral and medial involvement.

Each patient underwent surgical treatment using a midline-posterior skin incision, tendon was split at the line incision, full thickness, from posterior to anterior and is debrided removing all tendinopathic tissue. The Achilles tendon is released distally, and reflected medially and laterally, exposing the whole calcaneal tuberosity. The prominence is removed using the micro-sagittal saw and osteotome. Care is taken to chamfer off the medial and lateral sides of the calcaneus so as not to leave a prominence is palpable under the skin.

All the patients required reinsertion of the Achilles tendon with the Achilles Arthrex SpeedBridge, an innovative soft tissue fixation device used in the treatment of Achilles injuries that creates only a single point of compression directly over the anchor. The procedure consists of four-anchor construct enables a true knotless repair and a greater area of compression for the Achilles tendon on the calcaneus, improving stability and possibly allowing for earlier return to normal activities.

Postoperatively, 6 of 6 patients were able to return to work or routine activities by three months completely pain free.

Radiographic features (1)

Plain film:

- Loss of Kager triangle due to retrocalcaneal bursitis.
- Achilles tendon measuring over 9 mm, 2 cm above the bursal projection due to Achilles tendinopathy .
- convexity of the soft tissues posterior to the Achilles tendon insertion due to superficial tendo-achillis bursitis.
- prominent bursal projection of the calcaneum ("pump-bump").
- Chauveaux-Liet (CL) angle greater than 12°. CL angle is represented by the difference between the angle of verticalization (α) and morphologic angle (β) of the calcaneus (CL angle = α – β). Angle α is the calcaneal pitch angle or angle of verticalization of calcaneus described as the intersection of the baseline tangent to the anterior tubercle and the medial tuberosity with the horizontal surface. The angle β is formed between the vertical line tangent to the most posterior point of greater tuberosity and the straight line joining this point to the apex of the posterosuperior crest. A CL angle of more than 12° is considered abnormal, such as in Haglund syndrome.

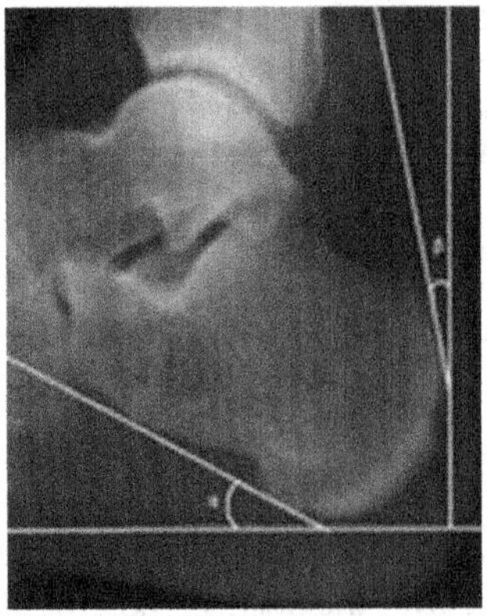

Figure 1. Normal Chauveaux-Liet angle.

Magnetic Resonance Imaging (MRI):

- Used in questionable cases.
- Focal enlargement and abnormal signal at Achilles tendon insertion segment.
- Retrocalcaneal and retro Achilles bursal fluid collection.
- Calcaneal bony spur better appreciated at T1 sagittal images.
- Marrow oedema of the posterior calcaneal tuberosity.

References

1. Sundararajan PP. Wilde TS. Radiographic, clinical, and magnetic resonance imaging analysis of insertional Achilles tendinopathy. J Foot Ankle Surg 2014; 53: 147-145
2. Weinfedl SB. Achilles tendon disorders. Med Clin North Am 2014; 98: 331-338

MUSCLE INJURIES: ANTIFIBROTIC THERAPY - EFFECTIVE HEALING - FASTER RETURN TO PLAY?

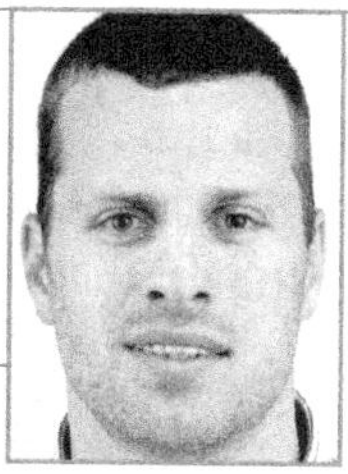

Kelc R, Vogrin M

Department of Orthopaedic Surgery, University Medical Center Maribor, Slovenia

Introduction

Injured skeletal muscle repairs spontaneously via regeneration; however, this process is often incomplete because of fibrotic tissue formation.
In our study we wanted to show improved efficiency of regeneration process induced by antifibrotic agent decorin in a combination with Platelet Rich Plasma (PRP)-derived growth factors.

Methods

A novel human Myoblast Cell (hMC) culture, defined as CD56 (NCAM)+ developed in our laboratory, was used for evaluation of potential bioactivity of PRP and decorin. To determine the effect on the viability of hMC we performed a MTT (3-(4,5-Dimethylthiazol-2-yl)-2,5-Diphenyltetrazolium Bromide) assay.
To perform the cell proliferation assay, hMCs were separately seeded on plates at a concentration of 30 viable cells per well. Cell growth medium prepared with different concentrations of PRP exudates (5%, 10%, and 20%) and decorin (10 ng/mL, 25 ng/mL, and 50 ng/mL) were added and incubated for seven days. After incubation we stained the cells with crystal-violet and measured the absorbance.
To study the expression of Transforming Growth Factor Beta (TGF-β) and myostatin (MSTN), two main fibrotic factors in the process of muscle regeneration we performed several Enzyme-Linked Immuno-Sorbent Assay (ELISA) assays in groups treated with all therapeutic agents (PRP, decorin and their combination).
Further we have studied the ability of these agents to influence the differential cascade of dormant myoblasts towards fully differentiated myotubes by monitoring step wise activation of single nuclear factors like MyoD and Myogenin via multicolor flow cytometry.
We stained the cells simultaneously with antibodies against CD56, MyoD and myogenin. We acquired cell images of 5,000 events per sample at 40 x magnification using 488 nm and 658 nm lasers and fluorescence was collected using three spectral detection channels. We analysed the cells populations according to expression of single or multiple markers and their ratios.
Finally, we examined the treated cell populations using a multicolour laser microscope after staining for desmin (a key marker of myogenic differentiation of hMC), α-tubulin, and nuclei. Optical images were acquired at the center of chamber slides where the cell density is at its highest using a Leica TCS SP5 II confocal microscope and analysed using Adobe Photoshop CS6, where a "Color Range" tool was used in combination with a histogram palette to count the pixels that correspond to desmin-positive areas in an image.

Results

The mitochondrial activity of cells, as determined by the MTT assay, was significantly increased ($p<0.001$) after exposure to tested concentrations of PRP exudate. Similarly, viability was elevated in all tested concentrations of decorin. PRP exudate enhanced the viability of cells to more than 400% when compared to the control ($p<0.001$). The viability of cells treated with PRP exudates was also significantly higher when compared to decorin ($p<0.001$).
Decorin did not show a significant effect on cell proliferation compared to the control; however, cultivation with PRP exudate leads to a 5-fold increase in cell proliferation ($p<0.001$).
Decorin was shown to down-regulate the expression of TGF-β when compared to the control by more than 15% ($p<0.001$)but significantly less than PRP exudate $p<0.005$). PRP significantly down-regulated TGF-β expression by more than 30% ($p<0.001$).
Similarly, the MSTN expression levels were significantly down-regulated by decorin and PRP. MSTN levels of cells treated with decorin were decreased by 28.4% ($p<0.001$) and 23.1% by PRP ($p<0.001$) when compared to the control group.
Using flow cytometry we detected a 39.1% increase in count of myogenin positive cells in the PRP-treated group compared to the control. Moreover, there was a 3.09% increase in cells positive only for myogenin, whereas no such cells were found in the control cell population. The population of cells positive only for myogenin is considered as fully differentiated and capable of fusion into myotubes as well as future mucle fibers and is thus of great importance for muscle regeneration. At the same time 20.6% fewer cells remained quiescent (positive only for CD56). Cells positive for both MyoD and myogenin represent the population that shifted significantly towards mature myocites during myogenesis but are not yet fully committed.
Finally, a statistically significant up-regulation of desmin expression ($p<0.01$ for the PRP treated group, $p<0.005$ for the decorin and PRP + decorin treated groups) was present in all therapeutic groups when compared to the control. While no significant difference was found between the PRP and decorin-treated groups, their combination led to a more than 3-fold increase ($p<0.005$) of desmin expression when compared to single bioactives.

Conclusions

PRP can be a highly potential therapeutic agent for skeletal muscle regeneration and repair, especially if in combination with a TGF-β antagonis decorin. Achieving better healing could likely result in faster return to play and lower reinjury rate.

REVISION OF ANTERIOR CRUCIATE LIGAMENT WITH LIGAMENT ADVANCED REINFORCEMENT SYSTEM

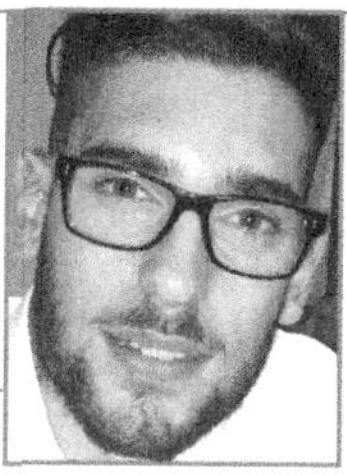

Picchetti F, Giannini E, Michelotti M

Kinetic Center, Pisa and Athena Srl, Firenze, Italy

Introduction

A 20-year-old professional football player (76 kg; 182 cm), play as goalkeeper on a Third League Italian team. Eighteen months after his first Anterior Cruciate Ligament (ACL) reconstruction of his left knee, he has a second injury on the same ligament. Our aim, through the second surgery with Ligament Advanced Reinforcement System (LARS) and a specific pre and post rehabilitation program, was to get the athlete back to playing in a short time.

Methods

We decided to postpone the surgery to undergo a three weeks rehabilitation program in preparation of the surgery. During this period the player underwent a rehabilitation protocol consisting of different exercises with/on/for: proprioception boards, tubing and lower quarters, squatting, leg press, hamstrings, core stability, treadmill, bike, and stretching.

After surgery (performed with LARS, with a re-absorbable screw for the fixation on the tibia and fixation in suspension for femur (Endobutton), we started with an intensified rehabilitative protocol which included two sessions per day for three weeks.

In the acute phase (8 days of duration) physical therapy with modalities (Electrotherapy, Magnetotherapy, Cryotherapy, Ultrasound Therapy) was administered, followed by rehabilitation exercises with/on/for: active knee flexion/extension, kinetic therapy with the therapist, progressive weight-bearing, recovery of walking and stepping, isometric and balance.

In the post-acute phase (7 days of duration) the player underwent hydrotherapy exercises on a rehabilitation pool, consisting of different exercises with/on/for: hydrobike, hip flexion/extension and abduction/adduction, walking with tools, knee flexion/extension, vascular tub, kinetic therapy with the therapist. Rehabilitation exercises were performed with/on/for: proprioception boards, kinetic therapy with the therapist, isometrics, tubing for lower quarters, treadmill, coordination on sand, core stability and balance, bike and massage and stretching at the end of the session.

In the functional phase (7 days of duration) the player underwent hydrotherapy with/on/for: hydrobike, stepping, proprioception boards, bouncer, walking, skipping with tools, and vascular tub. Rehabilitation exercises were performed with/on/for: proprioception boards, bike, bipodal squatting and on single leg, leg press, hamstrings, leg curl, tubing for lower quarters, core stability and balance, plyometrics on sand, treadmill, massage and stretching at the end of the session.

At the end of this period, the football player returned to his team working with his team's sport trainer.

The goalkeeper was periodically monitored with the following functional assessment tests:

- Range Of Motion (ROM), Fluidity of motion and Speed of motion test using an inertial sensor (Sensorize Freerehab, Rome, Italy).
- Isokinetic test to evaluate the force of lower limb (Biodex 3 System, New York, USA).
- Functional evaluation test using Y Balance Test for lower extremity (2) and Functional Movement Screening (FMS) (Functional Movement System, Danville, USA).

Visual Analogue Scale (VAS) 0-10 for pain was also applied during ROM assessment.

Results

ROM, Fluidity and Speed deficit (%) of the operated limb are reported in Table 1. Isokinetic test results are reported on Table 2. Y Balance Test and FMS are reported on Table 3.

ROM	Angle E	Angle F	Fluidity E	Fluidity F	Speed E	Speed F	VAS E	VAS F
Pre surgery	8	18	0	12	26	56	0	0
Post surg. 4 d.	18	35	20	29	74	80	5	4
Post surg. 6 w.	0	18	0	33	39	72	2	3
Post surg. 12 w.	0	8	0	0	13	21	0	0
Post surg. 24 w.	0	7	0	0	8	0	0	0

Table 1. Range Of Motion (ROM), Fluidity and Speed deficit of the operated limb expressed as percentage (%) of the ROM, Speed and Fluidity of the non-operated limb. E: knee extension; F: knee flexion. VAS is the Visual Analogue Scale for pain.

Isokinetic test	KExt R 90°/s	KExt L 90°/s	Diff %	KFlex R 90°/s	KFlex L 90°/s	Diff %	KExt R 210°/s	KExt L 210°/s	Diff %	KFlex R 210°/s	KFlex L 210°/s	Diff %
Pre surgery	229	110	52	125	80	36	141	129	9	77	70	10
Post surg. 6 w.	207	174	16	110	97	12	145	123	15	79	71	11
Post surg. 12 w.	248	215	14	135	116	14	170	150	12	96	84	12
Post surg. 24 w.	250	236	7	140	134	7	172	158	8	105	96	8

Table 2. Results of the Isokinetic test expressed in Nm. KExt: knee extension; KFlex: knee flexion; R: right; L: left (injured); Diff: difference between R and L.

Y Balance Test	Ant L	Ant R	Diff	Med R	Med R	Diff	Lat L	Lat R	Diff	Tot R	Tot L	Diff	FMS
Post surg. 22 d.	52.5	58.5	-6.0	97.0	102.0	-5.0	113.0	114.0	-1	87.5	91.5	-4.0	14/21
Post surg. 6 w.	54.5	58.0	-3.5	102.0	103.5	-1.5	113.0	115.5	-2.5	89.0	91.0	-2.0	16/21
Post surg. 12 w.	58.5	58.0	0.5	105.0	104.5	-0.5	115.5	116.0	-0.5	92.5	92.5	0.0	17/21
Post surg. 24 w.	59.0	59.0	0.0	108.0	107.0	1.0	116.0	119.0	-3	94.5	95.0	-0.5	17/21

Table 3. Results (expressed in cm) of the Y Balance Test. Ant: anterior; Med: medial; Tot: total score; Lat: lateral, L: left (injured); R: right; Diff: difference between L and R. The table shows also the score of the Functional Movement Screen (FMS) test.

The goalkeeper was able to train normally with his team eight weeks after the surgery.
He played his first official game, for 45 minutes, 11 weeks after surgery.

Conclusions

The surgical technique with LARS proved to be of primary importance in reducing complications (1), biological healing time and to avoid further structural damage to tissues which would have caused the removal of a second tendon using autograft.
The intensified rehabilitation program proposed proved efficient for the recovery in all aspects and it permitted the athlete to gradually and progressively increase muscle strength and functional exercises also on the football field.

References

1. Batty LM, Norsworthy CJ, Lash NJ, Wasiak J, Richmond AK, Feller JA. Synthetic devices for reconstructive surgery of the cruciate ligaments: a systematic review. Arthroscopy. 2015; 31(5): 957-968
2. Gribble PA, Hertel J, Plisky P. Using the Star Excursion Balance Test to assess dynamic postural-control deficits and outcomes in lower extremity injury: a literature and systematic review
3. J Athletic Training 2012; 47(3): 339-357

LATERAL COMPARTMENT OSTEOARTHRITIS IN A SOCCER PLAYER WITH VARUS KNEE: A CASE REPORT

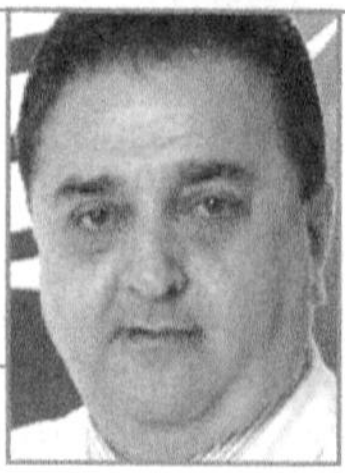

Cohen M[1], Debieux P[1], Gomes T[2]

[1]Universidade Federal de São Paulo, São Paulo; [2]Instituto Cohen, São Paulo, Brazil

Introduction

Osteoarthritis is a progressive degenerative joint disease. Usually, initial treatment must be non-operative. Different surgical procedures are available to treat this disease and osteotomies have extreme importance.
The purpose is to report a success case of a professional soccer player treated for an osteoarthritis of the lateral compartment of the right knee with a constitutional bilateral genu varus, caused by a wide lateral partial meniscectomy and surgically treated with distal femoral varus osteotomy.

Methods/Results

A 27-year-old man, professional soccer player with a constitutional bilateral genu varus, after few months of a wide lateral meniscectomy in December 2011 as a result of traumatic meniscal injury in right knee, experienced lateral compartment pain after running.
He noted an increase of the symptoms with pain in passive Range Of Motion (ROM). The athlete was incapacitated for professional sports activities by his symptoms. In addition, he exhibited an abnormal gait pattern with deficit valgus control on both knees.
After careful physical examination of the right knee, we could see a symmetrical and bilateral genu varus; range of motion between 0° to 140°; lateral joint pain; McMurray test positive during internal rotation, Appley and Steinmann tests positive for lateral pain; all stability tests were negatives. Radiographs of the knee evidenced reduction of the lateral joint space.
Initially, the patient was treated with non-operative protocol: physical therapy associated with oral analgesics and intra-articular injections with visco-supplementation. Also, the athlete was given complete rest and was not allowed to return to play or practice with the team.
He presented unsatisfactory clinical results due to its high physical demand after one year of non-surgical treatment and a distal femoral varus osteotomy was indicated. Once the patient was referred for surgery, treatment to increase muscle strength, especially the quadriceps muscle group, and ROM exercises of the knee were performed.
In August 2013, a standard arthroscopic of the right knee confirmed the isolated lateral compartment osteoarthritis. Micro-fracture was made to treat cartilage injuries. Finally, the distal femoral varus osteotomy with medial closing-wedge was done with tourniquet control. We performed a 10 cm knee medial approach and Vastus Medialis Obliquus (VMO) was exposed. The fascia was released posteriorly towards the attachment of the VMO on the medial intermuscular septum. A stable construction was realized by taking wedge from the medial supracondylar area, leaving the lateral cortex intact and closing the osteotomy with a 90° blade plate with the tensioning device applied. The patient was discharged from hospital in three days, when postoperative knee pain and effusion were minimal. We allow patients to walk with no weight bearing on the limb in proprioception training from the second postoperative day. The exercise program must also integrate the trunk, hip and ankle muscles to provide dynamic knee stabilization while addressing isolated Quadriceps Femoris deficiencies.

After six weeks, partial weight bearing was allowed. Full weight bearing was possible after nine weeks as long as we noted radiographic evidence that the bone had healed sufficiently. We adjusted his gait pattern during physical therapy to improve performance on high physical demand activities. The athlete was able to perform a 100 m sprint between 12.3 and 13.1 seconds at 100% intensity and kick a soccer ball without pain. Additionally, the athlete demonstrated full strength, measured with an isokinetic dynamometer Biodex System 4 (Biodex Medical Systems, Shirley, NY, USA) and functional tests. The results of peak torque of the right knee (normalized by the body weight) were 332% for extension and 188% for flexion, evaluated at 60°/s velocity. It was 8 % and 11 % lower for knee extension and flexion respectively, compared to the contra-lateral knee.
Our patient showed satisfactory absence of pain complaints, adequate muscle trophism, symmetrical full range of motion, and he returned to play in a professional football club on July 2015, about two years after surgery, after complete sports specific activities without pain or discomfort, maintaining correct technique.

Conclusions

It is known that Distal Femoral Osteotomy (DFO) is recommended for young and active patients. In our patient, we decided to make a DFO with a medial close-wedge, because he is a high performance athlete in need of aggressive rehabilitation for early return to sport, as this procedure presents less risk of non-union (1). There is a successful case report of a patient with lateral knee osteoarthritis after a medial close-wedge varus distal femoral osteotomy in order to prolong its professional sports activity.

References

1. Saithna A, Kundra R, Modi CS, Getgood A, Spalding T. Distal femoral varus osteotomy for lateral compartment osteoarthritis in the valgus knee. A systematic review of the literature. Open Orthop J 2012; 6: 313-319

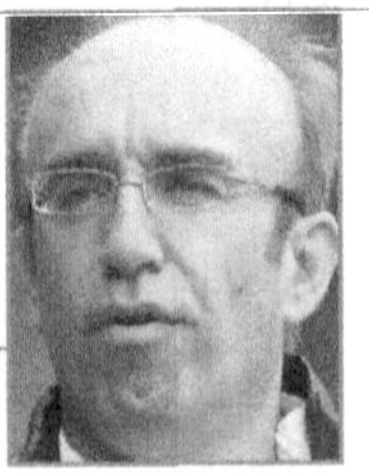

SERIOUS SHOULDER INJURY IN A HIGH LEVEL SOCCER PLAYER. RETURN TO PARTICIPATION AFTER SURGERY

Theos Ch[1], Kostas N[2], Koinis A[2]

[1]Olympiakós Sýndesmos Filáthlon Peiraiós and [2]Olympiacós FC Academy, Athens, Greece

Introduction

Shoulder injuries are not common in football but they are significant injuries and result in a significant absence from play (1, 2, 3). The surgical repair of shoulder instability in a high level goalkeeper seems to be a one-way ticket. During the training session the player has to come up against many falls and several exercises with the shoulder joint placed up to 90° that means full flexion, abduction and external rotation of the humerus. Considering the fact in a goalkeeper training session all the upper body joints and especially the joints of the shoulders are exposed in many loads, shoulder stabilization is a keystone for the proper rehabilitation.

Case report

A 18 years old male goalkeeper (178 cm height and 75 kg of weight), playing at Olympiacós FC Academy, had for a second time dislocation of his left shoulder. The first time of the injury underwent into a conservative treatment. The second time, seven months after the first injury, the player had a recurrent injury during a training session with the first team goalkeeper trainer. The result of the Magnetic Resonance Imaging (MRI) was Bankart and SLAP (Superior Labrum Anterior and Posterior) lesion at the left shoulder. We proceeded left shoulder arthroscopy for the surgical repair of the lesions. During the operation, we repaired Bankart lesion first, with two absorbable suture anchors (Linvatec Y-Knot, Conmed, USA) from the inferior to superior fashion and then the unstable SLAP lesion one absorbable suture anchor. The rehabilitation program based on modified rehabilitation protocols, giving emphasis in early mobilization of the shoulder, avoiding external rotation of the humerus, gains the Range of Motion (ROM) and proving proprioception stimuli after two weeks of the operation. Lower body and running exercises were started one month after the operation. The On the Field Rehabilitation (OFR) started after three and half months of the procedure performed sport specific exercises with the shoulder placed under 90° of flexion and external rotation. He started his rehabilitation program 7 days after his left shoulder surgery and after 4 months he started training with the team. One year after his operation he has no problems in following squad's program.

Conclusions

Shoulder injuries are not common in football but they are significant injuries and result in a significant absence from play. Early mobilization via manual therapy techniques of the humerus can provide better results in gaining ROM. Proprioceptive exercises can lead on muscular activation avoiding the risky loads in the joint.

References

1. Ekstrand J, Hagglund M, Waldén M. Injury incidence and injury patterns in professional football: the UEFA injury study. Br J Sports Med 2011; 45: 553-558
2. Hagglund M, Waldén M, Ekstrand J. UEFA injury study: an injury audit of European championships 2006 to 2008. Br J Sports Med 2009; 43: 483-489
3. Hawkins RD, Fuller CW. A prospective epidemiological study of injuries in four professional football clubs. Br J Sports Med 1999; 33: 196-203

Saturday 9th April 2016
POSTER AREA

FREE POSTER PRESENTATIONS

EPIDEMIOLOGY

Chairs

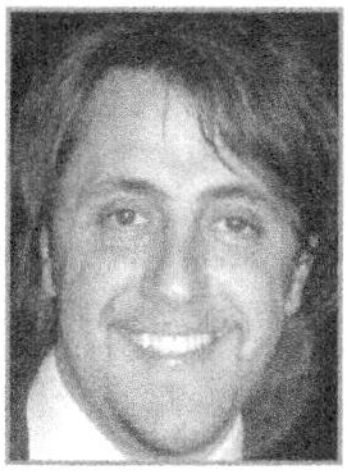

Marco Freschi
(Milan, Italy)

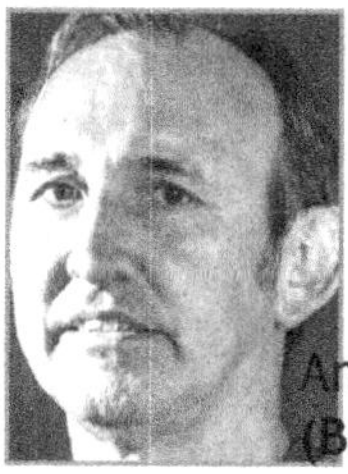

Antoni Turmo
(Barcelona, Spain)

PG01 Sleep disorders in Urugayan football players: pilot study
Pedemonte M, Barbosa E, Hurtado N (Maldonado and Montevideo, Uruguay)

PG02 Heterogeneity of risk assessment in sport medicine clinical practice: a pilot study **Weir A, Serner A, Wengensteen A, Steele RJ, Shirer I (Doha, Qatar; Montreal, Canada)**

PG03 Return to play after hamstring injuries: a qualitative systematic review of definitions and criteria **van der Horst N, van de Hoefer PA, Huisstede BMA, Reurnik G, Backx FJG (Utrecht and Rotterdam, The Netherlands)**

PG04 A meta-analytic review of the effects of soccer heading
Soni A, Musahl V, Braithwaite R, Chrisman SPD, McAllister Deitrick J, Lesniak B, Collins MW, Kontos AP (Pittsburgh, USA)

PG05 Epidemiological study on injuries and return to play in Italian young football players
Pisoni D, Danelon F, Gallo M, Barbieri L, Chianca A, Marinoni D, Scalise G (Milan, Italy)

PG06 Injuries in collegiate female football players in Japan
Oda K, Ogaki R, Murakami K, Yamaguchi T, Kurosawa T, Miyakawa S (Sendai and Tsukuba, Japan)

PG07 Prevalence of sports injuries in elite young Brazilian footballers
Herdy C, Simão R, Teixeira R, Ramos S, Vasconcellos F, Alkimin R, Pedrinelli A (Rio de Janeiro and São Paulo, Brasil)

PG08 Association between dietary habits, muscle damage and performance indices in youth soccer
Kotsis Y, Lambrou K, Sideris Y, Malagaris Y, Nomikos T (Athens, Greece; Galveston, USA)

PG09 Football (soccer) injury studies in China: a preliminary report
Xu J, Gao C, Gao Q, Ping H, Zhao J (Beijing, China)

SLEEP DISORDERS IN URUGUAYAN FOOTBALL PLAYERS: PILOT STUDY

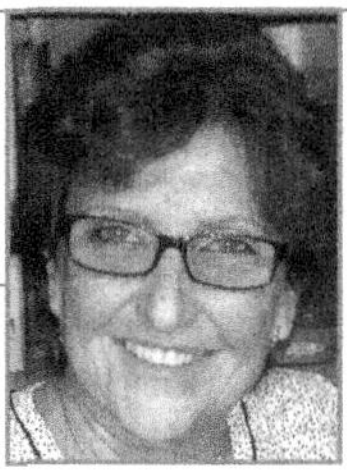

Pedemonte M[1], Barbosa E[2], Hurtado N[1]

[1]Centro de Medicina del Sueño. Facultad de Medicina, Instituto Universitario CLAEH. Punta del Este, Maldonado; [2]Asociación Uruguaya de Fútbol, Montevideo, Uruguay

Introduction

Sleep is not a function but a state, diverse from the waking one, where multiple physiological functions are processed: movements, cognition, autonomic and endocrinological functions, immunology, and emotions. Although in different ways, both states are essential. Sleep state occurs because of shifts in neuronal networks passing from waking mode to sleeping mode that may be organized by unknown hub neurons. For the physiological functions to develop at its maximum efficiency sleep must be qualitatively and quantitatively well organized. The hours of sleep that have been lost during one day must be compensated the following night to achieve optimal physiological conditions, such as learning and memories related to motor performance (1). Sleeping less than needed impacts negatively over all learning and memory mechanisms. The group of Dement (2) demonstrated that basketball players further improved their physical performance and mood following sleep extension. This research also shows that all the players tested where chronically sleep deprived.

Our aim is to determine disorders of sleep and chronobiology in the players and the worries that the coaches and physicians have about them. Our hypothesis is that sleep disorders are very frequent in football players and the impact on their performance during training, competition and in the time of recovery to return to the play are not been considered in its real dimension.

Methods

Two surveys were designed: i) for football players, 15 questions that explored sleep, chronobiology characteristics and repercussion during day time (it was applied in 28 Uruguayan football players under 15 years old, that belong to the Uruguayan National Football team); ii) for coaches and physicians, six questions to analyze how much they care about sleep disorders and what measures they take in order to prevent or improve them (applied in 10 coaches and physicians of the Uruguayan Football Association).

Results

In this pilot study the first survey showed that the 57% of the football players consider that they suffer from a sleep disorder.

The 82% have sleep deprivation, 71% have diurnal hipersomnia and 79% notices changes in mood and performance because of these disturbs.

Only 2 (7%) consulted with coaches or physicians on this matter.

The survey for the coaches and physicians showed that 100% realize the impact of sleep disorders on the players' performance but only 60% has applied sleep hygiene methods.

The 33% has sometimes used chronobiotics or Cognitive Behavioral Therapy.

Nobody has conducted sleep evaluations in football players.

Conclusions

While the impact of sleep on an athlete's evolution in their recovery is a general concern (3), there are still no well-designed studies analyzing its dimension.
These surveys are a tool to detect the state of art of sleep in football players as first step to take into consideration new methods to improve sleep disorders. This way, performance during training and competitions will improve, player will manage to recover better and faster from injuries, and return to play quickly.
While players, coaches and physicians show concerned about sleep disorders and their impact, actions are not taken. Therefore, besides developing a protocol to improve their sleep behavior, awareness should be raised amongst them.

References

1. Parmeggiani PL, Velluti RA (Eds). The physiologic nature of sleep. Imperial College Press, London, 2005
2. Mah CD, Mah KE, Kezirian EJ, Dement WC. The effects of sleep extension on the athletic performance of collegiate basketball players. Sleep 2011; 34: 943-950
3. Nédélec M, McCall A, Carling C, Legall F, Berthoin S, Dupont G. Recovery in Soccer. Part II Recovery Strategies. Sports Med 2013; 43: 9-22

HETEROGENEITY OF RISK ASSESSMENT IN SPORT MEDICINE CLINICAL PRACTICE: A PILOT STUDY

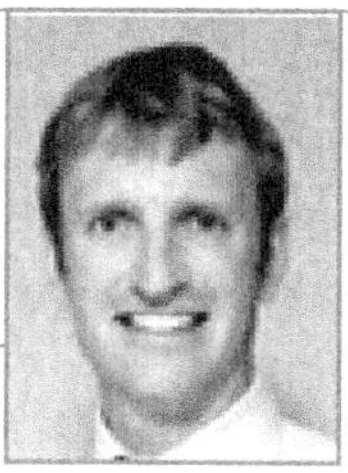

Weir A[1], Serner A[1], Wangensteen A[1], Steele RJ[3], Shrier I[2]

[1]Aspetar Orthopaedic and Sports Medicine Hospital, Doha, Qatar;
[2]Centre for Clinical Epidemiology, Lady Davis Institute, Jewish General Hospital, McGill University, Montreal, Canada;
[3]Department of Mathematics and Statistics, McGill University, Montreal, Canada

Introduction

Return To Play (RTP) decisions are an integral part of sports medicine, but different individuals may arrive at different decisions. The Strategic Assessment of Risk and Risk Tolerance (StARRT) model for return to play decision-making has been validated using only simulated clinical vignettes. Clinicians first assess the risk of an outcome based on a balance of tissue health and stress due to sporting activity, and then make a decision based on their tolerance of the risk. The different decisions clinicians reach may be a result of different risk assessments, or different risk tolerances. Although valuable in providing information on what clinicians believe they might do, clinical vignettes are limited by the amount of information that can be presented and the artificial setting. In addition, no study has yet attempted to elicit risk estimations for reinjury from different stakeholders in the same clinical context.
Purpose: To describe and compare risk assessments from sport medicine physicians, physiotherapists and athletes during routine care of injured athletes, and to elicit if there were factors that influenced their risk tolerance.

Methods

We recruited the physician and physiotherapist, and the athlete they were caring for ("triplet") to participate. Triplets were recruited from an acute groin injury study and an acute hamstring injury study at a at a specialized orthopedic and sports medicine hospital in Doha, Qatar. Each participant provided their own estimated probability distribution for risk of re-injury within the subsequent two months after RTP, based on the available knowledge from clinical care, the athlete chart with tests, and projected activity level. In addition, we asked participants about factors that influenced their risk tolerance for the particular case.

Results

Of the 15 athletes recruited, five were excluded because we obtained risk estimates from only one stakeholder. Of the remaining 10 cases, we obtained risk estimates from 7 triplets and 3 doublets. Despite the limited data set, there were clear and considerable differences in risk estimates among some of the comparisons. For example, one participant estimated the reinjury risk to be between 1-10%, another between 20-50%, and another between 30-40%. Factors that modified risk tolerance in at least three participants were: timing and season, pressure from athlete, and external pressure. Overall, risk modifiers influenced the decision in 13/27 possible cases.

Conclusions

Different stakeholders with access to the same information can have considerably different estimates for the risk of reinjury, which would be expected to influence RTP decisions. Risk tolerance in the real world is sometimes modified by factors identified in simulated clinical vignette studies.

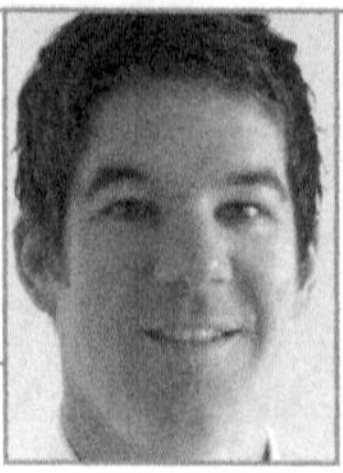

RETURN TO PLAY AFTER HAMSTRING INJURIES: A QUALITATIVE SYSTEMATIC REVIEW OF DEFINITIONS AND CRITERIA

van der Horst N[1], van de Hoef PA[1], Huisstede BMA[1], Reurink G[2], Backx FJG[1]

[1]University Medical Center Utrecht, Rudolf Magnus Institute of Neurosciences, Department of Rehabilitation, Nursing Science & Sports, Utrecht;
[2]Department of Orthopaedics, Erasmus Medical Centre, Rotterdam, The Netherlands

Introduction

"When will I be able to play again?" This question about Return To Play (RTP) in sports is of great importance for every athlete after a hamstring injury. The major concern of athletes, trainers, management, and other stakeholders is to start playing as soon as possible, but this might be in conflict with the athlete's actual physical fitness and readiness for match play (2). High hamstring recurrence rates are reported in soccer, of which 59% occur within the first month after RTP (1). A too early RTP after hamstring injury increases recurrence risk. Although there are numerous studies on RTP, comparisons are hampered by the multiple definitions of RTP used. Moreover, there is no consensus on which criteria should be used to determine when an athlete can start playing again.

Therefore, we conducted a systematic review of the literature on 1) definitions of RTP used in hamstring research, and 2) RTP-criteria after hamstring injuries.

Methods

Seven databases were searched for articles that provided a definition of, or criteria for, RTP after hamstring injury. There were no limitations on the methodological design or quality of articles. Content analysis was used to record and analyse definitions and criteria for RTP after hamstring injury (3).

In a content analysis, the first step is to create tentative labels for RTP definition and criteria within the articles, using an open coding procedure.

The second step was to perform axial coding in order to identify relationships among open codes. Axial coding, termed "axial" because coding occurs around the axis of a category, links categories at the level of properties and dimensions. In the third step, final content categories were identified by selective coding.

Results

Of 1303 articles retrieved, 608 were excluded as duplicate publications and a further 584 were excluded after screening of the title and abstract. The remaining full-text articles (n = 111) were checked for relevant content, based on eligibility criteria, by two researchers. Five articles were identified from the reference lists of retrieved articles. In total, 25 articles met the inclusion criteria. Thirteen of these 25 papers provided a definition of RTP and 23 of 25 papers described criteria to support the RTP decision. "Reaching the athlete's pre-injury level" and "being able to perform full sport activities" were primary content categories used to define RTP.

"Absence of pain", "similar strength", "similar flexibility", "medical staff clearance", and "functional performance" were core themes to describe criteria to support the RTP-decision after hamstring injury.

Conclusions

Only half of the included studies provided some definition of RTP after hamstring injury. A wide variety of criteria are used to support the RTP-decision, none of which have been validated. More research is needed to reach consensus on the definition of RTP and to provide validated RTP-criteria in order to facilitate hamstring injury management and reduce hamstring injury recurrence.

References

1. Brooks JH, Fuller CW, Kemp SP, Reddin DB. Incidence, risk, and prevention of hamstring muscle injuries in professional rugby union. Am J Sports Med 2006; 34: 1297-1306
2. Creighton DW, Shrier I, Schultz R, Meeuwisse WH, Matheson GO. Return-to-play in sport: a decision-based model. Clin J Sports Med 2010; 20: 379-385
3. Krippendorff K. Content analysis: an introduction to its methodology. 2nd ed; Thousand Oaks, California, Sage Publications, 2004

4

A META-ANALYTIC REVIEW OF THE EFFECTS OF SOCCER HEADING

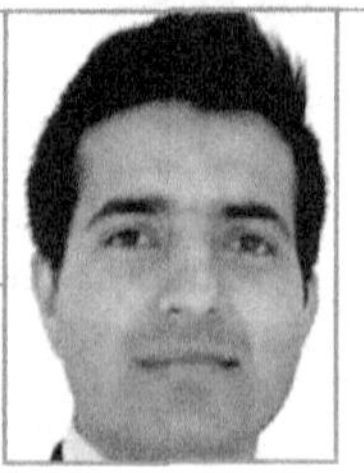

Soni A, Musahl V, Braithwaite R, Chrisman SPD, McAllister Deitrick J, Lesniak B, Collins MW, Kontos AP

University of Pittsburgh Medical Center, Department of Orthopaedic Surgery,
UPMC Rooney Sports Complex, Pittsburgh, USA

Introduction

Researchers and clinicians have raised concerns about the potential adverse effects of soccer heading. Surprisingly, during over four decades of research on the potential effects of soccer heading on symptoms, cognitive function and balance, there has not been a single meta-analytic review of the existent literature.
The purpose of the current study was to conduct a meta-analytic review of empirical research on the effects of soccer heading on neurocognitive performance, balance, and symptom reports. A secondary purpose of was to examine the role of potential moderating variables including age, gender, level of play, and soccer heading exposure.

Methods

A total of 1,436 studies were identified using the relevant search terms: concussion, mild Traumatic Brain Injury (mTBI), soccer, European football, soccer heading, header(s), concussion symptoms, cognitive impairment, and neurocognitive test/performance.
103/1,436 (7.1%) met the following study inclusion criteria: i) the study examined and reported on soccer athletes; ii) the population's age, sex, and sport position was described; iii) cognitive function, symptoms, balance, or other outcomes were quantitatively measured; iv) soccer heading exposure was quantitatively measured between at least two groups; and v) the study was written in the English language after December 1979. 21/1,436 (1.5%) contained necessary data to be included in the analysis (means, Standard Deviation, r, N).

Results

The results of a random effects model across all outcomes, groups and time points did not support an overall effect for soccer heading on cognitive, balance and other impairments ($k=21$; $g=-0.06$, 95% CI: -0.149-0.023; $p>0.05$).
Moderator analyses indicated that age/level of play was a potential moderating variable, with professional soccer players experiencing decreased outcomes associated with heading.

Conclusions

The results of this meta-analysis do not support an overall effect for soccer heading on cognitive, balance and other outcomes. Future studies need to be designed to establish clear relationships with soccer heading and concussion to protect our athletes.

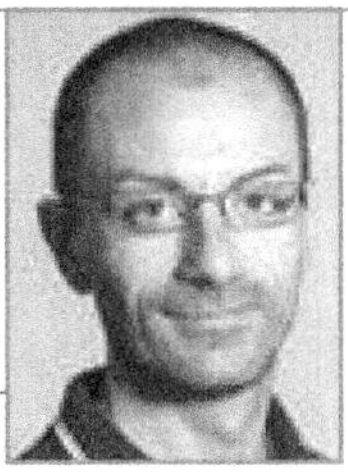

EPIDEMIOLOGICAL STUDY ON INJURIES AND RETURN TO PLAY IN ITALIAN YOUNG FOOTBALL PLAYERS

Pisoni D[1], Danelon F[1], Gallo M[1], Barbieri L[2], Chianca A[3], Marinoni D[4], Scalise G[5]

[1]Isokinetic Medical Group, Milan; [2]Suprema Calcio, Paderno Dugnano; [3]Accademia Internazionale, Milan; [4]Rozzano Calcio, Rozzano; [5]GS Concorezzese, Concorezzo, Italy

Introduction

An increasing Interest in injury epidemiology and prevention is evident in the football community. Injuries represent a social cost and can keep the players far from field for long time and even threaten long-term health of the player. The latter point is at most true when players are young. On the other hand football, being an organized physical activity, is encouraged and a prerequisite for the health of children and young people. In this context, prevention based on epidemiological evidence on injuries and average time for return to sports in the young players is mandatory.
Epidemiological data on juvenile football are lacking, even in country as Italy where football is really popular and participated among children. An isolated recent study on player younger than 13 years showed interesting results compared to adults at most on type of injuries, evidencing more bone-correlated injuries and upper limbs injuries, and evidenced an increasing incidence rate with increasing age of the players (3).
Aim of our study is to contribute to collect and share data on injuries in young football players in order to implement specific prevention strategy.

Methods

We are doing a survey on three male juvenile teams in and around Milan, Italy, monitoring 77 players in the Allievi category, mean(±SD) age is 15.5±0.7 years and applying the same injury definition and recording method used in adult players at professional level (1, 2).
We are presenting data over half season in Italy from the beginning of September till half of December. Exposure time for each player and injuries were reported by one coach of each team specifically instructed on reporting method before the start of the survey.

Results

Total exposure time of all players has been 8,150.5 hours, 6,229 of them in training and 1,921.5 of them in matches, with an average ratio training/match of 3.28, lower than in older football players. Injuries have been 25, with an overall incidence of injury of 3.07/1,000 hours; 5 injuries during matches and others during training sessions; injury incidence has been higher in matches than in training, respectively 3.5/1,000 hs and 2.8/1,000 hs (Table 1).

Teams	Players n°	Exposure in training (hours)	Exposure in matches (hours)	Exposure ratio Training/match	Incidence in traning (/1,000hs)	Incidence in matches (/1,000hs)	Total incidence (/1,000 hs)
1	23	1840	517.5	3.55	1.60	3.80	2.12
2	27	2020	747.0	2.70	2.30	4.98	3.02
3	27	2369	657.0	3.60	4.74	1.73	4.08
Totals	77	6229	1921.5	3.28	2.88	3.50	3.07

Table 1. Epidemiology of three teams of 15 years old players.

About Injuries location, nine of them (36%) involved the thigh, seven on the anterior thigh and two on posterior thigh.

Six injuries (24%) involved the knee, three injuries (12%) regarded the pubic area. Two injuries each for leg/ankle, lumbar spine and shoulder. Only one injury involved the wrist but it has caused the longest time to return to play (19 days).

Mean time needed to return to play has been 10.5 days.

About type of injury 16 (64%) have been classified as not caused by a unique trauma but by overload.

Conclusions

Examining our preliminary data injuries in young players appear to be less than among older people. Matches seem to be more dangerous for injuries, except in one team in which the ratio training/matches injuries incidence was inverted with more injuries during training. This data could be used by the technical staff of that single team as useful information to adopt specific strategy of prevention.

Mean absence from the field is shorter than in previous studies in younger players (3). The most common site of injuries has been the thigh, at most the anterior region of the thigh and classified as originated from muscle and tendon-bone overloads, perhaps related to kick movement.

These data could be used in programming specific prevention strategies for young players as improving warm-up and anterior thigh specific stretching strategy.

These data refers to the first half of the season and need to be confirmed in the second one to have a more complete database on which build up best prevention strategies.

References

1. Fuller CW, Ekstrand J, Junge A, Andersen TE, Bahr R, Dvorak J, Hägglund M, McCrory P, Meeuwisse WH. Consensus statement on injury definitions and data collection procedures in studies of football (soccer) injuries. Br J Sports Med 2006; 40: 193-201
2. Hägglund M, Waldén M, Bahr R, Ekstrand J. Methods for epidemiological study of injuries to professional football players: developing the UEFA model. Br J Sports Med 2005; 39: 340-346
3. Rössler R, Junge A, Chomiak J, Dvorak J, Faude O. Soccer Injuries in Players Aged 7 to 12 Years: A Descriptive Epidemiological Study Over 2 Seasons. Am J Sports Med 2015 Dec 8. [Epub ahead of print]

INJURIES IN COLLEGIATE FEMALE FOOTBALL PLAYERS IN JAPAN

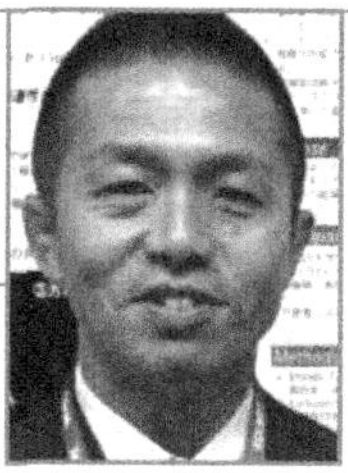

Oda K[1], Ogaki R[2], Murakami K[1], Yamaguchi T[1], Kurosawa T[1], Miyakawa S[3]

[1]Faculty of Sports Science, Sendai University, Sendai;
[2]Sports Research & Development Core, University of Tsukuba,
[3]Faculty of Health and Sports Science, University of Tsukuba, Japan

Introduction

Football is played worldwide by more than 265 million players, of whom, 26 million are female players.
The popularity of female football players in Japan has been rising since the winning of FIFA World Cup championship in 2011. The number of population continues to increase every year and exceeds approximately 30,000 today. Football requires physical contact, and therefore associates with a large number of injuries in both sexes. Injuries in male football have been the subject in many studies. However, the number of reports regarding female football injuries in adults is low and epidemiologic date in Japanese collegiate female football players is very rare.
The aim of this study was investigating the injuries in Japanese female collegiate football players in one season (March - January, 2014) using definitions established by the Federation International de Football Association (FIFA).

Methods

A total of 26 female collegiate football players (mean±SD age: 19.3±1.3 years; height: 159.3±7.1 cm; weight: 57.0±7.3 kg) participated in the study.
We investigated the injured situation (game or practice, contact or non-contact), type of injury (traumatic or overuse), location, severity, days until return to play, and a month that the injury occurs.
Injuries were classified into the following three categories according to FIFA severity:

- minimal (absence from training/games, 1 to 3days);
- mild (absence from 4 to 7 days);
- moderate (absence from 8 to 28 days);
- severe (absence > 29 days).

All injuries that resulted in absence from at least one scheduled practice session or game were recorded by athletic trainers.

Results

Overall, 30 injuries were documented in 14 players (53.8%).
80.0% of injuries were traumatic and 20.0% were overuse injuries.
40.0% of injuries were occurred during games and 60.0% were during practices.
56.3% of injuries were caused by the contact play and 43.7% were non-contact play.
Most injuries (86.7%) were located in the lower extremities with affecting ankle (36.7%), thigh (20%), and knee (16.7%).
The most frequent injury was the ankle sprain.
Of the injuries occurred during games, 41.7% were severe and 33.3% were moderate.
On the other hand, of the injuries occurred during practices, 44.4% were moderate and 22% were severe injuries.
The days taken until return to play with injuries during game and practice were 39.1±55.3 and 22.4±29.1 respectively. April was the predominant month for injuries (23.3%)

Conclusions

As with other studies, our results shows that the most injuries occurred in lower extremity and the ankle sprain was the most frequent injury in female football players. However, the days taken until return to play was longer in our study than its other studies.
The results suggest that, in addition to the rehabilitation that focuses on early recovery, reducing severity of injuries by applying the preventive intervention of lower extremity injuries is the crucial strategy to shorten the return to play in female football players.

References

1. Söderman K, Adolphson J, Lorentzon R, Alfredson H. Injuries in adolescent female players in European football: a prospective study over one outdoor soccer season. Scand J Med Sci Sports 2001; 11: 299-304
2. Yamamoto J. Epidemiology of professional soccer team injuries for three years. Football Science 2013; 11: 36-5

PREVALENCE OF SPORTS INJURIES IN ELITE YOUNG BRAZILIAN FOOTBALLERS

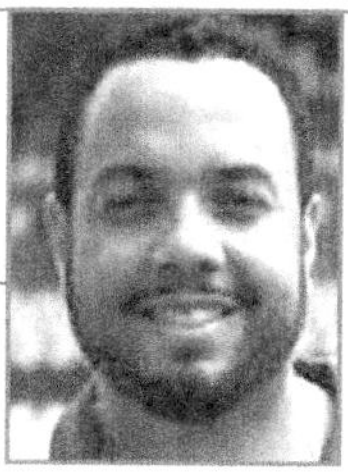

Herdy C[1,2], Simão R[1,2], Teixeira R[1], Ramos S[1,2], Vasconcellos F[3], Alkimim R[3], Pedrinelli A[4]

[1]Club de Regatas Vasco da Gama, Rio de Janeiro;
[2]Federal University of Rio de Janeiro, Rio de Janeiro;
[3]State University of Rio de Janeiro, Rio de Janeiro;
[4]São Paulo FIFA Medical Centre of Excellence, Sao Paulo, Brazil

Introduction

Football is a high performance sport which is practiced by more and more young athletes. This causes players to have greater demands regarding physical performance leading them to Early maturation and being more susceptible to injury. It is estimated that for every 1,000 hours of game play, the number of injuries is, on average, four to six times higher than the number of lesions that occur during training. FIFA (Fédération Internationale de Football Association), according to the Medical Assessment and Research Centre, defined as any injury occurring suffered by a player in competition or in training, which requires him or her to interrupt their activity and prevents them from participating in at least one practice or game. The aim of the study was to describe the profile of injuries in young football athletes in high performance categories.

Methods and Results

Data were collected from medical records of the medical department of 218 injured athletes belonging to a club in the first division of the Brazilian Championship.
The young athletes were evaluated in the following categories:

U-11, n = 30 (10.45 ± 0.5 years)
U-13, n = 34 (12.15 ± 0.3 years)
U-15, n = 23 (14.56 ± 0.4 years)
U-17, n = 24 (16.52 ± 0.5 years)
U-20, n = 32 (18.24 ± 0.6 years)

Data collection was conducted from January 2015 to November 2015 (11 months). The data were analyzed and classified according to the categories and the lesions identified as per the recommendations of the study group in injury FIFA Medical Assessment and Research Centre. The data were analyzed using IBM SPSS Statistics Version 21 and presented descriptively.

Results

The results showed that there was a total of 200 lesions in all categories, the teams U-15, U-17, U-20 stood out with the greatest occurrences of injuries. The overall incidence rate was 2.34 injuries per 1,000 hours of play/training.
It was observed that the prevalence and characteristics of lesions of young football players in different categories are higher according to the increasing number of games and that the older groups demonstrate a greater number of lesions more similar to that in adults. During the data collection period there was a total of 200 injuries (Table 1). There were a greater number and variety of injuries in older compared to younger age groups with 66 injuries in the U17 team and 61 injuries U-20 compared to 12 injuries in the U-11 and 15 injuries in the U-13 teams.
The commonest injuries were muscle stretch injuries (n=33) and contusions (n=32).
Ankle injuries (N=26) were more common than knee injuries (n=15).

Types Of Injuries	U-11	U-13	U-15	U-17	U-20	Total
Muscle Stretch	3 (25%)	1 (6%)	10 (22%)	9 (14%)	10 (16%)	33 (16%)
Myalgia	0	5 (33%)	7 (15%)	15 (23%)	4 (6%)	31 (15%)
Low Back Pain	0	2 (13%)	3 (7%)	1 (1%)	3 (5%)	9 (4%)
Trauma	2 (17%)	0	2 (5%)	12 (18%)	14 (23%)	30 (15%)
Contusion	5 (42%)	4 (27%)	13 (28%)	7 (11%)	3 (5%)	32 (16%)
Tendinopaties	0	1 (6%)	2 (4%)	3 (4%)	4 (7%)	10 (5%)
Sprain No Diagnosis	1 (8%)	1 (6%)	1 (2%)	4 (6%)	6 (10%)	13 (7%)
Knee Sprain	1 (8%)	0 (6%)	2 (4%)	3 (5%)	3 (5%)	9 (5%)
Ankle Sprain	0	1 (6%)	6 (13%)	11 (17%)	8 (13%)	26 (13%)
Anterior Cruciate Ligament	0	0	0	0	4 (7%)	4 (2%)
Posterior Cruciate Ligament	0	0	0	0	2 (3%)	2 (1%)
Herniated Disc	0	0	0	1 (1%)	0	1 (1%)
Totals	12 (100%)	15 (100%)	46 (100%)	66 (100%)	61 (100%)	200 (100%)

Table 1. Descriptive values of the types of lesions in the affected category U-11, U-13, U-15, U-17 and U-20. †U-11 until U-20, category aged 10 up to 20 years.

Table 2 displays the number of injuries and number of hours of exposure to matches and training. It is interesting to note that exposure to training was constant across age groups but exposure hours to match play increased as age increased. Generally the index of injury per 1,000/h exposure increased with age peaking at 6.31 in the U17 age group.
The overall incidence rate was 2.34 injuries per 1,000 hours of play / training.

	U-11	U-13	U-15	U-17	U-20	Total
N	30	34	23	24	32	143
Amount Injuries	12	15	46	66	61	200
Injuries for each athlete	0.40	0.44	2.00	2.75	1.91	1.40
Hours of game season	10.0	23.3	53.6	64.6	75.0	226.5
Hours of training	371.25	371.25	371.25	371.25	371.25	371.25
Incidence per 1,000/h	1.05	1.12	4.71	6.31	4.27	2.34

Table 2. Exposure and incidence of injuries by category.

Conclusions

The present study observed that the prevalence and incidence of characteristics of the injuries of young football players in different age categories are larger in older age groups and that the larger the number of games played the greater the number of injuries sustained to a level that is close to that found in adult players.

References

1. Consensus statement on injury definitions and data collection procedures in studies of football (soccer) injuries. Br J Sports Med. 2006; 40: 193-201
2. Junge A, Chomiak J, Dvorak J. Incidence of football injuries in youth players. Comparison of players from two European regions. Am J Sports Med 2000; 28: 47-50
3. Junge A, Dvorak J. Influence of definition and data collection on the incidence of injuries in football. Am J Sports Med 2000; 28: S40-S46

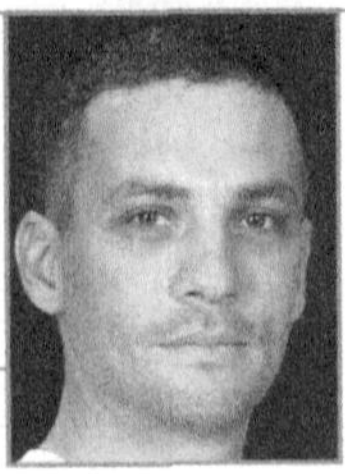

ASSOCIATION BETWEEN DIETARY HABITS, MUSCLE DAMAGE AND PERFORMANCE INDICES IN YOUTH SOCCER

Kotsis Y[1], Lambrou K[1], Sideris Y[1], Malagaris Y[2], Nomikos T[1]

[1]Faculty of Health Sciences and Education, Department of Nutrition and Dietetics, Harokopio University, Athens, Greece;
[2]University of Texas Medical Branch, Galveston, Texas, United States

Introduction

Soccer specific daily training requires balanced and healthy dietary habits in order to overcome the demanding nature of the game. The repetitive and eccentric nature of soccer specific movements can cause additional muscle damage which is accompanied by the leakage of muscle protein in the circulation, oxidative stress, inflammation and decline in muscle performance (2). In the case of the adolescent athlete, an adequate nutrition strategy becomes the key factor, either for improving the fuel replenishment process or for a healthier physical and mental development (3). However, few studies have examined the effect of dietary habits and the overall nutritional behavior of adolescent soccer players during the transition period and its impact on exercise-induced muscle damage indices (1).
The aim of this study was to evaluate the nutritional habits of Greek adolescent soccer players during the annual soccer transition period and correlate them with muscle damage and performance markers.

Methods

The sample of the study consisted of 56 adolescent soccer players (age: 16.8±2.7 years; height: 1.73±0.11 m; weight: 65.5±12.2 kg) participated in a four week football camp (20 x 90 minutes soccer specific training sessions) in order to increase their soccer skills and to maintain their athletic performance during the Transition Period (TP).
Blood samples were collected before the beginning and after the completion of TP in order to assess blood cell counts, classic biochemical markers such as glucose, total cholesterol, HDL, LDL, uric acid and markers of Exercise Induced Muscle Damage (EIMD), such as Creatine Kinase (CK), Lactate Dehydrogenase (LDH) and the antioxidant enzyme serum Glutathione Peroxidase (GPX-3) activity.
Performance assessment included jumping ability (squat and countermovement jump), speed testing (5, 10, 20 and 30 m), Repeated Sprint Ability (5 x 10 m) and Yo-Yo Intermittent Shuttle Run Test, Level 1.
Nutritional intake was assessed by a validated food frequency questionnaire, from which the index of adherence to Mediterranean Diet (Med Diet score) was assessed and five 24-hour dietary recalls.

Results

The estimation of the nutritional profile of our subjects revealed their preference to processed grains which led to a deficiency of dietary fibers intake. Energy intake averaged 2,322±491 kcal/day while protein, fat and carbohydrate intake was 18% (1.9 g/kg body weight), 36%, (1.8 g/kg body weight) 46% (5.3 g/kg body weight) of total energy intake, respectively.

Micro-nutrient intake was lower than the recommended for Ca, K, Mg, vitamins D and E. The Med Diet Score was 29.0±4.5 (range 0-55). Performance assessment revealed a decrease in time to complete 5 m (pre 1.06±0.06 s; post 1.01±0.06 s; p=0.001), 20 m (pre 3.18±0.10 s; post 3.12+0.11 s; p=0.008), 30 m (pre 4.45±0.17 s; post 4.37±0.20 s; p=0.009) and RSA (pre 12.53±0.44 s; post 12.26±0.38 s; p=0.004). No significant changes were observed in the measured biochemical indices pre- vs post-training period. However, the large variability of the percent changes between subjects allowed us to proceed to correlation analysis in order to investigate possible associations between nutritional habits and alterations of the biochemical and performance profile. The correlation analysis demonstrated the significant associations presented in Table 1.

Parameters	Pearson Correlation	p
CMJ (%) - Vegetables	0.771	0.001
CMJ (%) - Non Processed Cereal	0.578	0.030
CK (%) -Vit B6	0.518	0.040
LDH (%) - Starch	-0.897	0.006
LDH (%) - Folate	-0.863	0.012
SPRINT 30m (%) - Percent fat	-0.719	0.013
SQJ (%) - Calcium	0.764	0.006
CMJ (%) - Energy (Kcal)	0.757	0.007
CMJ (%) - Percent fat	0.755	0.007
CMJ (%) - Zn	0.844	0.001
CMJ (%) - MUFA	0.965	0.000
RSA (%) - Percent Fat	-0.735	0.010
RSA (%) - Vitamin A	-0.665	0.025
Yo-Yo stage (%)-Thiamin	0.770	0.006
Yo-Yo Distance(%)-Thiamin	0.791	0.004

Table 1. Correlation between dietary intake and Percent changes (%) of exercise induced muscle damage and performance. MUFA: monounsaturated fatty acids.

Conclusions

Soccer specific training during the transition period in adolescent players can increase exercise performance. Food intake with increased antioxidant and fiber content, such as fruits and vegetables, can promote exercise performance markers and attenuate EIMD parameters.
The key ingredients in those foods are Zn, Folic Acid, dietary fiber and antioxidant vitamins.
Changes to a healthier, supplement-free, nutritional habit can play a major role in fuel replenishment and in maximizing athletic performance in adolescent soccer players.

References

1. Garcia-Roves PM, García-Zapico P, Patterson AM, Iglesias-Gutiérrez E. Nutrient intake and food habits of soccer players: analyzing the correlates of eating practice. Nutrients 2014; 6: 2697-2717
2. Rampinini E, Bosio A, Ferraresi I, Petruolo A, Morelli A, Sassi A. Match-related fatigue in soccer players. Med Sci Sports Exerc 2011; 43: 2161-2170
3. Williams C, Rollo I. Carbohydrate nutrition and team sport performance. Sports Med 2015. 45, Suppl 1: 13-22

FOOTBALL (SOCCER) INJURY STUDIES IN CHINA: A PRELIMINARY REPORT

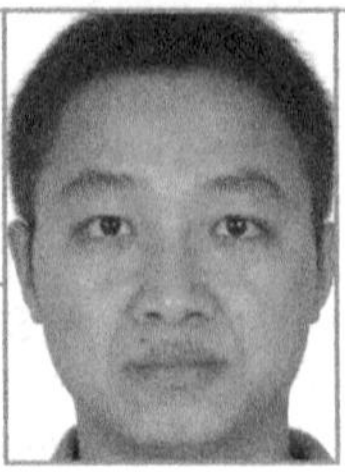

Xu J[1], Gao C[2], Gao Q[3], Ping H[1], ZhaoJ[1]

[1]Sport Biological Center, China Institute of Sport Science, Beijing;
[2]Sports Hospital, National Institute of Sports Medicine, Beijing;
[3]Department of Sport Rehabilitation, Beijing Sport University, Beijing, China

Introduction

A national football promotion Activity has been implemented in China since early 2015, covering not only professional football but also campus and grassroots football. Although football can serve as a health promotion sport, as a contact sport, it also has certain injury risks. To prevent football injuries and maximize health benefits of football, the first step is to know the epidemiological characteristics of injuries in football. Thus, the present report was written to investigate and summarize current researches on football injuries in Chinese players.

Methods

The MEDLINE and EMBASE databases were searched updated to December 8th 2015, using the following search term groups: 1) "football" and "soccer"; 2) "Chinese". Furthermore, the Chinese keyword of football (soccer) was also searched in Chinese Journal of Sports Medicine, the only specialty journal in sports medicine in China, updated to the same date as above. The literature search and screen were limited to articles published in English or Chinese. Only original reports on epidemiology, risks, or prevention of football injuries in Chinese football players were included in our final synthesis.

Results

In all, only one article in English and three ones in Chinese met the inclusion criteria. The English article was from Hong Kong, SAR, China, and followed the consensus statement on football injury definition and data collection procedures outlined by F-MARC. No English articles from Mainland China were found. All three Chinese articles were from Mainland China, however, none of them met the operational recommendations from the consensus statement mentioned above. The English article mainly reported prospective epidemiological data of training and match exposure, injury incidence (injuries per 1,000 player-hours), injury patterns, and injury severity in a Hong Kong male professional football league during 2010-2011 competitive season and compared the results to published data in European leagues. However, this study limited to only time-loss injuries and one competitive season in one city. No Chinese articles reported training and match exposure, and injury incidence (injuries per 1,000 player-hours). In all three Chinese articles, injury epidemiological data, if available, were mainly reported in injury numbers and percentages with respect to injury types, locations, severity, and occasions (training or match). Among the three Chinese articles, one only focused on Chinese female football players and the other two were on professional Chinese males. However, differences in definitions of injury or other aforementioned relevant terms, study design, and characteristics of players in these Chinese articles made it difficult to compare them with each other or other abundant injury data from European or other professional leagues.

Conclusions

Football injury studies in China are still at a preliminary level, especially in Mainland China. True injury risk or injury prevention studies in football are also lack. High quality football injury studies following the F-MARC consensus statement should be warranted to investigate the epidemiology, risks and injury prevention in Chinese football players.

Saturday 9th April, 2016 (afternoon)
FLEMING ROOM

INVITED SPEAKERS

RETURN TO PLAY FOLLOWING ACL INJURY

Chairs

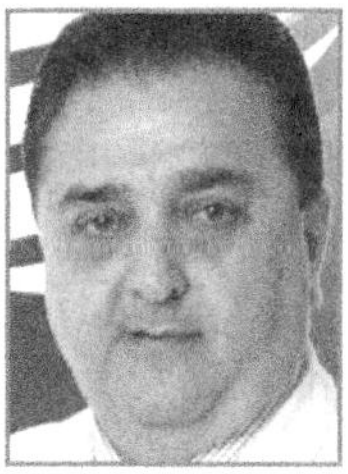

Moisés Cohen
(São Paulo, Brasil)

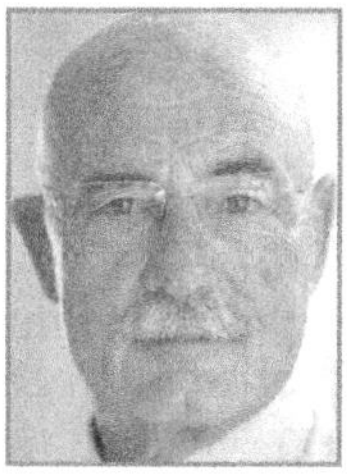

Maurilio Marcacci
(Bologna, Italy)

14:30	Return to play after anterior cruciate ligament repair in men's professional football **Marcus Waldén (Linköping, Sweden)**
14:45	Return to play in anterior cruciate ligament: criteria vs time **Richard Weiler (London, United Kingdom)**
15:00	Role of prehabilitation in accelerated return to play **May Arna Risberg (Oslo, Norway)**
15:15	Return to play after anterior cruciate ligament repair: outcome predictors analysis **Francesco Della Villa (Bologna, Italy)**
15:30	Prevention and management of anterior cruciate ligament repair complications **Freddie Fu (Pittsburgh, USA)**
15:45	Discussion
16:00	End of the session

RETURN TO PLAY AFTER ANTERIOR CRUCIATE LIGAMENT RECONSTRUCTION IN MEN'S PROFESSIONAL FOOTBALL

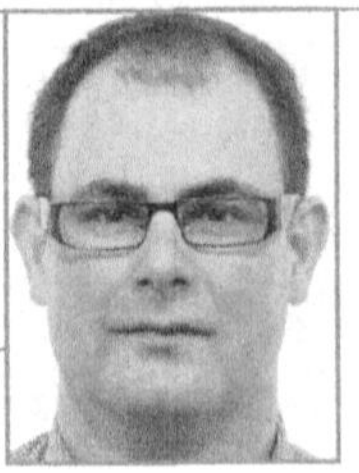

Waldén M

Division of Community Medicine, Department of Medical and Health Sciences, Linköping University, Linköping, Sweden

Introduction

It has previously been shown that the vast majority of Anterior Cruciate Ligament (ACL)-reconstructed male professional football players can return to the pitch within a year after surgery (1-3), but the continuous participation rate over time is unknown. Additionally, it is unclear whether re-rupture and further knee surgery in the final phase of the rehabilitation period or early after Return To Play (RTP) is a problem in this setting. The purpose of this study was therefore to evaluate knee complication rates before return to match play following ACL reconstruction and the influence of ACL injury on the subsequent playing career in male professional football players.

Methods

A total of 78 clubs with 4,443 male professional football players from the highest national leagues in 16 countries were followed over a varying number of seasons from January 2001 to May 2015. RTP was defined as the number of days from ACL reconstruction to full training with the team without restrictions (return to training) and to the first match appearance (return to match play). Players' club track records were followed for three years after RTP to evaluate the influence of the ACL injury on the short-term playing career.

Results

A total of 157 ACL injuries (140 total ruptures) in 149 players were recorded.
The majority of the total ruptures underwent ACL reconstruction (138/140; 98.6%).
RTP data were available for 134 players and all these returned to training (100%), 130 (97%) to the same playing level.
A majority of players were cleared for RTP within a year after surgery, 129 (96%) returned to training and 121 (90%) returned to match play.
The median lay-off times after ACL reconstruction were 202 days (6.6 months) to training and 225 days (7.4 months) to match play.
Five players (4%) re-ruptured their grafts during the rehabilitation or after return to training.
Four players (3%) had other knee surgery not related to the ACL during their rehabilitation or after return to training.
There were 3-year follow-up data available for 93 players: 81 players (87%) were still playing football 3 years after RTP, 60 (65%) at the same level.

Conclusions

All players who underwent ACL reconstruction for a total rupture returned to training, but the re-rupture rate and the rate of other knee surgery before return to match play were fairly high (7%).
The RTP rate within a year after ACL reconstruction was high (>90%), but only two-thirds played at the highest level 3 years later.

References

1. Erickson BJ, Harris JD, Cvetanovich GL, Bach BR, Bush-Joseph CA, Abrams GD, Gupta AK, Mccormick FM, Cole BJ. Performance and return to sport after anterior cruciate ligament reconstruction in male Major League Soccer players. Ort J Sports Med 2013: Jul 11; 1(2): 2325967113497189. doi: 10.1177/2325967113497189. eCollection 2013
2. Waldén M, Hägglund M, Magnusson H, Ekstrand J. Anterior cruciate ligament injury in elite fo-otball: a prospective three-cohort study. Knee Surg Sports Traumatol Arthrosc 2011; 19: 11-19
3. Zaffagnini S, Grassi A, Marcheggiani Muccioli GM, Tsapralis K, Ricci M, Bragonzoni L, Della Villa S, Marcacci M. Return to sport after anterior cruciate ligament reconstruction in professional soccer players. Knee 2014; 21: 731-735

RETURN TO PLAY AFTER ACLR: OUTCOME PREDICTORS ANALYSIS

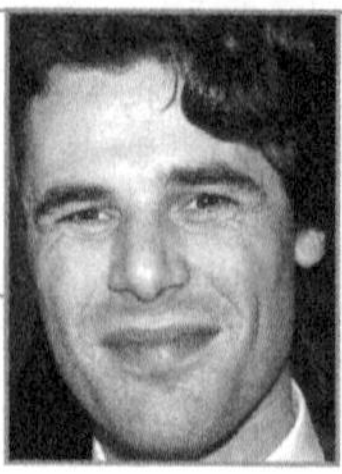

Della Villa F

Isokinetic Medical Group, FIFA Medical Centre of Excellence, Bologna, Italy

Anterior Cruciate Ligament Reconstruction (ACLR) and Return To Play (RTP) strategy after ACLR are probably one of the most discussed topics in the field of Sport Medicine and Orthopaedic rehabilitation. Safe and fast RTP and complete functional recovery, while avoiding re-injury, remain the key goals of the vast majority of the ACL injured athletes. Defining which pre-operative, surgical and post-operative care variables affect functional outcome and RTP rate of the patients may be helpful in targeting the recovery pathway (Spindler KP, Parker RD, Andrish JT, Kaeding CC, Wright RW, Marx RG, McCarty EC, Amendola A, Dunn WR, Huston LJ, Harrell FE Jr; MOON Group. Prognosis and predictors of ACL reconstructions using the MOON cohort: a model for comparative effectiveness studies. J Orthop Res 2013; 31: 2-9). In the recent years the growing interest in predictors and registry based research brought new evidence, supporting the fact that non-modifiable and moreover modifiable factors correlates with patients outcomes. Considering preoperative variables, young age, male gender, elite sport level and having a good psychological response have been demonstrated to correlate with a higher RTP rate (2, 3), while revision surgery and associated cartilage lesions correlates with worse results (1). Additionally to baseline variables, performance related factors were found to be correlated to RTP rate after ACLR (2), underlying the fact that a good post-surgery strategy may enhance a better result and that surgery and rehabilitation have to be considered parts of the same path. The importance of a comprehensive preoperative and post-operative rehabilitation program was highlighted from Grindem and colleagues, that reported better outcomes in an intensive rehabilitation cohort of patients if compared to the usual care (Grindem H, Granan LP, Risberg MA, Engebretsen L, Snyder-Mackler L, Eitzen I. How does a combined preoperative and postoperative rehabilitation programme influence the outcome of ACL reconstruction 2 years after surgery? A comparison between patients in the Delaware-Oslo ACL Cohort and the Norwegian National Knee Ligament Registry. Br J Sports Med 2015; 49: 385-389). Stating that we always need to respect the biological healing, it seems logical to think that, in order to RTP efficiently, the athlete have to achieve a complete functional recovery, defined also as the ability to perform during complex dynamic task. Defining and studying which features of the rehab protocol and which objective measurements correlate with better results may help to target the pre and post-surgical therapies in order to optimize outcomes of the patients and chances to RTP. We highlighted the importance of this approach building a rehabilitation based cohort after ACLR that we studied over a period of five years. The main purpose of our study was to look for possible independent predictors of functional outcomes and RTP following ACLR, in order to target the clinical strategy on patients features. Together with baseline variables, factors like recovery of muscle strength, patient compliance and other rehabilitation items could be analysed as possible predictors to improve patients outcome. Predictors research is a strong and growing reality in every field of medicine. In the Football Medicine Landscape ACL injury is well known to be potentially a career and life modifier injury for every athlete. The clinical application of what the current research tells us about predictors of RTP after ACLR may help the Sport Medicine team to target the recovery intervention and achieve better clinical results.

References

1. Andriolo L, Filardo G, Kon E, Ricci M, Della Villa F, Della Villa S, Zaffagnini S, Marcacci M. Revision anterior cruciate ligament reconstruction: clinical outcome and evidence for return to sport. Knee Surg Sports Traumatol Arthrosc 2015; 23: 2825-2845
2. Ardern CL, Taylor NF, Feller JA, Webster KE. Fifty-five per cent return to competitive sport following anterior cruciate ligament reconstruction surgery: an updated systematic review and meta analysis including aspects of physical functioning and contextual factors. Br J Sports Med 2014; 48: 1543-1552
3. Brophy RH, Schmitz L, Wright RW, Dunn WR, Parker RD, Andrish JT, McCarty EC, Spindler KP. Return to play and future ACL injury risk following ACL reconstruction in soccer athletes from the MOON group. Am J Sport Med 2012; 40: 2517-2522

5

PREVENTION AND MANAGMENT OF ANTERIOR CRUCIATE LIGAMENT RECONSTRCTION COMPLICATIONS

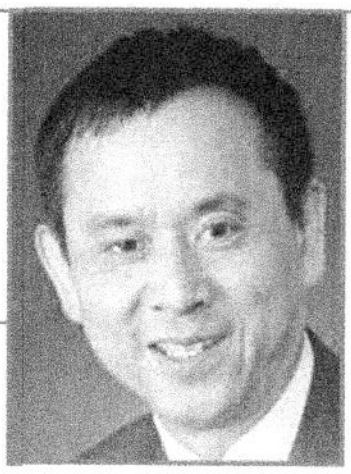

Fu FH

University of Pittsburgh, Department of Orthopaedic Surgery, Pittsburgh, USA

The goal of Anatomic Individualized Anterior Cruciate Ligament Reconstruction (ACL-R) is to achieve optimum results and early return to sports by respecting each patient's native knee anatomy.
The patient evaluation begins preoperatively, with a detailed history and physical examination.
The surgeon must consider a patient's age, type of activity, activity level, and cultural/personal preferences.
The evaluation continues intra-operatively when selecting the graft type (Bone-Patellar Tendon-Bone vs. Hamstring vs. Quadriceps Tendon) and tunnel drilling technique (Single Bundle vs. Double Bundle vs. One Bundle Augmentation vs. Over-the-Top).
Variation in anatomy is a major concern when performing an ACL-R, as the native insertion size and inter-condylar notch size are important parameters to consider when individualizing treatment.
An adequate rehabilitation protocol is equally important to decrease re-tears rates, with particular attention paid to the graft healing timeline so that the new graft is best able to tolerate the higher in situ forces experienced by anatomic reconstructions.
When an ACL-R fails, the surgeon must consider the cause of failure, avoiding mistakes that may have been made during the initial reconstruction.
3D Computed Tomography is invaluable here, allowing analysis of tunnel position and enlargement, both of which provide information about potential cause of ACL-R failure.
Graft and notch size mismatch is another common cause for ACL-R failure, predisposing to both limited range of motion and graft re-tear.

Saturday 9th April, 2016 (afternoon)
CHURCHILL AUDITORIUM

INVITED SPEAKERS

HOW TO MANAGE RETURN TO PLAY FOR HIP AND GROIN INJURIES

Chairs

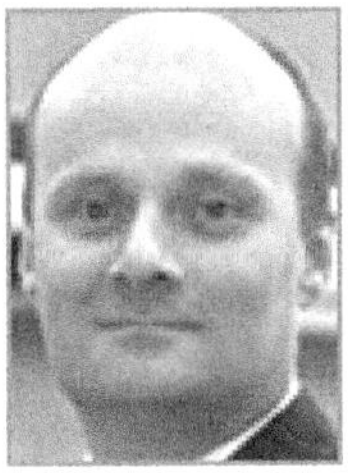

Damian Griffin
(Warwick, United Kingdom)

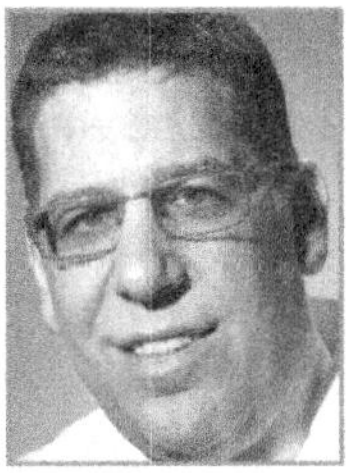

Ken Zaslav
(Richmond, USA)

14:30 Return to play in adductor-related groin pain
Peter Brukner (Melbourne, Australia)

14:45 Prevention of recurrence of adductor related groin pain
Adam Weir (Overveen, The Nederlands)

15:00 Return to play after groin surgery
Steve Kemp (St. George's Park, United Kingdom)

15:15 Return to play after adductor longus avulsion
Ernest Schilders (London, United Kingdom)

15:30 Return to play following hip arthroscopy
Per Holmich (Copenhagen, Denmark)

15:45 Discussion

16:00 End of the session

RETURN TO PLAY IN ADDUCTOR-RELATED GROIN PAIN

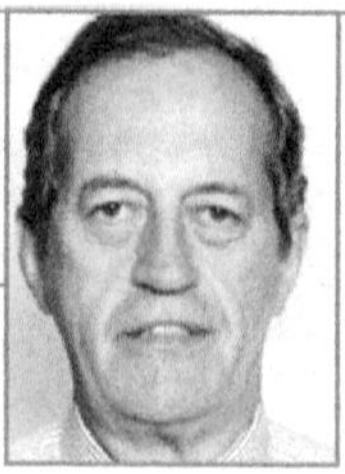

Brukner P

La Trobe University, Melbourne, Australia

A number of factors need to be considered when deciding on Return To Play (RTP) following an adductor-related groin injury.

These factors will are:

1. Ensuring adequate appropriate rehabilitation program.
2. Clinical assessment: Range of Motion, strength, pain-free.
3. Passive Range of Motions (PROMs), e.g. the Copenhagen Hip and Groin Outcome Score (HAGOS) are they relevant to the athlete.
4. Strength testing: hand held dynamometers, isokinetic adduction, abduction, hip flexion, groin squeeze.
5. Functional activities: cutting manoeuvres, zig zag running, high speed running (also monitored with Global Positioning Systems).
6. Completing full training at maximal intensity.
7. Workload acute/chronic: have they done enough to avoid a "spike".

The resultant decision about RTP takes into account some or all of these factors.

PREVENTION OF RECURRENCE OF ADDUCTOR-RELATED GROIN PAIN

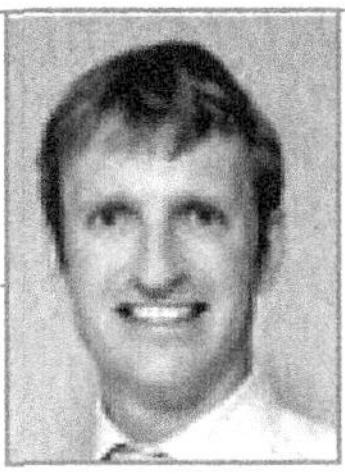

Weir A

Aspetar Orthopaedics and Sports Medical Hospital,
FIFA Medical Centre of Excellence, Doha, Qatar and Academic Medical Centre Amsterdam,
Centre for Evidenced Based Sports Medicine (ACES), Amsterdam, Nederland

Introduction

Adductor-related groin pain is the most common cause of groin pain in those participating in sports. It can be seen as in isolated entity and also commonly combined with other entities. There are two high quality randomised controlled clinical trials that have studied the possible treatment options (1, 3). A recent systematic review that included both these studies concluded that there is moderate evidence that active exercises are more effective than passive treatment modalities in improving the success of treatment and that multimodal treatment with manual therapy may shorten the time to return to play (2). Both of the randomised studies have also performed longer-term follow up studies of the cohorts included. The longer-term outcomes can be used in assisting clinical decision making regarding recurrence.

Methods

The randomised trial of Weir et al (3) included 54 athletes with long standing Adductor-Related Groin Pain (ARGP). They were randomised to either Mutli-Modal Treatment (MMT) with a forceful adductor manipulation and heat application followed by a stretching program and then a graded return to running and return to play program or Active Physical Therapy (AT).
The active physical therapy program comprised of an exercise program that was performed three times a week for a minimal of six weeks followed by a return to running program. They received instructions on the program on three occasions and the rest was performed without supervision at home.

Results

Three athletes in each group stopped during the study. 50% (13/26) for athletes in the MMT group had a full RTP in an average of 12.8±6.0 (SD) weeks and 55% in the AT group returned to full sports participation in 17.3±4.4 weeks.
The landmark study of Holmich et al. (1) randomised 68 athletes to either AT of Passive Treatment (PT) with Laser, massage, stretches and TENS. The AT group used the same program but was done in groups of 2-4 athletes under the supervision of a physiotherapist. 59 athletes completed the study. 79% in the AT group had RTP without pain in 18.5 weeks compared to 12% in the PT group.
Follow up of the cohort treated in the RCT by Weir et al. (3) after a mean time of 29 months examined the number of recurrences leading to time loss from sport. The rate of recurrence was 30% for the entire cohort and 22% in the MMT group and 36% in the AT group (difference not statistically significant).
Follow up 8-12 years of the RCT of Homich et al. (1) showed that there was no difference in activity level between the groups. There was a significant difference in the number of athletes reporting a good or excellent outcome (88% AT vs 78% PT) at this time. There was no reporting on recurrences as such over the follow up period or use of treatments after completion of the original study.

Conclusion

Current evidence supports that there is a real risk of recurrence in athletes after completing treatment for AGRP.
The traditional paradigm of injured vs. non-injured is an oversimplification of complex long-standing injuries and not useful in practice or research.
Continued active physical training, good education on expectations and attention to load monitoring with early intervention seem sensible options to consider to keep athletes on the field after Return To Play (RTP).

References

1. Hölmich P, Uhrskou P, Ulnits L, Kanstrup I-L, Nielsen MB, Bjerg AM, Krogsgaard K. Effectiveness of active physical training as treatment for long-standing adductor-related groin pain in athletes: randomised trial. Lancet 1999; 353 (9151): 439–443
2. Serner A, van Eijck CH, Beumer BR, Holmich P, Weir A, de Vos R-J. Study quality on groin injury management remains low: a systematic review on treatment of groin pain in athletes. Br J Sports Med 2015; 49 (12): 813. doi: 10.1136/bjsports-2014-094256. Epub 2015 Jan 29
3. Weir A, Jansen JACG, van de Port IGL, Van de Sande HBA, Tol JL, Backx FJG. Manual or exercise therapy for long-standing adductor-related groin pain: a randomised controlled clinical trial. Man Ther 2011; 16: 148-154

RETURN TO PLAY AFTER GROIN SURGERY

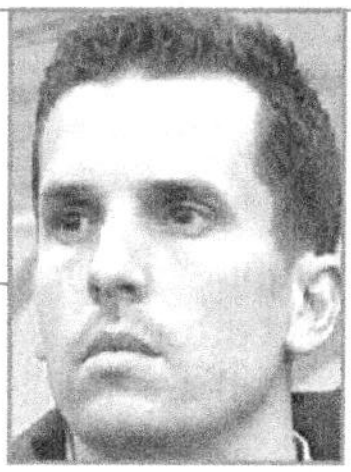

Kemp S

Perform Centre, St. Georges Park and St. Georges Park Senior Men's team, St. Georges Park, United Kingdom

Introduction

The Return To Play (RTP) considerations after groin surgery appear to lack structured clinical guidelines with limited levels of published evidence available. Currently, the majority of decisions on RTP appear to be based upon expert opinion and clinical experience rather than the evidence base. This was supported in a recent systematic literature review of 9 medical databases on the treatment of groin pain in athletes which included 72 studies, of which only 4 were deemed of high quality (1). The lack of high quality research is likely to be compounded by the complex nature of groin injuries which occur in numerous anatomical structures. The review paper also found that in the 72 studies 33 different diagnoses were used to describe the groin pain presented by the athletes. Such heterogeneous taxonomy has ultimately led to those using general temporal RTP prognoses to be inaccurate and often detrimental in the rehabilitation process, rather than taking into consideration all factors of this often multi factorial condition
To address these complexities, the Doha consensus statement (2) brought together 24 experts in the field of groin pain to agree on a classification system for groin pain in athletes. Now consensus for the clinical entities has been made it may now make return to play criteria for groin surgery be specific within its classification according to the Doha statement.
Whilst the consensus statement should be applauded in its attempt to clarify the terminology, it must also be recognized that it is merely one of the first steps on the journey to further develop the evidence base on groin pain and attempt to improve the lack of evidence highlighted in recent systematic reviews. Ultimately we should be looking to have valid and reliable objective outcomes for RTP criteria for all types of groin pain patients.
The purpose of this presentation is to provide a review of clinical practices used in a rehabilitation centre for elite athletes. It will highlight the return to play criteria used for football player's presenting groin pain.

Methods

A review of all clinical assessments used by clinicians at the Perform rehabilitation Centre is currently being carried out by the physiotherapy team. The aim is to standardize the way in which all groin injuries are assessed by all clinicians to ensure that they cover all aspects of rehabilitation (mobility, motor control, strength, work capacity). This will allow reliable and repeatable objective markers that could aid progressive rehabilitation and ultimately improve the RTP criteria following groin surgery.
The selection of clinical assessments has been based on the available evidence base, clinical experiences and discussions with experts in numerous sports. Once consensus has been gained on the assessments used, a literature search for each test will be carried out to look at the inter and intra tester reliability of each test, and where reliable tests are not available, offer alternative assessments which will require validation and reliability studies if they are to become part of the clinical assessment battery.

Conclusions

On initial review of literature, it would seem that the objective assessments in the RTP of groin injuries offer poor inter and intra rater reliability due to the lack of consensus in testing protocols. A battery of tests currently used for groin pain patients in an elite athlete rehabilitation centre can aid the rehabilitation process by using criterion based rehabilitation parameters. Once the clinical assessments can be shown to be repeatable and valid to the groin pain patient, the next step is to look to publish such tests to add to the evidence base and improve the RTP criteria for groin surgery patients using objective criterion based parameters.

References

1. Serner A, Van Eijck CH, Beumer BR, Hölmich P, Weir A, De Vos RJ. Study quality on groin injury management remains low: a systematic review on treatment of groin pain in athletes. Br J Sports Med 2015; 49(12): 813 http://doi.org/10.1136/bjsports-2014-094256
2. Weir A, Brukner P, Delahunt E, Ekstrand J, Griffin D, Khan KM, Lovell G, Meyers WC, Muschaweck U, Orchard J, Paajanen H, Philippon M, Reboul G, Robinson P, Schache AG, Schilders E, Serner A, Silvers H, Thorborg K, Tyler T, Verrall G, de Vos RJ, Vuckovic Z, Hölmich P. Doha agreement meeting on terminology and definitions in groin pain in athletes. Br J Sports Med 2015; 49: 768-774

RETURN TO FOOTBALL AFTER ADDUCTOR AVULSION

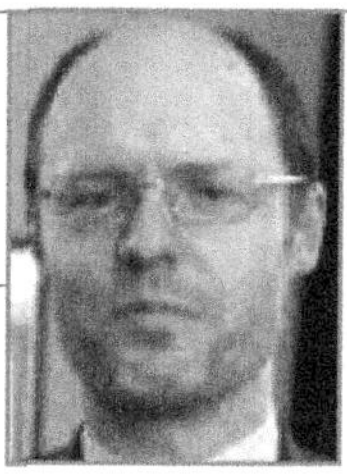

Schilders E

Fortius Clinic, London; Leeds Beckett University, Leeds, United Kingdom

Adductor Longus avulsion are significant injuries. Radiografically we can identify two groups: partial and complete avulsions. Complete avulsions are usually easy to diagnose; the players sustain an injury and experience sharp adductor related groin pain and are not able to continue.
The clinical presentation of a partial avulsions can be less obvious. The player can have a similar mechanism of injury as with complete avulsion but often the player can continue. The players with partial avulsions then follow a typical clinical pattern; following rehabilitation they can get to about 85-90% of their performance but not any higher. Pain restricts them with activities such as full sprint and striking long balls. This kind of scenario can easily continue for several months when the underlying partial avulsion is not picked up. Using the correct Magnetic Resonance Imaging (MRI) protocol is very important in order to pick up partial avulsions, which often go undiagnosed.
For both types the use of steroids is contraindicated: for athletes case of partial avulsions it increases the risk for further progress of the avulsion and a complete avulsion.
Chronic partial avulsions are treated with a partial release and players are able to return to competitive football between four to six weeks.
There is still controversy about treatment of complete displaced avulsions of the Adductor Longus. Steroid injections are contraindicated because it puts your athlete at risk for wound problems if it is decided to follow the surgical route.
Our recent cadaver study demonstrated the presence of the Pyramidalis-Aadductor Longus- Anterior Pubic Ligament complex.
It is more likely that the athlete has a severe injury when he also complains about lower abdominal pain. A hematoma can be seen over the pubic area and lower abdomen but never crosses the midline.
The literature reports good outcomes both with conservative and surgical reconstructions. In our experience in over 100 cases with partial and full avulsions, we found that 30% of the athletes with a complete avulsion had previously failed conservative management.
The return to football after a surgical reconstruction of the Pyramidalis-Aadductor Longus- Anterior Pubic Ligament complex is 12-14 weeks but some of the athletes returned to football as early as eight weeks postoperatively.
F-MARC center Fortius clinic is starting up a F-MARC endorsed study on acute Adductor Longus avulsions. Participants of other F-MARC centers and football teams will be able to login in a registry. Clinician will be explained how to perform clinical examination. MRI scans done following a specific protocol can be uploaded. All data will collected in a standardised way and will be anonymised. The participants will be given feedback about the injury. Participants will be notified if the injury is not a proximal adductor avulsion.

5

RETURN TOPLAY FOLLOWING HIP ARTHROSCOPY

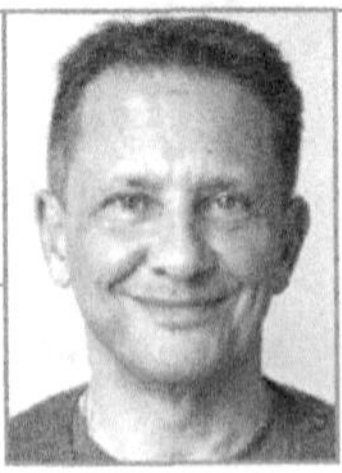

Holmich P

Amager Hospital, Copenhagen, Denmark

Introduction

Groin and hip injuries is a major problem especially in football and the other kicking sports. One of the main risk factors for groin injuries is previous injury. One reason for this could be that the Return To Play (RTP) is not managed sufficiently qualified. This can be caused by a number of factors like a wish for quick return from the club and/or the player. The damaged tissue needs time to heal and the general conditioning, strength and endurance should be re-established.

Methods

Evaluating if the player is ready for return to play during training and training matches is probably not in itself sufficient as epidemiological studies show that the risk of injury is several times higher during match than during training. With a scientific analysis of risk factors a number of parameters can be identified that are modifiable. These factors include strength of specific muscle groups, and the balance between the muscles on all sides of the joint. Range of motion of the hip joint could also be an important factor, however, it is not always easily modifiable as some it might be caused by cam and pincer deformities only modifiable by surgery.
In general the influence of the bony morphology of the hip joint is an interesting subject for ongoing and future research. Also the correlation of these bony changes to the soft tissue injuries that constitute the majority of hip and groin injuries in sport.
When training muscle strength it has in recent years been shown that there is a possibility to modify the structural changes that comes with increasing age and this might be a phenomenon that could be an important feature in future treatment and prevention of groin injuries. The ideal balance between the strength of the adductor muscle group and of the abductor muscle group is probably also a very crucial tool and we have some interesting research data to support this for future studies.
Monitoring the players during the season looking for warning signs of an upcoming groin or hip injury is also a possibility. Should the strength be used? And what types of measurement? Or should provocation tests looking for early signs of tenderness or pain be developed? Or maybe if the range of motion decreases?
The treatment and rehabilitation programmes used for treating groin and hip injuries are of cause essential to return the player free of injury and ready for play. However, the evidence for the ideal treatment is not available in many instances.

Conclusion

Return to play after groin and hip injuries is a complex problem.

Saturday 9th April, 2016 (afternoon)
PICKWICK ROOM

FREE ORAL PRESENTATIONS

REHABILITATION AND RETURN TO PLAY

Chairs

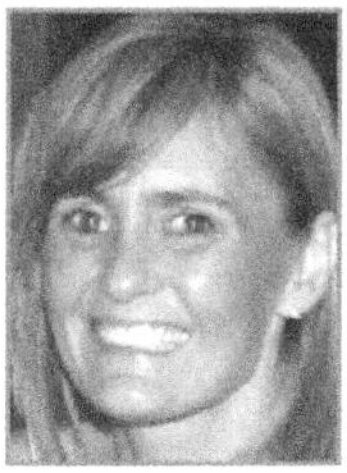

Diana Bianchedi
(Rome, Italy)

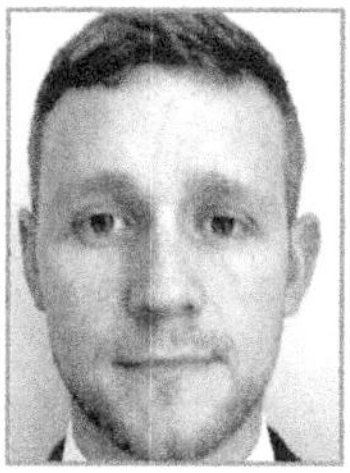

Christopher Jones
(London, United Kingdom)

14:30 Rehabilitation following ACL reconstruction in football players: an individualistic approach towards progressive results
Hoogendyk DJH (Los Angeles, USA)

14:40 The speedcourt system in rehabilitation after anterior cruciate ligament surgery **Fieseler G, Proeger S, Brehme K, Pyschik M, Schulze S, Delank KS, Schwesig R, Bartels T (Wuppertal and Halle, Germany)**

14:50 Return to sports training benefits self-reported knee function after anterior cruciate ligament reconstruction
Arundale A, Snyder-Mackler L (Newark, USA)

15:00 Return-to-competition after anterior cruciate ligament reconstruction: a multifaceted approach
Bloch H, Riepenhof H, Krutsch W (Hamburg and Regensburg, Germany; Rome, Italy)

15:10	Patella luxation in an adolescent soccer player **Herfert J, Bernecker R, Landkammer Y, Klampfer H, Wicker A (Salzburg, Austria)**
15:20	A rehabilitation protocol for conservatively and surgically managed ankle syndesmosis injuries **Urwin J, Broman D, Calder J, Rosenfeld P, Rolls A (London, United Kingdom)**
15:30	Two pictures, one result: return to play **Zahar M, Zerguini Y (La Marsa, Tunisia; Algier, Algery)**
15:40	Discussion
16:00	End of the session

REHABILITATION FOLLOWING ACL RECONSTRUCTION IN FOOTBALL PLAYERS: AN INDIVIDUALISTIC APPROACH TOWARDS PROGRESSIVE RESULTS

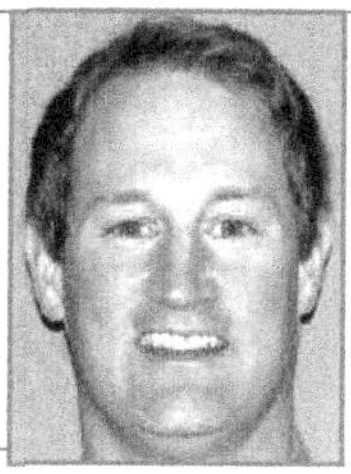

Hoogendyk DJH

SMART Performance Labs, Los Angeles, USA

Introduction

There is a correlation between traumatic injury involving the knee, specifically the Anterior Cruciate Ligament (ACL), faulty movement patterns, dysfunctional biomechanics, and neuro-musculature control in athletics, which involve cutting, jumping, and deceleration (1, 3). These movements are performed by football players at every level, and provide potential for injury to the knee. Those at risk are adolescent players, especially girls (3). If these patterns of movement dysfunction are not correctly addressed, the football player is susceptible to injury, re-injury and progression of a chronic injury state (1, 2).

The aim of this presentation is to show an on-patient tailored sport specific rehabilitation protocol after ACL reconstruction, with a particular focus on early development of neuromuscular pathway efficiency, biomechanical markers, movement pattern restoration, objective strength test ratios and qualitative testing parameters for Return To Sport (RTS).

Our protocol is based on establishing early, sport specific, rehabilitation biomechanical markers that culminate with a qualitative and quantitative return to football testing matrix at 4-6 months time, enabling the player to return to non-contact sports participation at 6-7 months and full football participation at 8-9 months time.

Case Report

We present the case of a 17 year old USA Olympic team female football player. She reported a non-contact ACL injury during competition. The Magnetic Resonance Imaging (MRI) confirmed the diagnosis of isolated left knee ACL injury. ACL-Reconstruction (ACLR) with Bone Patellar Tendon Bone (BPTB) autograph was performed after a three-week pre-rehabilitation programme, with the aim to reduce knee effusion and flogosis, restore Range Of Motion and strength of the involved limb. After surgery the patient immediately undertook rehabilitation, following the seven phases reported in table 1.

Phase	Time range	Program
1	Weeks 0-2	Normalizations of systems (ROM and pain) and avoid quadriceps atrophy
2	Weeks 3 to 7	Initiate DL strengthening, normalized gait, step up 8", hip strategy in frontal and sagittal planes, initiate trunk and pelvic stabilization
3	Months 2 to 3.75	Progress DL strengthening, initiate SL strengthening, progress forward step down 8", progressional running mechanics, DL hop and stick drills, advanced proprioception drills.
4	Months 4 to 5.75	Level 1 testing matrix (Table 2)
5	Months 6 to 7.25	RTS Testing matrix (table 3)
6	Months 7.5 to 9	Non-contact practice participation, sport specific drills with equipment, dissociation drills
7	Months 9 +	Sport drills performed 95%, single leg jumps performed 95%, triple jumps performed 95%, medical team consensus on return to play

Table 1. Program of the post-operative rehabilitation phases.

Four months after surgery the athlete undertook the Level 1 testing matrix. The testing matrix (Table 2) comprehend: 1) knee and hip muscles strength assessment, 2) movement patterns assessment. The strength assessment consisted of a isometric BTE Primus RS (BTE Technologies, Hanover, USA) knee extensor, hip extensor and hip abductor strength. Data are reported in Nm/kg and referred to reference values. Knee extensor strength is compared to the contralateral knee. The movements assessment consist in the evaluation of six functional movements (step down, drop down, lateral landing, deceleration, triple hop test and cut maneuver) that are evaluated through semi-objective criteria using a motion analysis software 2D/3D (Simi Reality Motion Systems GmbH, Unterschleissheim, Germany) and culminate in a score (0-50) based on patient movement. A score of 45/50 is considered as the threshold of low risk of re-injury. Each of the aforementioned movements is analyzed and graded to obtain the mentioned scoring criteria. Factors such as hip stability, hip strategy, shock absorption, and trunk stability are graded (0 poor, 1 moderate, 2 Excellent) in the frontal and sagittal plane during each of the movements and the score is tabulated.

Strength parameters	**Result**	**Reference**	**Deficit**
Knee extensor (Nm/kg)	2.10	1.92 (contralateral)	+8%
Hip extensor (Nm/kg)	1.91	2.35±0.38	-19%
Hip abduction (Nm/kg)	1.37	1.62±0.26	-15%
Ratio hip extension/knee extension	0.91	1.00	--
Movement parameters	**Result**	**Reference (1st level)**	**Observation**
Movement pattern score	18	20	High risk

Table 2. Level 1 testing matrix.

After the test the athlete undertook rehabilitation sessions to abolish the -19% and -15% hip extensor and abductor strength deficit with double limb and single limb exercise, progress dynamic balance tasks, progress movement training to incorporate single leg jumps and cutting mechanics. At six months after surgery the athlete undertook a repetition of the test to assess patient readiness to return to non-contact activity.

Strength parameters	Result	Reference	Deficit
Knee extensor (Nm/kg)	2.10	1.92 (contralateral)	0%
Hip extensor (Nm/kg)	2.35	2.35±0.38	0%
Hip abduction (Nm/kg)	1.47	1.62±0.26	-9%
Ratio hip extension/knee extension	1.10	1.00	--
Movement parameters	**Result**	**Reference (1st level)**	**Observation**
Movement pattern score (0-50)	47	50	Low risk of re-injury

Table 3. Return to Sport testing matrix.

The second test identified excellent movements pattern restoration but a mild deficit of hip abductors strength (-9%). The patient was anyway allowed to progress in the rehabilitation path to on field drills (Phase 6). Strength deficit was subsequently tested and no deficit was reported.
After completing the last phases of recovery, she was able to return to full football participation eight months after surgery. After meeting all the criteria: 1) Strength, 2) Movement, 3) Activation, 4) Balance and Running. She is currently playing at the same pre-injury level.

Conclusion

An individualistic approach to ACLR rehabilitation, based on hip and knee strength parameters and movement pattern restoration may be effective in allowing RTS and controlling the re-injury phenomena.

References

1. Meyer G, Ford K, Palumbo J, Hewett T. Neuromuscular training improves performance and lower-extremity biomechanics in female athletes. J Strength Cond Res 2005; 19: 51-60
2. Meyer G, Sugimoto D, Thomas S, Hewett TE. The influence of age on the effectiveness of neuromuscular training to reduce anterior cruciate ligament injury in female athletes. Am J Sports Med 2013; 41: 203-215
3. Hewett T, Myer G, Ford K. Biomechanical measures of neuromuscular control and valgus loading of the knee predict anterior cruciate ligament injury risk in female athletes. Am J Sports Med 2005; 33: 492-501

THE SPEEDCOURT SYSTEM IN REHABILITATION AFTER ANTERIOR CRUCIATE LIGAMENT SURGERY

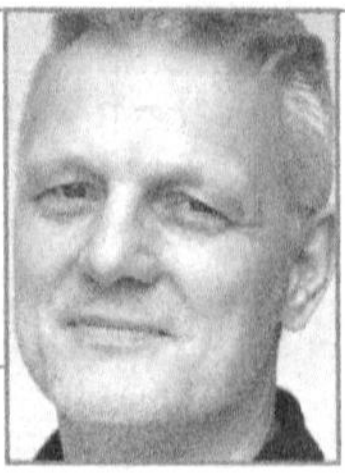

Fieseler G[1], Proeger S[2], Brehme K[2], Pyschik M[2], Schulze S[2], Delank KS[3], Schwesig R[3], Bartels T[2]

[1]OGAM Center for Orthopedics and Sports Medicine, Wuppertal; [2]SportsClinic Halle, Halle (Saale); [3]Department of Orthopedic and Trauma Surgery, Martin-Luther University Halle-Wittenberg, Halle (Saale), Germany

Introduction

Deficits in postural functions are known as predictors for successive injuries on the same Anterior Cruciate Ligament (ACL) and other impairments or injuries at the lower extremities (1). Therefore, athletes with a mechanically stable knee joints after ACL-reconstruction suffer on a high risk of ligament re-injuries for about 0-19% for the ipsilateral joint or 7-24% for the contralateral, primary uninjured knee joint (1). In addition, the time after surgery should not be the exclusive and single criterion to decide if the athlete is able to return to specific sports activities, even at the previous level (2).

It is first described experimentally, that delayed muscle reactions above 100 milliseconds (ms) as Long Latency Response (LLR) initiated after postural balance impulse were contributed to cortico-spinal control. So far, unconscious damage control happens in dimensions around 50 ms as Early Latency Response (ELR). Rehabilitation programs usually work with reaction times above 350 ms, so patients and athletes might adapt to slow motion responses for physical stress or disturbances. The ability to answer critical situations with fast and direct functional mechanism is reduced (3). Therefore, training with responses below 200 ms after stimulus seems to be more useful and advantageous. So far, Teichmann et al. evaluated significant improvements in the single-leg press, stand jump, 20 m sprint and single-leg balance test in professional athletes after ACL-reconstruction surgery with a training and exposure of unexpected disturbances, which causes muscular reactions below 200 ms of time latency. The percentage of numbers of return to sport increased and the ratio of re-injuries was reduced in this group of elite athletes (3).

The purpose of our study was to evaluate and find advantages of a programme with Unexpected Disturbances (UDP) (response time beyond 200 ms) in the late rehabilitation (5 months) after ACL-surgery compared to current sensomotoric based concepts.

Methods

Fifty athletic patients (14 female, 35 male; age: 32.7±10.0 years) were randomized and followed either a new training with the SpeedCourt (GlobalSpeed GmbH, Hemsbach, Germany) (28 athletes) or underwent a regular stabilisation programme (22 athletes; control group).

Training with the SpeedCourt consisted 5-6 exercises for about 15 to 30 seconds and three repetitions each. Practice included sprints, which were generated incidentally for directions and speed, different colours were used and attached with tasks.

Regular rehabilitation training (time: 30 minutes) was performed with different unstable grounds (i.e. Posturomed, Slashpipe, BOSU), 30 seconds for each exercise and 3 repeats. After a short break for 15 seconds the contralateral leg was exposed to the same setting.

A workout for strength was followed after every single training session.

Subjects were assessed at baseline and after three weeks, i.e. six sessions in total. The comparison of evaluations (pre- and post-training) was calculated with a two-factorial (time, group) univariate analysis with parameters for flexibility, reaction time, tapping, jump force (uni- and bilateral) and anthropometry.
For anthropometry, the comprehensive of the upper leg, knee and lower leg were measured, by metric tape 15 and 10 cm above, at, 15 and 10 cm below joint line.
The sports performance tests included: i) total range of motion in flexion and extension (tROM); ii) finger-ground distance; iii) ground reaction time; iv) time of contact; v) tapping; vi) jump height (uni- and bilateral); vii) jump width (bilateral).
Extension range of motion of the knee joint was measured in supine, flexion range of motion was assessed in abdomen down position. The finger-ground distance was evaluated with the athlete positioned upright on a step, straight leg and maximum flexion in the hip joint.
Ground reaction time, time of contact, tapping, uni-/bilateral jump height and width were determined with the SpeedCourt.

Results

Results are shown in table 1.

	SpeedCourt Group		Control Group	
	Pre Training	Post Training	Pre Training	Post Training
Knee joint without Surgery (m)	0.382±0.018	0.379±0.016	0.356±0.014	0.368±0.009
Knee joint with Surgery (m)	0.385±0.027	0.386±0.025	0.365±0.005	0.370±0.008
10 cm below joint Line, without Surgery (m)	0.385±0.031	0.386±0.033	0.363±0.015	0.362±0.014
10 cm below joint Line, with Surgery (m)	0.376±0.032	0.379±0.031	0.353±0.014	0.358±0.011
10 cm above joint line, without Surgery (m)	0.456±0.027	0.460±0.025	0.429±0.054	0.432±0.055
10 cm above joint line, with Surgery (m)	0.443±0.026	0.445±0.025	0.414±0.050	0.417±0.049
15 cm above joint line, without Surgery (m)	0.498±0.028	0.504±0.024	0.470±0.063	0.477±0.065
15 cm above joint line, with Surgery (m)	0.487±0.026	0.494±0.023	0.452±0.060	0.458±0.059
15 cm below joint line, without Surgery (m)	0.392±0.032	0.394±0.032	0.373±0.015	0.371±0.020
15 cm below joint line, with Surgery (m)	0.403±0.033	0.404±0.036	0.387±0.017	0.383±0.017
Jump height bilateral (cm)	24.5±6.80	25.7±7.00	27.5±6.40	27.7±6.70
Jump height unilateral without Surgery (cm)	15.5±4.70	17.5±5.10	15.1±3.20	17.4±4.90
Jump height unilateral with Surgery (cm)	11.0±5.3	13.8±5.2	12.2±2.9	13.4±4.0
Jump width bilateral (m)	1.38±0.29	1.46±0.25	1.49±0.21	1.57±0.25
Tapping (n/3 s)	32.0±2.8	34.0±2.4	32.0±2.4	31.6±5.9
Time of contact without Surgery (s)	0.37±0.12	0.30±0.11	0.44±0.04	0.37±0.086
Time of contact with Surgery (s)	0.33±0.08	0.29±0.09	0.37±0.09	0.33±0.08
Ground reaction tim without Surgery (s)	1.43±0.35	1.27±0.29	1.37±0.12	1.26±0.13
Ground reaction tim with Surgery (s)	1.38±0.33	1.26±0.31	1.38±0.11	1.33±0.08
Finger-ground distance (cm)	-2.5±8.9	-4.8±10.5	3.3±13.0	-0.6±10.9
Extension ROM knee joint without Surgery (°)	-0.3±1.1	-0.3±0.8	-1.1±1.9	-1.1±1.9
Extension ROM knee joint with Surgery (°)	1.0±1.6	0.3±1.1	0.0±0.0	0.0±0.0
Flexion ROM knee joint without Surgery (°)	127.8±7.8	127.0±7.8	128.7±6.3	128.6±9.2
Flexion ROM knee joint with Surgery (°)	124.8±8.0	127.5±8.9	126.1±5.8	127.9±6.7

Table 1. Mean±SD of anthropometry values of lower leg (with and without surgery) measured at different levels, and Mean±SD results of the functional assessment tests performed before and after training in both groups.

In between the two groups 7 out of 24 parameters (29%) showed significant influences, i.e. highest in the comprehensive of the non-surgical knee joint (η^2=0.694) and the surgical knee joint (η^2=0.229). Lower leg dimensions measured 10 and 15 cm below joint line were different (η^2=0.183; η2=0.200) significantly at the non-operated side.
Jump height unilateral (η^2=0.148) and reaction time (η^2=0.138) was improved on the operated leg. Differences in the outcome parameters like tapping, jump height and ground reaction time between the surgical and non-surgical knee were remarkably reduced in the SpeedCourt intervention group.

Conclusions

Interventional training programs with the SpeedCourt system seem to be advantageous in the late rehabilitation following ACL-knee surgery compared to current senso-motoric based concepts. We achieved improvements of anthropometric and functional parameters. Further studies with larger groups and longer periods of evaluation are necessary to support this data and to possibly establish a new innovative rehabilitation concept. Clinically, the demonstrated SpeedCourt system might help to determine the return to sports time for athletes more objectively and prospectively reduce the rate of ACL re-injuries.

References

1. Fulton J, Wright K, Kelly M, Zebrosky B, Zanis M, Drvol C, Butler R. Injury risk is altered by previous injury: a systematic review of the literature and presentation of causative neuromuscular factors. Int J Sports Phys Ther 2014; 9: 583-595
2. Petersen W, Taheri P, Forkel P, Zantop T. Return to play following ACL reconstruction: a systematic review about strength deficits. Arch Orthop Trauma Surg 2014; 134: 1417-1428
3. Teichmann J, Suwarganda EK, Lendewig C, Wilson BD, Yeo WK, Aziz RA, Schmidtbleicher D. Unexpected disturbance program for rehabilitation of high performance athletes. J Sport Rehabil 2015; Feb 6. [Epub ahead of print]

RETURN TO SPORTS TRAINING BENEFITS SELF-REPORTED KNEE FUNCTION AFTER ACL RECONSTRUCTION

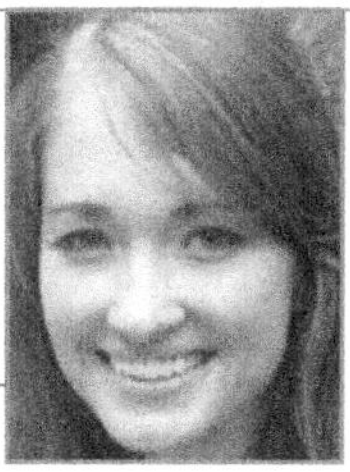

Arundale A, Snyder-Mackler L

The University of Delaware, Newark, USA

Introduction

There are many clinical commentaries on the terminal phases of rehabilitation after Anterior Cruciate Ligament (ACL) reconstruction, however there is very little research beyond expert opinion on specific interventions or programs. The purpose of this study was to examine if one year after ACL reconstruction athletes who undergo a specialized return to sports program (3) have higher self-reported knee function, participate more frequently in cutting/pivoting activity, are more likely to pass return to sports criteria (a proxy measure of function), and return to their pre-injury level of activity.

Methods

Forty three amateur soccer players (all positions) participated in this study (Table 1).
Eighteen athletes completed a specialized return to sports program (3) in the terminal phases of their rehabilitation after primary ACL reconstruction (Training group).
Twenty five athletes participated as a Control group, with no standardized return to sports rehabilitation.

Strength parameters	Training Group	Control Group
Age (yrs)	21.8±5.9	22.3±5.6
Sex	9 men and 9 women	19 men and 6 women
Height (m)	1.7±0.1	1.8 ±0.1
Weight (kg)	73.3±11.7	76.1±15.6

Table 1. Demographics and Anthropometrics

One year after primary ACL reconstruction, all athletes underwent quadriceps strength (Kincom, Chattanooga, TN, USA) and single-legged hop testing (single, cross-over, and triple hop for distance and the six meter timed hop) (2), and filled out the Knee Outcomes Survey-Activities of Daily Living (KOS), Global Ratings of Perceived Knee Function (GR), International Knee Documentation Committee 2000 Subjective Knee Form (IKDC), and Marx Activity Rating Scale (Marx).
Athletes also noted if they had returned to their pre-injury level of activity. The University of Delaware return to sports criteria were used as a proxy measure of function. According to these objective criteria, a passing score required ≥90% quadriceps strength limb symmetry, ≥90% limb symmetry on all four single-legged hop tests, and a score of ≥90% on the KOS and GR.
One athlete in the Training group did not participate in quadriceps strength or single-legged hop testing due to moving away, however they did complete the self-report measures.
Independent t-tests were used to determine if there were differences between groups in IKDC and Marx scores. Chi-squared tests were used to determine if there were differences between groups in the number of athletes who passed return to sport criteria and the number who returned to their pre-injury level of sport. Alpha was set a priori at $p<0.05$.

Results

There was a significant difference between groups in IKDC score ($p<0.01$), with the Training group having higher IKDC scores (97.9±3.3%) than the Control group (93.0±3.9%).
There was no significant difference in Marx score ($p=0.60$) between groups.
There was no significant difference between groups in the number of athletes who passed the return to sport criteria ($p=0.16$), or in the number of athletes who returned to their pre-injury level of activity (0.36) (Table 2).

	Training Group	Control Group
Returned to Pre-injury Level of Activity	14 (77%)	15 (60%)
Did not return to pre-injury Level of activity	4 (23%)	10 (40%)

Conclusions

This study indicates that specialized return to sport training (3) may be beneficial for athletes returning to soccer after ACL reconstruction. One year after primary ACL reconstruction those who received training had higher self-reported knee function and while there was no significant difference between groups in the number of athletes who returned to their pre-injury level of activity, 77% of those who received training returned to their pre-injury level of activity compared to 60% in the control group, and 65% among all athletes according to a recent meta-analysis (1).

References

1. Ardern CL, Taylor NF, Feller JA, Webster KE. Fifty-five per cent return to competitive sport following anterior cruciate ligament reconstruction surgery: an updated systematic review and meta-analysis including aspects of physical functioning and contextual factors. Br J Sports Med 2014; 48: 1543-1552
2. Noyes FR, Barber SD, Mangine RE. Abnormal lower limb symmetry determined by function hop tests after anterior cruciate ligament rupture. Am J Sports Med 1991; 19: 513-518
3. White K, Di Stasi SL, Smith AH, Snyder-Mackler L. Anterior cruciate ligament-specialized post-operative return-to-sports (ACL-SPORTS) training: a randomized control trial. BMC Musculoskelet Disord 2013; 14: 108

RETURN-TO-COMPETITION AFTER ACL RECONSTRUCTION: A MULTIFACETED APPROACH

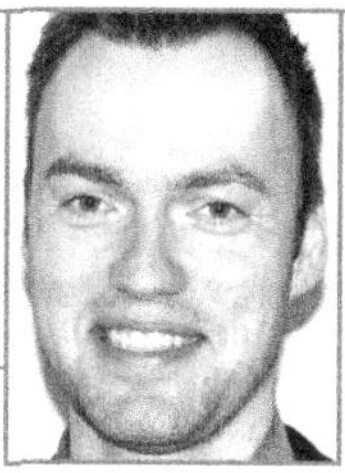

Bloch H[1], Riepenhof H[2,3], Krutsch W[4,5]

[1]VBG, German Social Accident Insurance Institution for the Administrative Sector, Hamburg, Germany; [2]BG Clinic Hamburg, Hamburg, Germany; [3]AS Roma, Rome, Italy; [4]University Medical Centre Regensburg, Regensburg, Germany; [5]FIFA Medical Centre of Excellence, Regensburg, Germany

Introduction

In football, especially before huge sport events, like the UEFA European Football Championship, time based forecasts about the return of important players after a serious injury appear in sports media. As a result of this, team physicians often are confronted with internal and public pressure asking for an early return of the player to the pitch (1). When analysing injuries in German professional soccer, injuries of thighs (19.9 %) and knees (17.7 %) are most frequent (2). Although the proportion of Anterior Cruciate Ligament (ACL) ruptures in the first three German professional football leagues seems to be low (approximately 1.0 % of all insurance cases), they are accompanied by high medical costs and days of absence. This is aggravated by the fact that a previous ACL injury represents the greatest risk factor of a recurrence injury (3). Until now standardised and practical progressive test methods for an optimal return to training and competition are missing. The VBG (Verwaltungs-Berufsgenossenschaft, i.e. German insurance company), as the statutory accident insurance institution for the semi- and professional sport in Germany, is searching for a more objective assessment after an ACL injury. Based on a multidisciplinary expert panel a standardised and consensus based algorithm should be fixed.

Methods

To obtain the goal of a consensus approach the VBG initialised a corporate project with the German Sports University Cologne. Within this project relevant German research groups and stakeholders of the medical staff of German elite team sports, including the highest leagues in football, basketball and ice-hockey, were identified. Thirty-five attendees followed the invitation to a consensus workshop. Five more experts weren't able to participate and were consulted afterwards. The expert panel included surgeons, team physicians, athletic coaches, physiotherapists, sport psychologists and scientists. Afterwards the discussed aspects of the expert panel were summarised in a final report. Based on the results of this consensus process and with additional input of the authors a test manual was generated.

Results

To classify the test manual, four essential steps of the rehabilitation process were defined (Return-to-Activity, Return-to-Sports, Return-to-Play and Return-to-Competition). The test manual should be used to assess, if the player is ready to return to unrestricted team training (Return-to-Play). To avoid that the test results were only compared between the injured and the non-injured leg, the test manual should also be used as a pre injury screening, to gain player specific norm values. Based on the consensus workshop minimal and maximal requirements in seven categories were defined. Within the manual the setup, the performance and the test evaluation for the minimal requirements are explained.

To assess postural control the modified star excursion balance test should be used as a minimal requirement. Side to side differences of the anterior reach distance should be smaller than 4 cm, while the total score should not fall below 94%. The hop test category consists of a bi- and unilateral drop jump, the counter movement jump, the side hop test and the single leg hop for distance. For the hop tests a Lower Limb Symmetry Index (LSI) greater than 90% is recommended. Within the speed category the tapping test (frequency speed) and a repeated sprint ability test (speed endurance) were explained. For the tapping test a tapping coefficient rated as 'good' (15.0-17.5) and for the repeated sprint ability test a 'good' fatigue index (0.85-0.89) should be achieved. If the technical requirements are not available, agility should be assessed in form of change of direction tasks (e.g. modified agility T-test, lower extremity functional test etc.). Two agility tests focusing on different tasks (e.g. change of direction, curves) should be chosen. For example, within the modified T-test the time difference between two runs should not be greater than 10%. For the lower extremity functional test a separate cut-off score for women (135 s) and men (100 s) exists. To provoke standardized fatigue and assess endurance a spiro-ergometry (maximum requirement) or minimal a field test (eg. YoYo IR 1) as a minimal requirement should be used.
The 3D-motion analysis applies to be the gold standard to assess motion quality in athletes. As a minimal requirement different tools to assess 2D-motion quality were described (real-time observational screening, (modified) landing error scoring system). These tests should be passed rated as 'good' or 'good control'. The ACL-RSI was found to be a practical psychological recommendation. 79 athletes (42 male, 37 female) with a mean age of 22.3±2.0 years were tested on an average of 6.5±1.44 (range 4-12) months after ACL reconstruction. The most frequent limitations which reject a return on the pitch after six months were inadequate results at the hop tests (n=12) especially under fatigued conditions (n=19) and agility tests (n=7). Even nine months after ACL reconstruction the hop tests under fatigued conditions remain the most critical factor for a return to play decision (n=12).

Conclusions

Progressive and assessment based criteria within a multifaceted test battery may help to reduce pressure on medical teams and athletes and thus prevent recurrence injuries. Further on a pilot implementation in form of a multicenter approach is initiated.

References

1. Best R, Bauer G, Niess A, Striegel H. Return to play decisions in professional soccer - A decision algorithm from a team physician's viewpoint. Z Orthop Unfall 2011; 149: 582-587
2. VBG Daten und Fakten zum bezahlten Sport. 12. Symposium Hochleistungssport. 16.11.2015 http://www.vbg.de/SharedDocs/Medien-Center/DE/Faltblatt/Pressemeldungen/151116_Daten_Fakten_bez_Sport_2014-fin.pdf?__blob=publicationFile&v=1
3. Paterno MV, Mitchell JR, Schmitt LC, Ford KR, Hewett TE. Incidence of second ACL injuries 2 years after primary ACL reconstruction and return to sport. Am J Sports Med 2014; 42: 1567-1573

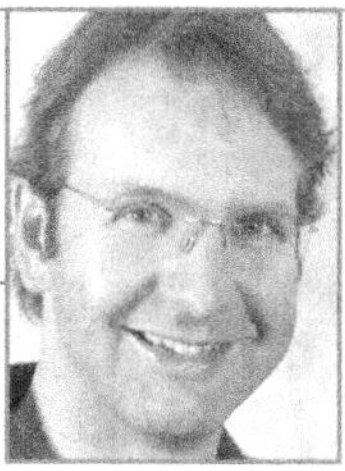

PATELLA LUXATION IN AN ADOLESCENT SOCCER PLAYER

Herfert J[1], Bernecker R[1], Landkammer Y[1], Klampfer H[2], Wicker A[1]

[1]Institute of Physical Medicine and Rehabilitation, Paracelsus Medical University, Salzburg;
[2]Institute of Traumatology, Paracelsus Medical University, Salzburg, Austria

Case report

A 17 years old male soccer player (172 cm, 70 kg) was presented after patella luxation.
He suffered his second traumatic patella luxation at the left knee and was successfully treated by Medial Patello Femoral Ligament (MPFL) reconstruction.
Beneath physiotherapy and rehabilitation training (knee brace; S: 0/0/60°, +15° every two weeks, total time six weeks; full body weight from day one after surgery, start with physiotherapy, lymphatic drainage and mobilization of lower extremity joints at the first four weeks, start with ergometer training and walking units at Alter G (Fremont, USA) in week 5, following core stability training, instability training, jumps, strength training, free running at week 9) the player received 25 isokinetic training sessions and 2 isokinetic tests between week 5 and 20 post surgery.
The soccer player started the isokinetic training at week 5 after surgery. He got 2 trainings per week and started with 120 and 90°/s, assistant mode 5 series with 15 repetitions (reps) each, knee extension and flexion in concentric mode. After two weeks he did the same protocol, but eccentric mode in extension. The protocol was boosted until he reached 60°/s without assistance in concentric and eccentric mode. The first isokinetic test at 16 weeks after surgery showed by comparing left (injured) and right side a lack of Peak Torque (PT) over three velocities (60, 180, 240°/s) in the knee extensor muscles on the injured side (17.9 - 34.1% deficit), no significant difference in the knee flexor muscles (-6 to -0.4% deficit).
PT within five repetitions at 60°/s the footballer reaches in the extension 169.9 Nm (left, injured) and 257.2 Nm (right), as well as 147.4 Nm (left, injured) and 153.0 Nm (right) in the flexion.
The second isokinetic test was performed a month later. The isokinetic retest still showed by comparing left-injured and right side a lack of PT over three velocities (60, 180, 240°/s) in the knee extensor muscles on the injured side (16.2- 19.8% deficit), no significant difference in the knee flexor muscles (-2.5 – 0.5% deficit). PT within five repetitions at 60°/s the footballer reaches in the extension 241.0 Nm (left/injured) and 287.8 Nm (right), as well as 170.3 Nm (left/injured) and 169.8 Nm (right) in the flexion. At week 21 after surgery, the athlete joined the team and started with individual training.

Conclusions

Isokinetic muscle training allows effective muscle training under a maximum of joint protection (1, 2). This training seems to be beneficial, especially in fast sports with high muscular demands during extremely varying and challenging tasks, like they are found in soccer. Referring to this case report and the literature, isokinetic training could be included into rehabilitation and even preventive training.

References

1. Froböse I, Nellessen-Martens G. Training in der Therapie. Urban & Fischer Verlag, München, 1998
2. Mayer F, Horstmann T, Röcker K, Heitkamp HC, Dickhuth HH. Normal values of isokinetic maximum strength, the strength/velocity curve, and the angle at peak torque of all degrees of freedom in the shoulder. Int J Sports Med 1994; 15 Suppl 1: S19-S25

A REHABILITATION PROTOCOL FOR CONSERVATIVELY AND SURGICALLY MANAGED ANKLE SYNDESMOSIS INJURIES

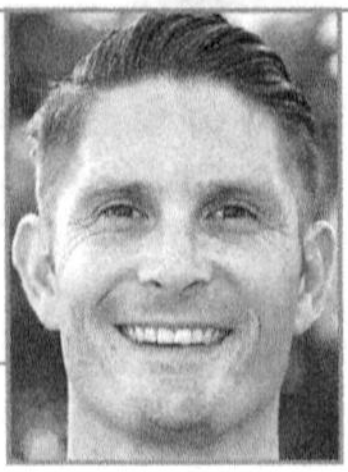

Urwin J, Broman D, Calder J, Rosenfeld P, Rolls A

Reading Football Club, Arsenal Football Club, West Ham United Football Club, Fortius Clinic, London, United Kingdom

Introduction

Ankle injuries in professional football are relatively common. Hagglund et al. (1) recorded that ankle injuries made up 13% of total injuries in sport. The prevalence of syndesmosis injuries themselves were noted as 3% of total ankle injuries in football (1). To the authors knowledge there is a dearth of quality literature surrounding the rehabilitation of both surgically and conservatively managed syndesmosis injuries. For this reason we describe the case reports of four individual professional footballers with significant ankle syndesmosis injuries. Two athletes were managed conservatively and two surgically with the implementation of specific rehabilitation protocols.

Case reports

Four male professional footballers sustained significant ankle syndesmosis injuries whilst, competing for their respective clubs and in one case country.

Player Characteristics	Level of Play	Mechanism	Able To Continue	Injury
Age: 26 Height: 183 cm Weight: 89 kg	International	External rotation of the foot with combined dorsi-flexion	Yes (for 3 minutes then removed from the field of play)	Grade II
Age: 20 Height: 190 cm Weight: 83 kg	English Football League Championship	External rotation of the foot with combined dorsi-flexion	Yes (for 20 minutes)	Grade II
Age: 25 Height: 191 cm Weight: 87 kg	International	External rotation of the foot with combined dorsi-flexion	No	Grade II
Age: 28 Height: 177 cm Weight: 77 kg	International	External rotation of the foot with combined dorsi-flexion	No	Grade II

Table 1. Characteristics of the players.

All athletes had no history of previous ankle syndesmosis injuries on the affected side. The mechanism of injury in all four cases was forced external rotation of the foot combined with dorsi-flexion. Two of the injuries were sustained through direct contact and two through non-contact change of direction.

The footballers were diagnosed with significant ankle syndesmosis injuries through clinical assessment and imaging (weight bearing X-ray and Magnetic Resonance Imaging). All four of the professional footballers were classified as grade II injuries using the West Point Ankle Grading System (2).

Rehabilitation protocols were devised and implemented for both the surgically and conservatively managed players.

Tightrope fixation was utilised in the surgically managed group with a four week period of immobilisation post-surgery.

The rehabilitation protocol was implemented daily over a 10-12 week period. The conservatively managed players were similarly immobilised in an Aircast boot for 3-4 weeks and were rehabilitated daily over a 6-9 week period.

Return to play was recorded as 51 and 63 days in the conservatively managed group, with 86 and 87 days being noted in the surgically managed players.

Follow-up for the conservative group was 6 months and 1 year for the surgically managed athletes.

Conclusions

This case series describes successful rehabilitation protocols for significant ankle syndesmosis injuries that were managed both conservatively and surgically. In all of the professional footballers described, return to play was under 13 weeks with no recorded re-injury or evidence of prolonged symptoms in the affected ankle. Our case series further raises the debate of conservative versus surgical intervention for grade 2 syndesmosis injuries.

References

1. Hägglund M, Waldén M, Ekstrand J. Risk factors for lower extremity muscle injury in professional soccer: the UEFA injury study. Am J Sports Med 2013; 41: 327-335
2. Gerber J, Williams G, Scoville C, Arciero R, Taylor D. Persistent disability associated with ankle sprains: a prospective examination of an athletic population. Foot Ankle Int 1998; 19: 653-660

TWO PICTURES, ONE RESULT: RETURN TO PLAY

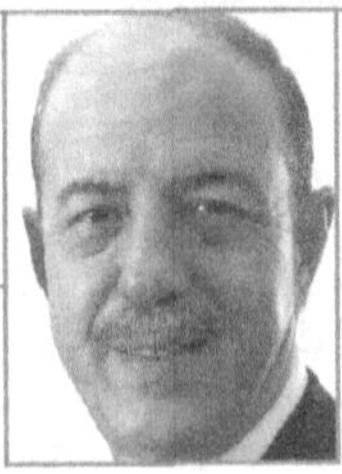

Zahar M, Zerguini Y

La Marsa, Tunisia; FIFA Medical Center of Excellence, Algier, Algery

After more than twenty years of practice in football medicine , we chose to present to my colleagues just two cases: one professional player(male, 28 years old) and one young player (male, 15 years old).
The professional player present an adductor pain, he cannot finish the games. The younger suffered from knee pain, my colleagues Physician tell him to stopped training and competition.
The two players have the same thinking: football is magic! How can I help them?
We have the same dental record for the players: picture of the dental occlusion and a Panoramic X-ray.

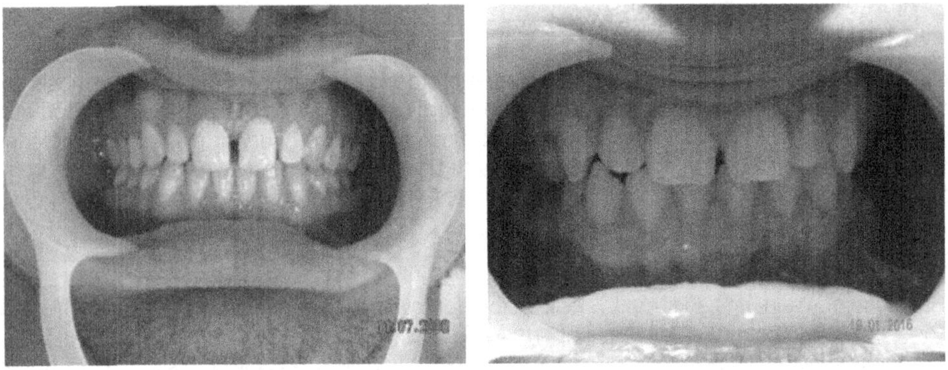

Figure 1. Pictures of the dental occlusion of case 1 (left) and 2 (right).

Our colleagues physician can also have just this two pictures into their medical record, which give them many information about the dental health. This picture give them enough information about the occlusal relationship and their impact on muscular balance.
We realize the same clinical exam for the two players.

Two different therapeutics protocols were done. For the professional player we prescribe the extraction of the third Molars. For the young player we decide to correct the dental relationship with an orthodontic appliance.

The players describe the same result: No adductor pain from more than five years, and no knee pain, and this player start again his football practice from more than three months, demonstrating the result of our conservative treatment.
Sports dentist can also help players to return to play.
An interdisciplinary approach (sports dentist and football doctor) can also help players to return to play.

Saturday 9th April, 2016 (afternoon)
FLEMING ROOM

INVITED SPEAKERS

IMPACT OF KNEE INJURIES ON RETURN TO PLAY

Chairs

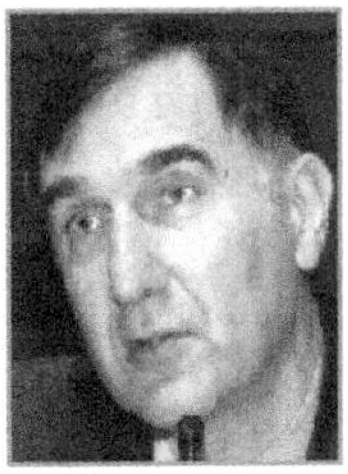

Andrea Ferretti
(Rome, Italy)

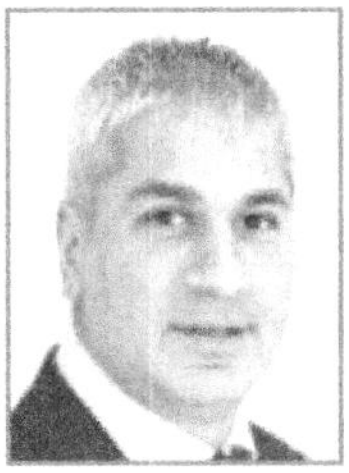

Dinesh Nathwani
(London, United Kingdom)

16:30	Return to play following conservative treatment of the medial collateral ligament **Edwin Goedhart (Haarlem, The Nederlands)**
16:45	Can postero-lateral corner surgery influence the outcome **Claudio Zorzi (Verona, Italy)**
17:00	Return to play after meniscal surgery **Cécile Batailler (Lyon, France)**
17:15	Return to play following cartilage surgery: time or criteria? **João Espregueira-Mendes (Porto, Portugal)**
17:30	Return to play after multiple ligament injuries **Matteo Denti (Milan, Italy)**
17:45	Discussion
18:00	End of the session

RETURN TO PLAY FOLLOWING MEDIAL COLLATERAL LIGAMENT CONSERVATIVE TREATMENT

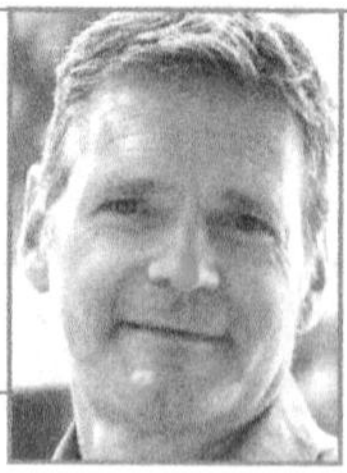

Goedhart E

Sport Medical Centre of the Royal Netherlands Football Association,
FIFA Medical Centre of Excellence, Haarlem, The Netherlands

Introduction

The challenge of the decision making in and around the process of Return To Play (RTP) originates in the field of tension between a good recovery and a fast recovery. This also applies for the conservative approach of the treatment a ruptured Medial Collateral Ligament (MCL) of the knee.
A good recovery implies a complete healing of the ligament, stable with valgus stress, without subjective complaints during functional loading and without increased risk for re-injury.
The need for a fast recovery depends on the status of the player, the time in the season, the pressure for results the players expectations and that of his environment.
Where the good recovery focuses predominantly on the physical aspects, the relevant aspects of a fast recovery are mainly environmental of origin. The decision on RTP is made easier, when the injured athlete and the surrounding system have adequate expectations of the possible time schedule to full recovery, the possible setbacks, the end points that are set in advance and the risks of accelerated RTP.
A proper prognosis on recovery time starts with a correct diagnosis. This will provide you with information on the expected recovery time, not the definite recovery time: each injured knee will follow its own course ultimately.

Relevance of the localization: anatomy, biomechanics and vascularisation

There is some agreement on the static stability. At the medial side of the knee, this is predominantly provided by the MCL complex consisting of the superficial layer of MCL (sMCL), the deep layer MCL (dMCL) en the Posterior Oblique Ligament (POL).
The sMCL is the most important stabilizer to valgus motion and has an additive function in stabilizing the knee for exorotation whereas the distal part contributes to stabilizing mainly exorotation, but also endorotation in flexion. The POL assists the sMCL in stabilizing endorotation and valgus motion mainly in extension. The main function of the dMCL (consisting of a proximal meniscofemoral and distal mensicotibial part) lies in stabilizing exorotation, besides valgus and endorotation depending on the angle of flexion, mainly supportive to the other structures.
The next assumptions are based on relatively few and older publications and should be carefully interpreted: 1) The distal insertion of sMCL seems to be the most strongest one, the proximal origin the weakest. 2) The tendency and quality of the healing process seems reduced at the insertion sites (especially the tibial insertion) compared to midsubstance injuries. 3) The vascularisation seems better proximally than distally.
Combining the available information leads to the following conclusions and assumptions: i) A lesion is expected more frequently in the proximal part of the sMCL. This location has a good tendency for repair. The better vascularization could be responsible for a better and faster healing. ii) A lesion of the distal part of the sMCL might have a lower tendency for healing due to lesser vascularization. A complication could be the presence of a Stener like lesion of the MCL where the anterior fibers of the superficial MCL are displaced over the pes anserinus tendon. iii) Lesions of POL are usually ruptured together with the sMCL and result in an increased valgus and rotational instability.

It remains unclear whether one should have any specific concerns regarding the healing of this ligament. This is also applicable for the dMCL, although there exist some concerns for the femoral attachment of the dMCL, when complaints remain present after the expected time for recovery. iv) Based on the fore mentioned information one might conclude that a lesion near the origin will heal the fastest with a shorter RTP.

Severity

After a rupture of the MCL complex the degree of increased gapping on valgus stress at 20° flexion indicates the grade of the lesion. Care should be taken with significant gapping in 0° flexion, indicating involvement of the Anterior Cruciate Ligament. The more severe the gapping, the longer the period for RTP. The estimated time for RTP of a grade 1-lesion is 2-4 weeks, grade 2 is 4-6 weeks and grade 3 is 6 weeks or more.

The focus of rehabilitation

Most isolated MCL lesions will respond well on conservative treatment. To ensure a good and fast recovery, early mobilization with the use of a hinged brace with a 0-90° of Range of Motion (ROM) is a very effective approach in the conservative treatment of MCL injury. It will enhance the formation of collagen at the ruptured site, but ensures the possibility to activate the muscles and other tissues and avoid the muscle wasting and decrease in motor control around the knee. The rehabilitation programs depends on the type of athletes and cultural backgrounds with regional preferences for certain applications. All focus on early mobilization with avoidance of valgus by the use of a hinged brace with full ROM. The subsequent phases are characterized by increasing loads for strengthening exercises, the transition from bicycle, crosstrainer, jogging, running towards all kind of agility drills and introduction of ball exercises with concomitant (outward) rotational stress. This ultimately results in the integration in full training.

The indicators for RTP

It is a continuous anecdotally based discussion whether strength and other skills should be at a certain pre-injury level before RTP or that the functional assessment (processing the training sessions) should be the key-factor. Above the general physical aspects should meet the criteria for entering the game. The athlete has not been able to fulfil the complete soccer specific demands during the rehabilitation. Data from Global Positioning Systems, Local Position Measurements and video may support that the player is ready for RTP. These criteria can even be made position specific, but the development in this field is slower than desired.
Anxiety for re-entering the game might be made objective by questionnaires, but the social pressure could well be influencing the way the athlete responds.
The expectations from staff and/or player are also factors to deal with. The unacceptable risks should be properly defined and carefully evaluated with all the persons concerned.

Conclusions

The management on RTP Following MCL conservative treatment contains both physical and psycho-social aspects. Managing the expectations starts with proper diagnosis and subsequent expected prognosis. The content of the rehabilitation program should be clarified and the possible setbacks noticed. The ligament healing, the physical skills and fitness, the mental status and the desires of the player and his surrounding system all have to be carefully assessed in order to prepare the right timing for the RTP decision.

RETURN TO PLAY AFTER MENISCAL SURGERY

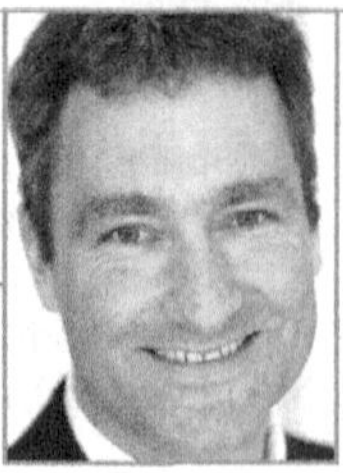

Schneider A[1], Batailler C[1], Wascher DC[2], Lustig S[1,3], Servien E[1,3], Neyret P[1,3]

[1]Centre Albert Trillat, FIFA Medical Center of Excellence, Hôpital de la Croix Rousse Lyon, France; [2]Department of Orthopaedics, University of New Mexico, Albuquerque, USA; [3]Académie Médicale de Football de Lyon, Lyon, France

Introduction

Football is a major provider of meniscal injuries. It represents 8% of all injuries sustained over a season in professional soccer (1). A meniscal lesion causes pain and effusion, which restrict sport practice by a real dysfunction of the knee-joint. An early diagnosis then a thoughtful treatment is primordial to a short Return To Play (RTP) at pre-injury level which is often the main concern of players and teams. Surgeons treating patients with Anterior Cruciate Ligament (ACL) injuries must be prepared to address concomitant meniscal injuries. Therapeutic decisions need a discussion between players, surgeon and club. The management of meniscal tears in athletes presents specific features.

Review of literature

Few studies report results about RTP after meniscal surgery in football players.

- The partial meniscectomy allows a faster RTP (without limitation during rehabilitation) than meniscal repair. In a study including 90 meniscectomized (Lateral M or Medial M) soccer players knee operated on, the median time to RTP was longer in the LM group than the MM group (respectively 7 and 5 weeks) and the probability to RTP was six times greater after MM (2). Moreover LM have showed more adverse events like residual pain, swelling or even chondrolysis (Mariani PP, Garofalo R, Margheritini F. Chondrolysis after partial lateral meniscectomy in athletes. Knee Surg Sports Traumatol Arthrosc 2008, 16: 574-580). Higher Osteo-Artritis (OA) risk was also described at long term after meniscectomy in (un)stable football player's knee (Chantraine A. Knee joint in soccer players: osteoarthritis and axis deviation. Med Sci Sports Exerc 1985, 17: 434-439).
- Alvarez-Diaz reported a 89.6% rate of players after meniscal repair which returned to the same level of competition (ACL reconstruction associated for 52% of them) (Alvarez-Diaz P, Alentorn-Geli E, Llobet F, Granados N, Steinbacher G, Cugat R. Return to play after all-inside meniscal repair in competitive football players: a minimum 5-year follow-up. Knee Surg Sports Traumatol Arthrosc 2014 Sep 27. [Epub ahead of print]).

Howewer evidence-based medicine remains poor concerning football players.

How make the most adapted decison ?

We will consider three main parameters to manage meniscal injuries in football players.

1. First we analyse the meniscal tear (location, delay, ability to be repair).
2. Then, the status of the ACL is critical when deciding whether or not to repair a meniscal tear. Warren described failure rate of 30% to 40% of meniscal repairs if the knee remains unstable (Warren RF. Meniscectomy and repair in the anterior cruciate ligament-deficient patient. Clin Orthop Relat Res 1990; 252: 55-63). In an ACL deficient knee, a simultaneous ACL reconstruction

must be discussed (Hanks GA, Gause TM, Handal JA, Kalenak A. Meniscus repair in the anterior cruciate deficient knee. Am J Sports Med 1990; 18: 606-611; Koukoulias N, Papastergiou S, Kazakos K, Poulios G, Parisis K. Mid-term clinical results of medial meniscus repair with the meniscus arrow in the unstable knee. Knee Surg Sports Traumatol Arthrosc 2007; 15: 138-143). Finally we have to consider the football player, his past medical history, his carreer, his expectations and despite the delay to recover, the increased risk to develop OA.

What is already known ?

The outcomes depend to many parameters. The associated lesions (chondral injuries, ACL rupture) and the therapeutic options change substantially the prognosis and RTP. Prevention of meniscus injuries is thus one of the reasons for ACL injury prevention (FIFA 11+).

- **Meniscectomy** allows a faster recovery than repair. Usually, this takes between two to eight weeks after arthroscopic surgery, depending on the tear and individual recovery. The LM seems have more difficult outcomes than MM and must be avoided as soon as possible. Isolated meniscectomy reduced the length of career in years (5.6 vs 7.0; P=0.03) and games played (62 vs 85; P=0.02) compared to college football athletes without history of injured knee (Brophy RH, Gill CS, Lyman S, Barnes RP, Rodeo SA, Warren RF. Effect of anterior cruciate ligament reconstruction and meniscectomy on length of career in National Football League athletes: a case control study. Am J Sports Med 2009; 37: 2102-2107). The reoperation rate is also lower that for meniscal repairs (1.4% versus 16.5% at short-term ; 3.9% versus 20.7% at long-term follow up (Paxton ES, Stock MV, Brophy RH. Meniscal repair versus partial meniscectomy: a systematic review comparing reoperation rates and clinical outcomes. Arthroscopy 2011; 27: 1275-1288).
- **After meniscal repair** Lateral meniscus heals better than medial meniscus (Beaufils P, Cassard X. Meniscal repair-SFA 2003. Rev Chir Orthop Reparatrice Appar Mot 2007; 93(8 Suppl):5 S12-13). The failure rate after repair may delay complete recovery, especially in elite athletes. Progressive return to low impact sport is possible after 2 to 3 months. The return to high-level football will be between 6 and 8 months. In youngest players meniscal conservation is highly recommended, to prevent OA, even if recovery and return to football lasts much longer.

In case of unstable knee, there is a high success rate for meniscal repairs done in conjunction with ACL reconstruction. Repair doesn't delay the recovery in association with ACL reconstruction. Some authors described also a significantly reduced loss of sports activity after repair (about 80 % RTP; Logan M, Watts M, Owen J, Myers P. Meniscal repair in the elite athlete: results of 45 repairs with a minimum 5-year follow-up. Am J Sports Med 2009; 37: 1131-1134) compared to partial meniscectomy).

Conclusions

The therapeutic strategy must consider the immediate career of players, but also long term clinical outcomes. RTP depends on numerous parameters (associated injuries, meniscal tear, ACL status, age, level of football) but above all player's and club's expectations. The best treatment for each individual patient much be decided even if pressure on team physicians is immense in quickly restoring injured elite players to a high level of performance. Meniscectomy allows a rapid RTP in professional player but results deteriorate with time. The onset of OA seems to be less frequent after isolated meniscal repair, but complications are more frequent and RTP often delayed. In youngest players Meniscus must be preserved particularly in ACL deficient knee (associated ACL reconstruction).

References

1. Chomiak J, Junge A, Peterson L, Dvorak J. Severe injuries in football players. Influencing factors. Am J Sports Med 2000; 28 (5 Suppl): S58-68
2. Nawabi DH, Cro S, Hamid IP, Williams A. Return to play after lateral meniscectomy compared with medial meniscectomy in elite professional soccer players. Am J Sports Med 2014; 42: 2193-2198

RETURN TO PLAY AFTER CARTILAGE SURGERY: TIME OR CRITERIA?

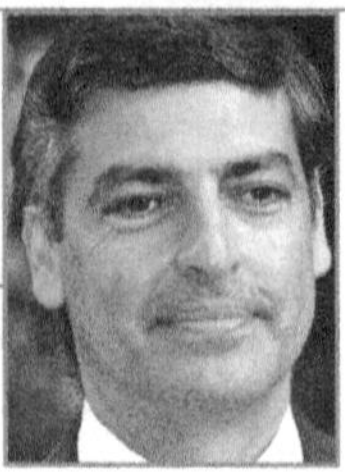

Espregueira-Mendes J

FC Porto; Orthopaedics Department of Minho University;
Clínica do Dragão, Espregueira-Mendes Sports Centre, FIFA Medical Centre of Excellence;
Dom Henrique Research Centre, Porto, Portugal

High demanding sports, including football, are associated with significant forceful, repetitive joint contact forces, which leads to temporary or permanent changes in the chondral and osteochondral homeostasis (3). These changes are often associated with concomitant pathologies which may lead to an early onset of osteoarthritis. In fact, these lesions often cause disabling symptoms, such as, pain, swelling, catching and locking of the knee. Still, in presence of local chondral defects, the player may be asymptomatic (2); still, if these defects are not treated properly, they might lead to longer periods of rehabilitation or even to an early career ending.

The management of articular cartilage lesions is complex and multifactorial, reason why it still remains a challenge for the orthopaedic community.

Return to competition within the same level is not always granted and there is evidence of increased prevalence of early osteoarthritis, especially in elite level athletes. In this sense, keystones for knee cartilage surgery in this specific population are restoring the hyaline cartilage tissue that can resist to the sports high mechanical demands, reestablish the knee normal range of motion and function, and repair the physiological properties of the osteochondral unit with integration of the regenerated cartilage tissue.

Several treatment algorithms have been emerging in order to better address these lesions and reestablish the cartilage surface. Nonetheless, a consensus has not been reached yet in which concerns the advantages between them in regard to the clinical and functional outcomes and return to sports.

Focusing into the football players, microfracture have showed good results with a successful return to demanding, high-impact football of athletes with knee articular cartilage defects. However, increased age, socioeconomic lifestyle, rehabilitation provided and delayed surgery have been pointed out as limiting factors for a faster return to sports. The Autologous Chondrocyte Implantation (ACI) / Matrix-Induced Autologous Chondrocyte Implantation (MACI) have also showed good results throughout the scientific literature in regard to the football players. It has been shown that it results in good to excellent outcomes for most of the football players, with increased results in the Tegner score. In fact, when compared to microfracture, it has been shown that it leads to higher clinical and functional scores and better quality of life; although microfracture deteriorates over time, it allows a faster rehabilitation. In this line, the mosaicplasty has also shown good to excellent clinical and functional outcomes in most of the players, especially for younger players who had smaller lesions.

In which concerns the return to competition, these surgical techniques result in similar rates of return to sports and divergent rehabilitation periods. While microfracture resulted in 80-95% of the players returning to sports (75-95% within the same level), mosaicplasty had a rate of 87% (67% same level) and the ACI procedure 86% (67% same level). Though, when applied to recreational players, the ACI procedure lead to a lower rate (33%).

The time to return to competition diverged considerably according the surgical technique used. Mosaicplasty procedure enabled the fastest period to return to sports, where within an average of 4.5 months the player returned to compete again. In this line, the microfracture lead to a longer period of rehabilitation, resulting in a mean period of 8 months till return to sports.

The ACI procedure resulted in the longest time until returning to competition, encompassing a total of 12.5-18.1 months of rehabilitation. In this sense, sport-specific rehabilitation protocols can hasten the return to competition and provide a safe and durable cartilage repair.
Regarding football players, we rely on the mosaicplasty procedure, using bone plugs autografts from the upper tibio-fibular joint (1). This technique provides good results just like another above mentioned surgical technique, however without significant comorbidities related to the donor site.
In conclusion, upon the choice of the surgical technique, several factors should be taken into account, such as, athlete specific factors, injury location and size, concomitant procedures, time into the season and career status, among others. Therefore, the surgeon must acknowledge all these factors and opt for the best technique for each single player.

References

1. Espregueira-Mendes J, Pereira H, Sevivas N, Varanda P, Da Silva MV, Monteiro A, Oliveira JM, Reis RL. Osteochondral transplantation using autografts from the upper tibio-fibular joint for the treatment of knee cartilage lesions. Knee Surg Sports Traumatol Arthrosc 2012; 20: 1136-1142
2. Gomoll AH, Filardo G, De Girolamo L, Esprequeira-Mendes J, Marcacci M, Rodkey WG, Steadman RJ, Zaffagnini S, Kon E. Surgical treatment for early osteoarthritis. Part I: cartilage repair procedures. Knee Surg Sports Traumatol Arthrosc 2012; 20: 450-466
3. Heijink A, Gomoll AH, Madry H, Drobnič M, Filardo G, Espregueira-Mendes J, Van Dijk CN. Biomechanical considerations in the pathogenesis of osteoarthritis of the knee. Knee Surg Sport Traumatol Arthrosc 2012; 20: 423-435

Saturday 9th April, 2016 (afternoon)
CHURCHILL AUDITORIUM

INVITED SPEAKERS

RETURN TO PLAY IN FOOT AND ANKLE INJURIES

Chairs

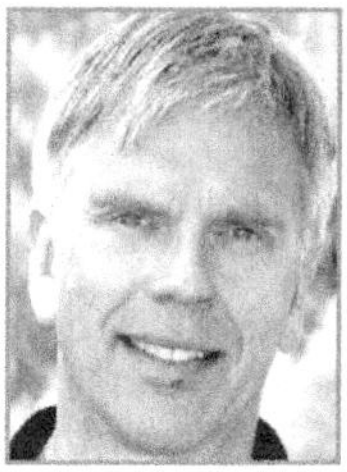

Thor Einar Andersen
(Oslo, Norway)

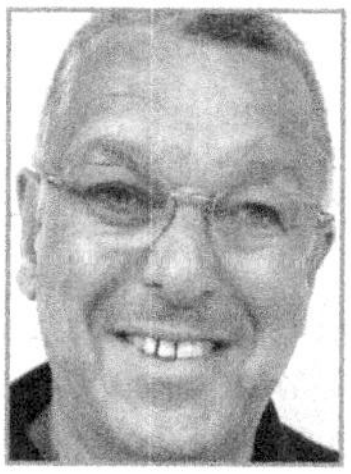

Graham Smith
(Glasgow, United Kingdom)

16:30 Return to play following conservative treatment of ankle sprain
Juan José Garcia Cota (Pontevedra, Spain)

16:45 Return to play for ankle injuries in professional football
Eva Carneiro (London, United Kingdom)

17:00 Return to play in stress fractures of ankle and mid foot
Pieter D'Hooghe (Doha, Qatar)

17:15 Return to play in V metatarsal fracture
Francesca Vannini (Bologna, Italy)

17:30 Return to play in retro-calcaneal bursitis: surgery or conservative treatments **Pereira Hélder (Porto, Portugal)**

17:45 Discussion

18:00 End of the session

RETURN TO PLAY FOLLOWING CONSERVATIVE TREATMENT OF ANKLE SPRAIN

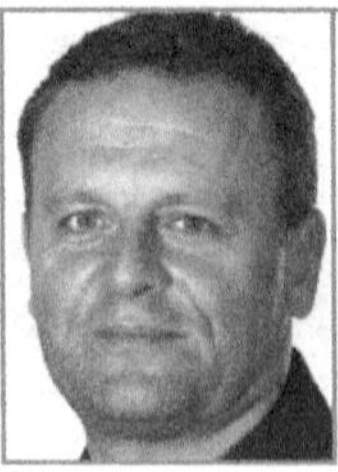

Garcia Cota J

Spanish National Team; Real Club Celta De Vigo, Medical Department;
Sport Trauma and Orthopaedic Surgery Department, Hospital Miguel Dominguez, Pontevedra, Spain

The ankle sprain is one of the most common injury in a lot of sports and particularly in football practice. The risk of injury during match play is around five times greater than during training, and the recurrence correlates with premature return to play and a prior ankle injury. For this reason the moment to take decision to allow the player to back the competition is very important in order to keep the player´s health and avoid bad results and recurrences

To take that determination some data are required but there are not guidelines widely accepted by the professionals who care the player´s health, so the return To Play (RTP) decision after ankle sprain is a real challenge for us. Therefore every team medical staff has to use his particular action plan in this kind of injury. Anyway, there are some objective and subjective data, which we can take them into account to decide.

First of all we need to consider the ligament injured. The healing time is different if the sprain is in lateral ligament (90%), medial ligament (deltoid) or if it is a syndesmosis injury.

Secondly, to know the correct diagnosis and the grade of the sprain will be hugely helpful to determinate the time needed to heal and estimate the time off competition for the player.

In clinical examinations, the range of motion must be completely recovered (specially dorsiflexion) aswell as the muscle strength and proprioception. Of course the one foot weight bearing, running or jump must be done without pain, at least with minor or slight discomfort that don't limit the activity on the pitch.

The swelling signs are not important to take a RTP decision because in most cases this signs remain a lot of time, and it not means a bad follow-up.

In addition to the clinical examination, there are some tests, which can give us evidence that everything is going well in the sprained ankle. A very important data is that the player be able to work with all the team in at least two normal training sessions, without limitations.

Also psychological factors play an important role in RTP deciding moment. So aspects such a player´s mental toughness or his sense of safety and trust should be considered.

Finally the treatment doesn´t finish when the player returns to play, so he must also keep training session to a complete recovery and to reduce the risk of recurrence or even a new injury. In this respect, it should be noted that the use of taping surely provides protection to the ankle.

RETURN TO PLAY IN (STRESS-) FRACTURES OF ANKLE AND MIDFOOT

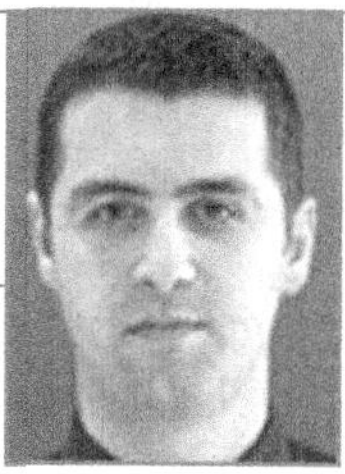

d'Hooghe P, Thompson A

Aspetar, Orthopaedic and Sports medicine Hospital,
FIFA Medical Centre of Excellence, Doha, Qatar and Belgian National Football Association Medical Committee

In competitive athletes, stress fractures of the distal tibia, foot and ankle are common and lead to considerable delay in return to play. The pathogenesis is multifactorial and usually involves repetitive sub-maximal stresses. Factors such as bone vascularity, training regimen and equipment can increase the risk of stress fracture. Intrinsic factors, such as hormonal imbalances, may also contribute to the onset of stress fractures, especially in women.

The classic presentation is a patient who experiences the insidious onset of pain after an abrupt increase in the duration or intensity of exercise. The diagnosis is primarily clinical, but imaging modalities such as plain radiography, scintigraphy, computed tomography, and magnetic resonance imaging may provide confirmation.

Most stress fractures are uncomplicated and can be managed by rest and restriction from the precipitating activity. Tensile forces and the relative avascularity at the site of a stress induced fracture often lead to poor healing. A subset of stress fractures can present a high risk for progression to complete fracture, delayed union, or nonunion. Management is based on the fracture site. In some athletes, metabolic workup and medication are warranted. High-risk fractures, including those of the navicular, proximal fifth Meta-Tarsal (5th MT), and medial malleolus, present management challenges and may require surgery, especially in high-level athletes who need to return to play quickly. Noninvasive treatment modalities such as pulsed ultrasound and extracorporeal shock wave therapy may have some benefit but require additional research. Fracture of the fifth metatarsal has the potential to be a career ending injury in male professional football. Complications such as re-injury and non-union are common. Little is known about the plantar loading parameters of football players who have sustained a 5th MT fracture as they return to full play. This project aims to improve the understanding of how plantar loading parameters are altered following 5th MT fracture when compared to matched healthy control participants.

Fifth Meta-Tarsal stress fractures mainly occur among young football players during the preseason and high-intensity training periods. 78% of all lower limb stress fractures in elite male football players occur at the fifth Meta-Tarsal bone (2).

Rehabilitation is challenging with delayed union or re-fracture being common complications leading to the injury being known as a potentially career-ending injury in male professional football players. In two recent large studies on elite male football players return to full play following 5th MT stress fracture averaged 80±22 days (2) and 95±44 days (3) respectively.

In a large study by Ekstrand & Van Dijk (3) examining 5th MT fractures among male professional football (soccer) players at sixty-four European elite teams from 2001-2012, prodromal symptoms were present in 45% of players who sustained a 5th MT fracture. These "warning" type symptoms suggest that load and bone stress play a role in the development of 5th MT stress fractures.
In-shoe plantar load is a proxy of ground reaction force experienced by the player when performing soccer-specific movements. While it is known that soccer shoes increased plantar loads in specific areas of the foot (1), it is not known how these plantar loading parameters are altered in those recovering from 5th MT stress fracture when compared to healthy un-injured matched participants. Improved understanding of plantar loading parameters post 5th MT injury may help improve return to play strategies and ultimately allow for identification of those players at risk of developing a stress fracture.

References

1. Bentley JA, Ramanathan AK, Arnold GP, Wang W, Abboud RJ. Harmful cleats of football boots: a biomechanical evaluation. Foot Ankle Surg 2011; 17: 140-144
2. Ekstrand J, Torstveit MK. Stress fractures in elite male football players. Scand J Med Sci Sports 2012; 22: 341-346
3. Ekstrand J, van Dijk CN. Fifth metatarsal fractures among male professional footballers: a potential career-ending disease. Br J Sports Med 2013; 47: 754-758

RETURN TO PLAY AFTER FIFTH METATARSAL FRACTURE

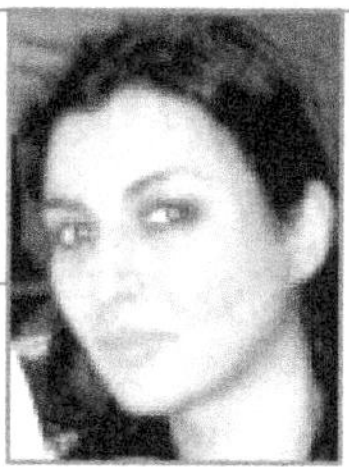

Vannini F, Mosca M, Massimi S, Giannini S, Faldini C

1st Orthopaedic Clinic, Rizzoli Orthopaedic Institute, Bologna, Italy

Introduction

Athletes are at risk for foot injuries, including fifth metatarsal fractures. Due to the peculiar nature of these fractures and the anatomical condition connected to the insertion of the Peroneus Brevis tendon on the fifth metatarsal bone, these fractures may be an issue capable to affect the future play and performance of athletes.

Purpose of this study is to evaluate how to avoid a decrease in performance on return to competition when compared with pre-injury in athletes.

Methods

A literature review on the topic was made; furthermore 12 athletes either professional or semiprofessional treated for a fifth metatarsal bone fracture were evaluated retrospectively.

Fracture type and treatment received were recorded and a correlation with return to play was attempted.

Results

From the literature review a relative high frequency of re-fracture (7.3%) was evident in professional athletes, and required revision with bigger screws. Return to progressive weight bearing was 6 weeks.

Return to previous level of competition was achieved by 85% of athletes.

Surgical treatment resulted the preferred treatment in high level athletes.

Elite athletes demonstrated no decrease in performance on their return to play, although this may be an ending career injury, especially in lower class athletes or either less motivated.

Conclusions

Fifth metatarsal bone fractures are well-studied injuries in terms of etiology, diagnosis, and management. However, the effect of these injuries on future performance of athletes is unknown. Maximizing initial fixation stiffness may decrease late failure rate.

Orthopaedic surgeons should be prepared to counsel and educate elite athletes who sustain this kind of injury.

RETURN TO PLAY IN RETROCALCANEAL BURSITIS: SURGERY OR CONSERVATIVE TREATMENTS

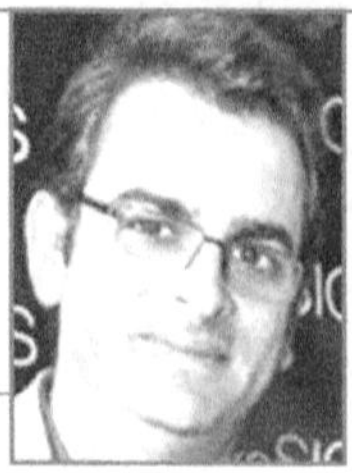

Pereira H

Ripoll y De Prado Sports Clinic, FIFA Medical Centre of Excellence, Murcia and Madrid (Spain); Life and Health Sciences Research Institute (ICVS), School of Health Sciences, University of Minho, Braga/Guimarães, Portugal

Insertional Achilles tendinopathy (IAT) refers to pathology at the insertion of the Achilles tendon onto the calcaneum.
One of the presentations of IAT is retrocalcaneal bursitis. This entity might limit sports activity in both high-level and amateur level.
Physiopathology involves recurrent stress placed upon the attachment site of the Achilles tendon, causing inflammation, micro tears, swelling and pain.
Overuse is an important etiologic factor, considering the high prevalence of this condition among long course runners.
Despite mechanical overload is considered a major risk factor, correlation with varus hindfoot malalignment, advancing age, dyslipidaemia, male gender and high body mass index has also been described (1).
The diagnosis of insertional Achilles tendinopathy is often clinical, based on a triad of symptoms: pain at the site of insertion of Achilles tendon, accompanied by swelling (which may be due to retrocalcaneal bursitis) and impaired performance of the diseased tendon (3).
Radiological findings might include Haglund's deformity which is an enlargement of the posterosuperior prominence of the calcaneum and/or calcaneal spurs.
The first line of treatment is usually conservative (physiotherapy, medication, shoe wear).
Patient's expectations and level of activity are very important in the choice of treatment.
When properly indicated, good outcome has been reported with endoscopic calcaneoplasty (2). This endoscopic approach has been growing in popularity when compared to open techniques. It enables addressing retrocalcaneal bursitis, bony deformity and/or Achilles tendon debridement. It favors faster return to high-level sports activity comparing to open surgery when conservative treatment fails.

References

1. Lim S, Yeap E, Lim Y, Yazid M. Outcome of calcaneoplasty in insertional achilles tendinopathy. Malaysian Orthopaedic Journal 2012; 6 (Suppl. A): 28-34
2. van Dijk CN, Niek C. Ankle Arthroscopy: techniques developed by the amsterdam foot and ankle school. Springer, Berlin-Heidelberg, 2014
3. Witt BL, Hyer CF. Achilles tendon reattachment after surgical treatment of insertional tendinosis using the suture bridge technique: a case series. J Foot Ankle Surg 2012; 51: 487-493

Saturday 9th April, 2016 (afternoon)
PICKWICK ROOM

FREE ORAL PRESENTATIONS

FUNCTIONAL ASSESSMENT

Chairs

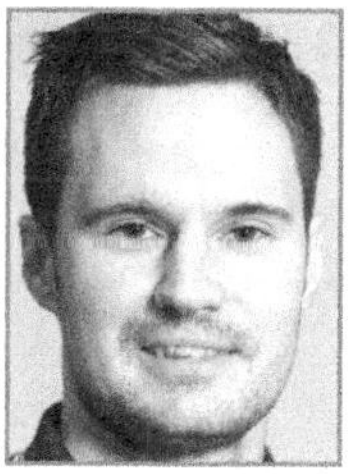

Matthew Buckthorpe
(London, United Kingdom)

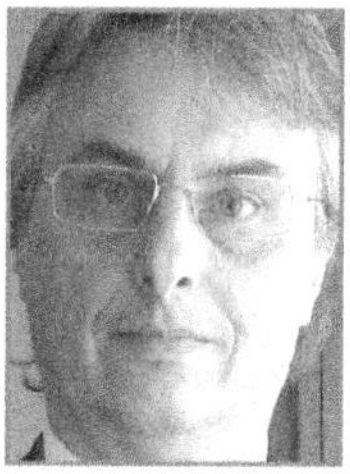

Davide Susta
(Dublin, Ireland)

16:30 Comparison of different ankle isokinetic strengthening program on strength of sedentary male
Kalaycioglu T, Yurt Y, Bayrakci Tunay V (Ankara, Mersin, Turkey)

16:40 Substantial inter-season variability in isokinetic strength in professional football **van Dyk N, Bahr R, Whiteley R, Eirale C, Tol JL, Kumar BD, Hamilton B, Farooq A, Witvrouw E (Doha Qatar; Oslo Norway; London, United Kingdom; Ghent, Belgium; Auckland, New Zealand; Amsterdam, The Netherlands)**

16:50 Effect of high intensity interval cycling training on soccer-specific fitness
Chan HCK, Ho WKY, Yung PSH, Chan KM (Hong Kong, China)

17:00 Gauntlet test performance and injury risk in collegiate female soccer players **Ness BM, Zimney K, Schweinle WE (Vermillion, USA)**

17:10 The biomechanics and EMG of the support leg during three types of football kicking **Ólafsson S, Gibbs S (Akureyri, Iceland; Dundee, United Kingdom)**

17:20 Use of wearable electromyography in rehabilitation processes from muscle injuries **Gasol-Santa X, Turmo-Garuz A, Díaz-Cueli D, Ruzza M, Hoffren-Mikkola M (Barcelona and Sant Cugat, Spain; Kuortane, Finland)**

17:30 Inter-season variability of a functional movement test in professional football **Bakken A, Targett S, Bere T, Eirale C, Farooq A, Tol JL, Whiteley R, Witvrouw E, Khan K, Bahr R (Doha, Qatar; Oslo, Norway; Vancouver, Canada)**

17:40 Discussion

18:00 End of the session

COMPARISON OF DIFFERENT ANKLE ISOKINETIC STRENGTHENING PROGRAM ON STRENGTH OF SEDENTARY MALE

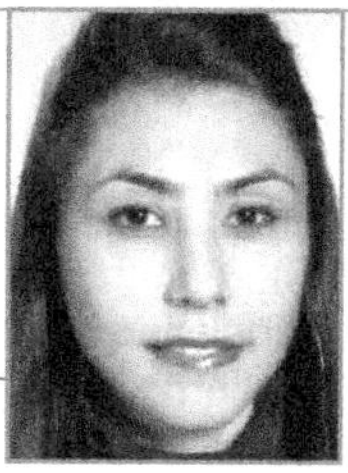

Kalaycioglu T[1], Yurt Y[2], Bayrakci Tunay V[1]

[1]Hacettepe University, Faculty of Health Sciences, Department of Physiotherapy and Rehabilitation, Ankara, Turkey; [2]Eastern Mediterranean University, Faculty of Health Sciences, Department of Physiotherapy and Rehabilitation, Mersin, Turkey

Introduction

Strength-training exercises are used to increase muscular development and to improve neuromuscular control (1, 2). Recently most researchers suggested that pure eccentric resistance training shows more improvement on muscular hypertrophy, acute concentric force ability than both pure concentric resistance training and traditional eccentric/concentric training (2, 3). The aim of this study was to investigate the effects of different isokinetic ankle invertors and evertors strengthening program on strength of university-level healthy sedentary males.

Methods

Forty- three males between 18 and 26 years of age participated in the study. None of the subjects had a history of lower extremity injury for at least six months, ankle or foot surgery or current neuromuscular disorder, had physical therapy or used orthosis for foot or ankle, participated in a regular strength training program.

The participants were randomly divided into two groups which were concentric isokinetic ankle strengthening (n=22; age: 21.3±1.7 yrs; BMI: 25.0±4.0 kg/m^2) and eccentric isokinetic ankle strengthening (n=21; age: 21.1±1.6 yrs; bmi: 24.6±4.1 kg/m^2).

These trainings were done three days a week, for eight weeks by using isokinetic dynamometer (CSMİ, Humac Norm, USA). Measurement for evaluating isokinetic muscle strength was repeated before and after trainings for each group at 60°/s, 120°/s concentric and 60°/s eccentric angular velocity with six repetitions. Maximum peak muscle torque of ankle invertor and evertor muscles groups were evaluated for both sides. Following 10 minutes treadmill warm-up, three isokinetic strength trials were completed when the participants supine position lying, knee and hip at 90° flexion and ankle neutral position. Strength measurement was done 20° eversion and 30° inversion range of ankle motion.

Strengthening programs procedures were progressively harder by using increasing number of repetition or set. Isokinetic trainings were performed with 10 repetitions, 2-3 set at 60°/s and 120°/s angular velocities. During training the eccentric group performed only eccentric exercises, the concentric group only concentric exercises. Significance of differences was set at $p<0.05$.

Results

There were statistically significant increases in evertor concentric strength at 60°/s and 120°/s angular velocities for both sides of the all groups after training program. The values at 60°/s of eccentric angular velocity showed improvement for eccentric group after training, but they were not statistically significant for both groups (Table 1).
After isokinetic training it was not shown significant differences in invertor muscles except in the concentric group at 120°/s in concentric mode (Table 1).

		Concentric Strengthening Group				**Eccentric Strengthening Group**			
		Dominant Mean±S.D.		**Nondominant**		**Dominant Mean±S.D.**		**Nondominant**	
Velocity	Movement	Pre	Post	Pre	Post	Pre	Post	Pre	Post
Con 60˚/s	Inversion	34.6±11.8	34.1±7.1	32±12.6	38.8±10.7	33±9.5	35.1±5.9	37±8.4	35.2±8.1
	Eversion	30.6±15.6	42.6±11.6	26.5±13.1	35.4±5.4	34.8±9.2	41.8±8.7	31±9.8	35.2±6.3
Conic 120˚/s	Inversion	26.6±9.2	29±5.3	23.9±9.3	31.4±8.5	27.2±6.8	29±5.3	29.7±6.4	29.2±7.2
	Eversion	20.4±10.7	35.1±9.3	19.6±9.5	29.5±4.6	26.8±6.5	32.5±6.5	25.1±9.1	28.1±4.8
Ecc 60˚/s	Inversion	37.9±13.4	37±9.5	44.7±19	43±14.9	37.6±15.6	40.1±11.8	40.5±9.9	39.4±13.1
	Eversion	38.2±10.7	41.9±11.8	36.6±13.8	39.9±12.5	39.8±17.6	46.7±15.4	40.2±17.5	43.1±13.2

Table 1. Mean±SD of peak muscle torque (Nm/kg) of ankle inversion and eversion in the dominant and nondominant lower extremities, before (Pre) and after (Post) training.

Concentric strengthening training was more effective than eccentric training for concentric muscle strength measurement.

Conclusions

Isokinetic training program was more effective for ankle evertor muscles than invertor muscle groups on both sides. This can improve muscle balance by this way, keep ankle stability and prevent ankle inversion sprains.
Strength training programs for ankle muscles may be applied to athletes after ankle injuries prevention especially returning to play after ankle injuries.

References

1. Isner-Horobeti ME, Dufour SP, Vautravers P, Geny B, Coudeyre E, Richard R. Eccentric exercise training: modalities, applications and perspectives. J Sports Med 2013; 43: 483-512
2. Uh BS, Beynnon BD, Helie BV, Alosa DM, Renstrom PA. The Benefit of a Single-Leg Strength Training Program For the Muscles Around the Untrained Ankle A Prospective, Randomized, Controlled Study. Am J. Sports Med 2000; 28: 568-573
3. Vogt M, Hoppeler HH. Eccentric exercise: mechanisms and effects when used as training regime or training adjunct. J. Appl. Physiol 2014; 116: 1446-1454

SUBSTANTIAL INTERSEASON VARIABILITY IN ISOKINETIC STRENGTH IN PROFESSIONAL FOOTBALL

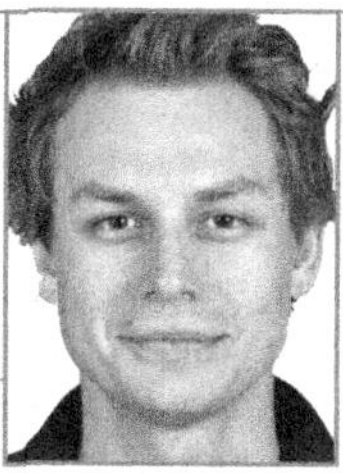

van Dyk N[1], Bahr R[1,2], Whiteley R[1], Eirale C[1], Tol JL[1,6,7], Kumar BD[3], Hamilton B[1,5], Farooq, A[1], Witvrouw E[1],

[1]Aspetar Orthopaedic & Sports Medicine Hospital, Doha Qatar; [2]Oslo Sports Trauma Research Center, Department of Sports Medicine, Norwegian School of Sport Sciences, Oslo Norway; [3]Institute of Sport Exercise & Health, University College London, London, United Kingdom; [4]Department of Rehabilitation Sciences and Physiotherapy, Ghent University, Ghent, Belgium; [5]High Performance Sport New Zealand / New Zealand Olympic Committee Associate Researcher, Sport Performance Research Institute New Zealand (SPRINZ), Millennium Institute of Sport and Health, Mairangi Bay, Auckland, New Zealand; [6]The Sports Physician Group, Department of Sports Medicine, St Lucas Andreas Hospital, Amsterdam, The Netherlands; [7]Amsterdam Center of Evidence Based Sports Medicine, Academic Medical Center, Amsterdam, The Netherlands

Introduction

Isokinetic strength tests are often utilized in preseason screening, clinical assessments or as criteria for Return To Play (RTP). Isokinetic evaluations are used to determine strength deficits compared to previous seasons or side-to-side differences. Prospective studies frequently report follow-up periods over more than one season without repeated measurements. However, the stability of isokinetic strength measurements and the potential influence of systematic and random errors on the variability of these findings are poorly understood, and no study has investigated the long-term consistency of isokinetic strength measures. Thus, the aim of this study was to investigate the stability of isokinetic strength of the hamstring and quadriceps muscles from one season to the next and over several seasons.

Methods

Professional football players from all teams in the first division of the Qatar Stars League performed an isokinetic evaluation of the knee flexors and extensors (System 3, Biodex, New York, USA) as part of their annual periodic health evaluation at Aspetar Sports Medicine Hospital during four consecutive seasons (2010-11 through 2013-14).

The pre-season testing included quadriceps and hamstrings concentric protocols at 60°/s and 300°/s, and hamstrings eccentric protocol at 60°/s.

To assess whether there were systematic differences between seasons, we used paired samples t-tests and calculated the mean difference between tests.

To determine random variability between season we calculated Intraclass Correlation Coefficients (ICC) and the Measurement Error (ME: the standard deviation of the difference between tests divided by the square root of 2), and also expressed this as a percentage of the baseline value. The Minimal Detectable Change (MDC) was also calculated for all the strength measurements.

Results

A total of 563 players performed 2136 isokinetic assessments during the four year follow up. We included 335 players in the analysis; 240 players were tested two consecutive pre-seasons (over 1 season), 86 players with two seasons between tests (over 2 seasons) and nine players with three seasons between tests (over 3 seasons).
The results for concentric quadriceps and hamstrings strength at 60°/s and concentric quadriceps strength at 300°/s were comparable (Table 1).
A small, systematic improvement was found in quadriceps concentric at 60°/s over two and three seasons, quadriceps at 300°/s and hamstrings concentric at 60°/s over one and two seasons, hamstring concentric strength at 300°/s over one and three seasons and hamstring eccentric at 60°/s over two seasons ($p<0.05$).
Similar results were found for eccentric hamstring strength at 60°/s (Table 1). The random variability in the measurements ranged from 10 to 30 Nm, which corresponds to 10-16%.

	MPT (Nm)	Mean difference (95% CI) (Nm)	MDC (Nm)	ICC (95% CI)	ME (Nm)	ME (%)
Q Conc 60°/s Over 1 Season	234.1±42.5	1.0 (-2.1, 4.2)	67.9	0.82 (0.78, 0.85)	24.5	10.5
Q Conc 60°/s Over 2 Season	225.2±40.3	13.3 (8.2, 18.4)	65.9	0.79 (0.68, 0.86)	23.8	10.6
Q Conc 60°/s Over 3 Season	239.4±43.7	14.5 (0.0, 28.9)	56.9	0.86 (0.61, 0.95)	20.1	8.4
Q Conc 180°/s Over 1 Season	131.9±24.6	4.4 (2.9, 6.0)	34.2	0.87 (0.82, 0.89)	15.7	12.7
Q Conc 180°/s Over 2 Season	129.2±25.7	5.9 (2.6, 9.1)	41.5	0.79 (0.71, 0.85)	13.3	10.9
Q Conc 180°/s Over 3 Season	139.8±25.0	18.2 (-1.6, 38.0)	78.0	0.28 (-0.63, 0.71)	17.9	14.4
H Conc 60°/s Over 1 Season	123.7±23.0	4.9 (2.9, 6.9)	43.5	0.73 (0.51, 0.68)	12.4	9.4
H Conc 60°/s Over 2 Season	122.4±22.8	6.1 (3.3, 9.0)	36.9	0.77 (0.67, 0.84)	15.0	11.6
H Conc 60°/s Over 3 Season	124.2±22.8	6.7 (-5.2, 18.6)	47.0	0.82 (0.53, 0.93)	29.8	21.3
H Conc 300°/s Over 1 Season	93.9±21.3	4.7 (2.9, 6.6)	47.4	0.32 (-0.19, 0.65)	14.5	15.4
H Conc 300°/s Over 2 Season	93.4±20.9	2.8 (-0.2, 5.9)	39.0	0.69 (0.58, 0.77)	14.1	15.1
H Conc 300°/s Over 3 Season	89.9±15.0	10.2 (3.3, 17.1)	27.3	0.68 (0.09, 0.88)	10.2	11.4
H Ecc 60°/s Over 1 Season	181.7±37.0	3.8 (0.4, 7.3)	73.7	0.68 (0.61, 0.73)	26.6	14.6
H Ecc 60°/s Over 2 Season	176.2±38.0	11.6 (5.9, 17.4)	73.4	0.66 (0.52, 0.75)	26.5	15.0
H Ecc 60°/s Over 3 Season	182.2±41.4	10.7 (-8.6, 30.1)	76.2	0.78 (0.43, 0.92)	29.2	16.0

Table 1. Comparison of isokinetic strength tests over different seasons. Q Conc: Quadriceps concentric; H Conc: Hamstrngs concentric; H Ecc: Hamstrings eccentric. Values of Maximal peak Torque (MPT) expressed in Nm, are shown as mean ± Standard Deviations (SD). MDC: Minimal Detectable Change; ICC: Intraclass Correlation Coefficient; ME: Measurement Error.

Conclusion

Substantial inter-season variability was observed for isokinetic testing of the quadriceps and hamstring muscles, and this stability of these measurements must be given consideration when interpreting isokinetic strength over different seasons.

EFFECT OF HIGH INTENSITY INTERVAL CYCLING TRAINING ON SOCCER-SPECIFIC FITNESS

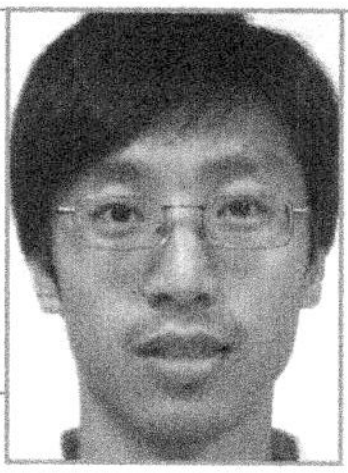

Chan HCK, Ho WKY, Yung PSH, Chan KM

Department of Orthopaedics and Traumatology, Prince of Wales Hospital,
Faculty of Medicine, The Chinese University of Hong Kong, Hong Kong, China

Introduction

Cycling exercise with continuous protocol is usually used as a reconditioning exercise during rehabilitation as cycling exercise is impact-free movement compared to running (2).
For reconditioning of soccer players, restoring both the aerobic endurance and explosive performance in running mode are critical. High Intensity Interval Cycling Training (HIICT) has been proven to significantly improve maximum oxygen intake ($V'O_{2max}$) and Peak Power Output (PPO) on stationary bike (1). HIICT may be a good training to implement which can speed up the reconditioning process. However, to date, no prospective studies have been performed to determine the effect of HIICT on soccer-specific fitness.
The purpose of this study was to examine the effect of high-intensity interval cycling training on soccer-specific fitness in terms of speed, agility, and aerobic endurance.

Methods

Seventeen sub-elite players (16 male, 1 female) were assigned to either the experimental group (HIIT group; n=9; age: 23.7±4.3 yrs; height: 172.2±4.6 cm; weight: 67.5±8.0 kg) or the control group (n=8; 35.1±11.5 yrs; 171.9±1.9 cm; 63.6±5.9 kg) in accordance to their demographics.
The HIIT group received 12 HIICT sessions, three times a week, for four weeks.
Initially, training session consisted of four sets of repeated 30 seconds all-out bout with four minutes active recovery, then it progressively increased by one set each week.
Assessment on i) $V'O_{2max}$ and PPO; ii) speed; iii) agility and iv) aerobic endurance were done at pre-test and post-test by adopting: a) the maximal oxygen consumption test; b) the linear 30 m sprint test; c) the pro-agility test and d) the yo-yo intermittent recovery test level 1 (YYIRT1) respectively.
Breath-by-breath gas analysis (Cardio 2, Medical Graphics Corp., St.Paul, MN, USA) and mechanically braked cycle ergometer (Monark Ergomedic 874E, Vansbro, Sweden) were used in maximal oxygen consumption test. Infra-red timing gate system (Smartspeed, Fusion sport, Summer Park, Australia) was used in 30 m sprint test and pro-agility test.
ANOVA (2x2) were used to determine the difference of all data between groups during pre-test and post-test assessments with the significance level set at $p \leq 0.05$.

Results

The results are shown in Table 1.

	Experimental Group (*n* = 9)		Control Group (*n* = 8)	
	Pre	**Post**	**Pre**	**Post**
30 m sprint time (s)	4.49±0.15	4.56±0.15	4.69±0.22	4.78±0.33
Pro-agility time (s)	5.22±0.23	5.21±0.11	5.27±0.17	5.29±0.19
YYIRT1 distance covered (m)	1426±611	1675±678 *	1045±595	1070±640
MHR during YYIRT1 (beat/min)	193±5	194±6	189±3	193±11
VO_{2max} (mL/kg/min)	49.6±8.1	53.7±9.2 *	45.1±11.0	45.1±9.8
$VO_{2absolute}$ (L/min)	3.30±0.49	3.57±0.47 *	2.83±0.54	2.81±0.58
MHR during $V'O_{2max}$ (beat/min)	183±6	183±5	183±14	182±11
Power output at $V'O_{2max}$ (W)	248±12	274±11*	243±12	231±12

Table 1. The effects of 4-week high-intensity interval cycling training program on physical performance measures Values are represented as mean ± SD. YYIRT1: Yo-Yo intermittent Recovery Test Level 1;
MHR: Maximum heart rate during $V'O_{2max}$ test.*Significant improvement in Experimental Group compared to Control Group

Compared to control group, significant improvement was found in $V'O_{2max}$, power output at VO_{2max}, and YYIR1 performance.
No improvement was found in 30m sprint test and pro-agility test.

Conclusions

The results showed that 4-week high-intensity interval cycling training have a beneficial effect on aerobic endurance in both cycling mode and running mode, no significant effect were found on speed and agility performance. HIICT is suitable for building up the aerobic endurance of soccer players as a reconditioning training. Speed and agility training should be supplemented based on the situation of the athlete.

References

1. Laursen PB, Jenkins DG. The scientific basis for high-intensity interval training: optimising training programmes and maximising performance in highly trained endurance athletes. Sports Med 2002; 32: 53-73
2. Woodward MI, Cunningham JL. Skeletal accelerations measured during different exercises. Proc Inst Mech Eng H 1993; 207: 79-85

GAUNTLET TEST PERFORMANCE AND INJURY RISK IN COLLEGIATE FEMALE SOCCER PLAYERS

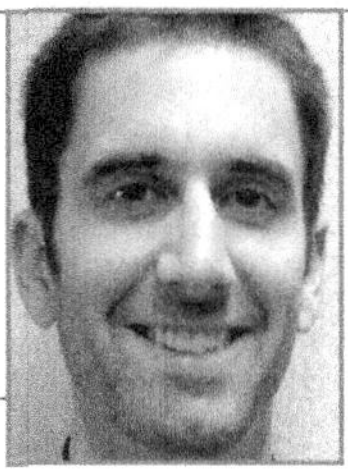

Ness BM, Zimney K, Schweinle WE

University of South Dakota; Vermillion, SD, USA

Introduction and Purpose

Women's participation in soccer has increased dramatically in recent years (2). However, women seem to be at greater risk for specific types of injuries than men (1). Modifiable injury risk factors and relevant assessments have been identified in this population. Among these, the convenient and inexpensive Gauntlet Test (GT) is used with soccer athletes to assess physical fitness, an intrinsic risk factor (3). However, there is little empirical support for the utility of the GT in this population to predict time loss injury during the competitive season. The purpose of the study was to investigate GT performance in intercollegiate Division I female soccer athletes, and determine if GT performance was predictive of injury.

Methods

GT trials were administered and recorded by the team's coaching staff during the pre-season testing period, approximately six weeks prior to any match play each season. Subsequent GT attempts were completed on successive days if any athlete was unable to complete the GT trial successfully. A GT trial was deemed successful if the athlete completed all five stages under the specified time limits (see Table 1).

Stage	Distance (m)	Run Time Allowed	Rest Time
1	1,600	6 minutes, 30 seconds	2 minutes
2	800	3 minutes, 30 seconds	1 minute, 30 seconds
3	400	1 minute, 30 seconds	1 minute, 30 seconds
4	200	45 seconds	1 minute, 30 seconds
5	100	18 seconds	

Table 1. Gauntlet Test

If an athlete was not successful on the GT at the initial attempt, the athlete's participation in team-based activities (practice, matches) was restricted until a successful GT trial. GT data was obtained via available fitness records and discussions with coaching staff.
GT results and demographic data, e.g., age, body mass index, and playing position, were retrospectively collected for intercollegiate Division I female soccer players over three consecutive seasons. Soccer-related injury characteristics that resulted in time loss from participation were obtained from the athletes' medical record maintained by the team's athletic training staff, and verbally verified.
Analyses using SAS 9.4 software (SAS Institute; Cary, NC; USA) include descriptive statistics and logistic regression with Receiver Operating Characteristic (ROC) analyses to define the relationship between GT results and subsequent injury.

Results

Seventy-one subjects met the inclusion criteria for data analysis, with mean age 19.6±1.2 yrs. Twelve lower body injuries and two head injuries occurred that resulted in time loss from participation. Eight of the lower body injuries were of minimal severity (1-6 days for return to play), while the remaining four injuries were severe in nature (return to play in 30+ days). The severity of injury (time to return to play) was not associated with GT performance (p=0.71). Logistic regression results are summarized in Table 2. Age, height, and weight were not predictive of time loss injury, either alone or in a predictive model including these predictors and GT results. Thus, results from a bivariate logistic regression using GT results to predict time loss injury are reported here.

Predictor	Bivariate OR	Multivariate OR
Age	1.30	1.286
Mass	0.996	1.015
Height	0.068	0.027
Gauntlet trials to success	3.578*	4.508*

Table 2. Logistic regression results. *P<0.02

ROC analysis results indicate that the Gauntlet Test has good diagnostic properties (AUC =0.714). The Youden index was 2 GT trials for success, at which sensitivity = 0.92 and specificity =0.46. For successive numbers of GT trials before success (1, 2, or 3), the predicted probabilities for injury were 0.063, 0.194, and 0.463.

Conclusions

The GT appears to be a convenient, affordable and predictive screen for potential lower body injury among female soccer athletes. With each unsuccessful GT attempt the odds that an athlete would sustain an injury increased significantly by a factor of 3.5. The majority of time loss injuries were of mild severity with relatively short duration for return to play.

References

1. Faude O, Junge A, Kindermann W, Dvorak J. Injuries in female soccer players: a prospective study in the German national league. Am J Sports Med 2005; 33: 1694-1700
2. FIFA Big Count 2006: 270 million people active in football. 2007; http://www.fifa.com/mm/document/fifafacts/bcoffsurv/bigcount.statspackage_7024.pdf. Accessed August 31, 2015
3. Wyss T, Von Vigier RO, Frey F, Mader U. The Swiss Army physical fitness test battery predicts risk of overuse injuries among recruits. J Sports Med Phys Fitness 2012; 52: 513-521

THE BIOMECHANICS AND EMG OF THE SUPPORT LEG DURING THREE TYPES OF FOOTBALL KICKING

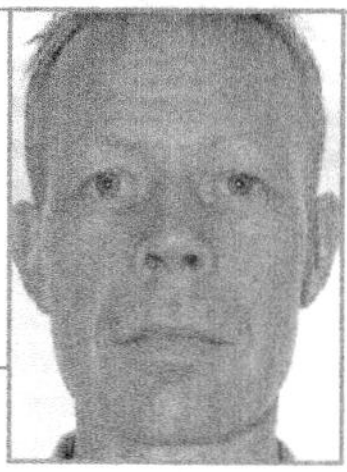

Ólafsson S[1], Gibbs S[2]

[1]Efling physical therapy, Akureyri, Iceland;
[2]University of Dundee, Dundee, United Kingdom

Introduction

Footballers start kicking at a young age while they are still growing. The effects of repetitive kicking on the support leg may potentially lead to overuse injuries and the long term effectsneeds further research. Most kicking studies have focused on the kicking leg, with limited investigation of the effects of kicking on the supporting leg, despite the majority of non-contact knee injuries occurring in single leg loading. No studies to date have examined the 3-D kinematics of the supporting hip, or Electromyography (EMG), of the role of the Adductor Longus, or compared the EMG of Biceps Femoris and Semitendinosus.

The objective of this study was to evaluate the biomechanics of the pelvis and the support leg, as well as to measure the EMG of the key muscles of the support leg, during kicking.

Methods

One group of experienced footballers, age 12-13 years, was compared to an elite group of players 18-19 years. Twelve players in each group performed Direct Kicks (DK) at 10°, Side-Foot Kicks (SFK) at 30° and Instep Kicks (IK) at 45° angles of approach. They all wore football boots (Adidas F3), and run up was three steps on artificial grass. The supporting hip, knee and pelvic angles were assessed using 27 reflective markers (eight Vicon cameras, Vicon, Oxford, UK).

The players landed on a force platform (AMTI, Watertown, USA) before kicking the ball into a net, and the EMG of eight lower limb muscles was recorded with eight Trigno wireless channels (Delsys Inc. Boston, MA, USA).

Results

The older players had 38% greater static knee varus. The mean measured Ground Reaction Forces (GRF) in three planes, were over 99 (X), 90 (Y) and 303 N/kg (Z). The vertical (Z) and posterior (X) breaking forces were greater at lower angles, but lateral forces (Y), with higher angles of approach. First Ground Contact (GC) was on the heel with a posterior lean of the torso, hip adduction and knee varus, coupled with high rotational loads on the pelvis, hip and knee (Figure 1).

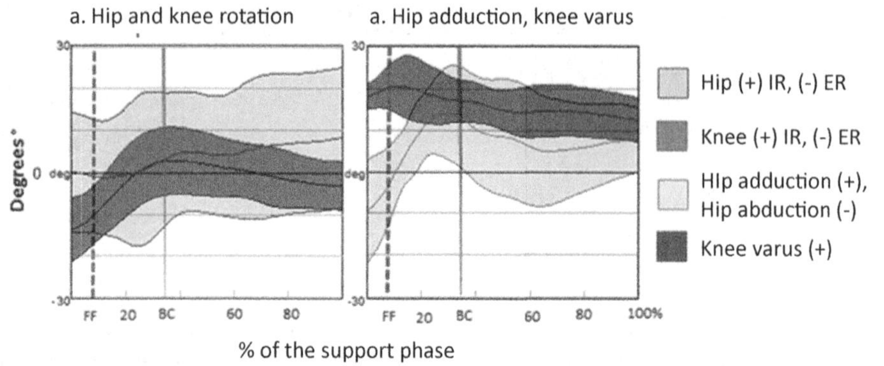

Figure 1. The hip and knee kinetics of an instep curved kick (U13s 8 kicks).

The peaks in GRF and joint forces, occurred at high velocities and loading rates. The vertical loading rate was over 200 times bodyweight per second, with the peak force near foot-flat.
At GC, the pelvis was in anterior pelvic tilt and maximum posterior rotation, with the support hip in relative external rotation and slight abduction.
At Ball Contact (BC) during all kicks, the hip was in adduction and knee varus and pelvic anterior rotation was only seen during DK and IK.
The Vastus Medialis exhibited the highest activity as a percentage of Maximal Voluntary Isometric Contraction (MVIC), at 214% in IK, followed by Vastus Lateralis.
The Biceps Femoris activity was greater than semitendinosus, with a similar pattern as the vasti and Gastrocnemius which peaked at BC.
Semitendinosus peaked earlier at GC.
Gluteus Medius was more active before BC, being 124% MVIC in DK, with lower activity in FT, during rotation of the pelvis.
Adductor Longus values, ranged from 82-92% MVIC, and tibialis anterior and gastrocnemius had important contributions to kicks.

Conclusions

The loading pattern in kicking puts strain on the supporting joints and may play a part in explaining the high incidence of Osgood-Schlatters in adolescence and hip and knee degeneration, in ex-football players.

USE OF WEARABLE ELECTROMYOGRAPHY IN REHABILITATION PROCESSES FROM MUSCLE INJURIES

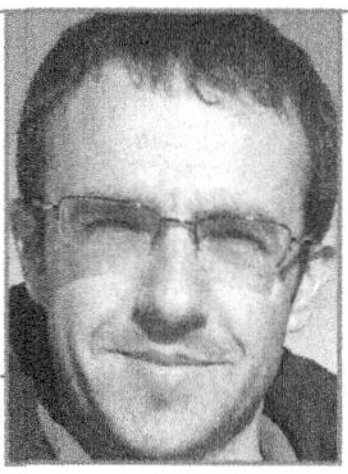

Gasol-Santa X[1], Turmo-Garuz A[1,2 3], Díaz-Cueli D[1], Ruzza M[3], Hoffren-Mikkola M[4]

[1]RCD Espanyol of Barcelona, Spain; [2]High Performance Center of Sant Cugat, Consorci Sanitari de Terrassa, Sant Cugat, Spain; [3]Professional Sports Medicine School, University of Barcelona, Spain; [4]Kuortane Olympic Training Center, Kuortane, Finland

Introduction

Due to huge burden caused by injuries and rehabilitation processes to professional football clubs, there is an increasing interest for objective monitoring of functional rehabilitation processes from muscle injuries. On the other side, there is an increasing development of wearable devices that are easy-to-use in many sport conditions. Time to return to play from injuries is critical and correct decisions about player's condition should be made in tight schedule. Unfortunately, the re-injury rate is high which highlights that additional methods to evaluate player's physical condition more precisely should be sought. Knapik et al. (2) reported a higher risk of injury in athletes with imbalances in knee flexor strength or hip flexibility greater than 15% between the right and left sides. With modern wearable electromyography (EMG) devices it is possible to monitor muscle imbalances in both laboratory as well as in field conditions including fast exercises that may better represent the real training and game conditions and requirements. This information may help football club professionals in decision making during functional rehabilitation processes and possibly therefore decrease and avoid further injuries. The objective of this study was to determine the use and importance of surface EMG (sEMG) data from wearable devices on decision making process during rehabilitation processes and return to play.

Methods

Subjects of the study were one elite goalkeeper and one elite midfielder of La Liga (Spain) aged 21 (193 cm, 91 kg) and 28 (174 cm, 72 kg) years, respectively, who had suffered grade II hamstring injuries affecting conjoint tendon. The goalkeeper's injury was located 12.0 cm from ischiatic tuberosity and was 5.0 cm long, without objective gap on muscle fibers. The midfielder's injury was located 9.5 cm from ischiatic tuberosity and was 4.5 x 2.0 cm in dimension involving muscle fibers of biceps femoris. In both cases diagnosis was made by ultrasound scan and magnetic resonance imaging two days after injury. According to Munich consensus of muscle injuries both of them were 3A type injuries (3).
Myontec's MBody Pro (Myontec Ltd, Kuopio, Finland) was used to monitor hamstring and quadriceps muscle groups sEMG in different gym and field exercises during the functional rehabilitation processes. The method has been validated against traditional sEMG and has been shown to be a reliable tool to assess EMG both in static and dynamic exercises (1). A follow-up evaluation was made based on Isometric Wall Squats (IWS) of 45 s of work and 15 s rest as well as four sets of 50 meters running at constant speeds (12 and 18 km/h) (Run12 and Run18, respectively). Tests were performed once a week.

Results

Results showed muscle activation asymmetries between injured and non-injured legs at various phases of rehabilitation processes. Asymmetries were reduced to the final phases of rehabilitation. Table 1 shows the relative sEMG in injured and uninjured leg for running and isometric wall squats at different measurement time points.

			Quadriceps			Hamstrings		
Player	week	Exercise	%EMG injured leg	%EMG uninjured leg	% diff	%EMG injured leg	%EMG uninjured leg	% diff
Goalkeeper	2	IWS	43.9	56.1	21.2	43.0	57.0	24.5
Goalkeeper	3	IWS	49.5	50.5	2.0	47.1	52.9	11.0
Goalkeeper	4	IWS	47.6	52.4	9.2	34.5	65.5	47.3
Midfielder	2	IWS	40.9	60.0	33.2	36.3	63.7	43.0
Midfielder	3	IWS	39.8	60.2	33.8	49.6	50.4	1.6
Midfielder	4	IWS	46.6	53.4	12.7	54.0	46.0	-14.8
Goalkeeper	3	Run12	44.1	55.9	21.1	32.8	67,2	51.2
Goalkeeper	4	Run12	44.3	55.7	20.5	41.6	58.4	28.8
Midfielder	2	Run18	41.4	58.6	29.6	37.7	62.3	39.5
Midfielder	3	Run18	60.8	39.2	-35.5	47.8	52.2	8.4
Midfielder	4	Run18	51.8	48.2	-6.9	51.1	49.9	-2.3

Table 1. Difference (% diff) between injured and uninjured leg sEMG during various phases of rehabilitation process. IWS: Isometric Wall Squats; Run 12: running at 12 km/h; Run 18: running at 18 km/h.

Conclusions

Clinical interpretation of sEMG data may be useful in monitoring the course of the injury.
sEMG registered in fatigue could help to show up asymmetries that could be otherwise undetectable in last stage of the rehabilitation process.

References

1. Finni T, Hu M, Kettunen P, Vilavuo T, Cheng S. Measurement of EMG activity with textile electrodes embedded into clothing. Physiol Meas 2007; 28: 1405-1419
2. Knapik JJ, Bauman CL, Jones BH, Harris JM, Vaughan L. Preseason strength and flexibility imbalances associated with athletic injuries in female collegiate athletes. Am J Sports Med 1991; 19: 76-81
3. Mueller-Wohlfahrt HW, Haensel L, Mithoefer K, Ekstrand J, English B, McNally S et al. Terminology and classification of muscle injuries in sport: the Munich consensus statement. Br J Sports Med 2013; 46:342-350

INTER-SEASON VARIABILITY OF A FUNCTIONAL MOVEMENT TEST IN PROFESSIONAL FOOTBALL

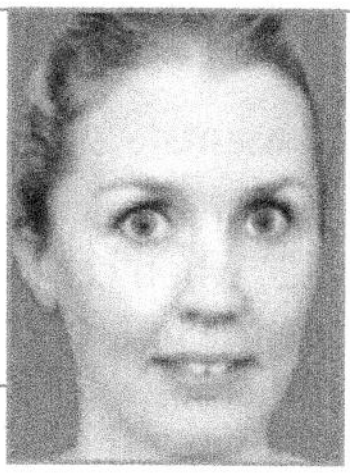

Bakken A[1,2], Targett S[1], Bere T[2], Eirale C[1], Farooq A[1], Tol JL[1], Whiteley R[1], Witvrouw E[1], Khan K [1,3], Bahr R[1,2]

[1]Aspetar Orthopaedic and Sports Medicine Hospital, Doha, Qatar; [2]Oslo Sports Trauma Research Center, Norwegian School of Sport Sciences, Oslo, Norway; [3]Center for Mobility and Hip Health, University of British Columbia, Vancouver, Canada

Introduction

Functional movement tests have become popular components of clinical examinations, intended to identify the player at risk for injury, to determine treatment response and also used in the return to play decision (2).

The Nine Plus screening battery test (9+) is a functional movement test intended to identify multiple movement factors predisposing the athlete for injury or re-injury (1). However, the inter-season variability of the 9+ test is unknown. To be able to meaningfully interpret differences in a test result, the normal variation, in the absence of any intervention, is important to document.

The purpose of this study was therefore to examine the stability of the 9+ test between two consecutive seasons in a group of professional male football players.

Methods

A total of 236 asymptomatic, Qatar Star League football players performed the 9+ as part of their annual pre-season musculoskeletal Periodic Health Evaluation (PHE) at the start of the 2013-2014 and 2014-2015 seasons.

Players were tested on eleven tests of the 9+: Squat, one-legged squat, the Norwegian squat, in-line lunge, hip flexion, straight leg raise, push-up, diagonal lift, rotation, shoulder mobility and drop jump.

Movement quality for each test was graded on a four-point scale (0-3) with a maximum total score of 33.

All players were blinded to their 9+ score from the previous season and no intervention was initiated from test 1 to test 2.

Information on time-loss lower extremity injuries in training and matches during the intervening football season was obtained from the Aspetar Injury and Illness Program.

Results

A significant increase in mean total score of the 9+ test battery was found at year 2 (+1.5±0.3, SE) when compared to year 1 (22.2±4.1 (SD); P<0.001); however, the stability was low (intraclass correlation coefficient (ICC (95%CI)): 0.26(0.13-0.38)).
Among the 236 players, 124 players had a ≥1 time-loss lower extremity injury (absence of >1 day) between the two 9+ test scores.
There was an improvement in mean total scores in both the injured (+2.0±0.4 (SE), P<0.001) and uninjured (+1.0±0.4, P=0.02) groups. However, the stability between year 1 and 2 was low in both the injured (ICC (95% CI): 0.30 (0.11-0.46)) and non-injured group (ICC (95% CI): 0.22 (0.04-0.38)). Players with a severe lower extremity injury (≥ 28 time-loss days; N=36) had the highest increase in mean total score between year 1 and year 2 (+3.0±0.8 (SE); P=0.001); again, stability was low in this group (ICC (95% CI): 0.22(-0.06-0.49)).

Conclusions

There is substantial intra-individual variability in mean total score of the 9+ test between two consecutive seasons irrespective of injury and severity of injury. Additionally, there is a small but systematic improvement from one season to the next.
The 9+ is therefore expected to have limited predictive value in terms of future injury risk. Also, usefulness of the test may be limited for other clinical purposes.

References

1. Frohm A, Heijne A, Kowalski J, Svensson P, Myklebust G. A nine-test screening battery for athletes: a reliability study. Scand J Med Sci Sports 2012; 22: 306-315
2. Hegedus EJ, Cook CE. Return to play and physical performance tests: evidence-based, rough guess or charade? Br J Sports Med 2015; 49: 1288-1289

Sunday 10th April, 2016 (morning)
FLEMING ROOM

INVITED SPEAKERS

CAN REGENERATIVE MEDICINE CHANGE RETURN TO PLAY OUTCOMES?

Chairs

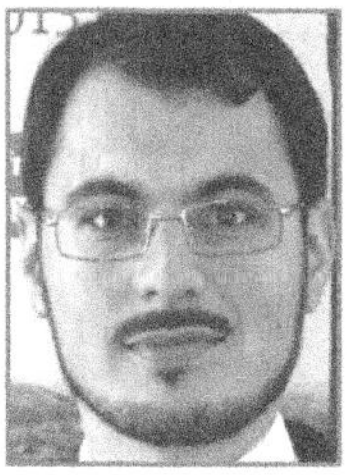

Giuseppe Filardo
(Bologna, Italy)

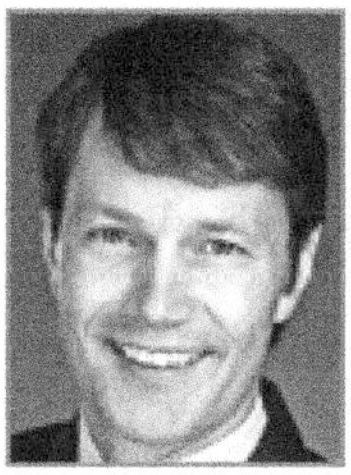

Kai Mithoefer
(Boston, USA)

8:00	Platelet rich plasma and return to play: scientific, clinical and ethical implications **Nicola Maffulli (Salerno, Italy)**
8:15	Future trends: are stem cells the answer? **Laura De Girolamo (Milan, Italy)**
8:30	Regenerative medicine role in return to play after muscle and tendon injuries **Ramon Cugat (Barcelona, Spain)**
8:45	How can regenerative medicine affect return to play after cartilage injuries? **Riley Williams III (New York, USA)**
9:00	A team's experience with regenerative medicine **Lluis Til y Perez (Barcelona, Spain)**
9:15	Discussion
9:30	End of the session

PLATELET-RICH PLASMA AND RETURN TO PLAY: SCIENTIFIC, CLINICAL AND ETHICAL IMPLICATIONS

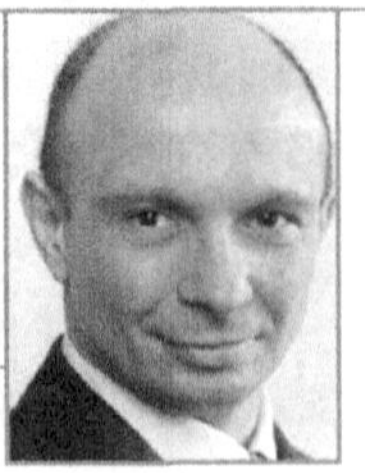

Maffulli N

Institute of health Science Education, Barts; The London School of Medicine and Dentistry, London, United Kingdom; Dipartimento di Medicina e Chirurgia, Università degli Studi di Salerno, Italy

Introduction

We critically review clinical studies after Platelet-Rich Plasma (PRP) therapy for tendinopathy, plantar fasciopathy, and muscle injuries. We review PRP formulations used across studies; and identify knowledge deficits that require further investigation.

Methods

After a systematic review in PubMed, we identified clinical studies assessing PRP efficacy in tendon and muscle during the past decade. We standardized data extraction by grouping studies based on anatomic location; summarized patient populations, PRP formulations, and clinical outcomes; and identified knowledge deficits that require further investigation.

Results

Overall, 1,541 patients had been treated with PRP in 58 clinical studies.
Of these, 26 addressed upper limb tendinopathies and 32 addressed the lower limb (810 patients and 731 patients treated with PRP, respectively).
The quality of research is higher for the upper limb than for the lower limb (23 controlled studies, of which 17 are Level I, v 19 controlled studies, of which 6 are Level I, respectively).
Patients have been treated mostly with leukocyte-platelet-rich plasma, except in the arthroscopic management of the rotator cuff.
The safety and efficacy of PRP for muscle injuries has been addressed in 7 studies including 182 patients.
Differences across results are mainly attributed to dissimilarities between tissues and different stages of degeneration, numbers of PRP applications, and protocols.

Conclusions

Given the heterogeneity in tendons and tendinopathies, currently, we are not able to decide whether PRP therapies are useful. Despite advances in PRP science, data are insufficient and there is a clear need to optimize protocols and obtain more high-quality clinical data in both tendinopathies and muscle injuries before making treatment recommendations.

FUTURE TRENDS: ARE STEM CELLS THE ANSWER?

de Girolamo L

Galeazzi Orthopaedic Institute, Milan, Italy

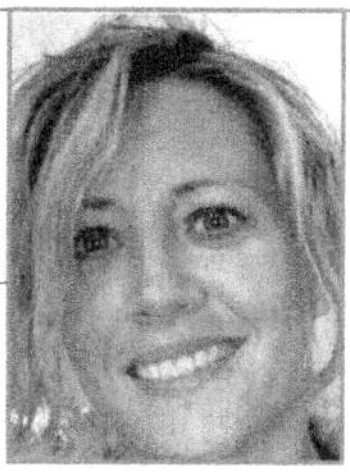

In the last decades, multipotent Mesenchymal Stem/Stromal Cells (MSCs) emerged as a possible powerful tool in the treatment of various disease related to tissue degeneration, inflammation and trauma. The documentation that MSCs are derived from perivascular cells, pericytes explains how MSCs can be isolated from almost every tissue in the body. However specific sites have been identified as particularly favorable in order to obtain a considerable number of cells to be used for tissue repair (1). In particular although bone marrow is still the most common source of MSCs, in the last two decades there has been a continuous effort to identify alternative sources of MSCs, mainly driven by a constant quest for a "more convenient" source (2). The subcutaneous adipose tissue has recently gained a great attention as a source of MSCs due to a simple and less invasive method of harvesting, and to a higher yield of MSCs if compared to bone marrow. Infrapatellar Hoffa fat pad has been also found to be a good source of MSCs, although his harvesting could be controversial. The potential of MSCs can be exploited by either using expanded cells or concentrated progenitor pools. The use of expanded stem cells allows a more reproducible treatment, as it is possible to isolate a purer MSC population and to know exactly the number of cells used in each treatment, making this approach more controlled. However, the treatment with autologous expanded cells is a two-step procedure, which makes it more invasive and of a higher cost. Furthermore, the need for extensive cell manipulation makes expanded cells as an Advanced-Therapy Medicinal Product (ATMPs) subjected to more complicated regulatory requirements for their use in clinical practice. As a result, a number of different devices for the intraoperative concentration of both bone marrow and adipose tissue-derived MSCs have been developed and are commercially available today. These progenitor cell concentrates are easier to use; they have all advantages of a one-step surgery procedure, though containing a lower number of MSCs in comparison to expanded cell suspension and differing markedly in composition. Although traditionally the regenerative capacity of MSCs was identified in their presumptive plasticity, their therapeutic effect seem to be particularly due to their paracrine function through the secretion of a broad range of bioactive molecules. Their potential is exploited through immunomodulation, angiogenesis, support of growth and differentiation of local stem and progenitor cells, chemo-attraction, anti-scarring and anti-apoptosis effects (3). This allows to consider MSCs as therapeutic agents even if they do not engraft or differentiate into tissue-specific cells, thus significantly increasing the range of MSCs therapeutic applications. Within this range, regenerative medicine and stem cell therapies hold much promise for the treatment of various injuries and diseases suffered by sportspeople. In particular, MSCs have been demnostrated to be effective in the treatment of cartilage, tendon and muscle injuries, either when used in combination with surgery or alone as injective treatment of cell concentrates. Thanks to their anti-inflammatory and immune-modulatory potential, MSCs can be an useful tool to accelerate the rehabilitation phase after surgery, promoting the return to a normal tissue homeostasis, and thus leading to a faster return to play. However, no high level study has investigated the real effectiveness of this approach in term of return to play so far. Nevertheless, the avoidance of surgery and long recovery times being replaced by immediate relief, the proved biological potential of these cells, their safety profile and their ease of use should make this approach to be considered a potentially useful tool acting in sinergy with all the other traditional rehabilitation techniques to allow athletes to return to sport as sooner as possible.

References

1. Caplan AI. Adult mesenchymal stem cells: when, where, and how. Stem Cells Int 2015; 2015: 628-767
2. Marmotti A, de Girolamo L, Bonasia DE, Bruzzone M, Mattia S, Rossi R, Montaruli A, Dettoni F, Castoldi F, Peretti G. Bone marrow derived stem cells in joint and bone diseases: a concise review. Int Orthop 2015; 38: 1787-1801
3. Murphy MB, Moncivais K, Caplan AI. Mesenchymal stem cells: environmentally responsive therapeutics for regenerative medicine. Exp Mol Med 2013; 45: e54

HOW CAN REGENERATIVE MEDICINE AFFECT RETURN TO PLAY AFTER CARTILAGE INJURIES

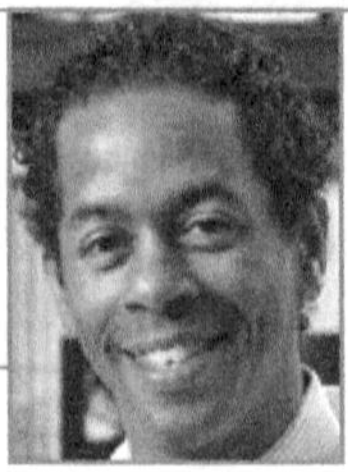

Williams RJ III

New York Red Bulls and Hospital for Special Surgery, FIFA Medical Centre of Excellence, New York, USA

Articular cartilage injuries can be devastating for the elite athlete. Such injuries typically occur in the knees and ankles of high level soccer players world wide. Unfortunately, there is exists no one standard method of regenerating normal functional articular cartilage repair tissue in affected athletes. However, current nonoperative and operative modalities are increasingly effective in restoring function and enabling a return to high level sports.

Nonoperative modalities including viscosupplemenation and Platelet Rich Plasma (PRP) injections have shown some promise in decreasing pain and increasing function in individuals affected by early osteoarthritis of the knee. Randomized trials comparing both visco-supplementation (hyaluronic acid) and PRP to placebo injection demonstrated significant short term functional improvement (Filardo G, Di Matteo B, Di Martino A, Merli ML, Cenacchi A, Fornasari P, Marcacci M, Kon E. Platelet-Rich Plasma intra-articular knee injections show no superiority versus viscosupplementation: A Randomized Controlled Trial. Am J Sports Med 2015; 43: 1575-1582; Patel S, Dhillon MS, Aggarwal S, Marwaha N, Jain A. Treatment with platelet-rich plasma is more effective than placebo for knee osteoarthritis: a prospective, double-blind, randomized trial. Am J Sports Med 2013; 41: 356-364). Such strategies can be employed to affected athletes in-season and in other circumstances where timing prevents a more definitive operative repair.

Long term functional recovery following articular cartilage injury is best achieved with operative repair. Historically, microfracture arthroplasty has been the most frequently used method for treating these injuries in high level athletes. Unfortunately, numerous studies have demonstrated that even in cases of good short term outcomes, most athletes experience a deterioration of function after 2-3 years.

Modern methods of articular cartilage repair now focus on the use of cell and tissue based repairs including autologous osteochondral transplantation, Autologous Chondrocyte Implantation (ACI), minced allograft tissue implantation (DeNovo NT), synthetic scaffold implantation and whole tissue allograft transplantation (1, 2, 3. These tissue based approaches provide athletes with a durable repair tissue that is superior to the fibrocartilaginous tissue characteristic of cartilage lesions treated with microfracture.

Cell and tissue based cartilage repair methods are best suited to regenerate articular cartilage lesions and should be used primarily to predictably and durably return high level soccer players to sport.

References

1. Crawford DC, DeBerardino TM, Williams RJ 3rd. NeoCart, an autologous cartilage tissue implant, compared with microfracture for treatment of distal femoral cartilage lesions: an FDA phase-II prospective, randomized clinical trial after two years. J Bone Joint Surg Am 2012; 94: 979-989
2. Kon E, Filardo G, Berruto M, Benazzo F, Zanon G, Della Villa S, Marcacci M. Articular cartilage treatment in high-level male soccer players: a prospective comparative study of arthroscopic second-generation autologous chondrocyte implantation versus microfracture. Am J Sports Med 2011; 39: 2549-2557
3. Krych AJ, Robertson CM, Williams RJ 3rd; Cartilage Study Group. Return to athletic activity after osteochondral allograft transplantation in the knee. Am J Sports Med 2012; 40: 1053-1059

Sunday 10th April, 2016 (morning)
CHURCHILL AUDITORIUM

INVITED SPEAKERS

LONG TERM CONSEQUENCES OF INJURIES

Chairs

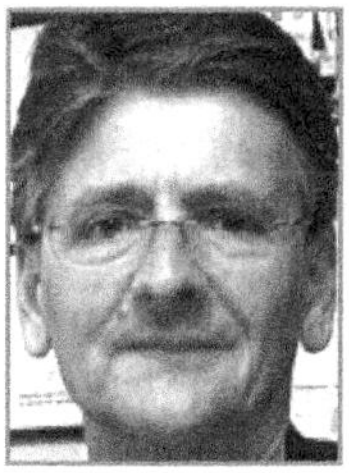

Mark Batt
(Nottingham, United Kingdom)

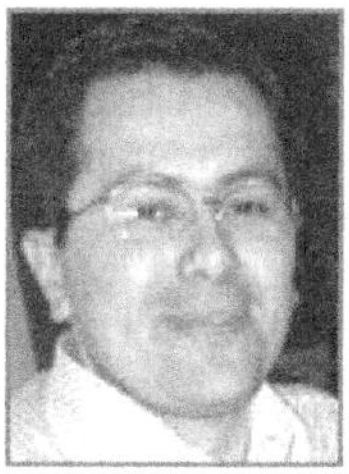

Emanuel Papacostas
(Thessaloniki, Greece)

8:00 Managing the last years of career of high injury risk players
Kristof Sas (Ronse, Belgium)

8:15 Most common medical problems in players after retirement
Luis Serratosa (Madrid, Spain)

8:30 Life after football: medical care for ex footballers
Charlotte Cowie (Burton, United Kingdom)

8:45 Mental health in current and retired players
Vincent Gouttebarge (Amsterdam, The Nederlands)

9:00 Long term management of osteoarthritis in the retired players
Ewa Roos (Odense, Denmark)

9:15 Discussion

9:30 End of the session

MANAGING THE LAST YEARS OF CAREER OF HIGH INJURY RISK PLAYERS

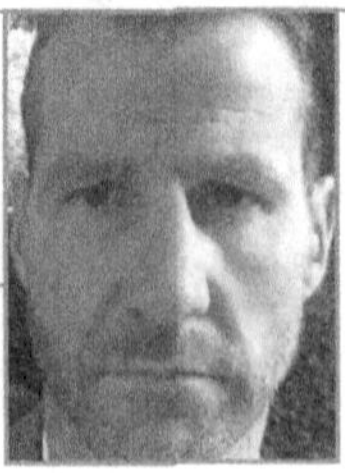

Sas K

AZ Glorieux, Ronse, Belgium

When working with elite footballers for a long time, you notice different kinds of careers:

1. The most frequent one: from ±18 up to ±34 years of age
2. The very long careers (which is rather rare): from ±18 years of age or younger until 38 years of age or even older (e.g. Ryan Giggs, Roger Milla, Teddy Sheringham, Javier Zanetti; but most of them are goalkeepers – cf. Buffon, Shilton, Mondragon, Brad Friedel, etc...)
3. In between type 1 and 2 you will find a lot of players who played until 32-34 at the highest level and who take things easier at a later stage or end in lower divisions.
4. The short careers with players rising very quickly but disappearing afterwards due to sports related or medical reasons (or even because they suffered from a sort of burn-out) (the best example is certainly George Best).

Filtering these different kinds of careers through the eyes of a doctor, we notice that the first type are often players regularly suffering from (small) injuries but who also played on a more than decent level. They consequently succeeded in coming back each time to their pre-injury level. We find type 2 amongst players who were rarely (seriously) injured and who really were top players (often even international level; i.e., the above mentioned examples). Type 3 are often players who were rarely injured but either reached the top at a later stage (they aren't exhausted mentally yet) or were less talented and accepted more easily to play on a lower level. In the group of short careers we find players who in an early stage had to quit football (due to several (re)injuries or one fatal injury), sometimes even before their career really began. But in this group we also find these young promising players not able to consolidate their status and who completely disappeared from the scene. They very often did not succeed in coping with the status and/or high expectations.

It is important to focus on how we can make sure that players will not end up in group 4, but in group 1 or 3. This is indeed one of the most important challenges for a team doctor: taking care of high injury risk players in a way that they are not or not often injured while still performing on the highest possible level.

Logically, we can't achieve this by our own! We therefore need an optimal cooperation between the coach/manager, the physical coach and the team doctor. In that respect I always speak in terms of a 'golden triangle': the coach/manager being on top of the triangle (he is after all taking the ultimate decisions) while the physical coach and the team doctor are at the baseline angles. They should ensure a good balance between load capacity and workload. The team doctor should make an accurate evaluation of the load capacity to avoid that the player's workload is higher than his load capacity which will ultimately result in 'underperformance' or even worse in an injury; the physical coach on the other hand is responsible for the workload. He should determine the right workload for every single player in order to prepare him for an optimal performance, avoiding 'undertraining' and thus 'underperformance', but also avoiding overtraining which will also result in 'underperformance' or even injuries. If both the team doctor and the physical coach are real experts in their jobs, each player will be able to perform in an optimal way, enabling the head coach/manager to go for the best possible team performance. This explains the 'golden triangle'.

But this triangle is obviously as strong as its weakest link. That's why a club should invest in each of these three areas to expect top performances (depending of course on the quality that is present in the selection).

This leads us to presumably the core business of a team doctor: managing high injury risk players. It is our task to evaluate the injury risks by using different test protocols.
For young players primary prevention is usually applied; for older players who might be ending their career soon secondary and even tertiary prevention will be more important. This means actually that young players who often only recently are exposed to the higher load and demands of professional football (the transition from youth to professional football) need to be protected against themselves. In this area scientific tools are nowadays available, making our decisions more easy to take: Creatine Phosphokinase (CPK), urine osmolality, heart rate, Rate of Perceived Exertion (RPE), Global Positioning Systems (GPS), etc... Regarding somewhat older players we will have to rely more on their 'feeling' and our experience. Very often these players suffer from a major injury from the past or a global joint damage. From the age of 30 on the majority of top level players suffer from cartilage damage in one or several joints, e.g., as a consequence of Anterior Cruciate Ligament reconstruction, joint instability, cam lesion, (partial) meniscectomy, etc... Mostly these players perfectly know how to cope with repetitive efforts. Our job is to monitor/supervise the process and when necessary communicate with/justify towards the coach/manager.
Despite the huge scientific progress of the past decade, our job remains (at least partially) a piece of art, where knowledge (science) and experience are completed by a kind of a 'sixth sense' or 'fingerspitsegefuhl'. That is what makes our job beautiful and exciting, but also very difficult.

MOST COMMON MEDICAL PROBLEMS IN PLAYERS AFTER RETIREMENT

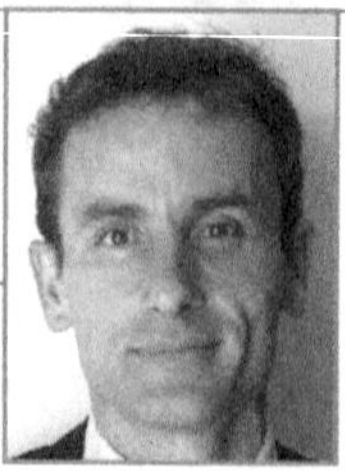

Serratosa L

Ripoll & De Prado Sports Clinic, FIFA Medical Centre of Excellence, Hospital Universitario Quiron, Madrid, Spain

It is widely accepted that exercise and sport have long-term health benefits for participants. But all physical activity carries also risks of injury and illnesses that occasionally may have long-term consequences. In the last decades there is an increased interest in the link between professional sports and the risk of future disease. The truth is that nowadays, data about the health status and health behaviour of former elite athletes is still scarce.

Football is the most popular sport worldwide with around 300 million registered players and a high injury incidence compared to other sports. Football injuries are more frequent at the elite level and some might have long-term consequences mainly related with increased risk of premature Osteo-Arthritis (OA) of the knees, hips and ankles. OA of the lower limbs is a common cause of pain and disability, may affect more than one joint and therefore have a negative impact in the Health Related Quality of Life (HRQL) of former football players (3). Knee is the most commonly affected joint and also the one that is more often associated with permanent disability in footballers (3). Some studies have shown that team sports athletes have lower mortality due to cardiovascular diseases than age-matched controls (2), but there also appears to be consensus in that the benefits of prior sports participation are not maintained unless the physical activity is continued. OA may decrease the level of physical activity and lead to obesity, worsening of the lipid profile, increased risk of developing hypertension and type II diabetes, and thereby increase the risk of cardiovascular disease in retired players.

OA has also been shown to interfere with employment opportunities, especially of physically demanding jobs such as football coaching/management and may as well have a negative impact in the psychological well-being and own health perception of former football players (3).

Anxiety and depression among other symptoms related to mental disorders appear to be more prevalent among retired professional footballers, and are correlated with history of severe injuries during the player's career (1).

In the last decades, we have also seen a growing interest in the possible neuro-psychological deficits associated with the cumulative effects of heading in football players.

Another aspect of concern may be the adverse long-term effects (gastrointestinal, cardiovascular, renal) associated with the overuse and abuse of Non-Steroidal Anti-Inflammatory Drugs (NSAIDs) and analgesics among professional football players.

Sports clinicians and all involved parties should dedicate more efforts to reduce the long-term physical and psychosocial consequences of football injuries as well as to develop supportive measures for retired players.

References

1. Gouttebarge V, Aoki H, Kerkhoffs GM. Prevalence and determinants of symptoms related to mental disorders in retired male professional footballers. J Sports Med Phys Fitness 2015 Mar 27. [Epub ahead of print]
2. Sarna S, Sahi T, Koskenvuo M, Kaprio J. Increased life expectancy of world class male athletes. Med Sci Sports Exerc 1993; 25: 237-244
3. Turner AP, Barlow JH, Heathcote-Elliott C. Long term health impact of playing professional football in the United Kingdom. Br J Sports Med 2000; 34: 332-336

MENTAL HEALTH IN CURRENT AND RETIRED PLAYERS

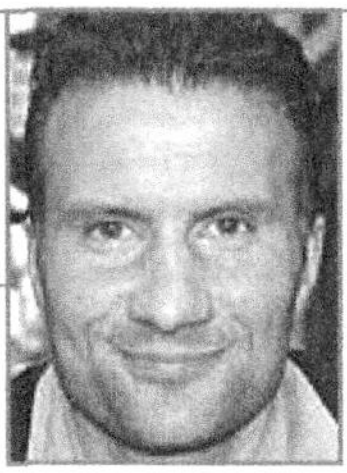

Gouttebarge V[1,2], Kerkhoffs G[2]

[1]World Players' Union (FIFPro), Hoofddorp;
[2]Department of Orthopaedic Surgery, Academic Medical Center, Amsterdam, Netherlands

Introduction

During their career, professional footballers are highly at risk for musculoskeletal injuries. Especially severe or recurrent injuries among professional footballers are considered to be major physical and psychosocial stressors as those induce long periods out of training or competition for players. In common with elite athletes from other sport disciplines, these physical and psychosocial stressors may predispose on short- and long-term to mental health problems such as distress and anxiety/depression. In the worst cases, severe or recurrent injuries may lead to early retirement from professional football, involuntary retirement being a potential risk for post-sport life mental health problems.

In contrast to the extensive amount of information available about severe or recurrent musculoskeletal injuries, scientific information about the occurrence of mental health problems among current and retired professional footballers is scarce. Whether severe musculoskeletal injuries during a football career are related to the occurrence of mental health problems among current or retired players remains unclear. Consequently, the aim of the study was to explore the potential relation of football-related severe musculoskeletal injuries with mental health problems (distress, anxiety/depression, sleep disturbance, adverse alcohol use) among current and retired professional footballers.

Methods

Cross-sectional analyses were performed on baseline questionnaires from an ongoing prospective cohort study among current and retired professional footballers. Inclusion criteria for the participants were: i) being between 18 and 45 years old; ii) being male; iii) being able to read and comprehend texts fluently in either English, French or Spanish; and iv) being a member of the national players' union either in Belgium, Chile, Finland, France, Japan, Norway, Paraguay, Peru, Spain, Sweden and Switzerland. Being a member of the national players' union means committing and/or have committed significant time to football training and competing at the highest or second highest professional football level.

The number of severe injury during professional football career was examined with a single question. In our study, severe injury was defined as one that affected the musculoskeletal system and occurred during team activities, leading to either training or match absence for more than 28 days. Assessed through validated scales, the outcome measures in our study were distress (Distress Screener), anxiety/depression (12-item General Health Questionnaire), sleep disturbance (PROMIS short form) and adverse alcohol use (AUDIT-C).

Based all variables included in the study, an electronic questionnaire was set-up in English, French and Spanish. Prevalence rates and 95% confidence interval (95% CI) were calculated. Univariate logistic regression analyses (expressed as odds ratio OR and related 95% CI) were used to explore the relation between severe injury and mental health problems.

Results

A total of 789 participants were included in the analyses: 540 current players (response rate of 37%) and 219 retired players (response rate of 69%). Current players were on average 27 years old and have been playing professional football for 8 years (54% in the highest leagues). Retired players were on average 35 years old (mean career duration of 12 years) and were retired from professional football for 4 years.
Of the current players, 45 % had incurred one or two severe musculoskeletal injuries during their career and 33% three or more. The number of severe musculoskeletal injuries during a football career was correlated with distress, anxiety/depression and sleep disturbance. Current players who had sustained one or more severe musculoskeletal injuries during their career were two to nearly four times more likely to report mental health problems than current players who had not suffered from severe musculoskeletal injuries.
Of the retired players, 44 % had incurred one or two severe musculoskeletal injuries during their career and 41% three or more. The number of severe musculoskeletal injuries during a football career was correlated with anxiety/depression and sleep disturbance but no statistically significant associations were found.

Conclusions

It can be concluded that the number of severe musculoskeletal injuries during a professional football career is correlated and associated with mental health problems, especially among the current players. These results emphasises the importance of applying a multidisciplinary approach to the clinical care and support of professional footballers facing lengthy periods without training and competition as a consequence of recurrent severe injuries. Also, supportive measures such as an end-career examination might be needed for retired players.

LONG TERM MANAGEMENT OF OSTEOARTHRITIS IN THE RETIRED PLAYERS

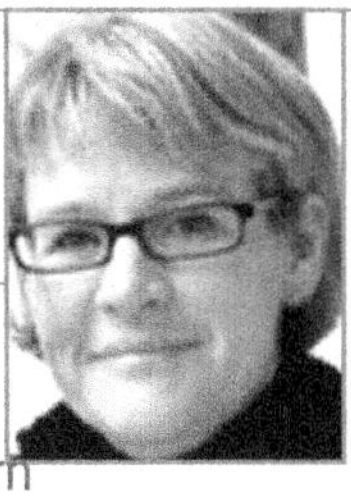

Roos EM

Department of Sports and Clinical Biomechanics, University of Southern Denmark, Odense, Denmark

Treatment goals for young patients with old knees include empowering patients to self-manage their symptoms to allow physical activity to promote good general health.
Upon presenting himself to the health care professional some 10-20 years after sustaining the major joint injury that significantly altered his career, the ex-athlete commonly express that he is suffering from a "sports injury". The health care professional, who notice pain, some stiffness and the ex-athlete not being able to participate in the physical activities he wants, diagnose the ex-athlete with Osteo-Arthritis (OA). Both perspectives are perfectly valid, but a common understanding of the diagnosis and of how to treat the symptoms and regain function is a pre-requisite for a long-term successful outcome. To merge the different views of the ex-athlete and health care professionals formalized education is indicated.
There are unfortunately few quick fixes with a sustainable long-term outcome. Outcome is deteriorating with additional number of surgeries, and joints are replaced at younger age is those with a prior injury.
Interestingly, and despite a background in sports, similar risk factors for worse outcome are seen in ex-athletes as in other populations. Increased body weight and lower education are risk factors for worse outcome also in ex-athletes. Muscle weakness is also a risk factor for symptoms and OA, and here ex-athletes have a more favorable situation since they are well aware of what it takes, and often are interested in improving muscle strength and function.
Unfortunately participating in soccer or other ball sports during the weekend and do nothing else during the week is rarely good for the OA knee. While physical activity is good for the general health, it may be deleterious for the OA joint and OA-specific exercise therapy is needed to optimize knee function. To achieve the best result, supervised exercise therapy is recommended to get going.

Sunday 10th April, 2016 (morning)
FLEMING ROOM

INVITED SPEAKERS

RETURN TO PLAY FOLLOWING MUSCLE INJURIES

Chairs

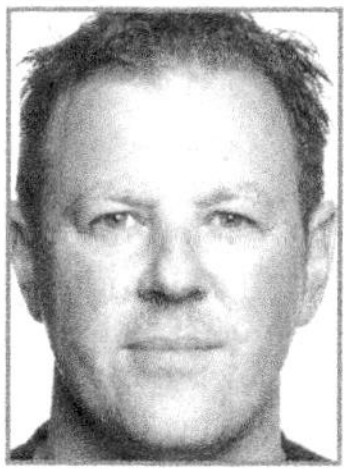

Colin Lewin
(London, United Kingdom)

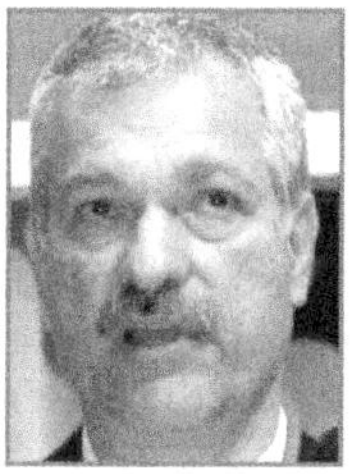

Nikos Malliaropoulos
(Thessaloniki, Greece)

9:30 Managing return to play in players with recurrent hamstrings injuries
Carl Askling (Stocholm, Sweden)

9:45 Return to play after quadruiceps injury
David Fevre (Blackburn, United Kingdom)

10:00 Return to play case history after adductor injury
Zafar Igbal (Beckenham, United Kingdom)

10:15 Calf injuries and return to play considerations
Seth O'Neill (Leichester, United Kingdom)

10:30 Return to play after compartment syndrome
Tony Edwards (Auckland, New Zeland)

10:45 Discussion

11:00 End of the session

1

MANAGING RETURN TO PLAY IN PLAYERS WITH RECURRENT HAMSTRING INJURIES

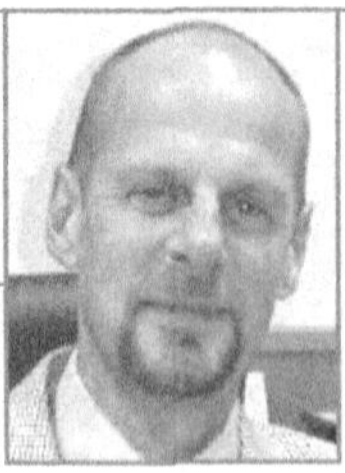

Askling CM

Swedish School of Sport and Health Sciences,
and Section of Orthopaedics and Sports Medicine, Department of Molecular Medicine and Surgery, Karolinska Institutet, Stockholm, Sweden

Introduction

Acute hamstring injuries are, year after year, the single most common injury in European professional football. Despite secondary prevention strategies, the recurrence rate seems not to decrease. The return to play from acute hamstring injury is a difficult multifactorial decision, and there is no consensus on a single clinical or functional test or imaging investigation that provides strict criteria for safe return.

Definition hamstring re-injury

Injury at the same anatomical location as the primary one. Classified as early, if the re-injury occur no more than 2 months after return or late, 2-12 months after return.

Previous hamstring injury - strongest riskfactor

The strongets risk factor for hamstring injury appears to be a previous history of hamstring injury. Some reasons for this increased risk could be incomplete tissue healing and/or low eccentric hamstring strength and/or between limb imbalance in eccentric hamstring strength.

Re-activiation of BFlh - a major problem

Approximately 80% of all acute hamstring injuries in elite football have their primary location in Biceps Femoris long head (BFlh) and typically occur during high-speed running actions. Almost all re-injuries also hit BFlh and the recurrence rate among BFlh is as high as 18% for European elite football. That indicates inadequate rehabilitation program or a premature return to football, in worst case, a combination of both.

It has been suggested that the cause of eccentric weakness in the commonly injured BFlh is prolonged neuromuscular inhibition of voluntary activiation, probably pain-driven in the early phase.

Since most hamstring injuries in football occurs when hamstrings is in a lengthened state, hipflexion combined with knee extension, rehabilitation protocols should be preferentially biased toward exercises that attempt to mirror that particular situation with high loads at long muscle-tendon lengths.

L-protocol & Askling H-test - eliminate re-injuries?

A recent study on Swedish elite football players, showed that a rehabilitation protocol consisting of lengthening type of exercises (L-protocol) was significantly more effective to promote return to full team training/match compared with a conventional protocol (C-protocol) after acute hamstring injuries (mean 28 days vs 51 days), respectively (1, 2).
An active ballistic hamstring flexibility test, Askling H-test, could provide useful additional information to the common clinical examination before allowing return to full team training and/or match. A combination of L-protocol and Askling H-test seems to be effective to both promote return and to avoid re-injuries (3).

References

1. Askling CM, Tengvar M, Thorstensson A. Acute hamstring injuries in Swedish elite football: a prospective randomized clinical trial comparing two rehabilitation protocols. Br J Sports 2013; 47: 953-959
2. Askling CM, Tengvar M, Tarassova O, Thorstensson A. Acute hamstring injuries in Swedish elite sprinters and jumpers: a prospective randomized clinical trial comparing two rehabilitation protocols. Br J Sports 2014; 48: 532-539
3. Askling CM, Heiderscheit BC. Acute hamstring muscle injury: types, rehabilitation, and return to sports. In: Doral MN, Karlsson J (EDS). Sports Injuries. Prevention, diagnosis, treatment and rehabilitation. Springer-Verlag, Berlin, 2015, pp. 2137-2147

RETURN TO PLAY AFTER QUADRICEPS INJURY

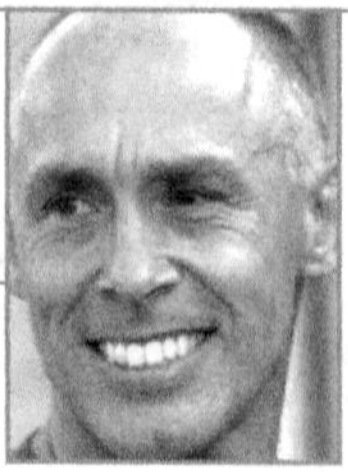

Fevre D

Sports Medicine, Blackburn Rovers FC, Blackburn, United Kingdom

Introduction

Quadriceps muscle injuries in sport are usually caused either by direct trauma, in the form of a blunt collision force, or indirect trauma following a powerful eccentric muscle contraction. The primary injury, often referred to as a 'dead leg' is a fairly conventional sports injury to rehabilitate, only occasionally leads to complications and very rarely leads to re-injury. The secondary injury type usually involves kicking or sprinting and the quadriceps strain accounts for 5.1% of total injury in male professional football (2) compared to 7% in female soccer players (NCAA 2012).
In isolated anatomy, the quadriceps femoris muscle group has four components of which the direct head of the central Rectus Femoris (RF) originates deep to tensor fascia lata and sartorius from the anterior inferior iliac spine of the pelvis. The indirect head originates from the superior acetabular ridge and travels deep and parallel to the direct head tendon. Due to its biarticular nature, the RF flexes the hip and extends the knee. The other three vasti (lateralis, medialis and intermedius) originate from various parts of the femoral shaft with all four components attaching to the patella via the quadriceps tendon. In the more functionally based myofascial anatomy pathway, RF is the key component of the superficial front line and its activity in the sagittal plane is closely linked to that of the rectus abdominis via the pelvis. All components are innervated by the femoral nerve.

Therapy

Non operative therapy in the majority of cases is the normal rehabilitation protocol. Injury that involves more than 15% of the RF cross-sectional area and/or is longer than 13 cm in length results in a prolonged recovery time (1). Injuries of the RF central tendon also results in a significantly longer rehabilitation interval than injury in the periphery of the RF and the vastus musculature (1). Surgical intervention may be necessary in complete tears, persistent pain with non-operative treatment, reattachment of displaced avulsion fractures and large haematoma collections (3).

Return to play

The Return to Play (RTP) rehabilitation programme for quadriceps injury begins before the injury occurs. In the professional world of sport this is more feasible than for the recreational sportsperson as baseline information can be obtained during various stages of the athlete's annual training calendar such as pre-season or as part of a transfer screening protocol. Key components related to quadriceps injury include assessment of the myofascial meridians such as the Superficial Back Line and Superficial Front Line (SBL and SFL), the Thomas Test and the Stride Flexibility Test (SFT) to assess specific hip flexor, RF and corresponding hamstring length.
Isokinetic muscle strength testing with conventional and functional, concentric and eccentric based test speeds also contribute to the individual player profile.
Information related to these individual multi-factoral components can help to minimise injury risk but does not totally eliminate the unexpected components which occur in sporting activity.
The therapist needs an appreciation of the healing process in order to design a safe, appropriate and functional based rehabilitation programme. As healing of the quadriceps injury occurs, several key rehabilitation goals must be achieved before the final stage rehabilitation phase can be entered into safely.
Functional movement in any sporting activity must incorporate maintained stability of the athlete in combination whilst successfully distributing resultant strain across the body during activity. A primary action muscle such as RF requires the complete myofascial components of the SFL to act to achieve the desired goal. The ability to recognise this process during rehabilitation is a key component in reducing the risk of re-injury in relation to all RTP pathway protocols.

References

1. Cross TM, Gibbs N, Houang MT, Cameron M. Acute quadriceps muscle strains: magnetic resonance imaging features and prognosis. Am J Sports Med.2004; 32: 710-719
2. Ekstrand J, Hägglund M, Waldén M. Epidemiology of muscle injuries in professional football (soccer). Am J Sports Med 2011; 39: 1226-1232
3. Waterman S. Section B: The thigh. In: DeLee JC, Drez D Jr, Miller MD (Eds). DeLee and Drez's Orthopaedic Sports Medicine. 3rd ed. Philadelphia: Saunders Elsevier; 2009: 1493-1497

CALF INJURIES AND RETURN TO PLAY CONSIDERATIONS

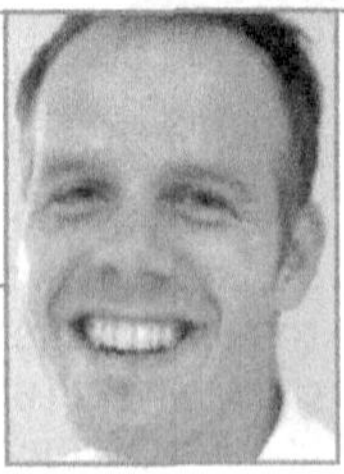

O'Neill S

University of Leicester, United Kingdom

Muscle injuries to the calf account for around 13% of all muscle injuries in professional football making it the 4th most injured group after hamstrings, adductors and quadriceps.

Despite the common occurrence of calf injuries little research has been undertaken into this area and most clubs employ variable Return To Play (RTP) strategies.

Current data predicts a squad of 25 players will have 15 muscle injuries within a season, equating to two calf injuries.

Most people assume that the gastrocnemius is most frequently injured, however new data suggests that the more common injury may be isolated soleus injuries or injuries combined with the gastrocnemius.

Calf injuries in particular seem to affect older players more frequently than younger players, this is an important consideration for clubs with older than average squads.

Calf injuries are not rapid to resolve, on average 15 days will be lost per calf injury, this is marginally more than per hamstring injury.

As we know the majority of muscle injuries are non-contact in nature suggesting that internal muscle forces may correspond to injury risk.

Due to the lack of primary research into calf injuries in elite football we have to draw on data from other posterior chain muscles (hamstrings) to understand how we might rehabilitate and prevent calf injuries.

RETURN TO PLAY AFTER EXERTIONAL COMPARTMENT SYNDROME

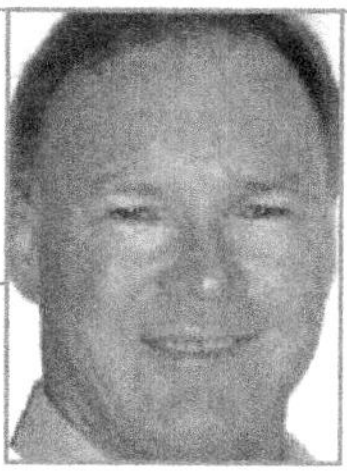

Edwards T

Axis Sports Medicine Specialists, FIFA Medical Centre of Excellence, Auckland, New Zealand

Exertional compartment syndrome is one of the three most common causes of exercise related lower leg pain in the player. It shares the honour with medial tibial periostalgia and stress fractures of the tibia or fibula. It is characterised by onset of pain and tightness after a period of pain free exercise and builds to a crescendo, usually stopping the player from exercising, at which point the pain settles quickly over a few minutes with rest. The pattern of pain differentiates this condition from the others, but the situation becomes blurred as the three conditions can frequently coexist. The differential diagnosis includes popliteal artery entrapment, referral from the lumbar spine, tumours such as osteoid osteoma and such anatomical variations as a low inserting soleus.

In the player with lower leg pain, our approach to management is initially conservative, with attention to the player's proximal stability, calf stretching, soft tissue treatments and podiatry intervention. If there are persistent symptoms despite intensive rehabilitation, then the diagnosis of compartment syndrome is made with post exercise pressure measurement of the affected compartments using the Stryker Intra-Compartment Pressure Monitor. Plain films along with Magnetic Resonance Imaging (MRI) or scintigraphy can help to rule out other pathologies. Some papers propose the use of MRI to make the diagnosis of exertional compartment syndrome (3), but in our hands it is primarily used to assess the presence of stress fracture or periosteal changes. Surgical fasciotomy is the treatment of choice if exertional compartment syndrome is the confirmed diagnosis, and this is combined with medial tibial periosteal debridement if indicated (1, 2).

The process of Return To Play (RTP) in our programme starts immediately post operatively. The player remains in hospital overnight with surgical drains in place to minimise haematoma formation and hence minimising fibrosis. In the first week post operatively the player rests, uses crutches as needed, and is reviewed at the seven to ten day mark and dressings removed. They start exercise biking at the two week mark depending on their wound repair, and then deep water running and beginning some progressive walking by week three-four. If the surgery only involves the anterior compartment then the player will begin a progressive running programme at the four-five week mark. This begins as steady state running, building from ten minutes in a stepwise fashion up to 30 minutes and then a progression into repeated sprint work. They are usually training at the six week mark with graduated loading. They will return to full training at eight weeks.

In those who have had superficial and deep compartment fasciotomy then the return to play is slower and they will bike and deep water run for up six to eight weeks, before the they start running. This can be slower if surgery involves periosteal elevation and debridement and is symptoms based. The player will likely return to full training at the 10-12 week mark.

In conjunction with the progressive loading programme their rehabilitation involves addressing their kinetic chain and especially posterior chain strengthening. Attention to their footwear and muscle balance is imperative.

References

1. McCallum JR, Cook JB, Hines AC, Shaha JS, Jex JW, Orchowski JR. Return to duty after elective fasciotomy for chronic exertional compartment syndrome. Foot Ankle Int 2014; 35: 871-875
2. Packer JD, Day MS, Nguyen JT, Hobart SJ, Hannafin JA, Metzl JD. Functional outcomes and patient satisfaction after fasciotomy for chronic exertional compartment syndrome. Am J Sports Med 2013; 41: 430-436

Sunday 10th April, 2016 (morning)
CURCHILL AUDITORIUM

INVITED SPEAKERS

MEDICAL AND PSYCHOLOGICAL ISSUES IN RETURN TO PLAY

Chairs

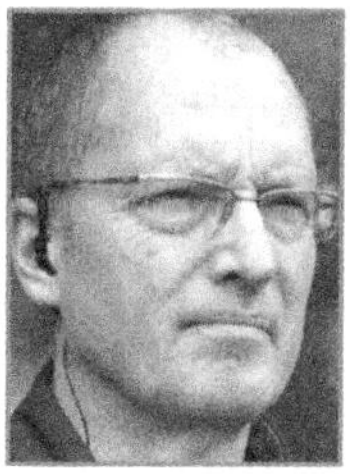

Ian Beasley
(London, United Kingdom)

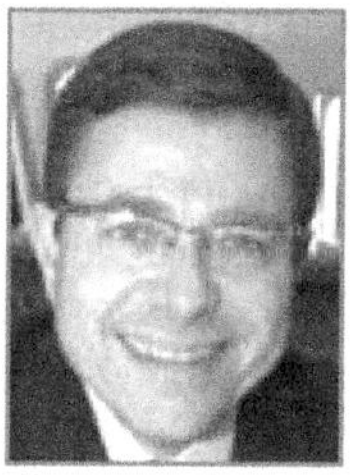

Fabio Pigozzi
(Rome, Italy)

9:30 Return to play criteria following concussion
Matt Perry (Albrighton, United Kingdom)

9:45 Heart disease and the complications for return to play
Sanjay Sharma (London, United Kingdom)

10:00 Return to play following medical illness
Martin Schwellnus (Pretoria, Republic of South Africa)

10:15 Nutrition support during injury and return to play
Ronald Maughan (Aberdeen, United Kingdom)

10:30 Cognitive behavioural therapy and fear of re-injuries
Thomas Marcacci (Bologna, Italy)

10:45 Discussion

11:00 End of the session

RETURN TO PLAY CRITERIA FOLLOWING CONCUSSION

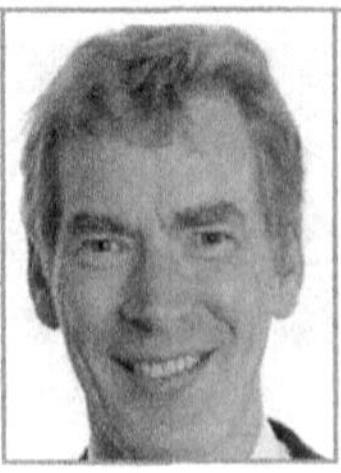

Perry M

English Premier League, London and Wolverhampton Wanderers FC, Wolverhampton, United Kingdom

When an apparently concussed player remains on the pitch, or returns to competition too soon this behaviour places a player at risk of further, potentially catastrophic injury. This event may reflect poor knowledge amongst players, poor standards amongst doctors, poor safety systems within clubs or poor regulation within football (2).
In April 2015 the Football Association (FA) convened a panel of national and international experts to develop new national concussion guidelines. In November 2015 the FA Concussion Guidelines were published. They include clear Return to Play (RTP) criteria and define a Graduated Return to Play Protocol (GRTP). The standard GRTP lasts a minimum of 19 days (adults) and 23 days (ages 17-19) following complete resolution of symptoms.
An Enhanced Care Standard (ECS) is defined. The ECS definition establishes medical criteria which permit a shorter timeframe for the GRTP. If the medical criteria are met, and following complete resolution of symptoms, RTP may occur after a minimum of 6 days (Adults) and 12 days (ages 17-19).
The FA guidelines (3) differ from the Zurich Consensus Guidelines (1) and consider the implications for medical provision and player safety in English Football.
The FA's Concussion Guidelines are a very powerful statement of best practice for the grassroots and the professional game. They are an important public health document concerning:

- The Criteria for the Enhanced Care Setting.
- The role of Clinical Guidelines in RTP decisions in Professional Football.
- The legal and ethical duty of care owed by doctors (Good Medical Practice, Non Maleficence, Beneficence, Confidentiality) to players/patients returning to play following concussion.
- The legal duty of care owed by clubs/employers to employees returning to work following injury (Health and Safety at Work Act, Health Surveillance, Risk Assessment).
- The rights of a player wishing to return to play (autonomy, mental capacity) when considering subjective measures of recovery, objective measures of recovery and time based criteria.
- The challenges these guidelines raise for the leagues, the clubs and their medical staff.

To achieve effective change the guidelines need to improve knowledge amongst players, standards amongst doctors and safety systems within clubs. Accordingly they should be supported by an implementation program that includes education both at grass roots level (Parents, Children, Teachers, and Coaches) and at professional level (Clinicians, Officials, Coaches, Players and Club Directors)
The duty of professional clubs and leagues is to provide an appropriate clinical environment in which to assess support and protect players (employees) recovering from this potentially serious work related injury.

Whilst clinical guidelines are not binding, doctors working in professional sport will recognise that the legal requirements on the doctor and employer are closely aligned. Both share a duty to protect the welfare and long term wellbeing of their patient and employee.
A Club Doctor's responsibility must now include:

- The measurement of baseline neurocognitive function allowing objective assessment of recovery.
- Study of the different manifestations of concussion and their associated recovery and treatment trajectories.
- Provision of education programs for players and coaches within the club.
- An understanding of Occupational Health regulations.

References

1. Consensus Statement on Concussion in Sport issued by the 4th International Conference on Concussion in Sport, Zurich 2012. http://bjsm.bmj.com/content/47/5/250.full
2. Fuller C W. Implications of health and safety legislation for the professional sports person. Br. J. Sports Med 1995; 29: 5-9
3. The FA's Concussion Guidelines. http://www.thefa.com/my-football/coach/concussion

RETURN TO PLAY FOLLOWING ACUTE MEDICAL ILLNESS

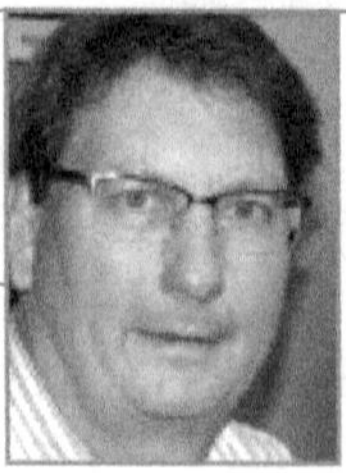

Schwellnus M

Institute for Sport, Exercise Medicine and Lifestyle Research, Faculty of Health Sciences, University of Pretoria, South Africa

Acute illness affects about 1 in 10 athletes during periods of competition, but there is some evidence that this is more common during periods of intense training.
The majority of these acute illnesses affect the respiratory tract, followed by the gastro-intestinal tract and the cause is attributed to infective illness in most cases.
Participation in exercise training or competition whilst suffering from an acute illness is not only associated with reduced exercise performance, but can also increase the risk of acute medical complications, including serious life-threatening medical complications.
The current Return To Play (RTP) guidelines for acute respiratory tract illness are largely based on the clinical tool, known as the "neck-check".
However, there are very few research data validating the use of the "neck-check" as the RTP guide following acute illness.
Recent data do indicate that athletes with acute illness that is associated with systemic symptoms or signs, who return to competition, have a 2-3 times higher risk of reduced exercise performance.
There are also data indicating that these athletes, participating with an acute illness that is associated with systemic symptoms or signs, have an increased risk of medical complications during exercise.

NUTRITION SUPPORT DURING INJURY AND RETURN TO PLAY

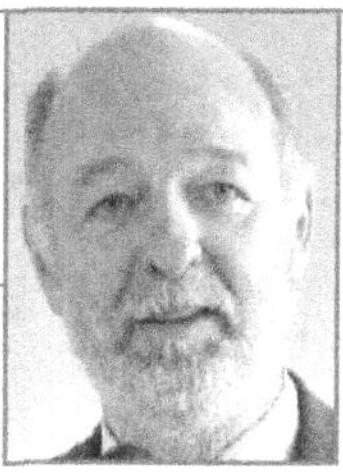

Maughan RJ[1], Shirreffs SM[2]

[1]University of Stirling, Stirling;
[2]St Andrews University, St Andrews, United Kingdom

The nutritional demands of intensive training and competition require athletes to adopt specific strategies to ensure that their energy intake is appropriate to their nutrition goals and that a sufficient amount of all of the essential macro-and micro-nutrients is consumed.

During periods of reduced training, and especially during enforced inactivity caused by injury, the daily energy expenditure is reduced by the amount normally expended during training plus any further reduction caused by curtailment of the activities of daily living. When the normal training load is substantial, this may mean a reduction of up to 50% in the habitual energy expenditure. This in turn means a substantial reduction in the total amount of food eaten each day if an unwanted increase in body mass, and more especially in body fat content, is to be avoided. Nevertheless, an adequate intake of energy and protein must be maintained to limit the muscle wasting that normally accompanies a period of inactivity.

To achieve this reduction in energy intake while still meeting all nutrient needs will likely require increased attention to the selection of the foods that are eaten. While it might be necessary to reduce the intake of fat and carbohydrate, the intake of protein should be maintained during the recovery and rehabilitation phases.

It may also be useful to review the distribution of the protein intake over the day to ensure an adequate intake in the early part of the day: breakfast and lunch should each provide at least 20-25 g of protein and high-protein snacks may be useful if there is a long gap between the main meals.

Where total energy intake is severely restricted, a broad-spectrum multi-vitamin, multi-mineral supplement may be prescribed: provided this is obtained from a reputable manufacturer and supplier (and ideally has been approved by one of the recognised supplement testing programs) it is a low-risk solution to any concerns over micronutrient intake.

A number of supplements are advertised as promoting tissue repair after injury, but the evidence for most is limited or even non-existent.

Protein is undoubtedly important, but food sources are a preferred option.

There is some evidence that creatine supplementation may limit loss of muscle tissue and may promote muscle growth and strength development after injury or immobilisation.

An adequate intake of a number of nutrients - including anti-oxidants, iron, zinc, essential fatty acids and others - is important, but again food sources can provide adequate amounts and supplementation with excessive amounts may even be harmful in some cases.

5

COGNITIVE BEHAVIOURAL THERAPY AND FEAR OF RE-INJURIES

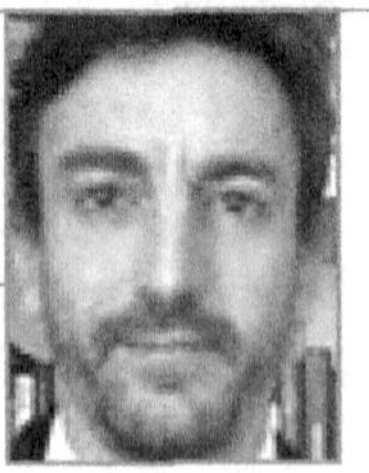

Marcacci T, Raboni D, Berti Ceroni F

Mood, Centre for the Study and the Cure of Mood Disorders, Bologna, Italy

Introduction

An injury is a particularly stressful event in a football player's career and it impacts on the person as a hole, on his sense of integrity, continuity and self-efficacy. Sensations, body experiences, emotions related to actions and representations changes deeply during the rehabilitation, compared to the period before the injury. Mood deflection, anxiety related to the course and the outcome of the rehabilitation, concerns about personal identity are reactions to expect in the normal path of the rehabilitation and therefore it is worth to treat them always to sustain the path toward the return to play and to prevent problems.

Issue

Our experience has been matured in Bologna, since 2009, within a collaboration between different healthcare professionals i.e, psychologists (Mood, Center for the Cure and the Study of the Emotional Distresses), sports physicians (Isokinetic Medical Group), orthopaedic surgeons (Rizzoli Orthopaedic Institute) and several coaches and trainers (sport clubs).

On the base of case reports and descriptive researches' data, several perspectives of psychological work with football players during rehabilitation can be considered, with particular attention to the critical moment of the return to play, through the different phases of reacquisition of the athletic gesture, resume of the contact with the ball, return to team and to competitions.

Several techniques of intervention can be utilised, set on the base of an evaluation of the patient's psychological need, in consideration of his psycho-physical state and of the career-moment when the injury occurs. Our work is exemplified in a setting of both individual and small group, showing the integrated use of several methodologies, aimed to tailoring the psychological intervention: psychoeducation, techniques of management of the psycho-physical tension, imagery, cognitive behavioural techniques, expressive therapy.

Furthermore, as an integration of the case reports, data descriptive of the psychological characteristics are collected from a sample of football players and other athletes through standardized questionnaires like the Profile of Mood State and the Tampa Scale of Kinesiophobia.

Conclusions

An injury is a particularly stressful event in a football player's career. The psychological dynamics which are intrinsically bounded to it, if left to chance, could lead to difficulty respect to the return to play even in a situation of a good physical resume.

The clinical and theoretical experience matured within the collaboration between different healthcare professionals shows the benefit to take care of the psychological aspects through all the rehabilitation path, both to prevent possible problems and to foster psychological competencies related to sport which enable an optimal return to play.

Sunday 10th April, 2016 (morning)
PICKWICK ROOM

FREE ORAL PRESENTATIONS

ORTHOPAEDIC SURGERY

Chairs

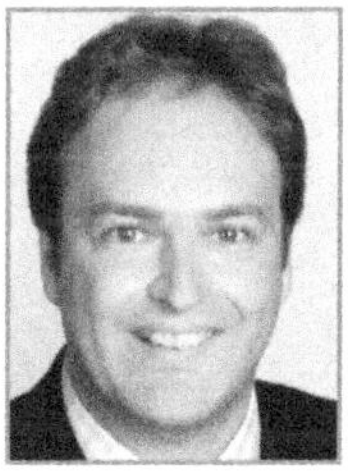

Peter Angele
(Regensburg, Germany)

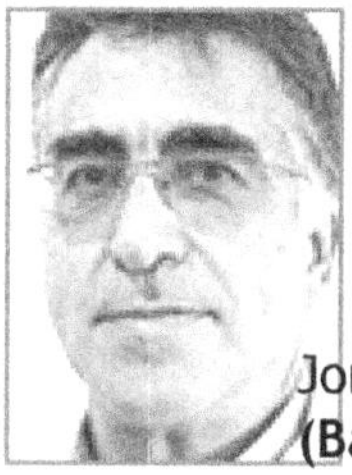

Jordi Ardèvol Cuesta
(Barcelona, Spain)

9:30 National ACL registry in football: the direct way for injury prevention and safe return to play **Angele P, Krutsch W (Regensburg, Germany)**

9:40 Dynamic functional ratio for scheduling return to play after anterior cruciate ligament reconstruction **Monnot D, Vigne G, Sonnery-Cottet B, Thaunat M, Fayard JM, Rogowski I (Lyon and Villeurbanne, France)**

9:50 The additional lateral tenodesis of the knee: early results in soccer players **Karachalios GG, Tamviskos A, Krinas G, Pavlides E, Milionis G (Pireus, Greece)**

10:00 Is sport activity possible after arthroscopic meniscal allograft transplant? **Marcheggiani Muccioli GM, Grassi A, Roberti di Sarsina T, Raggi F, Nitri M, Tsapralis K, Nanni G, Della Villa S, Marcacci M, Zaffagnini S (Bologna, Italy)**

10:10 Chronic pubalgia in footballers treated with a pyramidalis muscle release **Dimitrakopoulou A, Schilders E, Kartsonaki Ch, Cooke C (London and Oxford, United Kingdom)**

10:20 Prevalence of Cam morphology is higher in academy football players compared with a control population **Palmer AJR, Gimpel M, Fernquest S, Wotherspoon M, Birchall R, Newton J, McNally E, Arden N, Javaid K, Carr AJ, Glyn-Jones S (Oxford and Southampton, United Kingdom)**

10:30 Acutrak screw fixation for fifth metatarsal stress fracture in Japanese footballers **Katori Y, Matsunaga R, Sando T, Yamamoto K (Tokyo, Japan)**

10:40 Return to play football following surgical treatment for acute avulsion of adductor longus enthesis
Schilders E, Dimitrakopoulou A, Kartsonaki Ch, Cooke C (London, Leeds and Oxford, United Kingdom)

10:50 Discussion

11:10 End of the session

NATIONAL ACL REGISTRY IN FOOTBALL: THE DIRECT WAY FOR INJURY PREVENTION AND SAFE RETURN TO PLAY

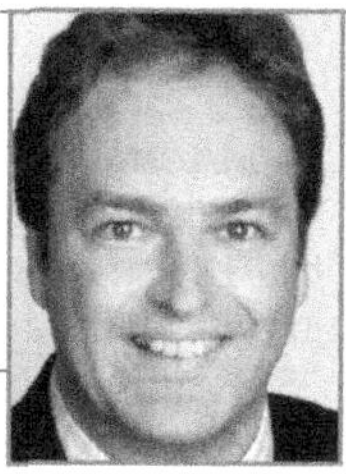

Angele P[1,2], Krutsch W[1]

[1]Department of Trauma Surgery, University Medical Centre Regensburg, FIFA Medical Centre of Excellence, Regensburg; [2]Sporthopaedicum Straubing, Regensburg, Germany

Introduction

Anterior Cruciate Ligament (ACL) injuries in football are common and main reason for frequent time out in football for more than six months. For an adequate injury prevention strategy, a detailed knowledge about influencing factors of ACL injuries is necessary. In the season 2014-2015 the ACL Registry in German Football was founded and a continuous monitoring of ACL injuries in professional and amateur football was started.

Methods

In a prospective investigation of ACL injuries in German football, a data documentation about incidence and influencing factors of ACL injuries in football is based on four column. The media screening of online and print media, the collaboration with the national football associations, the collaboration with the football clubs and the support of the health insurances are the fundament of the ACL football data. After registration of an ACL injured football player, two standardized questionnaire were filled out by the player. Topics of the two questionnaire are football exposure, pre-injuries, other influencing factors, performed treatment and return to play issues.

Results

One-hundred-fifty-three in seven specifically investigated Football Divisions were registered over one season in the national professional football and the amateur football of the Bavaria region. Additionally more than 400 ACL injuries in amateur player of other parts of Germany were also registered.

Average age in male players was 24.3 (range: 12-45) years, and 21.6 (range: 13-35) in female players.

A high rate of professional ACL injured athletes were of international level (57% of the First Division players) and 68% of the injuries in professional player happened in the pre-season period.

The male professional players revealed 33 ACL injuries in three Divisions (First, Second and Third) over one season, while 66% occurred in the first round of the season.

The First Division (n=14) showed more ACL injuries than the Second and Third Division.

The female First Division presented 11 ACL injuries, with two-thirds in defenders. ACL injuries were in general seen mainly as match injury (85.5%), as non-contact injury (71.1%) and had indication for surgical reconstruction (93.5%).

A little previous-injury was seen in two-thirds of the injuries as main influencing factor for the occurrence of ACL injuries, while these injuries happen on other body regions or represented overuse complaints in thigh, foot or back.

Weak training programs were seen in the majority of cases, where important exercises like jumping or balancing exercises (<40%) or trunk stability (<20%) were only performed in the minority of all teams with an ACL injured player.

Short-term changes on the football player are well known as influencing factor for ACL Injuries (1). Typical short term changes on the player with occurred ACL injury were presented in the registry by: 1) rise of a the team, 2) change of a team, 3) change of the team coach directly before ACL injury (50%).
33.3% of all ACL injured players changed their football shoes directly before the injury.
The Return To Play (RTP) after ACL injury showed no professional player in male football back on field within six months.

Conclusions

In the presence of still high rates of ACL injuries in amateur and professional football, injury prevention strategies should have highest priority for team coaches, clubs, football associations and players.
For an improvement of the prevention of ACL injuries, the preseason period as vulnerable period should be considered. Also massive short-term changes on player during the season should be avoided and replaced by step-for-step adaption, which is important for training issues.
In presence of successful prevention programs in the football medicine literature, the scientific data should transferred to football basis by teaching programs of the football associations.

References

1. Krutsch W, Zeman F, Zellner J, Pfeifer C, Nerlich M, Angele P. Increase in ACL and PCL injuries after implementation of a new professional football league. Knee Surg Sports Traumatol Arthrosc. 2014 Oct 8. [Epub ahead of print]

DYNAMIC FUNCTIONAL RATIO FOR SCHEDULING RETURN TO PLAY AFTER ANTERIOR CRUCIATE LIGAMENT RECONSTRUCTION

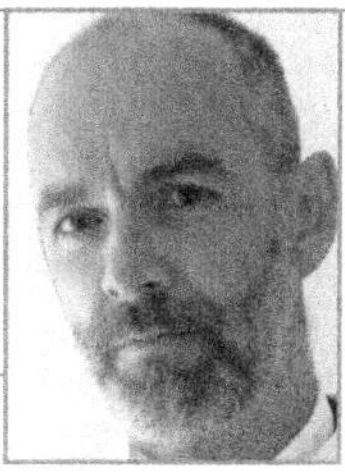

Monnot D[1], Vigne G[2], Sonnery-Cottet B[1,3], Thaunat M[1,3], Fayard JM[1,3], Rogowski I[4]

[1]Centre Orthopédique Santy, Lyon; [2]Athletic France, Lyon ; [3]Hopital privé Jean Mermoz, Lyon; [4]Université de Lyon, Centre de Recherche et d'Innovation sur le Sport-EA 647, Villeurbanne, France

Introduction

Anterior Cruciate Ligament (ACL) injury has the longest disability time and is the most costly injury in soccer players. After ACL reconstruction, the decision-making for return-to-play is commonly based on the functional isokinetic ratio, computed between the maximal torques produced by the Hamstrings during eccentric extension (Hecc) and by the Quadriceps during concentric extension (Qcon). Normal knee function is described by a ratio ranged between 0.9 and 1.0 (1). A major limitation of this ratio is however that the coincidence of maximal Quadriceps and Hamstrings torques do not arise during functional motions, as the maximal torques occur at different knee joint angles. It could be then helpful for return-to-play scheduling to assess this ratio during the course of knee joint extension, especially as Pataky (2) has interestingly proposed a methodology, called Statistical Parametric Mapping (SPM), to compare biomechanical behaviors for continuous field. Using SPM method, this study aimed at comparing the dynamic functional isokinetic ratio between healthy knees and knees after LCA reconstruction in soccer players.

Methods

1,894 patients, undergone LCA surgery between 2011 and 2015 by three surgeons, were bilaterally assessed isokinetically during the full 0-118° range of motion (Contrex MJ, Dübendorf, Switzerland) at six-month (±20 days) after surgery.
From this database, the results for 270 knees of 176 male soccer players (24.8±7.4 years old) were extracted and assigned into four groups. The healthy group (HG, n=95) included knees without history of surgery, and for which peak torques during isokinetic concentric extension and flexion at 90°/s were higher than 2.2 Nm/kg and 1.1 Nm/kg, respectively, and peak torques during eccentric extension at 30°/s was higher than 1.4 Nm/kg.
Other patients were assigned into three groups according to the type of autograft for the ACL reconstruction: Gracilis Tendon Graft (GTG group, n=34), Semitendinosus and Gracilis Tendon Graft (SGTG group, n=119), and Patellar Tendon Graft (PTG group, n=22).
The repetition including the maximal torque value of the isokinetic test was extracted from four repetitions of eccentric extension at 30°/s (Hecc), and from 20 repetitions of concentric extension at 240°/s (Qcon), then sampled into continuum position for the range of motion 90°-30° flexion angle (common range of knee joint flexion angle values for constant velocity).
The Dynamic Functional Isokinetic Ratio (DFIR) was then computed by divided each torque value of Hecc by Qcon. SPM for two independent groups was applied to compare DFIR between the healthy group and GTG, SGTG or PTG groups. Significant difference was set at $p<0.01$.

Results

The results showed that DFIR was significantly lower for 90-54° flexion range of motion in GTG (p=0.001) and for 90-71° flexion range in SGTG (p=0.01) than in HG, while DFIR was significantly higher for 90-40° flexion range in PTG than in HG (p<0.001).
The lower DFIR in GTG and SGTG groups suggested a muscular deficit in antagonist muscle, whereas the higher ratio in PTG group may reveal a muscular deficit in agonist muscle. Furthermore, such deficits mainly occurred in flexed knee position, and their effects on DFIR lasted on a shorter range of motion for SGTG than for GTG or SGTG groups.

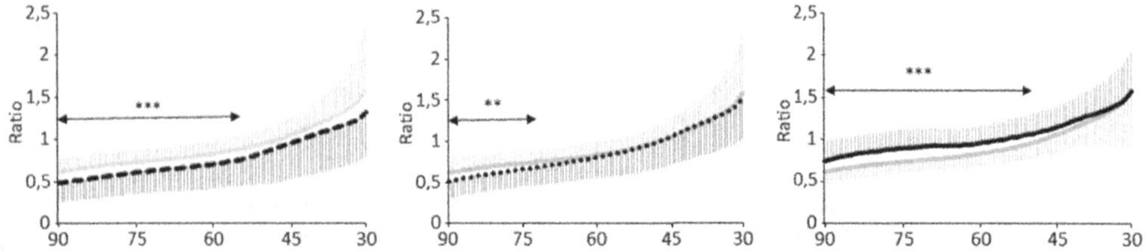

Figure 1. Mean (± standard deviation) DFIR for healthy group (grey line) and GTG (dotted line, left), SGTG (small-dotted line, center), or PTG (black line, right) over the course of knee joint flexion (in degrees), with ** for p=0.01 and *** for p≤0.001.

Conclusions

These findings revealed that the 6-months rehabilitation process did not allow the same recovery of knee function for all types of autografts used for ACL reconstruction. Such differences involved that the return-to-play may schedule strengthening exercises at specific angulations in order to recover the optimal knee function.
The dynamic functional isokinetic ratio brings new knowledge for rehabilitation and return-to-play scheduling, and its use by clinicians and fitness coaches may open up new opportunities to optimize the recovery time.

References

1. Coombs R, Garbutt G. Developments in the use of the hamstring/quadriceps ratio for the assessment of muscle balance. J Sports Sci Med 2002; 1: 56-62
2. Pataky TC. Generalized n-dimensional biomechanical field analysis using statistical parametric mapping. J Biomech 2010; 42: 1976-1982

THE ADDITIONAL LATERAL TENODESIS OF THE KNEE: EARLY RESULTS IN SOCCER PLAYERS

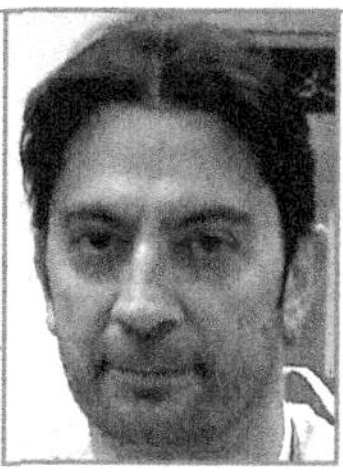

Karachalios GG[1], Tamviskos A[1], Krinas G[1], Pavlides E[2], Milionis G[2]

[1]Arthroscopic Surgery and Sports Injury Department, Metropolitan Hospital, Pireus;
[2]Laertion Rehabilitation Center, Pireus, Greece

Introduction

The residual pivot shift after an Anterior Cruciate Ligament (ACL) reconstruction is the main prognostic factor for athlete's satisfaction , functional stability and the protection of the knee from menisco-cartilage injuries (1).
The anterolateral stability is not fully restored using the intra-articular reconstruction (2), but could be improved by the addition of an extra-articular lateral tenodesis (3).
The aim of this study is to present our experience with this combined procedure regarding the time of return to play , the special issues during rehabilitation, the stability of the knee and an early follow-up.

Methods

Our study includes 37 patients who underwent this combined procedure, during 2014.
All they were male football players aged 16-34 years old: 3 playing in first division, 16 in second/third division and 18 amateurs. The inclusion criteria where: high demanding athletes, age <20, and clinical and signs of anterolateral instability: pivot shift and/or lateral compartment bone oedema in Magnetic Resonance Imaging (MRI). Twenty players had a concomitant meniscal injury: 8 we repaired, 7 trimmed and in 5 we proceeded to partial meniscectomy.
No chondral injury needed any special treatment.
The surgical technique consists in intra-articular ACL reconstruction using a 4-strand autologus hamstring tendon graft, retaining and, if possible, pulling out-the remnants of the torn ligament, notchplasty and monoloop, lateral tenodesis with a staple.
We fixed the iliotibial band initially with the knee in 90° flexion and after the tenth athlete in 20°-30° and the tibia in external rotation.
After surgery the patients followed the formal rehabilitation program by a high experienced physiotherapist in cooperation with a rehabilitation performance trainer. Special attention was given in early recovery of full extension.

Results

All the players, except one, returned to unrestricted training in less than seven months.
Twenty athletes had a flexion deficit of less than 5° and five had a minimal extension deficit without anterior knee pain.
One needed an arthroscopic reoperation due to symptomatic lack of extension.
During the latest assessment two had an anterior translation of 2 mm more than the contralateral knee (Rolimeter Knee Tester, Aircast Europa, Neubeuern, Germany), none had pivot sign and none reported subjective instability.
So far there is no any re-rupture of the graft , meniscal repair failure or secondary chondral injury.
21 footballers continued playing for the same team and five dropped to lower level.

Conclusions

Our early result concerning the addition of a lateral tenodesis to the intra-articular ACL reconstruction showed improved stability and protection of the knee without slowing down the rehabilitation time.

Finally, for athletes with high demanding pivot activities (such as footballers) this methods provides a more stable knee and offers an unrestricted return to play.

References

1. Ayeni OR, Chanal M, Tran MN, Sprague S. Pivot shift as an outcome measure for ACL reconstruction: a systematic review. Knee Surg Sports Traumatol Arthrosc 2012; 20: 767-777
2. Georgoulis AD, Ristanis S, Chouliaras V, Moraiti C, Stergiou N. Tibial rotation is not restored after ACL reconstruction with a hamstring graft. Clin Orthop Relat Res 2007; 454: 89-94
3. Monaco E, Labianca L, Conteduca F, De Carli A, Ferretti A. Double bundle or single bundle plus extraarticular tenodesis in ACL reconstruction? A CAOS study. Knee Surg Sports Traumatol Arthrosc 2007; 15: 1168-1174

IS SPORT ACTIVITY POSSIBLE AFTER ARTHROSCOPIC MENISCAL ALLOGRAFT TRANSPLANT?

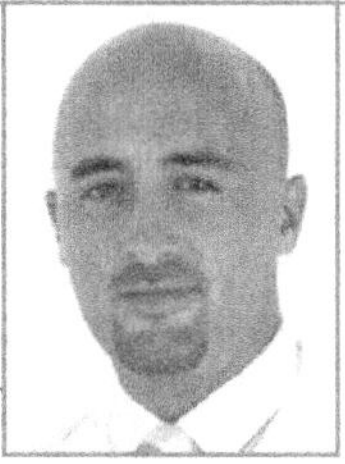

Marcheggiani Muccioli GM[1], Grassi A[1], Roberti di Sarsina T[1], Raggi F[1], Nitri M[1], Tsapralis K[2], Nanni G[2], Della Villa S[2], Marcacci M[1], Zaffagnini S[1]

[1]Istituto Ortopedico Rizzoli, Bologna; [2]Isokinetic Medical Group, FIFA Medical Centre of Excellence, Bologna, Italy

Introduction

Meniscal Allograft Transplantation (MAT) has produced good to excellent results in the general population (2); however, few investigations have examined MAT in athletes and sport-related outcomes.
Purpose: To report midterm clinical outcomes of MAT and the rate of return to sport in a physically active population.

Methods

The study included all physically active patients who underwent arthroscopic MAT without bone plugs (1) between June 2006 and March 2013 at a single institution and had a minimum of two years of follow-up.
Clinical evaluation was performed pre-operatively and at final follow-up with the Knee injury and Osteoarthritis Outcome Score (KOOS), the Tegner activity scale, and a 0- to 100-point subjective scale for knee function and satisfaction. Outcomes evaluated included ability to return to sport (Tegner score of 10), time to return to sport, level of sport activity upon return compared with pre-injury level, and level of decrease in sport participation or reasons for not returning to sport participation. Comparisons were made between patients who did or did not return to sport and between patients who returned to the same level or a decreased level. Regression analysis was performed to determine the variables affecting the outcomes.

Results

Eighty-nine (74 male; 15 female) patients whose mean±SD age at surgery was 38.5±11.2 years, were evaluated to a mean follow-up of 4.2±1.9 years.
Total KOOS improved from a mean±SD of 39.5±18.5 preoperatively to 84.7±14.8 at the latest follow-up ($p<0.001$).
Pain (measured as part of the KOOS) improved from 36.6±23.1 preoperatively to 89.6±14.1 at the latest follow-up ($p<0.001$).
The Tegner score improved significantly from a median of 2 (interquartile range [IQR], 1-4) preoperatively to a median of 4 (IQR, 3-6) at the latest follow-up ($p<0.001$), although it did not reach the pre-injury level of 6 (IQR, 5-7) ($p<0.001$).
Patient rated their knee function 83.9±18.0 and satisfaction 84.5±22.0 measured by a 0- to 100-point subjective scale.

Older age at surgery was correlated with the worst clinical results.
Sixty-six patients (74%) were able to return to sport 8.6±4.1 months after surgery.
Forty-four patients (49%) returned to the same level as pre-injury.
Twenty-three patients (26%) were unable to return to sport, the main reason was pain during high level activity.
Thirthy-six patients of the population study (40%) were soccer players: 23 of them (64%) were able to return to play soccer, 20 of them (55%) at the same level as pre-injury.
Patients who did not return to sport activity and those who reduced their activity level at follow-up had inferior subjective outcomes compared with those who returned to sport and those who returned to their pre-injury levels, respectively.
Only 11 patients (12%) underwent a surgical procedure during the follow-up period. Three patients underwent graft partial meniscectomy for a new traumatic lesion, three underwent arthroscopic debridement for knee pain, and one underwent peroneal nerve release due to scar entrapment after high tibial osteotomy. All these patients successfully returned to sport after the procedure. The other five patients (one unicompartmental knee arthroplasty, three hardware removal, and one patellar tendon repair) did not return to sport.

Conclusions

Arthroscopic MAT without bone plugs improved knee function and reduced pain, allowing sport resumption in 74% of patients and return to the pre-injury activity level in 49% of patients at midterm follow-up.

References

1. Marcacci M, Zaffagnini S, Marcheggiani Muccioli GM, Grassi A, Bonanzinga T, Nitri M, Bondi A, Molinari M, Rimondi E. Meniscal allograft transplantation without bone plugs: a 3-year minimum fol- low-up study. Am J Sports Med 2012; 40: 395-403
2. Verdonk PC, Demurie A, Almqvist KF, Veys EM, Verbruggen G, Verdonk R. Transplantation of viable meniscal allograft: survivorship analysis and clinical outcome of one hundred cases. J Bone Joint Surg Am 2005; 87: 715-724

CHRONIC PUBALGIA IN FOOTBALLERS TREATED WITH A PYRAMIDALIS MUSCLE RELEASE

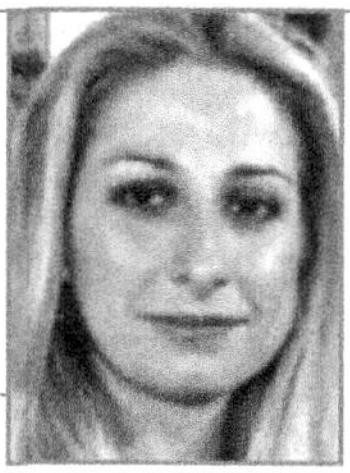

Dimitrakopoulou A, Schilders E, Kartsonaki Ch, Cooke C

The London Hip Arthroscopy Centre at The Wellington Hospital, London; Fortius Clinic; Leeds Beckett University, Leeds; and University of Oxford, Oxford, United Kingdom

Introduction

Pubalgia is a known cause of groin pain in athletes and represent a challenging entity in diagnosis and treatment. The complexity of the groin anatomy and the overlapped symptoms from different pathologies that may co-exist leading to chronic lower abdominal pain and disability in athletes. The purpose of this study is to report the clinical outcomes together with a new surgical technique and to determine if athletes could return to the same high level of performance promptly.

Methods

We included professional footballers who presented with chronic groin pain, pubalgia, pain resistant to non-operative treatment. Patients with associate sports' hernia (or inguinal disruption), osteitis pubis, adductor enthesopathy or hip pathology were excluded.

Demographic data and type of sports were noted. Medical history, clinical examination of the lower abdomen, groin and hip joint, imaging investigation and strength testing measurements were recorded.

All athletes were assessed for pain using a Visual Analogue Scale (VAS) and if they returned to sports at the same level as preoperatively.

Results

We assessed 18 footballers; 13 were professional and five were non-professional. All of them were males with a mean age 28.0±7.6 (SD) years old.

All of the athletes (100%) had constant pain during acceleration and some of them while striking a ball. The pain was localised on supra-pubic area radiating to midline 2-3 cm below the umbilicus (linea alba) and adductors area affecting their level of performance. Duration of symptoms was 7.5±6.8 months (range: 2-24 months).

Seven athletes had a pubic cleft injection (2, 3) prior to the surgery with short-term partially improvement of symptoms.

All athletes (100%) underwent bilateral Pyramidalis muscle release and Rectus Abdominis fascioplasty (1). The pain was improved and ranged from 0 to 3 postoperatively.

All of the patients (100%) returned to full training at a mean of 8.3±1.5 weeks (range: 6-12 weeks) and at their previous level of sporting activity 12 weeks post surgery but one athlete elected to stop playing due to ageing.

Conclusions

Pyramidalis muscle may cause long-standing pubalgia in footballers leading to disability and potential career-ending for the athlete.
A bilateral pyramidalis muscle release associated with rectus abdominis fascioplasty is a promising technique when prior non-operative treatment has failed.
Athletes have a prompt recovery and return to the same level of sports with this technique.

References

1. Martens MA, Hansen L, Mulier JC. Adductor tendinitis and musculus rectus abdominis tendopathy. Am J Sports Med 1987; 15: 353-356
2. Schilders E, Bismil Q, Robinson P, O'Connor PJ, Gibbon WW, Talbot JC. Adductor-related groin pain in competitive athletes: role of adductor enthesis, magnetic resonance imaging, and entheseal pubic cleft injections. J Bone Joint Surg Am 2007; 89: 2173-2178
3. Schilders E, Talbot JC, Robinson P, Dimitrakopoulou A, Gibbon WW, Bismil Q. Adductor-related groin pain in recreational athletes: role of adductor enthesis, magnetic resonance imaging, and entheseal pubic cleft injections. J Bone Joint Surg Am 2009; 91: 2455-2460

PREVALENCE OF CAM MORPHOLOGY IS HIGHER IN ACADEMY FOOTBALL PLAYERS COMPARED WITH A CONTROL POPULATION

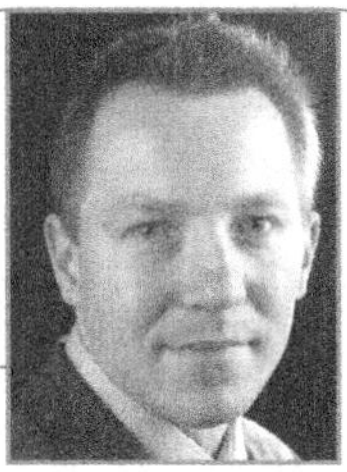

Palmer AJR[1], Gimpel M[2], Fernquest S[1], Wotherspoon M[2], Birchall R[2], Newton J[1], McNally E[1], Arden N[1], Javaid K[1], Carr AJ[1], Glyn-Jones S[1]

[1]Nuffield Department of Orthopaedics, Rheumatology, and Musculoskeletal Sciences, University of Oxford; [2]Southampton Football Club, Southampton, United Kingdom

Introduction

Femoroacetabular Impingement (FAI) is a common cause of hip pain and injury. The pathogenesis of the condition remains poorly understood and this significantly limits our ability to develop strategies for prevention, treatment, and rehabilitation. The prevalence of cam morphology is particularly high amongst professional footballers and is thought to develop in association with intense sporting activity during adolescence.

The purpose of this study is to understand how hip development differs between academy football players and a control population.

Methods

Players at an English Premiership Football Club Academy were invited to participate using a randomisation algorithm within each age group. The cross-sectional cohort was loaded towards the youngest age groups to enhance a future longitudinal study.

Twenty players were selected from the U10 and U11 teams, and 10 players from the U12, U13, U14, U15, U16, and U18 teams (n=100).

An age-matched population of volunteers from local schools were recruited as a control population (n=100). The control group comprised 50 males and 50 females.

Assessments were performed mid-season and morphological measurements were performed on Magnetic Resonance Imaging (MRI) of both hips (Achieva 3.0T, Philips Healthcare, Amsterdam, The Netherlands).

Participants completed questionnaires that included anthropometric data, past medical history, patient reported outcome measures, and validated activity scores. Assessments also included clinical examination, urine collection and physiological MRI. Morphological measurements were performed on 30 degree radial slices using in house software and the primary outcome was maximum alpha angle on radial slices.

Results

Maximum alpha angle measured on all radial slices increased with age (footballers r^2=0.403, p<0.0001; controls r^2=0.228, p<0.0001).
Mean maximum alpha angle in footballers was 82.68 degrees (95% CI: 77.98-87.39) for those with a closed physis compared with 58.65 degrees (95% CI: 56.42-60.87) for those with an open physis.
Mean maximum alpha angle in the control population was 63.54 degrees (95% CI: 61.06-66.01) for those with a closed physis compared with 56.25 degrees (95% CI: 54.46-58.05) for those with an open physis.
Within the control population, mean alpha angles were higher in males at 62.06 degrees (95% CI: 59.47-64.66) compared with females at 58.45 degrees (95% CI: 56.41-60.49).
Defining cam morphology as a maximum alpha angle greater than 60 degrees in any radial position, cam deformity was present in 93% footballer hips and 50% control hips in individuals aged over 16 years of age.
In footballers, the alpha angle is negatively correlated with internal rotation of the hip (r2=0.337; p<0.0001).
There was no statistically significant different in alpha angle between the dominant and non-dominant leg or playing position.

Conclusions

Cam morphology develops during adolescence and there is an extremely high prevalence amongst footballers compared with a general population cohort. Our general population cohort has a greater prevalence of cam morphology compared to other published studies and this is likely to reflect our use of maximum alpha across all radial slices and the increased likelihood of individuals who participate in sport to volunteer for our study.
Cam morphology is present in the vast majority of academy football payers by 16 years of age. When considering the treatment of hip and groin injuries it is important to identify whether cam morphology is an aetiological factor or an incidental finding.
Even when cam morphology is not the aetiological factor, rehabilitation programmes should take into account the co-existence of this condition, which is likely to represent a physiological response to loading rather than a pathological event.

ACUTRAK SCREW FIXATION FOR FIFTH METATARSAL STRESS FRACTURE IN JAPANESE FOOTBALLERS

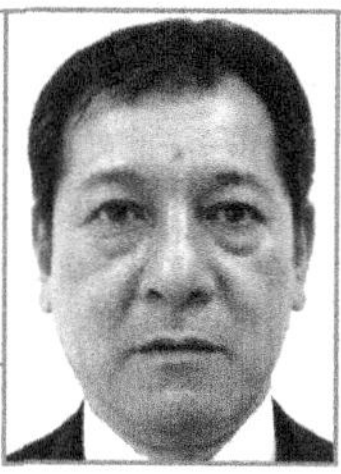

Katori Y, Matsunaga R, Sando T, Yamamoto K

Orthopedic Surgery, Tokyo Medical University, Tokyo, Japan

Introduction

Intramedullary screw fixation is an adequate option for treatment of proximal fifth metatarsal stress fracture in athletes to return to sports earlier and avoid recurrent fracture. However, non-union or delayed-union might be occurred in some cases even after operative treatment (2). Although Cannulated cancellous screw fixation is widely selected for fixation implant, several complications like screw head irritation or recurrent fracture after screw fixation were reported. On the other hand, Acutrak screw (Acumed Inc, Beaverton, Oregon, USA) has characteristic figure for preventing from screw head irritation by headless shape, and stabilization of fifth metatarsal bone with compression force and intramedurally occupancy by tapered shaped design. Yet, optimal implant selection for surgical treatment has not been determined. The aim of this study is to evaluate clinical results of Acutrak screw fixation for proximal fifth metatarsal stress fracture in Japanese football players.

Methods

Twenty four male competitive soccer players were treated with Acutrak screw for symptomatic proximal fifth metatarsal stress fracture. Patients mean age was 18.2 (range: 15-21) years old, and mean follow up period was 60.0 (range: 40-360) weeks.
Patients consisted of one professional footballer, thirteen college footballers, twelve professional club youth team footballers and three high-school footballers.
All patients were classified into Torg classification type II.
Nineteen patients were treated with Acutrak screw 4/5 and five patients were treated with Actruk screw Plus for internal fixation, and mean length of screw were 47.7 (range: 45-50) mm.
Low intensity pulsed ultrasound was applied postoperatively for all patients.
After one weeks of cast immobilization, patients were allowed to be weight bearing as tolerated. Running were allowed with personally modeled insole after six weeks unless tenderness of fracture site and pain on toe gait were found. Partially joining to the training was allowed after ten weeks, and full recovery for the training was aimed in twelve weeks after surgery. We evaluated radiologic findings and clinical results including duration to return to football retrospectively.

Results

Twenty three patients obtained primary bone union.
Non-union was occurred in one patient and recurrent fracture was seen in four patients.
Two patients underwent reoperation for screw exchange with an autogenous bone graft harvested from the iliac crest, one is for non-union and one is for recurrent fracture who were professional footballer.
Bone union could be obtained by conservative treatment in three recurrent fracture cases.
Twenty three patients except non-union case returned to the same level mean 12.6 weeks after primary surgery.
In radiographic evaluation, bone union was obtained in mean 10.0 weeks in twenty three patients.

Conclusions

Clinical failure of Acutrak screw fixation were relatively rare in former studies (3), as Acutrak screw can avoid screw head irritation with keeping compression force because of its structure, and has better intramedullary occupancy compared with other fixation method.
Our results shows four recurrent fractures and one non-union, overall 20.8% of clinical failure in twenty four patients. Approximately 20% of failure rate is relatively higher than previous reports which used other fixation methods (1). However, higher failure rates of conservative treatment were commonly reported, therefore operative treatment should be indicated to return to football earlier for high level footballers.
In our study, clinical failure might be caused by not only implant selection, but also inadequate operative technique and postoperative treatment.
Further study might be expected to determine the best implant selection, and adequate operative technique for establishing standard operation method.

Characteristic	Value
Time to bone union (weeks)	10
Nonunion (n)	1
Delayed union (n)	1
Refracture (n)	4
Reoperation (n)	2
Return to running (weeks)	6.7
Return to full activity (weeks)	12.6
Screw diameter 4/5 (n)	19
Screw diameter Plus (n)	5
Screw length 45 mm (n)	11
Screw length 50 mm (n)	13

Table 1. Characteristics of the Acutrak Screw fixation in the 24 patients.

References

1. Granata JD, Berlet GC, Philbin TM, Jones G, Kaeding CC, Peterson KS. Failed surgical management of acute proximal fifth metatarsal (jones) fractures: a retrospective case series and literature review. Foot Ankle Spec. 2015; 8: 454-459
2. Larson CM, Almekinders LC, Taft WE, Garrett WE. Intramedullary screw fixation of Jones fractures. Analysis of failure. Am J Sports Med 2002; 30: 55-60
3. Nagao M, Saita Y, Kameda S, Seto H, Sadatsuki R, Takazawa Y, Yoshimura M, Aoba Y, Ikeda H, Kaneko K, Nozawa M, Kim SG. Headless compression screw fixation of jones fractures: an outcomes study in Japanese athletes. Am J Sports Med 2012; 40: 2578-2582

RETURN TO PLAY FOOTBALL FOLLOWING SURGICAL TREATMENT FOR ACUTE AVULSION OF ADDUCTOR LONGUS ENTHESIS

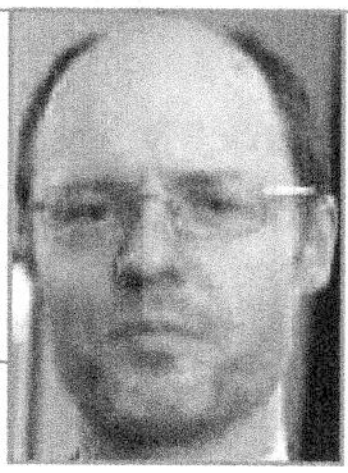

Schilders E[1], Dimitrakopoulou A[2], Kartsonaki Ch[3], Cooke C[4]

[1]The London Hip Arthroscopy Centre at The Wellington Hospital, London;
[2]Fortius Clinic, London;[3]Leeds Beckett University, Leeds;
[4]University of Oxford, Oxford, United Kingdom

Introduction

Adductor injuries are a common problem in football resulting in days of absence from sports and in high reinjury rate. Acute avulsion of the Adductor Longus through its fibrocartilagenous enthesis is an uncommon injury. The purpose of this study is to highlight the injury of the Adductor Longus at its enthesis, be it complete or partially avulsed, and to report the functional outcome and return to play following surgical treatment.

Methods

We included footballers who presented with an acute injury of the Adductor Longus origin. Demographic data, clinical examination, strength testing measurements, imaging features and level of sports were recorded. The time and the level to return to play football following selective partial adductor release (for partial avulsion with minimal displacement) (2) or Adductor Longus reattachment (for complete avulsion) (1) were documented.

Results

We included 58 out of 73 football players with acute adductor injury; 43 were professional players with a mean age at the time of operation 25±5 (range: 18-36) and 15 were non-professional with a mean age 38±7 (range: 23-48) yrs.
There were 32 professional and nine non-professional footballers with complete avulsion, 11 professional and six non-professional with partial avulsion with minimal displacement.
Previous history of adductor enthesopathy was noted in 31 professional of which 21 had undergone more than two corticosteroid injections and in seven non-professional, all of them had undergone corticosteroid injections. All of the athletes returned to play football but one player with incomplete tear at 8 weeks sustained a complete avulsion and underwent surgical reattachment.
The footballers with reattachment returned to full training at a mean 11.8±6.5 weeks and returned to play at a median 13 weeks (IQR 8). The footballers with selective partial adductor release returned to full training at a mean 6.4±2.1 weeks and returned to play at a median 8 weeks (IQR 4).

Conclusions

This study demonstrates that acute avulsion of the Adductor Longus should be treated taking into account the degree and type of injury. Surgical treatment be it reattachment of the enthesis or selective partial adductor release provides a significant clinical improvement and allows athletes to return to play promptly and at the same level.

References

1. Dimitrakopoulou A, Schilders EM, Talbot JC, Bismil Q. Acute avulsion of the fibrocartilage origin of the adductor longus in professional soccer players: a report of two cases. Clin J Sport Med 2008; 18: 167-169
2. Schilders E, Dimitrakopoulou A, Cooke M, Bismil Q, Cooke C. Effectiveness of a selective partial adductor release for chronic adductor-related groin pain in professional athletes. Am J Sports Med 2013; 41: 603-607

Sunday 10th April, 2016 (morning)
FLEMING ROOM

INVITED SPEAKERS

RETURN TO PLAY FOLLOWING TENDON INJURIES

Chairs

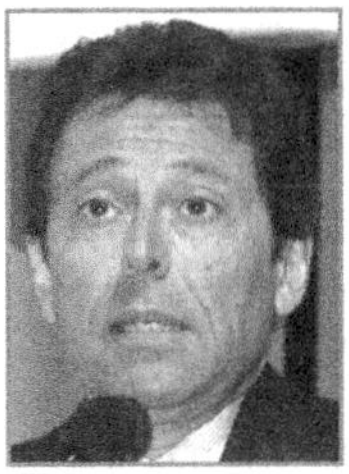

Franco Benazzo
(Pavia, Italy)

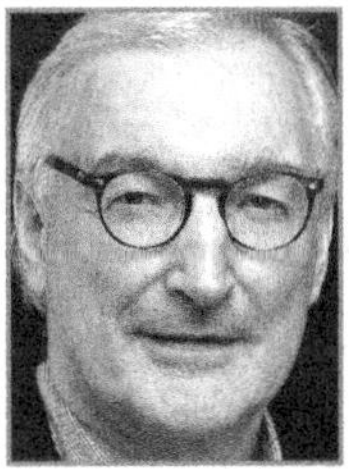

Lars Engebretsen
(Oslo, Norway)

11:30	Healing of tendon structure and restoration of function **Lorenzo Masci (London, United Kingdom)**
11:45	Return to play in conservative management of anterior knee pain **Karim Khan (Doha, Qatar)**
12:00	Surgical choiches for patellar tendon injury **Hakan Alfredson (Umea, Sweden)**
12:15	Return to play in conservative management of ankle tendon pathology **Jon Fearn (Finchampstead, United Kingdom)**
12:30	Surgical choiches for ankle tendon injuries and implications for return to play **James Calder (London, United kingdom)**
12:45	Discussion
13:00	End of the session

HEALING OF TENDON STRUCTURE AND RESTORATION OF FUNCTION

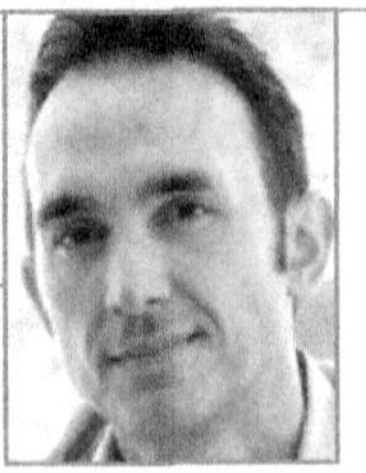

Masci L

Institute of Sports Exercise and Health (ISEH),
and Pure Sports Medicine, London, United Kingdom

There is no doubt that tendinopathy is associated with abnormal tendon structure. In fact, a generally accepted theory of tendon pathology, the tendon continuum, proposes that tendinopathy is based on progressive structural pathology as seen on ultrasound imaging. These microscopic changes include disorganization of collagen fibers, infiltration of vessels and nerves and a change in the size of proteoglycans in the extracellular matrix.
While there is general agreement that tendon pain responds to loading or therapeutic exercise, a term referred to as mechano-transduction, there is a discrepancy between clinical improvements in pain, restoration of function and structural improvements in conventional imaging.
Some practitioners advocate that improvements in clinical response occur without improvements in tendon structure. A recent meta-analysis suggests that structural change may not explain improvements in pain and that other mechanisms such as neural, biomechanical or myogenic may be more important (1). However, reasons for discordance between improvements in tendon pain and structure may be due to the limitations in conventional imaging techniques rather than an absence of a direct relationship. Ultrasound demonstrates fiber heterogeneity and detects ingrowth of vessels by power-Doppler. Magnetic Resonance Imaging (MRI) demonstrates increased signal in a tendon representing alteration in fibrillar alignment and increased water content. Both imaging modalities have limitations in reproducibility and lack objectivity in describing tendon changes over time. Recently, novel imaging modalities have been used in tendinopathy that have improved reproducibility and objectivity. Ultrasound Tissue Characterisation (UTC) semi-quantifies the stability of the grey scale images over the length of a tendon into 4 different echotypes. Degree of stability corresponds to different tissue types in histopathology of equine tendons. The ability to standardise attainment of ultrasound image of tendon addresses limitations of objectivity in conventional ultrasound (3). Ultrasound elastography is a novel technique that evaluates the mechanical properties of tendon. A specific type of elastography called Shear Wave provides quantitative values of tendon elastic properties at selected areas of interest in the tendon. It measures the velocity of the propagated shear waves and estimates tissue stiffness by calculating Young's elastic modulus. It provides an objective measure of stiffness of the tendon (2).
By using novel imaging modalities with improved objectively and reproducibility, a clearer relationship might emerge between tendon pain, function and structure. These modalities could provide supplementary information in conjunction with subjective clinical features (such as tendon pain) to guide loading programs in tendinopathy. Further research is required to assess the validity of these novel imaging modalities in the return to play management of tendinopathy.

References

1. Drew B, Smith T, Littlewood C, Sturrock B. Do structural changes (eg, collagen/matrix) explain the response to therapeutic exercises in tendinopathy: a systematic review. Br J Sports Med 2012; 48: 966-972
2. Ooi CC, Malliaras P, Schneider ME, Connell DA. Soft, hard, or just right? Applications and limitations of axial-strain sonoelastography and shear-wave elastography in the assessment of tendon injuries. Skeletal Radiol 2014; 43: 1-12
3. van Schie HTM, Bakker EM, Jonker AM, van Weeren PR. Computerized ultrasonographic tissue characterization of equine superficial digital flexor tendons by means of stability quantification of echo patterns in contiguous transverse ultrasonographic images. Am J Vet Res 2003; 64: 366-375

3

SURGICAL CHOICES FOR PATELLA TENDON INJURY AND IMPLICATIONS FOR RETURN TO PLAY

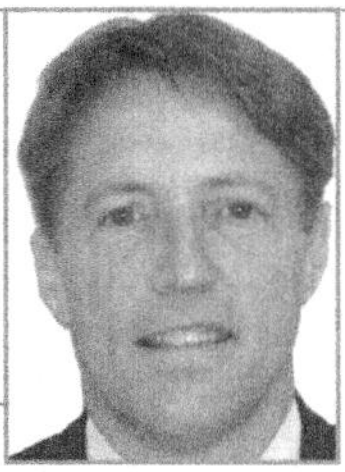

Alfredson H

Sports Medicine Unit, University of Umeå and Alfredson Tendon Clinic, Umeå, Sweden; Institute of Sport, Exercise and Health (ISEH), University College London Hospitals (UCLH), London, and Pure Sports Med Clinic, London, United Kingdom

Introduction

Proximal patellar Tendinopathy-Jumper´s knee is well known to be a troublesome injury, often not responding to the traditional conservative and surgical treatment alternatives. In sports with high demands on the knee extensor mechanisms, such as jumping and leg explosive sports, a high number of the participants suffer from patellar tendinopathy. It has been stated that as much as 50% of all high level volleyball players suffer from this condition.

First line of treatment is conservative-noninvasive, including biomechanical adjustments and different types of loading regimens, such as eccentric, concentric/eccentric and lately also isometric loading. The success rates from these regimens varies, but no convincing high success rate has been shown using any of these methods.

Second line of treatment often includes injection treatment, such as cortisone, Platelet Rich Plasma (PRP) and sclerosing polidocanol injections. Ultrasound (US) and Doppler (DP)-guided polidocanol injections outside the tendon have been shown to be beneficial, but is technically difficult-operator dependent, and time consuming because multiple injections are needed. Cortisone inside the tendon is being questioned because of its tissue destroying side effects and PRP inside the tendon is heavily questioned.

Many athletes manage to train and play with patellar tendinopathy throughout their career, but the ones with severe disabling pain are often treated surgically. For many years the golden standard procedure has been open tenotomy and revision, combined with a 6-12 months rehabilitation period. However, the results have not been good, and in a randomized study (1) similar results as with eccentric training, and only 50% good results, was achieved with this inside the tendon revision procedure.

Research on the tissue pathology and innervation patterns during the last 15 years has clarified that the nerves responsible for the pain in this condition are localized outside, and not inside, the tendon, and has led to the invention of a new type of surgical treatment-Ultrasound and Doppler-guided arthroscopic shaving.

Surgical treatment with Ultrasound and Doppler-guided arthroscopic shaving

Background: immunohistochemical staining of tissue biopsies from patients with proximal patellar tendinopathy have shown that the nerves are located in close relation to blood vessels outside the dorsal side of the proximal tendon, and can be found via US and Doppler examination. Local anesthetic injections targeting the region with high blood flow and nerves outside the tendon temporarily cures the pain.

Surgical treatment. The US+DP examination guides the arthroscopic surgical procedure (US examination together with arthroscopy in the operating room), that can be kept to be minimally invasive outside the proximal patellar tendon.

Rehabilitation. Because no intra-tendinous surgery is performed, the following rehabilitation can start immediately and be relatively aggressive and quick. Range of movement exercises and innervation training, immediate weight-bearing loading, biking, and low-load strength training within the first 3 weeks. Then there is a gradual increase of the loading and start of more sport specific training depending on swelling and pain.

Research. This new method has been evaluated in several scientific studies, including a Thesis and a 4-5 year follow-up (2, 3). The method has been shown to be safe, the results have been shown to be very good and stable, with more than 85% satisfied athletes returning to full sport activity within 3-4 months.

Altogether we have operated more than 700 athletes with this method, including rugby, football, volleyball and track and field athletes. The results have been good and stable.

In patients that previously have been treated with tenotomy and revision, the US+DP-guided procedure has been less successful.

Conclusions

Based on the poor clinical results with intra-tendinous surgical approaches, and the new research findings considering the innervation patterns, intra-tendinous surgical revision treatment of proximal patellar tendinopathy seems questionable.

Surgical treatment outside the tendon, such as US and DP-guided arthroscopic shaving, has been shown to have a high potential to allow for a pain-free return to high level patellar tendon demanding sports after a relatively short rehabilitation period.

References

1. Bahr R, Fossan B, Løken S, Engebretsen L. Surgical treatment compared with eccentric training for patellar tendinopathy (Jumpers knee). A randomized controlled trial. J Bone Joint Surg Am 2006; 88: 1689-1698
2. Willberg L, Sunding K, Forssblad M, Fahlstrom M, Alfredson H. Sclerosing polidocanol injections or arthroscopic shaving to treat patellar tendinopathy/jumper's knee? A randomised controlled study. Br J Sports Med 2011; 45: 411-415
3. Sunding K, Willberg L, Werner S, Alfredson H, Forssblad M, Fahlstrom M. Sclerosing injections and ultrasound-guided arthroscopic shaving for patellar tendinopathy - good clinical results and decreased tendon thickness after surgery - a medium term follow-up study. Knee Surg Sports Traumatol Arthrosc 2015; 23: 2259-2268

RETURN TO PLAY IN THE CONSERVATIVE MANAGEMENT OF ANKLE TENDON PATHOLOGY

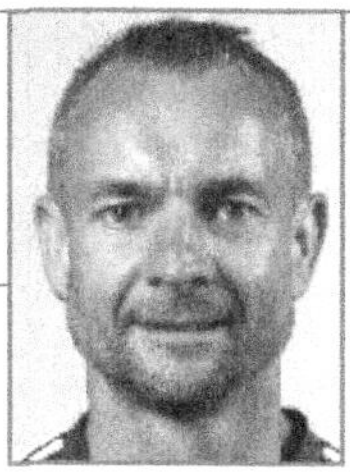

Fearn J

Chelsea Football Club Medical Team, London, United Kingdom

Tendon injuries are not a common problem in football and only make up 7% of injuries a team sustains in a season (UEFA study past five year average). A team's tendon injury profile depends on many factors including the playing personnel (age and past injury history) and the match and training intensity. Any changes such as coaching philosophies, playing surfaces, boot design, etc..., can have an influence on tendon homeostasis. At Chelsea football club, the first team squad have had only two ankle tendon injuries (Achilles tendon) over the past five seasons. Interestingly these were both more senior players but they had had no significant history of tendon problems. One player's injury was sustained following a direct contusion to the tendon during a tackle and the other following a sudden excessive load resulting in a reactive response in the tendon. In both cases the injury was isolated to the paratenon. It is essential to identify the type of tendon injury sustained (reactive/acute or chronic/degenerative), the cause (aetiology) and the tissue involved (e.g., paratenon or intra-substance). This will dictate the management that is undertaken. In the case of a reactive tendon due to a contusion resulting in a paratenonitis, the injury is treated as an inflammatory problem and treated accordingly, whereas a more chronic problem may require a longer term approach. Although investigations such as ultrasound scans and Magnetic Resonance Imaging (MRI) scan are useful in identifying the site and extent of the pathology it is worth noting that tendon pain can be present in pathologically unremarkable tendons and, conversely, a tendon with extensive pathology (for example intra-substance hypo-echoic changes on ultrasound scan together with significant neovascularisation on Doppler) can in fact be symptom free. The level of pathology present does not always indicate the extent of the pain present. In our recent experience all the ankle tendons injuries we have seen, have involved the Achilles paratenon. Following a few days of low load, pain-free activity and emphasis on not aggravating the problem and progressive increase in functional 'football-like' load is undertaken. This is the main management principle and other additional interventions such as tendon loading via exercise, electrotherapy and manual therapy are carried out if indicated. Progressive functional load is initially carried out in a partial weight bearing environment. We use a Hydroworx water treadmill (Middleton, USA) commencing at shoulder level and progressing to waist level as pain allows over a period of days. It is important to analyse the tendon's response to treatment over days as the pain response can be delayed. A player is then progressed in terms of functional ability and increasing load via the stretch-shortening cycle (i.e., ability to jog initially and later execute jumping and hopping movements). It is important to build low level volume of work (over time) and only when able go onto progress performing higher intensity movements (jumping, accelerating, decelerating, etc...). This approach of functional 'football-like' movement drills is continued outside on the field, building low level of work over time (volume) and then gradually increasing intensity and demand on the tendon involved.
Return to training is dependent on when a player is able to execute all functional movements to a training level and intensity pain-free and has no delayed reaction of tendon pain (i.e., no morning soreness or stiffness), the player have full strength capability in the region (maybe supported by laboratory based objective data such as isokinetics or jump tests) and, most importantly, the player's feedback that they feel ready. With respect to tendon pathology, clinical signs such as local tenderness and swelling and abnormal findings on imaging is not useful indication of the tissues ability to sustain load and no relied upon in isolation.

[illegible]

Tendon injuries are not a common [illegible] [illegible]

[illegible]

Sunday 10th April, 2016 (morning)
CHURCHILL AUDITORIUM

INVITED SPEAKERS

RETURN TO PLAY AND THE NIGHTMARE OF RE-INJURIES

Chairs

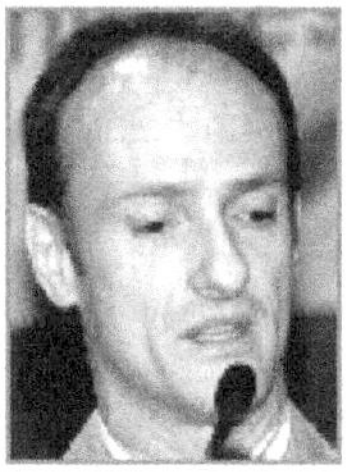

Massimo Berruto
(Milan, Italy)

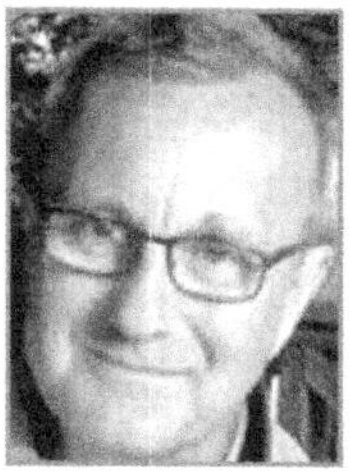

Magnus Forssblad
(Stockholm, Sweden)

11:30 Re-injuries in the UEFA Elite Club Injury Study
Jan Ekstrand (Linköping, Sweden)

11:45 Secondary prevention following knee surgery
Holly Silvers-Granelli (Santa Monica, USA)

12:00 Secondary prevention for muscle and tendon injuries
Erik Witvrouw (Doha, Qatar)

12:15 Managing return to play in players with history of recurrence
Cristiano Eirale (Doha, Qatar)

12:30 Training load and injury risk: can technology help to navigate in the perfect storm? **Tim Gabbett (Brisbane, Australia)**

12:45 Discussion

13:00 End of the session

RETURN TO PLAY AND RE-INJURIES IN UEFA CHAMPIONS LEAGUE

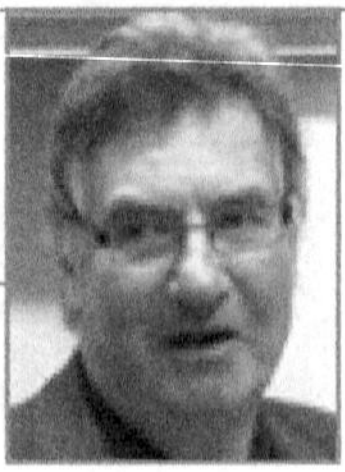

Ekstrand J

Football Reserach Group, Linköping University, Sweden

Introduction

The UEFA Champions League injury study is a prospective survey ongoing since 14 years (2). The database, consisting of 13,000 injuries is the world's largest concerning male elite level football. A large database from a homogenous material provides robust information of the risk of specific injuries, their consequences in form of lay off days Return To Play (RTP) and the risk of recurrence etc.

Methods

A total of 2,593 players comprising 56 teams from 16 countries in Europe were followed prospectively between 2001 and 2015. Team medical staffs recorded individual player exposure and time loss injuries.

All injuries resulting in a player being unable to fully participate in training or match play (i.e., time loss injuries) were recorded. The player was considered injured until the team medical staff allowed full participation in training and availability for match selection. A re-injury was defined as an injury of the same type and at the same site as an index injury occurring no more than two months after a player's return to full participation from the index injury.

Results

The mean age was 25±5 (range 16-43) years, mean height was 182±7 (range 160-205) cm, and mean body mass was 78±7 (range 56-110) kg.

11% of the players were goalkeepers, 32% defenders, 36% midfielders and 21% forwards. 75% were rightfooted.

The average re-injury rate was 11.1% but differed between clubs and countries. The injury rate has decreased for ligament injuries over the last 11 years, but overall training, match injury rates and the rates of muscle injury and severe injury remain high (1, 3).

Conclusions

Since a player was considered injured until the team medical staff allowed full participation in training and availability for match selection, a re-injury would either indicate a misjudgement of the medical team or a refusal of the coaching team to follow advices from the medical team or a failure of a calculated risk taking from all parties involved in the RTP decision.

References

1. Ekstrand J, Askling C, Magnusson H, Mithoefer K. Return to play after thigh muscle injury in elite football players: Implementation and validation of the Munich muscle injury classification. Br J Sports Med 2013; 47: 769-774
2. Ekstrand J, Hägglund M, Kristenson K, Magnusson H, Waldén M. Fewer ligament injuries but no preventive effect on muscle injuries and severe injuries: An 11-year follow-up of the UEFA champions league injury study. Br J Sports Med 2013; 47: 732-737
3. Hallén A, Ekstrand J. Return to play following muscle injuries in professional footballers. J Sports Sci 2014; 32: 1229-1236

RETURN TO PLAY AND THE NIGHTMARE OF RE-INJURY

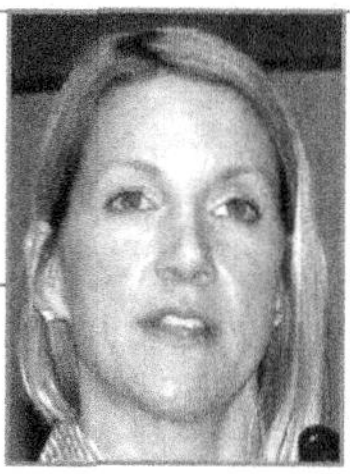

Silvers-Granelli H

University of Delaware, Newark, USA

Athletes who wish to return to sport after sustaining an Anterior Cruciate Ligament (ACL) injury face a difficult decision. Medically, a multidisciplinary approach for medical clearance; including the expert opinions of the orthopaedic surgeon, sports physician, physical therapist, certified athletic trainer, sports psychologist, and, most importantly, the goal of the athlete at hand should be paramount. The primary goal of an ACL reconstruction is to establish joint stability and decrease the risk of subsequent injury to the menisci and the articular cartilage surfaces. Many studies have established that a vast majority of patient who opt to have an ACL Reconstruction (ACLR) (65–88%) are able to return to sport within 18 months of undergoing an ACLR and subsequent rehabilitation (1, 2, 3). Reconstructive surgery and proper neuromuscular rehabilitation has been deemed effective in allowing injured athletes to resume to sport in a majority of patients. However, how do we address the conundrum of re-injury?

A major caveat with delineating return to sport after ACLR is that the re-injury rate to the involved joint, the uninvolved joint, and to other concomitant structures may be adversely elevated. Several studies have examined re-injury rates, which historically range from 2.3% to 30% (Paterno MV, Rauh MJ, Schmitt LC, Ford KR, Hewett TE. Incidence of Second ACL Injuries 2 Years After Primary ACL Reconstruction and Return to Sport. Am J Sports Med 2014; 42:1 567-1573). A study by Wasserstein et. al reported a significant difference in the re-injury rates in patients under the age of 25 (9% and 25%, respectively; $p<0.0001$). It was the first to demonstrate the high incidence of ACL re-injury in young, highly active patients who received allografts (Wasserstein D, Sheth U, Cabrera A, Spindler KP. A Systematic Review of Failed Anterior Cruciate Ligament Reconstruction With Autograft Compared With Allograft in Young Patients. Sports Health 2015; 7: 207-216). An additional study in young athletes reported that the re-injury rate in either lower extremity was 62% in men and 40% in women after the patients had resumed sports activities (Shelbourne KD, Gray T, Haro M. Incidence of subsequent injury to either knee within 5 years after anterior cruciate ligament reconstruction with patellar tendon autograft. Am J Sports Med 2009; 37: 246-251).

Another issue to contend with is the elevated prevalence of osteoarthritis after sustaining an ACL injury. The occurrence of an ACL injury is correlated directly to the incidence of OA (Lohmander LS, Saxne T, Heinegard DK. Release of Cartilage Oligomeric Matrix Protein (COMP) into joint fluid after knee injury and in osteoarthritis. Ann Rheum Dis 1994; 53: 8-13). Osteochondral bone bruises are present in 80-90% of ACL injuries, however the sequelea for dysfunction is not inherently clear (Engebretsen L, Arendt E, Fritts HM. Osteochondral lesions and cruciate ligament injuries. MRI in 18 knees. Acta Orthop Scand 1993; 64: 434-6).

When patients were longitudinally followed for 10-20 years after sustaining and ACL injury, 50% of those patients presented with osteoarthritis, associated joint arthralgia, and functional impairment (Lohmander LS, Englund PM, Dahl LL, Roos EM. The long-term consequence of anterior cruciate ligament and meniscus injuries: osteoarthritis. Am J Sports Med 2007; 35: 1756-1769).
Despite the earnest efforts of medical researchers, there currently is no clear consensus on return to play assessment or clearance. Several researchers have been examining the validity and reliability of return to play criteria, but the early findings seem to be mixed and inconclusive. Criteria such as rate of force development, jump landing mechanics, analysis of gait patterns, utilization of virtual reality immersion and analysis of joint contact force asymmetry are some of the variables that have been utilized for return to play criteria (Ardern CL, Taylor NF, Feller JA, Webster KE. Return-to-sport outcomes at 2 to 7 years after anterior cruciate ligament reconstruction surgery. Am J Sports Med 2012; 40: 41-48). Continued research must be advocated to standardize post-operative care and to determine the assessment tools and functional outcomes scores that can clearly assess an individual's readiness to return to play in order to mitigate the risk of future injury.

References

1. Corry IS, Webb JM, Clingeleffer AJ, Pinczewski LA. Arthroscopic reconstruction of the anterior cruciate ligament. A comparison of patellar tendon autograft and four-strand hamstring tendon autograft. Am J Sports Med 1999; 27: 444-454.
2. Feller JA, Webster KE. A randomized comparison of patellar tendon and hamstring tendon anterior cruciate ligament reconstruction. Am J Sports Med 2003; 31: 564-573
3. Siegel MG, Barber-Westin SD. Arthroscopic-assisted outpatient anterior cruciate ligament reconstruction using the semitendinosus and gracilis tendons. Arthroscopy 1998; 14: 268-277

MANAGING RETURN TO PLAY IN PLAYERS WITH HISTORY OF RECURRENCE

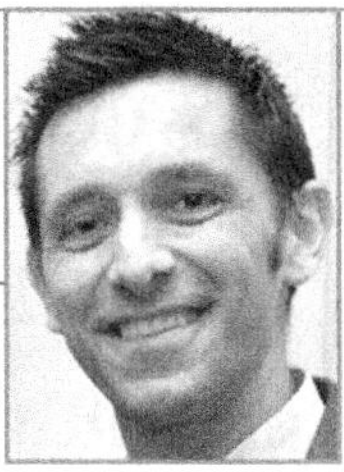

Eirale C

Aspetar, Qatar Orthopedic and Sport Medicine Hospital,
FIFA Medical Centre of Excellence, Doha, Qatar

Introduction

Return to play decision is arguably one of the most difficult challenges in Sport Medicine, especially at the professional level. A high injury rate for a team is often attributed to mismanagement by the technical or the performance staff, while the re-injury rate is commonly seen as a performance indicator for the medical staff. With limited evidence based protocols for deciding return to play currently existing, the decision on return to play is usually based on the personal experience of the clinicians.

Return to play

Managing the return to play of an athlete with a history of recurrent injuries is more difficult because previous injury and age are known risk factors in football. The athlete is therefore exposed to a higher hazard. Based on the literature review and our personal experience, we tried assess the differences in return to play strategies between players with index and recurrent injuries.

Different models for return to play have been proposed; we have utilised the Creighton decision-based model (1) which identifies the variables that may differ in cases of footballers with multiple re-injuries.

Among the medical factors determining return to play, the psychological state of the athlete has emerged to be of the upmost importance, and psychological factors may become crucial for the return to play decision. Also, the return to sport decision may be more heavily influenced by some external modifiers such as the pressure from the athlete and from the coach/managers. Particularly at the professional level, medico legal matters, and the fear of litigation in case of a new recurrence, may lead the clinician to treat in a conservative and defensive manner. At the elite level, pressure from the media may also play an important role.

The medical staff should carefully review the previous return to play strategies in a footballer with recurrent injuries, address identified mistakes and try different protocols.

Finally, it may be possible that an athlete was reinjured because potential risk factors, in addition to age and past history, were not corrected. Therefore, a cautious assessment of the risk factors is warranted as a crucial part of the return to play strategy.

Conclusions

Managing return to play in footballers with a history of multiple re-injuries may be challenging, especially at the elite level.

Particular attention should be paid to specific risk factors and to the correction of protocols that previously lead to failed rehabilitation

References

1. Creighton DW, Shrier I, Shultz R, Meeuwisse WH, Matheson GO. Return-to-play in sport: a decision-based model. Clin J Sport Med 2010; 20: 379-385

TRAINING LOAD AND INJURY RISK: CAN TECHNOLOGY HELP TO NAVIGATE IN THE PERFECT STORM?

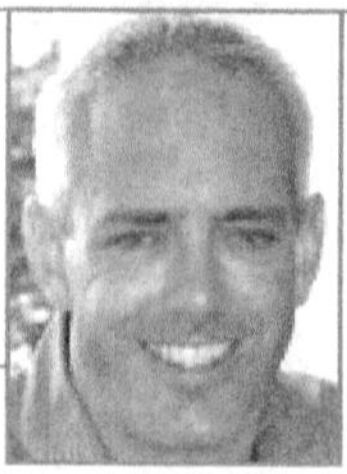

Gabbett TJ[1,2], Blanch P[3,4]

[1]School of Exercise Science, Australian Catholic University, Brisbane; [2]School of Human Movement Studies, The University of Queensland, Brisbane; [3]Essendon Football Club, Melbourne; [4]School of Allied Health Sciences, Griffith University Gold Coast, Australia

Introduction

The concept of progressive overload is well understood by practitioners (i.e., medical, physiotherapy, and strength and conditioning staff) involved in the rehabilitation of athletes. However, when returning athletes to competition following injury, there is often a disconnect between theory and practice, with practitioners having varying methods of assessing the readiness of an athlete to return to play.

Recently, we have described the acute:chronic workload ratio as a method of safely progressing training loads and quantifying injury risk (1, 2, 3). The acute:chronic workload ratio quantifies the workload that the athlete has performed relative to the workload they have been prepared for. An obvious, yet understated point in the return to play discussion, is that it is impossible to determine i) subsequent injury risk, and ii) whether the athlete is prepared for competition demands if workload is not accurately and reliably monitored.

Secondly, the metrics that provide the greatest insight into injury risk will differ from sport to sport (e.g., high-speed running may be important to football players, while balls bowled is likely to be more important for cricket fast bowlers). In this presentation, we discuss the acute:chronic workload ratio and describe how technology (specifically microsensors) can be used to quantify workloads and safely return injured athletes to competition.

Methods

We quantified the training and competition workloads of elite rugby league (mean ± SD age, 23±4 yr; n=53) and Australian football (24±4 yr; n=46) players, and cricket fast bowlers (26±5 yr; n=28). Locomotor (i.e. total distance, high-speed distance) and accelerometer loads were used to quantify workloads in rugby league and Australian football while balls bowled and session-Rating of Perceived Exertion (RPE) were used to quantify workloads of cricket fast bowlers. One-week data, along with four-week rolling average data were calculated for all workload variables. The one-week data represented the acute workload (i.e., fatigue), and the four-week rolling average data represented the chronic workload (i.e., fitness). The acute-chronic workload ratio was calculated by dividing the acute workload by the chronic workload (2).

Results

Irrespective of the workload measure used (i.e., total distance, high-speed running distance, accelerometer load, balls bowled, or session-RPE), an acute:chronic workload ratio >1.5 was consistently associated with an increased risk of injury.

Case reports

We also present two cases studies detailing successful and unsuccessful return to play. In case study 1, we present data on high-speed running distance. When the acute:chronic workload ratio was 1.6, the athlete sustained a low grade hamstring strain. On returning to training, the athlete's acute:chronic workload ratio was spiked from 0.2 to 1.9 (in one week), resulting in re-injury of the same hamstring. A delay of seven days existed between the spike in workload and subsequent injury.

In case study 2, the athlete sustained a shoulder injury, resulting in minimal training for a 3-week period. In the fourth week, the acute:chronic workload ratio was spiked from 0 to 4.0 (i.e., the acute load was four times greater than what the athlete was prepared for). The athlete sustained a low grade hamstring injury three weeks following the spike in workloads. When workloads were increased progressively and the acute:chronic workload ratio was maintained below 1.5, the athlete was able to successfully return to play.

Conclusions

Our data show that a high acute:chronic workload ratio is associated with increased injury risk in a wide range of sports. Importantly, following a spike in workload (i.e., acute:chronic workload >1.5), the risk of injury is elevated for 7-21 days.

Technology can assist practitioners to safely return athlete's to competition, but only when there is an understanding of competition demands and the athlete's current (i.e., acute) and previous (i.e., chronic) workloads.

References

1. Blanch P, Gabbett TJ. Has the athlete trained enough to return to play safely? The acute:chronic workload ratio permits clinicians to quantify a player's risk of subsequent injury. Br J Sports Med 2015 Dec 23. pii: bjsports-2015-095445. doi: 10.1136/bjsports-2015-095445. [Epub ahead of print]
2. Gabbett TJ. The training-injury prevention paradox: should athletes be training smarter and harder? Br J Sports Med, 2016; in press
3. Gabbett, TJ, Hulin BT, Blanch P, Whiteley R. High training loads alone do not cause sports injuries: how you get there is the real issue. Br J Sports Med, 2016; in press

Sunday 10th April, 2016 (morning)
PICKWICK ROOM

FREE ORAL PRESENTATIONS

MEDICAL ISSUES AND PREVENTION

Chairs

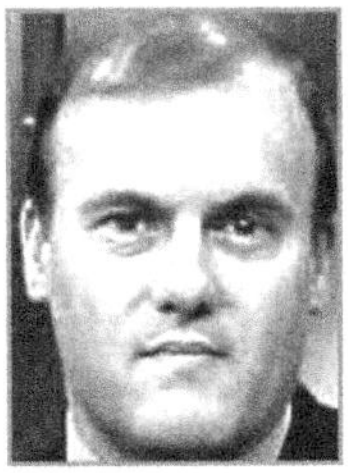

André Pedrinelli
(São Paulo, Brasil)

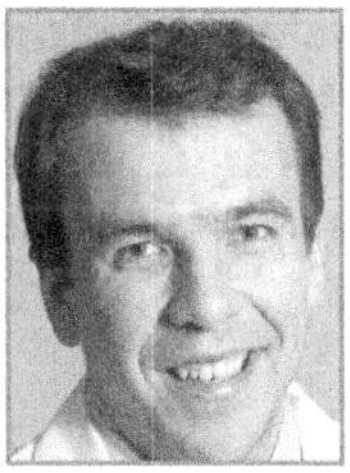

Matthew Stride
(London, United Kingdom)

11:22 Managing fatigue and early infection in football: a novel approach
Knight J, Stride M, Webster S, Purdue J (Plymouth and London, United Kingdom)

11:30 What does return to pre-injury risk mean?
Shrier I, Zhao M, Piche A, Slavchev P, Steele RJ (Montreal, Canada)

11:38 Shock absorbing studs in prevention of football injuries. A preliminary report **Ferretti A, Mapelli C, Gruttadauria A, Barella S, Ciuffini AF, Mombelli D, Calderaro C, Mazza D (Rome and Milan, Italy)**

11:46 Head injuries in children´s football
Feddermann-Demont N, Rössler R, Beaudouin F, aus der Fünten K, Chomiak J, Verhagen E, Junge A, Dvorak J, Faude O (Zurich and Basel Switzerland; Saarbrücken and Hamburg, Germany; Prague, Czech Republic; Amsterdam, The Netherlands)

11:54 Return to play after severe football injuries in children aged 7 to 12 years
Rössler R, Junge A, Chomiak J, Dvorak J, aus der Fünten K, Verhagen E, Faude O (Basel and Zurich Switzerland; Hamburg and Saarbrücken, Germany; Prague, Czech Republic; Amsterdam, The Netherlands)

12:02 Longterm health problems in former elite female football players: prevalence and risk factors
Prien, A, Prinz, B, Dvorak, J, Junge, A (Hamburg, Germany; Zurich, Switzerland

12:10 Inverse relationship between playing level and re-injury rates in men's football
Hägglund M, Waldén M, Ekstrand J (Linköping, Sweden)

12:18 Why female footballer players quit football. Polish survey results
Grygorowicz M, Piontek T, Dudzinski W (Poznan and Pila, Poland)

12:26 Prevention and return to play of injuries in elite football: the team coaches` view
Krutsch W, Zantop T, Angele P (Regensburg, Germany)

12:34 Injury prevention in children's football "FIFA 11+ kids": a cluster randomised controlled trial
Faude O, Rössler R, Bizzini M, Dvorak J, Chomiak J, aus der Fünten K, Verhagen E, Lichtenstein E, Junge A (Basel and Zürich, Switzerland; Prague, Czech Republic; Saarbrücken and Hamburg, Germany; Amsterdam, The Netherlands)

12:42 Discussion

13:15 End of the session

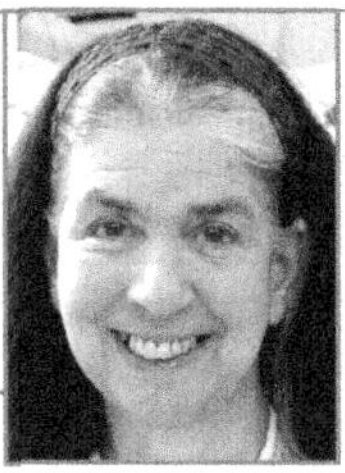

MANAGING FATIGUE AND EARLY INFECTION IN FOOTBALL: A NOVEL APPROACH

Knight J[1], Stride M[2], Webster S[1], Purdue J[3]

[1]Knight Scientific, Plymouth; [2]Isokinetic Medical group, FIFA Medical Centre of Excellence, London; [3]Brentford Football Club, London, United Kingdom

Introduction

There is always a risk of fatigue leading to overtraining in football where performance at the required work rate must be sustained for long periods of time. Normal strategies of balancing intensity of training with sufficient rest, are often denied players by demands of competition and the requirement to play many games within short periods of time. The aim of the project was to develop a sensitive management tool that could be used to identify the physiological and psychological state of the players. In this way the response to various training strategies and dietary interventions could be assessed using the same tool.

The immune system is extremely sensitive to both physiological and psychological stress thus making variables of immune function targets as markers in which to monitor the consequences of sustaining intense exercise for 90 minutes of football match-play. Such intense exercise is likely to induce muscle damage and inflammation characterised by invasion of neutrophils into muscle and release of inflammatory mediators. There have been a number of studies that have investigated the effects of short term intense training on resting immune functions and on immune-endocrine responses to endurance exercise. Individual measures of immune function, on their own however cannot really distinguish between Over Reaching (OR), Over Training (OT) and the Over Training Syndrome (OTS) from infection or post-viral fatigue. However, these investigations have led to an understanding that training load can lead to depressed leucocyte function such as: poor interactions with bacteria, depressed neutrophil and monocyte oxidative burst activity, reduction in T cell interferon-γ, low T cell $CD4^+/CD8^+$ ratios, poor antibody production and natural killer cell cytotoxicity. Salivary IgA for infection, C-Reactive Protein (CRP) for inflammation, ratios of testosterone/cortisol for stress and many blood parameters are also tested. These are helpful in determining health status of the athlete and for possible exclusion diagnoses but are less useful as management tools for the medical and coaching teams. Monitoring tools that can explain decrements in physical capacity, identify as well as predict a player's risk of injury or OR or OT as well as identify an infection in time to take remedial action are in great demand.

We present here details of the ABEL-Sport test that provides immediate results, utilizing only a small drop of capillary blood.

Methods

The ABEL-sport test (ABEL = Analysis By Emitted Light) was performed on a portable luminometer (ABEL-meter). The test incorporates the bioluminescent protein Pholasin which reacts with Reactive Oxygen Species (ROS). Capillary blood collected in EDTA tubes, diluted 1:1000 with buffers, light enhancer and Pholasin, after warming, was placed in the ABEL-meter. After one minute, fMLP (formyl-Methionyl-Phenylalanine) was added to activate the NADPH oxidase (the respiratory burst) via receptors to produce ROS. Light emitted by Pholasin in the test was recorded as light response graphs, quantifying changes in the rate of production and magnitude of the ROS generated. The results of the test were semi-automatically classified by shape against a library of abnormal curves (B – L) compared to normal reference curve A. Bar charts of the amount of light emitted were compared to Reference Curve A ± 1 standard alongside previous results.

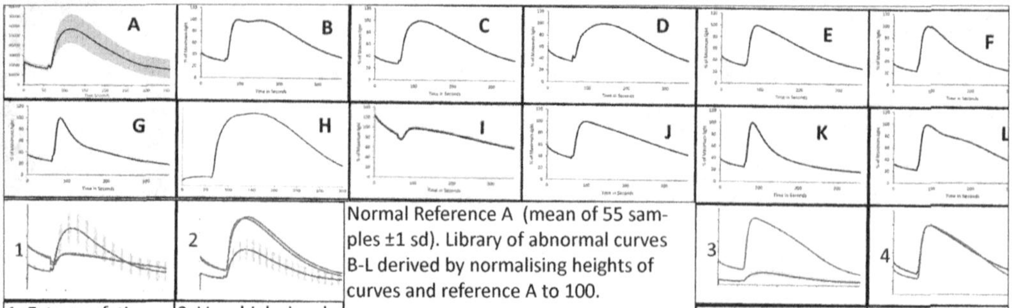

Normal Reference A (mean of 55 samples ±1 sd). Library of abnormal curves B-L derived by normalising heights of curves and reference A to 100.

1. Extreme fatigue compared to A

2. Very high signal likely infection

3. Response compared to A

4. Shape of 3 classified as Curve E

Assays were usually performed weekly by the clubs' staff on match-day + 2 on 1st team squads from 2013-14 and 2014-15 seasons, from the Premier League, Championship, League One and League Two with the recent level of play for each player tested recorded. Players identified with infections, inflammation (light response above the upper range) and/or various states of fatigue were treated accordingly with the test repeated one to two days later to assess the response to therapy. The supplement (Empower Sport Recovery Max) which contains 200 mg of reduced Glutathione (GSH) together with L-cysteine and anthocyanins was taken orally twice daily for at least two weeks but as long as was required for the light response to return to a normal height and shape. Players whose fatigued response was attributed to depression were counselled privately. Training load was modified to reflect the fatigue identified by those players exhibiting depressed respiratory burst activity and demonstrating symptoms of various states of fatigue. Dietary supplements with strong antioxidant polyphenol content were used for inflammation and infection for as long as was required, on average five days.

Results

Collation of the results from the individual clubs involved amounted to over three thousand tests carried out. From these the formulation of reference data and a library of response curves was possible. Curve shapes of interest: B = over reaching; E, I and J = fatigue; G = infection (probable viral) and fatigue; H = bacterial infection. Curve shapes morph one into the other, reflecting conditions of the players. Variation was noted in terms of light response, with the majority of players consistently mounting a heightened response, although many also showed a consistent depressed response. There were frequent changes in an individual's responses reported as well.

Figures left depict a series of light response curves super-imposed on the Reference curve. The magnitude of these responses is further presented as bar charts. The start of GSH supplementation is indicated by the arrow.

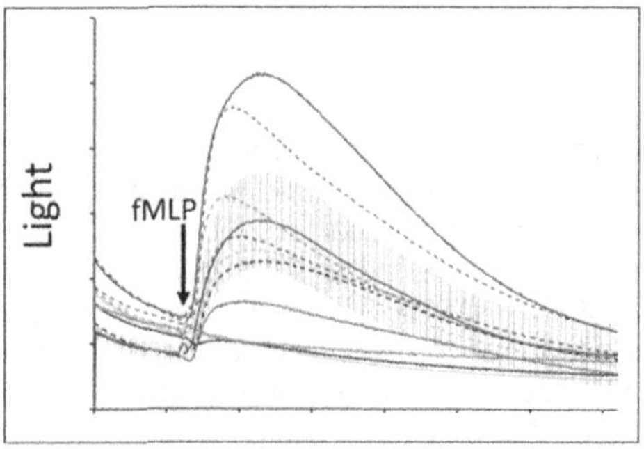

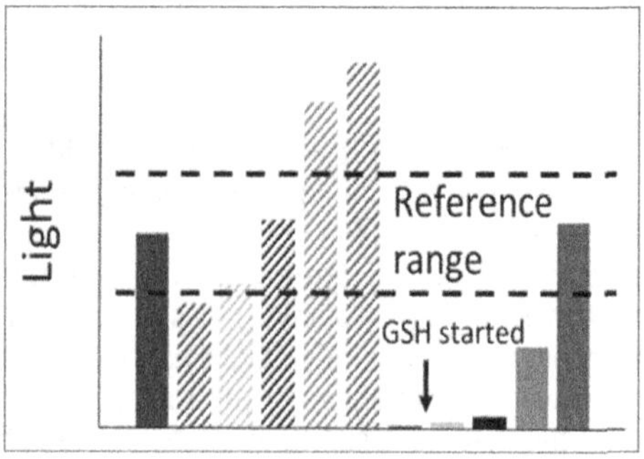

Conclusions

The results identified various responses during training such as OR (Curve B) as well as early infections often with no symptoms, degrees of fatigue, mental depression and more advanced infections (viral and bacterial). Collation and monitoring of the data over the course of the season allows for an individual's characteristics to be formulated. Intervention was carried out based on change in responses above or below reference range and/or change in shape. The high polyphenol supplement reduced the symptoms of infection. Players showing fatigue responded to GSH supplementation with increased respiratory burst activity correlating to feeling less fatigued.

As oxidation of GSH stimulates increased production of NADPH used in the recycling of GSH we propose the theory that the NADPH produced, is also used by the NADPH oxidase with concomitant increase in light.

2

WHAT DOES RETURN TO PRE-INJURY RISK MEAN?

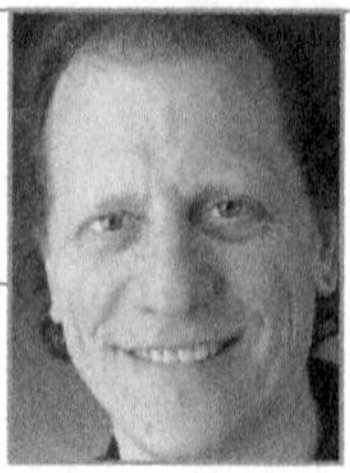

Shrier I[1], Zhao M[2], Piche A[2], Slavchev P[2], Steele RJ[2]

[1]Centre for Clinical Epidemiology, Lady Davis Institute,
Jewish General Hospital, McGill University;
[2]Department of Mathematics and Statistics, McGill University, Montreal, Canada

Introduction

Return To Play (RTP) decisions are often based on an assessment of risk factors for subsequent injury. These analyses usually follow the same statistical methodology as risk factors assessment for first injury. However, there are important differences in the underlying assumptions required for injury and re-injury risk factor analysis. In fact, the common analyses used in re-injury studies would end up concluding that previous injury is a risk factor for future injury, even if the athlete's risk had returned to pre-injury risk. Further, these analyses usually compare injury risk on returning to play versus baseline or pre-season risk, which is different than pre-injury risk (defined as the risk had the person never been injured).
Purpose: To describe the limitations of the commonly used analyses assessing previous injury as a risk factor, and to describe analyses that distinguish between the different "return to pre-injury risk" meanings.

Methods

We simulated data to mimic the context where the true risk of injury increases over the course of a season, as would be expected with mid-season fatigue and as teams approach post-season play-offs. We use standard regression and stratification to mimic the results that would be obtained through standard analyses.

Results

Simply using previous injury as a variable in a regression model to assess risk of subsequent injury will always show previous injury as a risk factor, even if the athlete's physical and psychological states have returned to baseline.
Even when investigators compare an athlete's risk after injury to their risk before injury, the investigators fail to account for differences in risk that occur over calendar time. Consider the context where a changing environment and style of play create a higher risk for every athlete as the season progresses. One can construct examples where even though an athlete has returned to his/her own immediate pre-injury state, the risk of injury is actually increased compared to both their baseline state at the beginning of the season, and the immediate pre-injury state due to factors external to the athlete.

Conclusions

Developing interventions based on flawed risk factor analyses from published studies will likely yield ineffective treatments. RTP decisions that are partly based on these published studies may not be optimal.

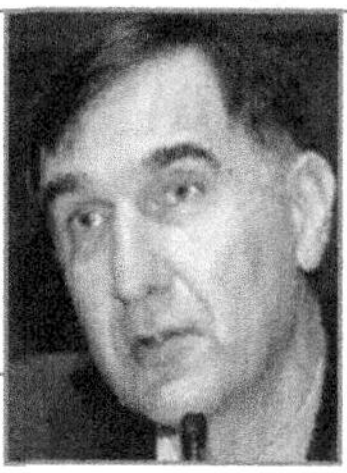

SHOCK ABSORBING STUDS IN PREVENTION OF FOOTBALL INJURIES. A PRELIMINARY REPORT

Ferretti A[1], Mapelli C[2], Gruttadauria A[2], Barella S[2], Ciuffini AF[2], Mombelli D[2], Calderaro C[1], Mazza D[1]

[1]Orthopaedic Unit, S. Andrea Hospital, Sapienza University, Rome;
[2]Department of Mechanics, Politecnico, Milan, Italy

Introduction

Football is generally considered to be a safe sport. However the risk of injury (especially at professional level) is substantial as the overall risk has been estimated to be about 1000 times greater than that of a typical high risk industrial occupation. Despite increasing interest towards injury prevention, little attention has been drawn to athletes equipment such as boots and studs, whose role in player performance and safety has been considered crucial. Recently, a new type of flexible studs (SASspik, Camparilab, Parma, Italy), designed to reduce risk of injuries in football and other outdoor sports (american football, rugby, field hockey, etc.) has been developed. These studs should allow the dissipation of the energy involved in the motion performed by athletes, resulting in a lower stress on various anatomical structures as muscle, tendon, ligaments and bone (1, 2, 3).

Methods

Saspik studs were preliminary tested in the laboratory with an universal traction/compression machine (MTS Alliance RF/150) equipped with dedicated devices built to allow vertical and oblique compression forces. Vertical and oblique forces were applied to either hindfoot and forefoot with a 2 KN force at a speed of 10 mm/min while the deformation of the inner sole was measured with four extensometers. First clinical on field trial was conducted on 15 players (12 men, 3 females) participating in football (N=14) or rugby (N=1) at various level (from amateur to professional) followed for a minimum of four months since they started using Saspik technology during practice and matches.

Results

In all the tested conditions the deformation of the inner sole was statistically lower when the shoe was equipped with SASspik studs as compared with standard, commercially available round studs. At follow up no player reported major traumatic or overuse injury or had discontinued Saspik due to discomfort or reduced performance. The rate of wear after a mean follow up of six months was acceptable and comparable with standard studs.

Conclusions

On the basis of these very preliminary data, use of flexible studs could result in a significant reduction of stress absorbed by athletes during sports activity, possibly reducing actual rate and severity of injuries, increasing comfort and no detrimental effect on athletic performance.

References

1. Ferretti A, Mapelli C, Barella S, Gruttadauria A, Mombelli D, Ciuffini AF, Calderaro C, Mazza D. Flexible studs in prevention of football injuries. A preliminary laboratory study. SCITEPRESS, Science and Technology Publications, Setubal, 2015
2. Ferretti A. Boots, studs and Injuries in football. UEFA Medical Matters 2015; 23: 2-7
3. Gehring D, Rott F, Stapelfeldt B, Gollhofer A. Effect of soccer shoe cleats on knee joint loads. Int J Sports Med 2007; 28; 1030-1034

HEAD INJURIES IN CHILDREN´S FOOTBALL

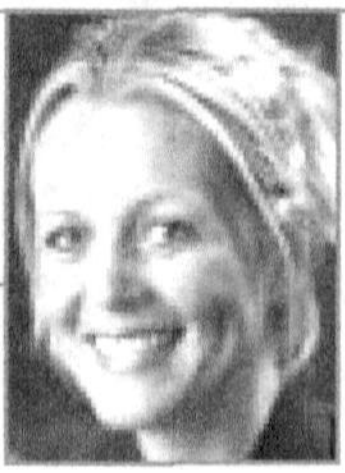

Feddermann-Demont N[1,2,3], Rössler R[4], Beaudouin F[5], aus der Fünten K[5], Chomiak J[3,6], Verhagen E[7], Junge A[2,3,8], Dvorak J[2,3], Faude O[4]

[1]Department of Neurology, Interdisciplinary Center for Vertigo and Neurological Visual Disorders, University Hospital Zurich, Zurich, Switzerland;
[2]Swiss Concussion Centre (SCC), Schulthess Klinik, Zürich, Switzerland;
[3]FIFA – Medical Assessment and Research Centre, Zurich, Switzerland
[4]Department of Sport, Exercise and Health, University of Basel, Switzerland;
[5]Institute of Sports and Preventive Medicine, Saarland University, FIFA – Medical Centre of Excellence, Saarbrücken, Germany;
[6]Department of Orthopaedics, 1st Faculty of Medicine, Charles University and Hospital, FIFA Medical Centre of Excellence, Prague, Czech Republic;
[7]Department of Public and Occupational Health, EMGO Institute for Health and Care Research, VU University Medical Center, Amsterdam, The Netherlands;
[8]Medical School Hamburg, Germany

Introduction

During recent years, concerns about the potential effects of sports-related head injuries, and particularly of concussion, on brain development of children have been raised. To date, prospectively collected data relative to football exposure time in young children are scarce.
This prospective cohort study aimed at analysing head and neck injuries occurring while playing organised football in 7 to 12 years old children in four European countries.

Methods

The study took place in Czech Republic, Germany, the Netherlands, and Switzerland over a period of 3 years. An injury was defined as any physical complaint sustained by a child during a scheduled football training session or match resulting in: a) the inability to complete the current training session or match, and/or b) the absence from subsequent training sessions or matches, and/or c) requiring medical attention. For this particular analysis, we refer to all injuries located to the head or neck. One person per participating club documented exposure time for each player as well as all injury characteristics and mechanisms through an online database according to an established consensus. Subsequently, detailed information regarding the injury as well as medical follow-up was retrieved from coaches, children and parents.

Results

A total of 39 head and one neck injuries (5% of all injuries) were documented during 9,933 player-seasons and a total exposure of 662,247 hours of playing football.
Three players had recurrent head injuries (nose bleeding and contusion).
The overall incidence was 0.25 (95% CI: 0.15-0.35) head/neck injuries per 1,000 hours of match play (N = 23 match injuries) and 0.03 (95% CI: 0.02-0.03) per 1,000 training hours.
The average age at injury was 10.4±1.6 (SD) years.

Eleven injuries (27.5%) were categorized as concussions, 9 (22.5%) as head contusions, 8 (20%) were lacerations or abrasions and 4 were fractures or dental injuries (N = 5% each).
The remaining 8 injuries were of minor severity and consisted mostly of nose bleeds in players of the youngest age category (under-9). Two injuries (one nose fracture and one concussion) resulted in a lay off time ≥ 28 days (incidence 0.02; 95% CI: 0.00-0.05). Six injuries led to 8 to 28 days lay off and 32 to less than one week. 26 (65%) injuries were medically treated (25 x physician, 1 x physiotherapist). Most injuries (55%; N = 22) resulted from collision or body duels, 12.5% (N = 5) from ball contact and 10% (N = 4) from heading duels. Table 1 shows the individual characteristics of the documented concussions. 82% (N = 9) concussions were due to contact with another player, mostly in duels or unexpected collisions.The concussions with longer lay off times resulted predominantly from head-to-head contact at the back of the head.

ID	Training/ match	Lay off (days)	Medically treated	Situation/ mechanism	Region of contact	Consequences
1	match	0	yes	ball contact	occiput	
2	match	0	no	collision/foot-to-head contact	face	dizziness
3	training	0	no	duel/elbow-to-head contact	occiput	
4	match	0	no	duel	face	headache/nose bleeding
5	match	2	yes	collision	occiput	
6	training	4	yes	ball contact	forehead	headache; several days rest and no school
7	training	4	no	collision/head-to-head contact	face	headache; several days rest
8	match	15	yes	duel	occiput	two weeks rest; no long-term effects
9	match	15	yes	collision/head-to-head contact	occiput	two weeks rest; no long-term effects
10	training	17	yes	duel	occiput	headache and dizziness; two weeks rest
11	match	38	yes	duel/head-to-head contact	occiput	several days in hospital for surveillance

Table 1. Individual characteristics of concussions.

Conclusions

The incidence and severity of head injuries in children´s football is generally low. Only two head injuries with a lay off time longer than one month occurred during the 3-year study period during a total exposure of nearly 700,000 hours of football.
Head injuries including concussion are considered as potentially harmful particularly in children due to the developing brain. Thus, compared to adults a more conservative treatment is recommended. Our results show that n ot all concussions receive the medical attention, which is essential for a safe management and return-to-play and -school, respectively.
Information and education of coaches and parents with regard to head injuries in children and Fair Play might help to raise awareness for this issue.

Acknowledgements
The authors gratefully acknowledge the financial support of FIFA.

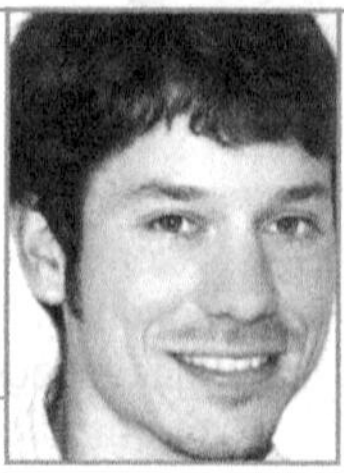

RETURN TO PLAY AFTER SEVERE FOOTBALL INJURIES IN CHILDREN AGED 7 TO 12 YEARS

Rössler R[1], Junge A[2,3,4], Chomiak J[2,5], Dvorak J[2,3,6], aus der Fünten K[7], Verhagen E[8], Faude O[1]

[1]Department of Sport, Exercise and Health, University of Basel, Basel, Switzerland; [2]FIFA-Medical Assessment and Research Centre (F-MARC), Zürich, Switzerland; [3]Schulthess Clinic, Zürich, Switzerland; [4]Medical School Hamburg, Germany; [5]Department of Orthopaedics, 1st Faculty of Medicine, Charles University and Hospital, FIFA-MCOE, Prague, Czech Republic; [6]Fédération Internationale de Football Association (FIFA), Zürich, Switzerland; [7]Institute for Sports and Preventive Medicine, Saarland University, Saarbrücken, Germany; [8]Department of Public and Occupational Health, EMGO Institute for Health and Care Research, VU University Amsterdam, The Netherlands

Introduction

Following a risk management approach, sound epidemiological data of football injuries in children have to be assessed prior to the development of a prevention programme. It has been shown that epidemiological data concerning younger children are lacking (2). Therefore, we prospectively collected epidemiological data on injuries in 7 to 12 year old child footballers. We observed that injury characteristics differ from those of high school players (3).
The objective of the present study was the analysis of lay off times resulting from severe football injuries in children aged 7 to 12 years.

Methods

The observation period covered three seasons (August 2012 to August 2015). Football teams (age categories under-9 to under-13) of officially registered football clubs from Czech Republic, Germany, Switzerland, The Netherlands were recruited.
A physical complaint sustained during a scheduled training session or match play was categorised as a severe injury if the player was (as a consequence) absent from sport for at least 28 days.
Data collection was accomplished using an internet-based registration platform. Coaches entered exposure data weekly into the system. In case a player sustained an injury, coaches entered corresponding information. The study coordinators were instantly informed about injury events and contacted parents and injured children via telephone to clarify open questions. In case of a medically treated injury, parents were asked to obtain the diagnosis from the physician.
Birth date and anthropometric baseline data were acquired from the parents and/or coaches. Players and parents signed an informed consent prior to the study.

Results

In total, 7,867 player seasons were recorded. Mean age of injured players was 10.7±1.5 (SD) years and 3.3% were girls. Players' mean height was 1.47±0.10 m, and players' weight was 37.8±9.8 kg. During the study period 150 severe injuries (23% of all injuries) occurred and led to median lay off time of 46 days (range 28-238). Most frequent severe injury locations were the upper limbs, knee, and ankle, with one fifth each (Table 1).

Location	N	(%)	Median	Min	Max
Head/face/neck	2	1.3	43	38	48
Shoulder/clavicle	8	5.3	56	37	115
Upper limbs	32	21.3	42	28	65
Trunk	2	1.3	110	39	180
Hip/groin	15	10.0	43	29	136
Thigh	7	4.7	50	30	163
Knee	29	19.3	47	28	238
Lower leg/Achilles tendon	9	6.0	42	35	160
Ankle	29	19.3	51	29	137
Foot/toe	17	11.3	47	29	110
Total	**150**	**100.0**	**46**	**28**	**238**

Table 1. Location of severe injury and lay off time in days

Regarding injury type, bone injuries were by far most frequent. Joint/ligament injuries accounted for one quarter (Table 2).

Type	N	(%)	Median	Min	Max
Bone injury	61	40.7	46	28	163
Joint/ligament injury	37	24.7	43	28	169
Muscle/tendon injury	22	14.7	45	30	150
Haematoma/contusion/bruise	5	3.3	44	38	110
Concussion	1	0.7	-	-	-
Other	24	16.0	50	30	180
Total	150	100.0	46	28	238

Table 2. Type of severe injury and lay off time in days

Ankle sprains (18% of all severe injuries) led to a median lay off time of 39 days (range 29-91) and ankle fractures (4%) to 78 days (31-137). Fractures of the clavicle (4%) led to 59 days (37-115) of absence. Knee pain with gradual onset (unspecified knee pain and M. Osgood Schlatter) accounted for 13% of all severe injuries and resulted in an average lay off time of 44 days (29-238). Sever's disease (4%) led to 47 days (30-92) of absence. With regard to injury mechanism most severe injuries were due to overuse (15%, 43 days, 29-238), growth (12%, 59 days, 30-180), and falling (12%, 46 days, 29-160). Running-related injuries (11%) showed a median lay off time of 51 days (30-136) and foul-related injuries (7%) of 48 days (42-163).

Conclusions

Severe injuries mainly affected the upper limbs, ankle, and knee. Long layoff times were seen for shoulder/clavicle, ankle, and thigh injuries. Bone injuries happened to be the most frequent type of severe injuries, which goes in line with data from high school football. The proportion of joint/ligament injuries was comparable to older players (1). Highest lay off times were reported for other (mainly growth-related) injuries, bone injuries, and muscle/tendon injuries. The amount of foul-related injuries was relatively low. Effective injury prevention programmes especially aim at specific injury types and mechanisms. Based on our epidemiological data, we developed a tailored injury prevention programme (FIFA 11+ Kids) which specifically aims at reducing the most common and severe injuries in children's football.

References

1. Darrow CJ, Collins CL, Yard EE, Comstock RD. Epidemiology of severe injuries among United States high school athletes: 2005-2007. Am J Sports Med 2009; 37: 1798-1805
2. Faude O, Rössler R, Junge A. Football injuries in children and adolescent players: are there clues for prevention? Sports Med 2013; 43: 819-837
3. Rössler R, Junge A, Chomiak J, Dvorak J, Faude O. Soccer injuries in players aged 7 to 12 years: A descriptive epidemiology study over two seasons. Am J Sports Med, 2015 Dec 8. pii: 0363546515614816. [Epub ahead of print]

Acknowledgements
The authors gratefully acknowledge the financial support of FIFA.

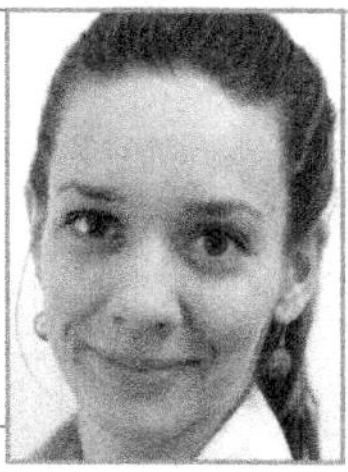

LONGTERM HEALTH PROBLEMS IN FORMER ELITE FEMALE FOOTBALL PLAYERS: PREVALENCE AND RISK FACTORS

Prien A[1], Prinz B[1], Dvorak J[2,3,4], Junge A[1,2,3]

[1]Medical School Hamburg (MSH), Hamburg, Germany; [2]FIFA Medical Assessment and Research Centre (F-MARC), Zurich, Switzerland; [3]Schulthess Clinic, Zurich, Switzerland; [4]Fédération Internationale de Football Association (FIFA), Zurich, Switzerland

Introduction

Women's football has gained considerable popularity in recent years. Between 2000 and 2006 FIFA reported a 50% increase of the total number of female players worldwide. While most research on the epidemiology of injuries in professional football was conducted with male players, some scientific information on female players has become available in recent years (2). However, very few studies have evaluated the long-term health consequences of a professional football career, particularly in female football (3). Thus, the aim of the study was to assess the prevalence of long-term health problems and associated risk factors in former elite female football players.

Methods

For the purpose of this study a quantitative, cross-sectional research design was implemented. Information on participant characteristics, career details, football-related injury history and perceived long-term health consequences was gathered using an anonymous online self-report questionnaire.

Results

152 (response rate: 62%) former First German League players answered the survey.
Around 70% described their current health as good or very good.
Over half reported knee problems during the last four weeks while exercising, and a third during normal daily activities (Table 1).
The second most common location for current complaints was the head (53.3%).
Almost one quarter (23.7%) of players suffered from Osteoarthritis (OA).
Regression analysis showed that OA in knee/ankle and other Physical Complaints (PC) in knee/ankle/head were significantly ($p<0.05$) predicted by number and severity of previous injuries. Further, older age, higher training volume and level of play were associated with an increased likelihood of OA ($p<0.05$), but not of PC.

	None	Minor	Moderate	Severe	Very Severe	Total with Complaints*
Rest	77.0	12.5	5.9	3.9	0.7	23.0
Right	84.2	8.6	4.6	2.0	0.7	15.8
Left	83.6	9.9	3.9	2.6	0	16.5
Stand	66.4	19.1	7.2	6.6	0.1	33.6
Right	75.7	14.5	5.9	3.3	0.7	24.3
Left	75.0	15.8	5.3	3.9	0.0	25.0
Walk	62.5	19.7	10.5	4.6	2.6	37.5
Right	71.7	16.4	7.9	2.0	2.0	28.3
Left	74.3	14.5	7.9	2.6	0.7	25.7
Stairs	54.6	17.8	15.1	9.2	3.3	45.4
Right	65.1	17.8	9.9	5.9	1.3	34.9
Left	67.1	13.8	11.8	5.3	2.0	32.9
Exercise	42.1	24.3	17.8	10.5	5.3	57.9
Right	54.6	22.4	13.2	6.6	3.3	45.4
Left	59.9	18.4	11.8	7.9	2.0	40.1

Table 1. Severity of knee complaints during the last four weeks in % of participants. *Percentage of participants with minor to very severe complaints.

Conclusions

German former elite female football players report a higher prevalence of PC and OA in knee and ankle, poorer subjective health, and increased pain medication use compared to the general population. Identified risk factors for long-term health problems included number and severity of previous injuries, age, training volume and level of play.
In light of these results the use of injury prevention measures and a cautious approach to return to play, particularly after knee, ankle and head injury, should be furthered in elite female football. Structured warm-up programs and proprioceptive training have proven effective in this context (1). Finally, it is evident that elite female football players need specific medical care during and beyond their career, with a focus on early diagnosis and treatment of OA. Future studies are needed to clinically assess prevalence rates of OA and possible neurocognitive changes.

References

1. Gilchrist J, Mandelbaum BR, Melancon H, Ryan GW, Silvers HJ, Griffin LY, Watanabe DS, Dick RW, Dvorak J. A randomized controlled trial to prevent noncontact anterior cruciate ligament injury in female collegiate soccer players. Am J Sports Med 2008; 36: 1476-1483
2. Junge A. Epidemiology in Female Football Players. In: Volpi P (Ed). Football Traumatology. Springer International Publishing, Heidelberg, 2015, pp. 21-27
3. Lohmander LS, Ostenberg A, Englund M, Roos H. High prevalence of knee osteoarthritis, pain, and functional limitations in female soccer players twelve years after anterior cruciate ligament injury. Arthritis Rheum 2004; 50: 3145-3152

Acknowledgements
The authors gratefully acknowledge the Fédération Internationale de Football Association (FIFA) for funding this study

INVERSE RELATIONSHIP BETWEEN PLAYING LEVEL AND REINJURY RATES IN MEN'S FOOTBALL

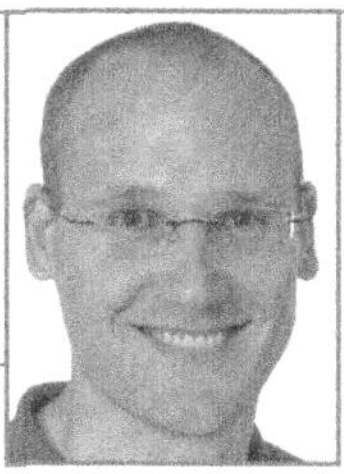

Hägglund M[1,2], Waldén M[2,3], Ekstrand J[2,3]

[1]Division of Physiotherapy, Department of Medical and Health Sciences, Linköping University, Linköping; [2]Football Research Group, Linköping; [3]Division of Community Medicine, Department of Medical and Health Sciences, Linköping University, Linköping, Sweden

Introduction

Recent studies have shown stable or even increasing injury rates in men's elite football in the last decade (1), highlighting the need for preventive measures. Previous injury is probably the strongest and well-documented risk factor for injury (2), increasing the risk of new injury up to 11-fold for hamstring injury, 7-fold for groin injury, and 5-fold for knee and ankle sprains. Thus, lowering re-injury rates may substantially impact on the total injury burden. The purposes of the study were to compare re-injury proportions, incidences and patterns between three different football playing levels, and to study time-trends in re-injury incidence in elite football.

Methods

Time-loss injuries were collected from injury surveillance of 43 top-level European professional teams (240 team-seasons), 19 Swedish elite premier division teams (82 team-seasons) and 10 Swedish amateur teams (10 team-seasons). Data were collected between 2001 and 2015, and participation ranged 1-14 years for the included teams. Re-injury was defined as an injury of the same type and at the same site as an index injury within the preceding year, with re-injury <2 months defined as an early recurrence, and >2 months as a delayed recurrence. Seasonal trend for re-injury incidence, expressed as average annual percentage of change, was analysed using linear regression

Results

13,050 injuries were registered, 2,449 (18.8%) being re-injuries, with 1,944 early (14.9%) and 505 delayed recurrences (3.9%).

Re-injury proportions differed between playing levels, with 35.1% in the amateur cohort, 25.0% in the Swedish elite cohort, and 16.6% in the European top-level cohort ($\chi2$ overall effect, $p<0.001$). The lowest re-injury proportions were consistently seen during pre-season and the highest in the second half of the competitive season in all cohorts (Figure 1).

A decreasing trend was observed in re-injury incidence in the European top-level cohort, with -2.9% average annual change over the 14-year study period (95% CI -5.4% to -0.4%; $p=0.026$). Similarly, a decreasing tendency was also seen in the Swedish elite cohort.

Hamstring injury was the most frequent re-injury diagnosis in the European top-level and Swedish elite cohorts, together with muscle injuries to the adductors and quadriceps.

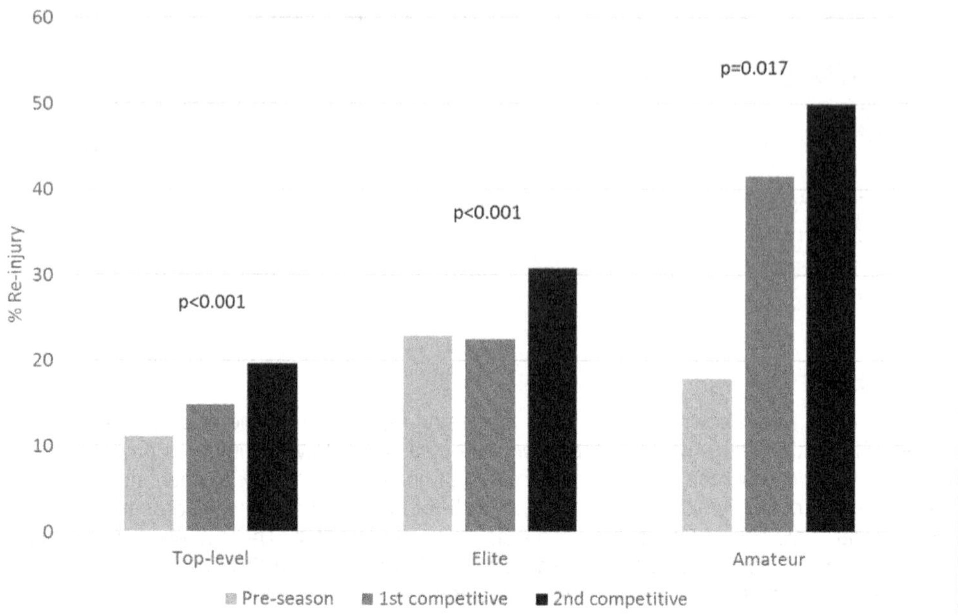

Figure 1. Re-injury proportion as a function of part of season.

Conclusions

- An inverse relationship was found between the playing level and re-injury rates in men's football. High manpower of medical staffs, high-quality rehabilitation and support in the Return To Play (RTP), and larger competitive squads allowing for sufficient rehabilitation time, are possible factors speaking in favour of top-level clubs.
- A decreasing trend in re-injury incidence was observed in European top-level clubs and in the Swedish premier division over the last decade.
- Re-injury proportions were higher in the second half of the competitive season compared with the first half of the season and pre-season, suggesting higher risk tolerance in RTP decisions towards the final stages of league play and cups.
- The high rate of early recurrences within two months shows that avoiding premature RTP is a crucial component to decrease the overall re-injury incidence. Strict adherence to rehabilitation protocols and graded RTP throughout the entire season, and ensuring respect for such protocols from all stakeholders within the club from the player, medical staff, fitness staff, and coaches to the members of the board, may help reduce the re-injury burden.

References

1. Ekstrand J, Hägglund M, Kristenson K, Magnusson H, Waldén M. Fewer ligament injuries but no preventive effect on muscle injuries and severe injuries: an 11-year follow-up of the UEFA Champions League injury study. Br J Sports Med 2013; 47: 732-737
2. Hägglund M, Waldén M, Ekstrand J. Previous injury as a risk factor for injury in elite football - a prospective study over two consecutive seasons. Br J Sports Med 2006; 40: 767-772

WHY FEMALE FOOTBALLER PLAYERS QUIT FOOTBALL. POLISH SURVEY RESULTS

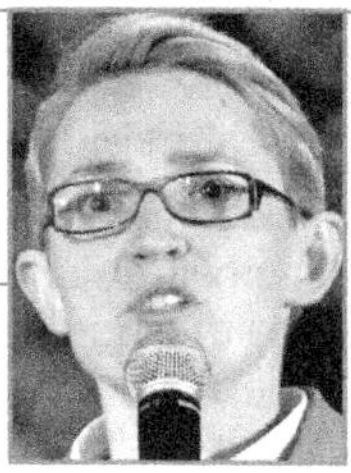

Grygorowicz M[1,2], Piontek T[1], Dudzinski W[1]

[1]Rehasport Clinic, FIFA Medical Centre of Excellence, Poznan;
[2]Stanislaw Staszic University of Applied Sciences, Pila, Poland

Introduction

Women's football is one of the most dynamically developing disciplines, and the popularity of football among women in Poland is similar to other team sports, like basketball or handball (1, 2). Over 5,000 active female footballers are registered in our county. However, there has been no research on the reasons why female football players quit training or on the physical condition of former players. Therefore, we focused on finding the actual reasons behind the decision to end one's football career, and on learning how the past career affects the player's health today.

Methods

Sixty-five Polish former female football players (aged 18-over 50 years old, whose football career lasted from 2 to over 15 years) completed the survey "The reasons of quitting or ending football career" through the Internet site: http://www.naukowastronafutbolu.pl/ankieta.html.

The survey consisted of 10 parts: 1) personal data, 2) current living status, 3) information about the main reasons and respondent's personal situation at the end of her football career, 4) data about the level of football competition, 5) character traits, 6) information about medical and specialist testing, 7) data about training/matches, 8) additional questions, 9) career abroad and 10) factors that contributed to the end of respondent's football career.

To express the relationship between different variables and to analyse which factors are related to the decision to end one's sports career we performed a statistical analysis using the nonparametric the χ^2 test for r $\times$c tables (Pearson's Chi-square test). The level of significance was set at $p<0.05$. PQStat 1.8.4.322 software was used in the statistical analysis.

Results

We noted a relationship between financial difficulties, fear of injury, the need to change the place of residence and the resignation from the game. Financial difficulties and the need to change the place of living did not affect the decision to end one's football career (χ^2 test: $p<0.005$ and $p<0.001$, respectively).

However, fear of injury had a very big impact on resignation and having to one's career (χ^2 test: $p<0.002$). 35% of all female football players who participated in the study had to end their careers as a result of long-term treatment of injury. Over 35% of players stated that they would have liked to play longer, but their health problems had made it impossible (χ^2 test: $p<0.001$).

There was a relationship between the main cause of resignation from the game and the type of health insurance the players held during their careers (χ^2 test: $p<0.025$).

37% of participants were covered only by the obligatory health insurance (at school, college or work) and 65% of them had to end the careers due to injury (probably as the result of the non-sport specific standards of treatment offered in Poland under the obligatory health insurance).

97% of athletes stated they had never been subjected to injury screening, and biomechanical testing. What is more, 68% of respondents said they wish to have known more about prevention. In 40% of athletes' current health status influences physical activity, 22% experience difficulties while changing the direction of movement and 36% of former footballers have knee problems.

Conclusions

The survey revealed the significance and urgency of addressing the medical aspect in women's football: injuries not only force women to quit playing football prematurely, but also affect their health long after their careers are over.
The main actions to allow female footballers enjoy longer and healthier careers should involve the introduction of broad, player-focused educational programmes on injury prevention, and the implementation of screening or testing as the possible way to identify and help players with high risk of injury.
Also, introducing additional, obligatory health insurance, covering the high-level medical and rehabilitation care in case of injury, could help athletes return to full sports activity and prevent them from having to quit the game.

References

1. FIFA Big Count 2006. FIFA. Retrieved July 10, 2008
2. Jakubowska H. The (un)changeable status of women's football: the case of Poland Women's football: played, watched, talked about! International research conference, Denmark, 21-22 June 2013. http://www.free-project.eu/documents-free/Working%20Papers/Jakubowska%20The%20%28un%29changeable%20status%20of%20women%27s%20football%20the%20case%20of%20Poland.pdf

PREVENTION AND RETURN TO PLAY OF INJURIES IN ELITE FOOTBALL: THE TEAM COACHES` VIEW

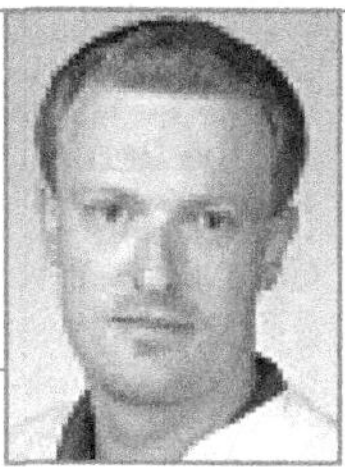

Krutsch W[1], Zantop T[2], Angele P[1,2]

[1]Department of Trauma Surgery, University Medical Centre Regensburg, FIFA Medical Centre of Excellence;
[2]Sporthopaedicum Straubing, Regensburg, Germany

Introduction

The performance and quality of injury prevention in football depends on the experience of the team staff, in which the team coach is the most important person in elite football. Team coaches are in majority former football player with high experience in the game. This study analysed the attendance and knowledge of football coaches in elite football about injury prevention and return to play issues after injuries.

Methods

In the context of an overall project about primary and secondary injury prevention in elite football in Germany, the team coaches were investigated in the beginning of the study period. They were investigated by standardized online questionnaire regarding own experiences and ideas about injury prevention and return to play after football injuries.

Results

Ninety-five team coaches of the elite football levels were analysed. 98.1 % of the coaches were retired football player, 20% played in professional football and 55% in the highest amateur levels. 100% of coaches assumed that prevention of football injuries is possible and 88.5% assumed the injury rates as a big problem in football.
The knee is well-known as most affected body region by severe injuries, particularly the ACL rupture (43%). Long time out of football (21%) and the severe long-term consequences after injuries (51%) were seen as the main reason for necessary injury prevention. For the team planning of the season, the team coaches calculate with in the mean 21 player and 7 injured player in the run of a season.
The analysis of the team coach estimation about risk factors for injuries in elite football revealed to slight regeneration time during the season (67%), low fitness level of the player (54%) und previous not recovered injuries (51%).
Direct influence on injury prevention was specified by the team coaches with the warm up program (75%), trunk stability (70%), neuromotor exercises (58%) and regeneration training (56%). Further improvement for injury prevention was seen by the team coaches with frequent preventive care by the physical therapist (76%), medical screening examinations (62%) or performance diagnostic (55%).
Training time was 90 minutes and 18 minutes was the provided time by the team coaches for the players' warm-up program before training or matches.
The currently performed training topics by these coaches are: warming-up exercises (98%), ball exercises (85%), shooting exercises (62%) and stretching (59%). Balance exercises (11%) and jumping exercises (16%) were rarely performed.

For the Return To Play (RTP) decision after football injuries is the medical doctor the man in charge (84%).
Only 20% of the team coaches want to have the last decision about the RTP time after injuries.
87% of the team coaches have experiences with the situation of football player with not recovered injuries on field against medical advice.
71% experienced not recovered player on field with a subsequent re-injury.
94% of the football coaches may believe in RTP testing to avoid re-injuries in football, and 100% want to use these testing, if they are available for them. 98% team coaches will use screening tests in the beginning of the season and a mean of 28 minutes is offered by the team coaches for such testing in the preseason period.
46% of the teams are currently using performance diagnostic or medical screening tests to the beginning of the season, mainly by lactate tests or the Cooper test.

Conclusion

As conclusion, this study revealed a high acceptance and knowledge about prevention of injuries in elite football coaches. Improvement of injury prevention and implementation of RTP testing are possible and should be a fundament of a frequent exchange between team coaches and medical staff.

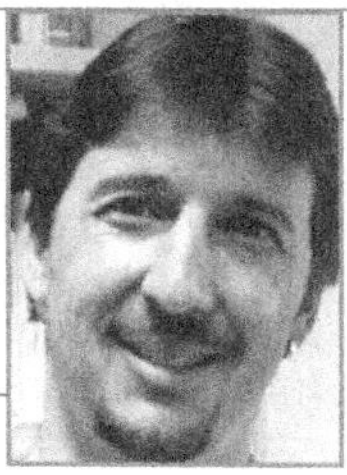

INJURY PREVENTION IN CHILDREN'S FOOTBALL "FIFA 11+ KIDS": A CLUSTER RANDOMISED CONTROLLED TRIAL

Faude O[1], Rössler R[1], Bizzini M[2,3], Dvorak J[2,3,4], Chomiak J[2,5], aus der Fünten K[6], Verhagen E[7], Lichtenstein E[1], Junge A[2,3,8]

[1]Department of Sport, Exercise and Health, University of Basel, Basel, Switzerland; [2]FIFA-Medical Assessment and Research Centre (F-MARC), Zürich, Switzerland; [3]Schulthess Clinic, Zürich, Switzerland; [4]Fédération Internationale de Football Association (FIFA), Zürich, Switzerland; [5]Department of Orthopaedics, 1st Faculty of Medicine, Charles University and Hospital, FIFA-M.C.O.E, Prague, Czech Republic; [6]Institute for Sports and Preventive Medicine, Saarland University, Saarbrücken, Germany; [7]Department of Public and Occupational Health, EMGO Institute for Health and Care Research, VU University Amsterdam, The Netherlands; 8Medical School Hamburg, Germany

Introduction

Football is the world´s most popular sport. The majority of officially registered players (58%) is younger than 18 years of age. Football is a high-intensity and high-impact contact sport bearing a risk of injury. Therefore, it is necessary to implement preventive measures starting at a young age to reduce the risk of injury and to optimize the health benefits associated with playing football (2). Based on own epidemiologic data (3) we developed a new injury prevention program for children (FIFA 11+ Kids). FIFA 11+ Kids has proven to beneficially affecting motor performance (1). The objective of the present study was to assess the effectiveness of FIFA 11+ Kids with regard to injury prevention.

Methods

Football teams (age categories under-11 to under-13) of officially registered clubs from Switzerland, Czech Republic, The Netherlands, and Germany were recruited, randomised to an Intervention (INT) or a Control group (CON), and followed-up for one season (August 2014 to August 2015). INT teams performed FIFA 11+ Kids as their warm-up, while CON teams warmed-up as usual.

A physical complaint sustained during a scheduled training session or match was recorded as an injury if the player: i) was unable to complete the current session or match, and/or ii) was as a consequence absent from the subsequent session or match, and/or iii) sought medical attention. Data collection was internet-based (injury registration platform). Coaches entered exposure data weekly. In case of an injury, coaches entered complementary information. The study coordinators were promptly informed and contacted parents and injured children via telephone to clarify remaining questions. In case of a medically treated injury, parents were asked to obtain the diagnosis from the physician. Injury incidence was calculated as number of injuries per 1,000 player-hours. Rate ratios of injury incidences between INT and CON and z-statistics were calculated.

Results

In total, 3,895 player seasons with a total of 292,749 hours of football exposure were recorded. The mean age of the injured players was 11.2±1.1 (SD) years, 3.8% were girls. During the study period 374 injuries occurred. The mean lay off time was of 16.6 (range: 0-160) days.
Injury incidence in INT was reduced by 25% to 56% compared to CON (Table 1).

	INT	CON	Rate ratio	p value
Overall	0.94 (0.80-1.11)	1.52 (1.34-1.73)	0.62 (0.50-0.76)	<0.001
Match	3.96 (3.14-5.00)	5.78 (4.82-6.94)	0.69 (0.51-0.92)	0.012
Training	0.52 (0.41-0.67)	0.89 (0.74-1.06)	0.59 (0.44-0.79)	<0.001
Severe	0.14 (0.09-0.22)	0.32 (0.24-0.43)	0.44 (0.26,0.73)	0.002
Lower extremity	0.71 (0.58-0.85)	1.20 (1.04-1.39)	0.59 (0.46-0.75)	<0.001
Non-contact	0.30 (0.22-0.40)	0.67 (0.55-0.81)	0.45 (0.28-0.74)	<0.001
Contact	0.62 (0.50-0.76)	0.83 (0.70-0.98)	0.75 (0.57-0.98)	0.032

Table 1. Injury incidences with 95% confidence intervals as well as corresponding rate ratios.
INT: intervention group; CON: control group.

Conclusions

The new injury prevention program FIFA 11+ Kids is effective in reducing injuries in children's football. There were considerable reductions in overall, match, training, severe, lower extremity, non-contact and contact injuries.
The overall injury reduction is comparable to the effects of prevention programmes observed in several studies in older youth football players (2).
The reduction of injury incidence might be due to an improved motor performance, an effect the FIFA 11+ Kids showed in an earlier study (1).
Based on this study the FIFA 11+ Kids can be recommended for children's football. A broad implementation may help to reduce injuries starting at a young age and thus to support the health benefits of football in the long term.

References

1. Rössler R, Donath L, Bizzini M, Faude O. A new injury prevention programme for children's football - FIFA 11+ Kids - can improve motor performance: a cluster-randomised controlled trial. J Sports Sci 2015 Oct 27: 1-8. [Epub ahead of print]
2. Rössler R, Donath L, Verhagen E, Junge A, Schweizer T, Faude O. Exercise-based injury prevention in child and adolescent sport: a systematic review and meta-analysis. Sports Med 2014; 44: 1733-1748
3. Rössler R, Junge A, Chomiak J, Dvorak J, Faude O. Soccer Injuries in Players Aged 7 to 12 Years: A Descriptive Epidemiological Study Over 2 Seasons. Am J Sports Med 2015 Dec 8. [Epub ahead of print]

The authors gratefully acknowledge the financial support of FIFA.

Sunday, 10th April, 2016
POSTER AREA

FREE POSTER PRESENTATIONS

FUNCTIONAL ASSESSMENT

Chairs

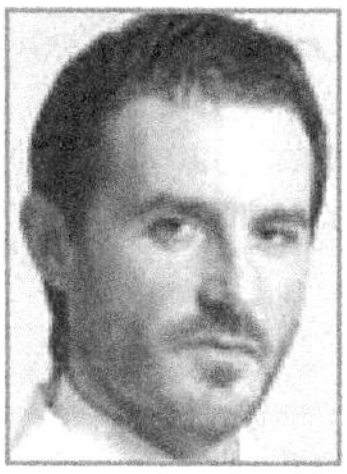

Emanuele Brotto
(Verona, Italy)

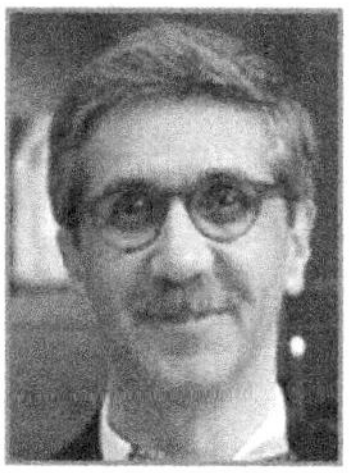

Giulio Sergio Roi
(Bologna, Italy)

PB01 Reference centile curves for screening body mass index and body postural stability in football players aged 8-18 years
Alberti G, Rossi A, Roi GS (Milan and Bologna, Italy)

PB02 Hip mobility and strength ratios of young football players
Gibbs S, Ólafsson S (Dundee, United Kingdom; Akureyri, Iceland)

PB03 Aerobic and anaerobic thresholds in rehabilitation: considerations by five hundred incremental running test
Baroli M, Castagnetti A, Roi GS, Lanza M (Verona, Italy)

PB04 Dermatoglyphics: a tool to observe the neuromotor potential of feet laterality
Souza R, Sosa MOV, Pratto AL, Buhringer W, Cardoso A, Frank B, Alberti A, de Jesus JA, Sartori G, Fin G, Nodari Júnior RJ (Joaçaba, Brazil)

PB05 Isokinetic thigh muscles evaluations of female high level soccer players
Grazzini G, Zuppardo S, Pellegrini F, Rosini V, Martelli G (Florence, Grosseto and Brescia, Italy)

PB06 Reactive agility profile and change of direction speed by playing position in u-16 elite soccer players **Trecroci A, Della Bella S, Alberti G (Milan, Italy)**

1

REFERENCE CENTILE CURVES FOR SCREENING BODY MASS INDEX AND BODY POSTURAL STABILITY IN FOOTBALL PLAYERS AGED 8-18 YEARS

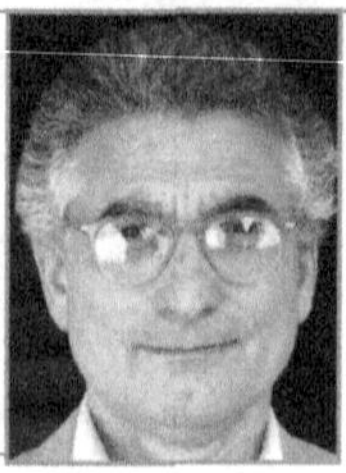

Alberti G[1], Rossi A[1], Roi GS[2]

[1]Università degli Studi di Milano, School of Exercise Sciences, Department of Biomedical Sciences for Health, Milan; [2]Isokinetic Medical Group, FIFA Medical centre of Excellence, Education and Research Department, Bologna, Italy

Introduction

Since birth, children grow up in terms of height and body weight, and subsequently in terms of the maturation of the nervous, endocrine, muscular, and cardiovascular systems. These adaptations lead to alterations in neuromuscular performances (3). The increase of Body Mass Index (BMI) can cause a reduction in the postural stability and then increase the risk of falls, particularly when combined with low muscular mass which can generate biomechanical failure of muscular responses and loss of stability mechanisms (2).
The aim of this study was to analyse the BMI and Body Postural Stability (BPS) in football players across childhood and adolescence, thus developing reference centile curves, and to investigate their relationship.

Methods

512 males from 8 to 18 years were recruited from Italian football teams. It was performed a cross-sectional study. BMI was calculated measuring height and weight [body mass (kg) / height (m2)]. BPS were taken by means of a Libra seesaw balance board (Libra, Easytech, Florence, Italy). Reference centile curves were created by Lambda-Mu-Sigma (LMS) method. To assess the difference among ages, Kruskal Wallis test was performed.
The correlation between BMI and BPS was evaluated by Pearson correlation coefficient controlled by age (partial correlation). In addition, a stepwise multiple regression analysis was used to determine the effect of age and BMI on BPS, and the effect of age and BPS on BMI. Finally, Pearson correlation coefficient or Sperman Rho were performed in order to detect the correlation between BMI and BPS in each age group. The assumption of normal data distribution was verified by Shapiro-Wilks' Normality test.

Results

Significant improvement in BMI ($\chi^2(1,10)=106.383$, $p<0.001$) and BPS ($\chi^2(1,10)=272.141$, $p<0.001$) were found across age (Figure 1).

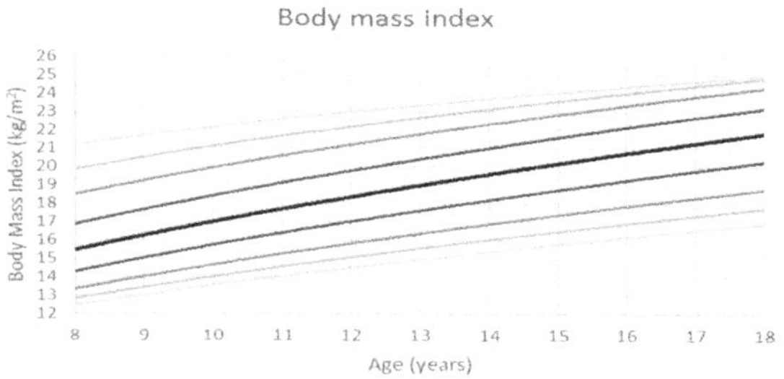

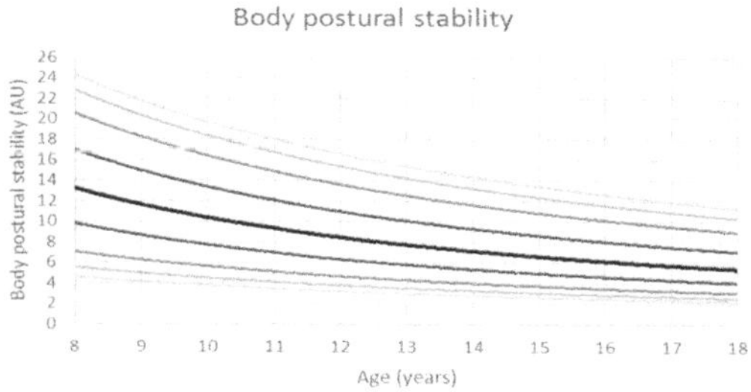

Figure 1. Reference centile curves for Body Mass Index and Body Postural Stability in football players across childhood and adolescence.

Significant partial correlation ($r=0.304$; $p<0.001$) was found between BMI and BPS.
The multiple regression revealed that age and BMI accounted for 47.5% and 4.8% of the variance of BPS ($F(_{2,510})=208.092$, $p<0.001$), respectively, and age and BPS accounted for 18.8% and 7.5% of the variance of BMI ($F(_{2,510})=90.915$, $p<0.001$), respectively.
Finally, the correlation were significant in each age group ($r>0.251$, $p<0.05$) except for football players of 11, 14, and 15 years old.

Conclusion

The football players increase BMI and improve their BPS during the growth. The reference centile curves provided in this study could help trainers to assess the levels of their football players. Previous studies found that the accumulation of fat tissue can reduce postural stability and contribute towards falls (1). Accordingly, we found a direct relationship between BPS and BMI across childhood and adolescence. The lower is the BMI, the better is the body postural stability during the growth, because high BMI demands more neuromuscular control to maintain postural stability (1). However, our results showed improvements on BMI and BPS were mostly affected by the body development during growth and barely affected by their relationship.
A greater limitation of this investigation is that this study have a cross sectional design. Future longitudinal study is needed to better investigate this topic.

References

1. Greve J, Alonso A, Bordini ACPG, Camanho GL. Correlation between body mass index and postural balance. Clinics 2007; 62: 717-720
2. Maffiuletti NA, Agosti F, Proietti M, Riva D, Resnik M, Lafortuna CL, Sartorio A. Postural instability of extremely obese individuals improves after a body weight reduction program entailing specific balance training. J Endocrinol Invest 2005; 28: 2-7
3. Roemmich JN, Rogol AD. Physiology of growth and development. Its relationship to performance in the young athlete. Cli Sports Med 1995; 14: 483-502

HIP MOBILITY AND STRENGTH RATIOS OF YOUNG FOOTBALL PLAYERS

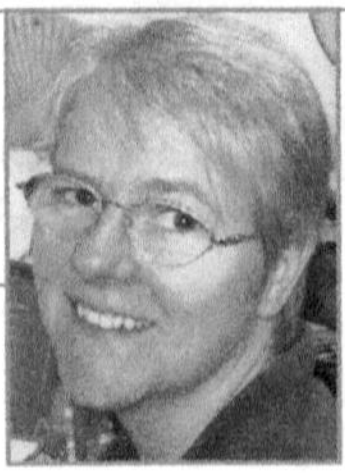

Gibbs S[1], Ólafsson S[2]

[1]University of Dundee, Dundee, United Kingdom;
[2]Efling Physical Therapy, Akureyri, Iceland

Introduction

A loss of hip mobility has been reported in adult football players, and been related to hip and groin pain (3), and may as well have relation, the development of knee varus and bony changes of the femoral neck in young footballers (1).
Lack of mobility may increase torsional strain at the lumbo-pelvic and knee joints. This may cause injury and secondary osteoarthrosis when subjected to repeated high loads in the frontal and transverse planes, in football. Secondly, movement pattern of kicking, may lead to the development of football specific adaptive muscle strength ratios, and these abnormal strength ratios may lead to groin or hip dysfunction and injury. The purpose of this study was to examine the relationships between kicking and muscle imbalance around the hip.

Methods

The hip Internal Rotation (IR), External Rotation (ER) and abduction Range Of Motion (ROM) were measured using an inclinometer (Patterson, Medical Ltd, Nottingham, UK). Hip strength ratios of IR/ER, and adduction/abduction were measured with a Hand-Held Dynamometer (HHD) (Lafayette Instruments, Indiana, USA).
The participants were from two teams of under 13 players (Group 1: mean 43.8±6.1 kg, 153.2±6.2 cm; Group 2: 44.7±8 kg, 155.8±8.1 cm), training at different intensities, and one group of elite under 20 players (Group 3: 76.5±7.3 kg, 78.2±5.6 cm). Of the under 13's, Group 1 was Non-Elite (NE) (n=15) training once per week and Group 2 was Elite players (E) (n=13) training 5 times per week.
The elite U20s team (n=18), Group 3, trained 5-6 times per week.
This is the first study of its kind on non-injured footballers, where mobility and strength ratios were tested. The method of HHD in prone position is introduced for testing adduction/abduction strength ratios.

Results

The U20s players had significant hip rotational mobility deficiency compared to reference values of 45°, with significantly less mobility on the support hip of IR ($p<0.003$) and ER ($p<0.001$) (Figure 1).

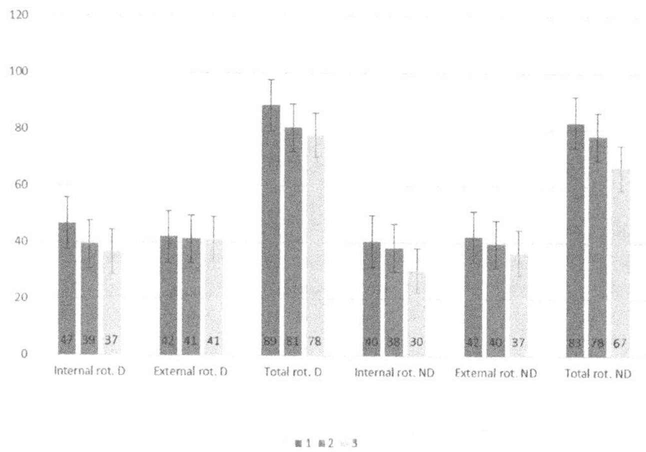

Figure 1. Hip mobility of all groups of the dominant (D) and non-dominant (ND) side.

The U20s had also significantly less ($p<0.05$) rotational and abduction mobility than the NE U13s group on both hips.
The elite (E) U13s had significantly less abduction and total rotation than the NE U13s ($p<0.05$) showing greater loss of IR.
There was not a side difference in strength, but the IR/ER strength ratios exhibited relative weakness of the internal rotators in all groups ($p>0.05$) with the greatest mean ER dominance in the U20´s as 0.68 on the non-dominant side.
The mean adductor/abductor ratio did favour adductor strength with values over one (>1). These were highest as 1.29 on the non-dominant side in Group 1, and on the dominant side in Group 2. This was higher than data of non-football athletes (2).

Conclusions

This study suggests that the reduced mobility and musculoskeletal changes of the hip may affect movement patterns in footballers, at a younger age than previously reported.
The study implies that imbalance is related to load as well as age, and the support leg may need more attention.
The results indicate a need for rotational and abductor training to protect the hip and knee in adolescent players, and to prevent hip and knee degeneration, as reported in ex-footballers.

References

1. Agricola R, Heijboer MP, Ginai AZ, Roels P, Zadpoor AA, Verhaar JA, Weinans H, Waarsing JH. A cam deformity is gradually acquired during skeletal maturation in adolescent and young male soccer players: a prospective study with minimum 2-year follow-up. Am J Sports Med 2014; 42: 798-806
2. Thorborg K, Petersen J, Magnusson SP, Hölmich P. Clinical assessment of hip strength using a hand-held dynamometer is reliable. Scand J Med Sci Sports 2010; 20: 493-501
3. Verrall GM, Slavotinek JP, Barnes PG, Esterman A, Oakeshott RD, Spriggins AJ. Hip joint range of motion restriction precedes athletic chronic groin injury. J Sci Med Sport 2007; 10: 463-466

AEROBIC AND ANAEROBIC THRESHOLDS IN REHABILITATION: CONSIDERATIONS BY 500 INCREMENTAL RUNNING TEST

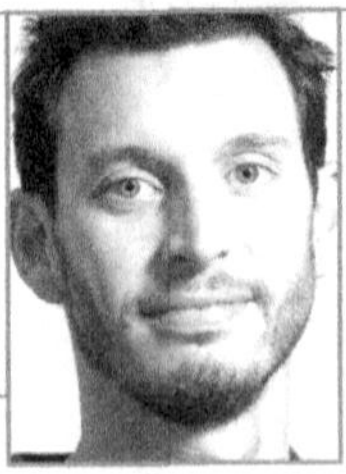

Baroli M, Castagnetti A, Roi GS, Lanza M

Isokinetic Medical Group, FIFA Medical Centre of Excellence, Verona and Department of Neurological, Biomedical and Movement Sciences, University of Verona, Verona, Italy

Introduction

Heart Rate (HR) monitoring is one of the most popular systems to monitor the intensity of the exercises during sporting activities. The improvement of this type of systems allows to use them also in rehabilitation, to derive information on the quantity of aerobic and anaerobic exercise carried by the patient. As an example, a monitoring system of HR via Wireless Fidelity (WiFi) (Polar Flow; Polar Electro, Kempele, Finland) can be utilized at very low cost to monitor the HR of every patient for the entire session.
The aim of this study is to analyse the reference heart rates to be utilized to monitor the aerobic and anaerobic intensity of the exercises.

Methods

509 consecutive Incremental Running Test (IRT) made in the last for years in our clinic were analysed. The IRT was carried out as soon as the patient was able to run for almost 10 minutes at 8 km/h. Patients were affected by different conservative and surgical orthopedic pathologies, most of them were involved in amateur or professional sporting activities.
Patients have been split in homogeneous groups according to sex and training level i.e. Sedentary (Sed) and Sport subjects (Sport).
The HRs corresponding to aerobic and anaerobic thresholds of each patient were detained through an IRT, starting at 7 km/h with speed increments of 2 km/h every three minutes until the anaerobic threshold is reached (1). At the end of every three minutes step, measurements of the Heart Rate (HR) (Heart Rate Monitors, Polar Electro, Kempele, Finland), and blood lactate concentration (Lactate Analyzer YSI 1500 Sport, Yellow Spring Corp., Yellow Spring, USA) from capillary samples from an ear lobe were taken.
Aerobic Threshold (T2) and anaerobic Thresholds (T4) conventionally settled at 2 and 4 mmol/L of lactate respectively, were then calculated in terms of speed (km/h) and HR (bpm) from the relationships between speed and lactate and between speed and HR; these thresholds are used to individualize the intensity of the training sessions in healthy players.
The maximum HR (HRmax) was calculated from the formula 220-year of age, then T2 and T4 were expressed also as % of HRmax.

Results

435 Males (M), age 32±12 yrs and 74 Females (F), age 34±13 yrs completed the IRT. The results are shown in Table 1.

	N	T2 km/h	T2 HR	T2 % MaxHR	T4 km/h	T4 HR	T4 % MaxHR
F Sed	22	6.6±1.0	153±9	83±5	8.9±1.0	172±8	93±4
F Sport	47	9.8±1.0	163±10	89±6	11.8±0.9	179±9	98±5
F All	69	8.2±1.0	158±10	86±5	10.3±1.0	176±8	96±5
M Sed	83	6.7±1.0	143±11	79±6	9.6±1.0	169±9	94±5
M Sport	350	10.2±2	162±11	88±6	12.8±1.5	178±10	97±6
M All	433	8.5±1.2	152±11	84±6	11.2±1.3	174±9	95±5

Table 1. Incremental Running Test (IRT); M: males; F: females; N: number of subjects; T2: aerobic threshold; T4: anaerobic threshold; MaxHR: maximum heart rate.

No significant differences were found between Females and Males ($p>0.05$).
Sedentary patients tends to show lower thresholds speeds and lower thresholds HR compared to Sports patients.
Older patients (>40 yrs) tend to have higher % MaxHR compared to younger.
An equation was made to calculate the % MaxHR corresponding to aerobic and anaerobic thresholds:

$$T2\ \%\ MaxHR = 0.0065 \times age\ (yrs) + 0.6564\ (R^2 = 0.519)$$
$$T4\ \%\ MaxHR = 0.0057 \times age\ (yrs) + 0.7648\ (R^2 = 0.4893)$$

Conclusions

The data of the present study can be utilized to indirectly calculate the HR corresponding to T2 and T4 from the age of the patient. However there is a certain variability around the average values, which can affect the correct intensity of training during rehabilitation. Furthermore it is important to consider also the fact that the % of MaxHR corresponding to T2 and T4 tend to increase with age. As a consequence, IRT seems to be the most precise and suitable test for a direct calculation of HR corresponding to T2 and T4 in all the patients.

References

1. Bosquet L, Léger L, Legros P. Methods to determine aerobic endurance. Sports Med 2002; 32: 675-700

DERMATOGLYPHICS: A TOOL TO OBSERVE THE NEUROMOTOR POTENTIAL OF FEET LATERALITY

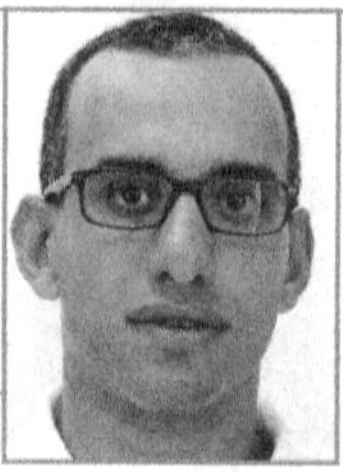

Souza R, Sosa MOV, Pratto AL, Buhringer W, Cardoso A, Frank B, Alberti A, de Jesus JA, Sartori G, Fin G, Nodari Júnior RJ

Universidade do Oeste de Santa Catarina, Joaçaba, Brazil

Introduction

The laterality is related to the personal internal system that enables him to use one side of the body more effectively than the other one for performing activities that require skills, characterized by a functional asymmetry, in which the right and left side space neuromotor are not homogeneous. The lateral preference for child development may indicate the genetic factors action, however the skilled motor behaviour acquirement through practical experience may indicate the laterality development. The use of genetic testing has been a more common tool to predict the success of children and teenagers in sport. One of the genetic and fetal development research possibilities, associated with the sport is the Dermatoglyphics.

Purpose: to analyse the right and left handed fingerprints characteristics related to the pedal dominance through the Dermatoglyphics.

Methods

To evaluate the teenagers' lateral pedal dominance, was used the measure handedness tool through gestural tasks proposed by Negrine (2).

The sample consisted of 394 adolescents, aged 11-17 years, males and females in Brazil. The protocol chosen to analyse the genetic potential and fetal development was the Dermatoglyphic, proposed by Cummins and Midlo (1). For capturing, processing and analysing the fingers' fingerprints, was used the computerized process for Dermatoglyphics reading, so, a reader comprising an optical scanner bearing which collects, interprets the image and builds it in binary code, a design, which is captured by specific treatment and reconstruction software of real images through the Leitor Dermatoglífico (Dermatoglyphic Reader, Salus Dermatoglifia, Luzerna, Brazil) validated by Nodari Junior (3).

Statistical analyses were processed in Statistical Package for Social Sciences (SPSS), version 20.0, and established the significance level of $p<0.05$. Comparing the groups and their quantitative variables, to observe the normality's distribution, was used the Kolmogorov-Smirnov test. The observation of non-normal distribution, applies to the inference Nonparametric Mann-Whitney test for comparisons between numeric variables. To compare categorical variables: Arc (A), Loop Radial (LR), Loop Ulnar (LU), Whorl (W), the chi-square test was used, and when found significant differences, applied to residue analysis adjusted.

Results

For the rare brands analysis between the two groups (right and left-footed), referring to qualitative variables (so, the figure type) there are significant differences in the Finger Minimum Left Hand (MET5, p=0.008), with larger quantity of LR in left-footed group and Raj value of 3.3, since the analysis of adjusted waste was considered as the mean values above the standard of 1.96.

Finger	**Foot Dominance**	**Fingerprint Figure Type**			
			LR	LU	W
MET5	Right	1.0	-3.3	-0.2	0.2
	Left	-1.0	3.3*	0.2	-0.2

Table 1. Rare brands analysis according to foot dominance. A: Arc; LR: Loop Radial; LU: Loop Ulnar; W: Whorl. *Significant difference p<0.05 between right and left.

Conclusions

In this study, was observed the presence of a predisposition brand that differentiates righties and lefties groups in relation to foot dominance, i.e. the LR in MET5 is the capability of left foot laterality.

References

1. Cummins H, Midlo CH. Finger Prints, Palms and Soles an Introduction to Dermatoglyphics. Dover Publications, New York 1961
2. Negrine A. Educação Psicomotora: a lateralidade e a orientação espacial. Pallotti, Porto Algre 1986
3. Nodari Junior RJ, Heberle A, Ferreira-Emygdio R, Knackfuss MI. Dermatoglyphics: correlation between software and traditional method in kineanthropometric application. Rev Andal Med Deporte 2014; 7: 60-65

ISOKINETIC THIGH MUSCLES EVALUATIONS OF FEMALE HIGH LEVEL SOCCER PLAYERS

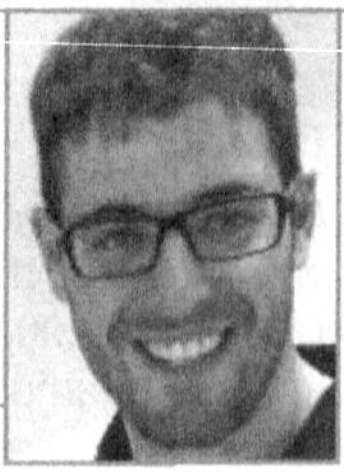

Grazzini G[1], Zuppardo S[2], Pellegrini F[3], Rosini V[1], Martelli G[1,2]

[1]Medicine and Surgery Faculty, Department of Motor Sciences, University of Florence;
[2]Pegaso Medical and Rehabilitation Centre, Grosseto;
[3]Female Soccer Team, Brescia, Italy

Introduction

Isokinetic evaluations of thigh muscles in professional soccer players are commonly used for a functional assessment during training, to highlight possible individual Hamstring/Quadriceps (H/Q) imbalances (1). These differences are often related only to variations in H/Q ratios, especially using the functional Hamstring eccentric / Quadriceps concentric ratio (H ecc/Q conc), an index particularly important for the prevention of muscle and joint injuries (1, 2). Almost all studies were performed on professional male athletes, but very few papers were dedicated to the isokinetic assessment of female soccer players (2, 3). The purpose of the present study was to detect the isokinetic H/Q ratios in a group of top level female soccer players.

Methods

Sixteen professional female soccer players were selected for this study: 1 goal-keeper, 5 defenders, 5 midfielders and 5 strikers, all belonging to an Italian First Premier League team (Female Soccer Team Brescia; weekly training: 6 sessions and 1 match on Saturdays).
Isokinetic tests, performed during the winter holidays in the 2015-2016 competitive season, consisted of Dominant (D) and Not Dominant (N) knee extensors (Q) and flexors (H) muscles evaluations by a Genu 3 isokinetic device (Easytech, Florence, Italy).
The test protocol consisted of H and Q concentric exertions (three repetitions at 90°/s and 15 repetitions at 240°/s), followed by three eccentric H exertions at -30°/s.
For each athlete, conventional concentric H/Q peak torque ratios (90°/s and 240°/s) were calculated for D and N legs, together with functional ratios relating the H eccentric peak torque at -30°/s and the Q concentric peak torque at 240°/s.
The nature of the deficit was determined by using statistically selected cut-offs: at 90°/s concentric H/Q ratio <0.55; at 240°/s concentric H/Q ratio <0.65 and a functional (H ecc / Q conc) ratio <1.0.

Results

Table 1 shows all anthropometric values and isokinetic H/Q ratios in our study group.
All H/Q ratios resulted within the normal range and only three athletes showed values lower than at least two cut-off indexes.
All statistical comparisons between dominant and not dominant legs were found not statistically significant and, at the same time, no differences were observed on isokinetic ratios among playing roles.

Age (yrs)	Height (cm)	Weight (kg)	BMI (kg/m²)	H/Q D 90 (%)	H/Q N 90 (%)	H/Q D 240 (%)	H/Q N 240 (%)	H/Q E30/C240 D (Nm)	H/Q E30/C240 N (Nm)
21.3±3.1	167±5	59.7±4.2	21.4± 1.1	66±6	63±8	72±9	69±10	1.68±0.26	1.67±0.31

Table 1. Anthropometric and isokinetic values in female professional soccer players (mean±SD).
BMI: Body Mass Index; H: hamstrings; Q: quadriceps; H/Q: hamstrings/quadriceps ratio; D: dominant limb; N: non dominant limb; E30: eccentric torque at -30°/s; C240: concentric Torque at 240°/s.

Conclusions

Isokinetic ratios values in our professional female soccer players were all normal and agreed with the other few papers in literature (2, 3). These data reinforce the assumption that isokinetic measurements could greatly help the medical and training staff to monitor the individual and team training programs.
High mean values in all H/Q ratios, in this group of top level soccer players, are probably related to the great attention dedicated to the strengthening of H muscles, in order to prevent muscle and joint injuries during training (1).

References

1. Croisier JL, Ganteaume S, Binet J, Genty M, Ferret JM. Strength imbalances and prevention of hamstring injury in professional soccer players: a prospective study. Am J Sports Med 2008; 36: 1469-1475.
2. Grazzini G, Martelli G. Isokinetic leg flexors/extensors evaluation of male and female soccer players. In: Roi GS, Della Villa S (Eds). Football medicine strategies for player care. Calzetti e Mariucci Editore, Perugia, 2015, pp 158-159
3. Jenkins NDM, Hawkey MJ, Costa PB, Fiddler RE, Thompson BJ, Ryan ED, Smith S, Sobolewski EJ, Conchola EC, Akehi K, Cramer JT. Functional hamstring:quadriceps ratios in elite women's soccer players. J Sports Sci 2013; 31: 612-617

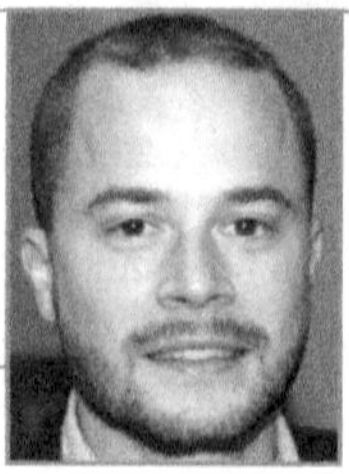

REACTIVE AGILITY PROFILE AND CHANGE OF DIRECTION SPEED BY PLAYING POSITION IN U-16 ELITE SOCCER PLAYERS

Trecroci A[1], Della Bella S[1], Alberti G[1]

[1]Università degli Studi di Milano, School of Exercise Sciences, Department of Biomedical Sciences for Health, Milan, Italy

Introduction and Purpose

Agility represents an essential training tool to improve neuromuscular control, injury reduction and power level (1). Agility is commonly defined as a rapid whole body movement with Change Of Direction or Speed (CODS) related to decision-making factors (e.g. reaction skills), which are crucial components at increasing scoring opportunities during a soccer match. Since attacking and defending soccer maneuvers occur performing CODS in response to a stimulus (3), it would be worthy to investigate changes in the opponent-based agility profile and changing of direction skills linked to the individual position. Thus, the purpose of the present study was to assess possible differences in reactive agility and CODS performance according to the playing position and to investigate their relationship in young elite soccer players.

Methods

Forty-four elite soccer players were enrolled in the study (mean±SD; age: 15.6±0.5 years, weight: 65.4±8.3 kg, height: 175.8±5.5 cm). All players had a minimum of five years of soccer training at baseline. Three playing positions were classified: Defenders (DF, n=16), Midfielders (MF, n=16) and Forwards (FW, n=12). Participants were tested using the Y-shaped reactive agility test based on the movements of an experimenter (RAT) and the sprint test with 90° turns (S90). The players were asked to perform three trials for each test and the fastest trial was taken into account within the analysis. As regards the RAT, it was examined only the total time rather than decision time. A one-way ANOVA was used separately to examine RAT and S90 differences among the playing positions.

Results

The analysis revealed that FW tended to be the best performers in the RAT and S90 (2.30±0.12 s and 6.50±0.16 s) compared to DF (2.35±0.17 s and 6.65±0.25 s) and MF (2.33±0.15 s and 6.60±0.28 s) respectively. In spite of that, no statistical differences were found among playing positions in both tests ($p>0.05$). Additionally, a non-significant correlation was found between RAT and S90 ($r=0.20$; $p=0.192$).

Conclusions

The ability to accelerate, decelerate and change direction reacting to a stimulus is a critical skill in soccer and it is considered discriminant for predicting inter-individual differences (2). Nevertheless, our findings did not showed performance changes according to the soccer roles. A probably explanation was due to the fact that the players involved in the study were at the initial stage of specialization, from age 15 to age 18 years. Hence, specific physical and cognitive abilities essential for all DF, MF and FW positions may not be fully developed.
Lastly, a significant correlation between reactive agility and CODS with 90° turn was not found, suggesting that their performance are independent skills, as previously demonstrated (3). The main limitation of the present study was the use of total time as the only variable to assess differences in the RAT performance. Further studies are needed to examined further time variables (e.g. decision time) to highlight potential variation between DF, MF and FW.

References

1. Milanović Z, Sporiš G, Trajković N, Sekulić D, James N, Vučković G. Does SAQ training improve the speed and flexibility of young soccer players? A randomized controlled trial. Human Movement Sciences 2014; 38: 197-208
2. Valente-dos-Santos J, Coelho-e-Silva M, Duarte J, Pereira J, Rebelo-Gonçalves R, Figueiredo A, Mazzuco MA, Sherar LB, Elferink-Gemser MT, Malina RM. Allometric multilevel modelling of agility and dribbling speed by skeletal age and playing position in youth soccer Players. Int J Sports Med 2014; 35: 762-771
3. Young WB, Dawson B, Henry GJ. Agility and change-of-direction speed are independent skills: implications for training for agility in invasion sports. Int J Sports Science and Coaching 2015; 10: 159-169

Sunday, 10th April, 2016
POSTER AREA

FREE POSTER PRESENTATIONS

RETURN TO PLAY IN OTHER SPORTS

Chairs

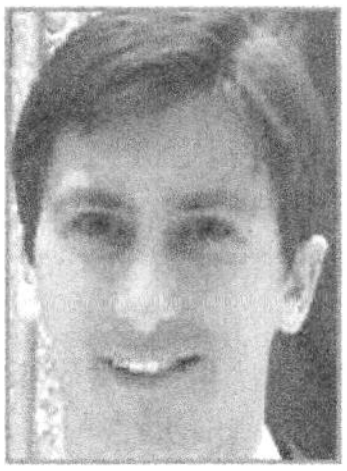

Daniel Broman
(London, United Kingdom)

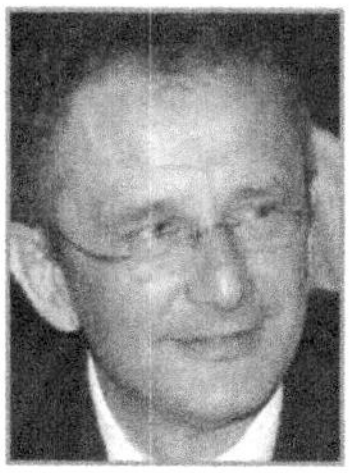

Pierpaolo Zunarelli
(Bologna, Italy)

PF01 Elite futsal athletes: dermatoglyphic profil
Nodari Júnior RJ, Panizzi Junior C, de Jesus JA, Alberti A, Souza R, Sartori G, Fin G (Joaçaba, Brazil)

PF02 Return to play of an amateur tennis player after extensor carpi radialis brevis rupture
Kekelekis A, Drakonaki E (Crete, Greece)

PF03 Conserxvative treatment after acute axillary nerve injury in a professional rugby player
Vittadini F, Gasparre G, Frizziero A (Padua, Italy)

PF04 Physiological response to whole body cryotherapy in professional rugby players
Banfi G, Lombardi G, Zani V, Bonomi FG, Sanguin G (Milan, Orzinuovi, Bergamo, and Rome, Italy)

PF05 Effect of a return to play circuit on Biceps Femoris activation in elite hockey players **Andrews CJ, Neill MC, Tejani SR, Manolas L, Graus KSC, Appleby B, Rosalie SM, Netto KJ (Perth, Australia; Florence, Italy)**

ELITE FUTSAL ATHLETES: DERMATOGLYPHIC PROFIL

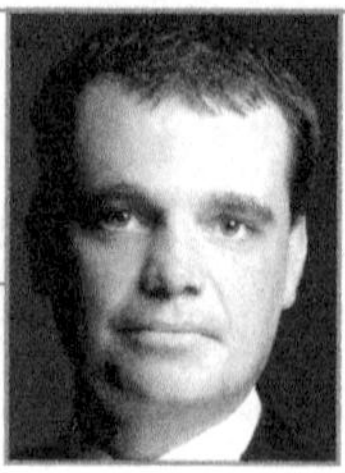

Nodari Júnior RJ, Panizzi Junior C, de Jesus JA, Alberti A, Souza R, Sartori G, Fin G

Universidade do Oeste de Santa Catarina, Joaçaba, Brazil

Introduction

Studies based on Dermatoglyphics state that the complexity of fingerprints drawings can observe genotype and fetal development characteristics, so this method can be an important tool in observing neuromotor potential characteristics (3).
Purpose: To analyse the dermatoglyphic profile of elite futsal athletes compared to non-athletes group.

Method

The sample was composed by 340 male individuals, divided into two groups: Group A (GA) composed by 170 professional Futsal athletes (26.7±4.6 yrs) and Group B (GB) composed by 170 non-athletes (22.4±3.8 yrs).
The GA is composed by the three best teams in the Italian and Portuguese Cup, Spanish King's Cup and the Brazilian Futsal League's 2011 season.
The protocol chosen was the Dermatoglyphic proposed by Cummins & Midlo (1), and for the capture, processing and fingerprint analysis, was used the Leitor Dermatoglífico (Dermatoglyphic Reader, Salus Dermatoglifia, Luzerna, Brazil) validated by Nodari Junior (2).
For the statistical analysis was established the level of significance $p<0.05$. In comparing the amounts of lines between GA and GB, to observe the normality distribution, was used the Kolmogorov-Smirnov test. The observation of non-normal distribution, applies to the inference Nonparametric Mann-Whitney Test for comparisons between numeric variables. To compare categorical variables: Arc (A), Loop Radial (LR), Loop Ulnar (LU), Whorl (W), the chi-square test was used, and when found significant differences, applied to Waste Analysis adjusted ($R_{aj}>1.96$).

Results

For the numeric variables comparison, the result shows that the number of ridges of six possible variables in the fingerprint, is significantly higher in GA compared to GB in the line summation of the respective fingers (Table 1).

Fingers	Abbreviation	Group A	Group B	p
Finger Thumb Left Hand	MESQL1	14.8±5.0	12.1±5.4	0.000
Ring Finger of the Left Hand	MESQL3	11.6±5.6	10.0±5.6	0.006
Finger Minimum Left Hand	MESQL5	13.0±5.9	11.2±6.2	0.016
Finger Thumb of the Right Hand	MDSQL1	16.5±21.5	14.3±21.6	0.000
Sum of Total Number of Left Hand Lines	SQTLE	62.0±4.6	54.9±4.9	0.006
Sum of the Total Number of Lines	SQTL	124.6±40.8	112.8±41.7	0.020

Table 1. Numeric variables comparisons between groups A and Groups B.

For the rare marks analysis between GA and GB, referring to qualitative variables, i.e., the figure type noted significant differences in the following fingers GA: Finger Thumb Left Hand (MET1; p=0.22), with higher amount of W (R_{aj}=2.1235); Finger thumb Right Hand (MDT1; p=0.07), with higher amount of W (R_{aj}=2.8398); Ring finger of the right hand (MDT3; p=0.024), with higher amount of LR (R_{aj}=2.1173); Minimum and Finger of Right Hand (MDT5; p=0.040), higher amount of LR ($_{Raj}$=2.5408).

Conclusions

The results reflect the Dermatoglyphic profile of the high performance futsal athlete has significant differences compared to non-athlete population, so the Dermatoglyphic can be able to serve as a guidance tool for sports talents.

For the quantities of lines the following indicators must be observed being the data presented characteristics of high performance athletes (Table 2):

Fingers	Abbreviation	Lines
Finger Thumb Left Hand	MESQL1	14.8±5.0
Ring Finger of the Left Hand	MESQL3	11.6±5.6
Finger Minimum Left Hand	MESQL5	13.0±5.9
Finger Thumb of the Right Hand	MDSQL1	16.5±21.5
Sum of Total Number of Left Hand Lines	SQTLE	62.0±4.6
Sum of the Total Number of Lines	SQTL	124.6±40.8

Table 2. Indicators of high performance athletes.

With regard to rare marks should be noted the presence of the following figures: W in MET1 and MDT1 and LR in MDT3 and MDT5.

References

1. Cummins H, Midlo CH. Finger Prints, Palms and Soles an Introduction to Dermatoglyphics. Dover Publications, New York 1961
2. Nodari Junior RJ, Heberle A, Ferreira-Emygdio R, Knackfuss MI. Dermatoglyphics: correlation between software and traditional method in kineanthropometric application. Rev Andal Med Deporte 2014; 7(2): 60-65
3. Serhiyenko LP, Lyshevska VM. A dermatoglyphics of foot in the prognosis of sporting gift: differential distinctions of dermatoglyphics of foot for sportsmen and people which do not go in for sports. Pedagog Psychol Med-Biol Probl Phys Train Sports 2013; 2: 66-69

RETURN TO PLAY OF AN AMATEUR TENNIS PLAYER AFTER EXTENSOR CARPI RADIALIS BREVIS RUPTURE

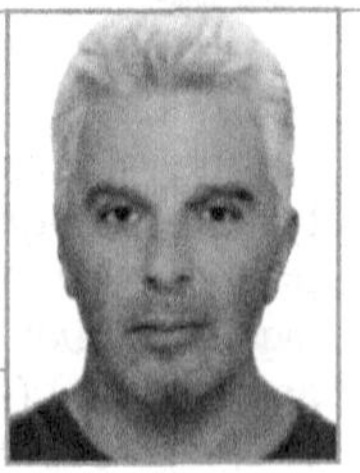

Kekelekis A[1], Drakonaki E[2]

[1]Sports Injury Clinic for Prevention and Rehabilitation, Agios Nikolaos, Crete;
[2]Diagnostic Clinic, Heraklion, Crete, Greece

Introduction

Lateral Epicondylitis, (LE), or tennis elbow as it is better known, is a painful musculoskeletal condition, the most common cause of elbow pain, and affects almost 1-2% of the general population each year. Up to 50% of all tennis players experience some type of elbow pain, and approximately 80% of these complaints attributed to tennis elbow. Additionally, LE is a common work-related medical condition, with a prevalence of 15% in working environments such as meat and fish industry. The duration of a typical episode of LE has been reported to be from 6 months to 2 years. LE is an overuse injury, characterized by degenerative changes and repetitive stress, causing microtrauma and microtearing of the common extensor origin at the attachment to the lateral epicondyle. The treatment of LE varies, from NSAIDs, bracing, electrotherapeutic modalities, acupuncture, manual therapy technique, injection therapies, and surgery. Injections were first introduced during the 50's, mainly glucocorticoids. However, the last decade new injection therapies have been presented. These include autologous Platelet Rich Plasma (PRP), autologous blood, prolotherapy, botolinum toxin, polidocanol, glycosaminoglycan polysulfate and, hyaluronic acid.
This case study highlights the return to play strategy followed after a successful hyaluronic acid injection therapy to 45-year-old male recreational tennis player due to a partial rapture of the Extensor Carpi Radialis Brevis (ECRB) tendon.

Case report

The subject, a 45-year old recreational tennis player, in great shape, good physical condition, and excellent general medical status, presented to the sports injury clinic reporting pain at the lateral site of his right (dominant) arm each time he was attempting to grab a subject, or to extend his wrist and inability to perform any hand and elbow activities. Similar symptoms were also reported a few weeks ago, however, after ice application and an anti-inflammatory medication therapy the condition improved. According to the subject's history, this was the second time he was facing a similar condition, however, the symptoms were stronger in volume and intensity. The subject reported an unpleasant sensation after a heavy backhand was performed on the lateral site of his dominate arm, (right arm), followed by a very painful feeling that forced him stopping tennis immediately.
The clinical examination followed, concluded, injury at the extensor tendon origin. Due to the clinical findings and the musculoskeletal history of the patient (re-injury), the subject was suggested to perform an ultrasound. The Ultra Sounds (US) imaging indicated a partial (0.8 cm) rupture of the ECRB tendon.
An US-guided injection therapy with Hyaluronic Acid was performed. After the injection, a plastic (removable) cast was applied for 10 days, in a slight wrist extension, in order to prevent any excessive movement and to allow the tissue to regenerate. By the end of the 10-days of immobility, the patient followed a specific 2-month rehabilitation program for 4 times a week, consisting of: i) isometric exercises of the wrist flexors and extensors; ii) stabilization exercises of the scapular

musculature; iii) isotonic exercises of the shoulder musculature; iv) manual mobilization of the shoulder and elbow joint and the wrist; v) deep tissue soft tissue mobilization; vi) aerobic training (45-60 minutes).
The isometric exercises were carried out in 4 sets of 12 repetitions of 10 s hold, pain free.
The isotonic exercises performed in 4 sets of 12 repetitions against 70% of 1RM resistance.
Treadmill and static bicycle were preferred for endurance exercises (3 times/week).
Volume and intensity were progressively increased every week, avoiding any isotonic activity of the wrist.
A second US imaging was executed after 8 weeks. The imagine findings indicated a 0.4 cm rupture, suggesting significant improvement. A second US-guided Hyaluronic Acid injection was performed.
The subject continued the same rehabilitation program for the following 8 weeks, with several modifications: i) isotonic exercises of the wrist flexors, pain free; ii) core stability and core strengthening exercises in all sagittal planes; iii) pattern of movements that mimic the tennis strokes, resistance free.
The isotonic exercises carried out according to the low volume/high repetition protocol, at 50% of 1RM resistance. Related to the core stability and core strength, different exercises were performed in all three sagittal planes (plank, both-side plank, and rotational exercises against resistance with the use of a 4kg-medicine ball).
After the end of the 8-week period, the patient executed a third US imaging. The imagine findings reported total healing of the tear, suggesting the effectiveness of the hyaluronic acid injection to the tendon's rapture.
The subject followed a 4-week rehabilitation program improving shoulder and arm strength. Additionally, resistance was increased progressively, and at the end of the 20th week an on-court tennis training was performed. By the 24th week the subject was ready to enjoy a competition game of tennis.

Conclusions

This case study clearly reports the effectiveness of US guided Hyaluronic Acid injection on the partial rupture (0.8 cm) of the ECRB. The athlete followed a specific rehabilitation program and returned to play a competition tennis game in 24 weeks after the incident.
Unfortunately, the scientific research is very limited, and not safe conclusions can be established related to the effectiveness of the hyaluronic injection in different tendon injuries (rotator cuff injury, Achilles tendon injury, or patellar tendon injury) in athletes. Further study is required, in order to provide sufficient results related to the effectiveness of the Hyaluronic Acid injection to tendon injuries.

References

1. Bisset L, Paungmali A, Vicenzino B, Beller E. A systematic review and meta-analysis of clinical trials on physical interventions for lateral epicondylalgia. Br J Sports Med 2005; 39: 411-422
2. Krogh TP, Bartels EM, Ellingsen T, Stengaard-pedersen K, Buchbinder R, Fredberg U, Blittal H, Christerseen R. Comparative effectiveness of injection therapies in lateral epicondylitis. Am J Sports Med 2013; 41: 1435-1445

CONSERVATIVE TREATMENT AFTER ACUTE AXILLARY NERVE INJURY IN A PROFESSIONAL RUGBY PLAYER

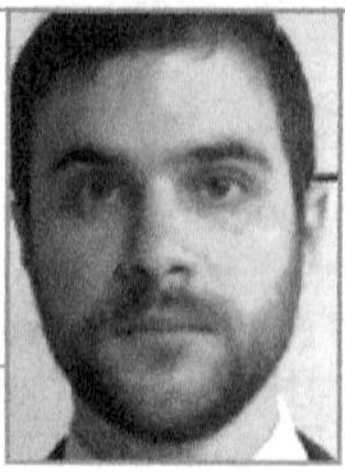

Vittadini F, Gasparre G, Frizziero A

Department of Physical Medicine and Rehabilitation, University of Padua, Italy

Post-traumatic axillary nerve injuries are common peripheral nerve injuries in athletes who participate in contact sports. Deltoid muscle paralysis is secondary to nerve trauma which occurs following shoulder dislocation or direct trauma to the deltoid muscle. Compression neuropathy has been reported to occur in quadrilateral space syndrome as the axillary nerve crosses this anatomic compartment. The axillary nerve is also extremely vulnerable during any operative procedure involving the inferior aspect of the shoulder, and iatrogenic injury to the axillary nerve remains a serious complication of shoulder surgery. Accurate diagnosis of axillary nerve injury is based on a careful history and physical examination as well as an understanding of the anatomy of the shoulder. Inspection, palpation and neurological testing provide the bases for diagnosis. A clinically suspected axillary nerve injury should be confirmed by electrophysiological testing, including Electro-Myography (EMG) and nerve conduction studies (Electro-Neurography: ENG). We observed a case of axillary nerve injury in a 27-years old national male rugby player (height 184 cm; mass 103 kg). The player sustained a traumatic anterior gleno-humeral dislocation with Hill-Sachs lesion, associated to subscapular and supraspinatus tendinopathies and tenosynovitis of long head biceps brachialis. As a consequence, he complained localized pain spreading from right shoulder to the back of the hand associated with paresthesia/anesthesia in deltoid area. Diagnosis was taken after trauma with both rehabilitative and orthopedic clinical observation and confirmed by EMG every two months, brachial plexus -upper limb magnetic resonance and dynamic cervical Magnetic Resonance Imaging. At the first clinical evaluation patient presented deltoid atrophy, positive rotator cuff tests and electromyography evidenced suffer of axillary nerve (assonotmesic-neutotmesic sufferance) causing right total denervation deltoid muscle. He began rehabilitation at a rate of 1 session a day, 5 days a week. These sessions were performed in a pool for aquatic exercise and in the gym of Rehabilitation Department of Padua University Hospital. The specific rehabilitation program was based on: strengthening exercises of deltoid muscle and shoulder stabilization (isometric and isotonic exercises for the rotator cuff, scapulae fixators and external rotators muscles; proprioception and functional exercises; recovery of speed, endurance, and kinetic coordination of the shoulder; neuromuscular electrical stimulation of the deltoid and medium-lower trapezius using balanced biphasic triangular waves (200-10 ms, 2 Hz, 0-30 mA). After seven months was observed deltoid normal muscular trophy, negative rotator cuff tests and signs of progressive re-innervation at EMG. Eight months after the injury, the player fully returned to active sport participation and to an official competitive match. At that time sensibility, stability and strength were completely regained as well the sport-specific gesture. In conclusion, post-traumatic axillary nerve injuries are frequent conditions affecting athletes. The correct diagnosis and a timely specific rehabilitation protocol allows to a full return to professional sport activity and may prevent the recurrence rate.

References

1. Atef A, El-Tantawy A, Gad H, Hefeda M. Prevalence of associated injuries after anterior shoulder dislocation: a prospective study. Int Orthop 2015 Jul 2. [Epub ahead of print]
2. Kuhlman GS. The "Burner". A Common Nerve Injury in Contact Sports. Am Fam Physician 1999; 60: 2035-2040
3. Safran MR. Nerve injury about the shoulder in athletes. Part 1, Suprascapular Nerve and Axillary Nerve. Am J Sports Med 2004; 32: 803-819

PHYSIOLOGICAL RESPONSE TO WHOLE BODY CRYOTHERAPY IN PROFESSIONAL RUGBY PLAYERS

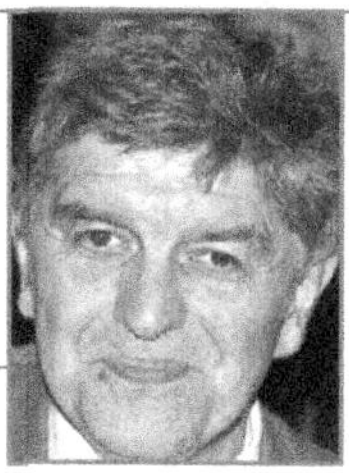

Banfi G[1,2], Lombardi G[1], Zani V[3], Bonomi FG[3,4], Sanguin G[5]

[1]IRCCS Istituto Ortopedico Galeazzi, Milano; [2]Vita-Salute San Raffaele University, Milano; [3]Centre of Systemic Cryotherapy, Poliambulatorio Bongi, Orzinuovi; [4]OU Interventional Cardiology, Humanitas Gavazzeni, Bergamo; [5]Federazione Italiana Rugby, Rome, Italy

Introduction

Cold-based therapies are widely used in relieving pain symptoms, particularly in case of inflammatory diseases, injuries and overuse symptoms, and in these two latter cases, mainly in the field of sports medicine.

A peculiar form of cold therapy or stimulation, namely Whole Body Cryotherapy (WBC), was proposed forty years ago for the treatment of rheumatic diseases: it consists of a brief exposure (two to three minutes) to very cold air (−110 to −160 °C), preceded by a 30 seconds-long preconditioning at −60 °C, in special temperature- and environmentally-controlled cryo-chambers (2). In sports medicine, WBC has gained wider acceptance as a method to improve recovery from muscle injury (1, 3).

Aim of this study was to evaluate the effects of WBC on various physiological and biochemical parameters in professional rugby players during a training camp.

Methods

Twenty seven males professional rugby players, belonging to the Italian National Rugby Team participating in a summer training camp, at the end of the competitive season, were enrolled (median age: 24.8 years; range 21.4-31.9).

WBC consisted of two sessions per day (in the morning, before the morning training session, and in the evening, after the afternoon training session) for seven consecutive days.

Training consisted of two sessions/day, two hours each. In the first 3 days, the morning session consisted of: i) warm-up; 2) strength training; 3) plyometrics; the afternoon session consisted of: i) warm-up; 2) rugby skills; 3) interval training.

On the 4th day, players were submitted to two light sessions of interval training. The 5th day was off. On the 6th day there were two sessions of free sport activities. On the last day, there were two sessions of endurance exercises.

Diet regimen was strictly defined. Blood and saliva were collected twice, in the morning at the beginning of the camp, prior the first WBC, and the day after the end of the camp. An additional saliva collection was performed in the evening of the first day of the camp (after the second WBC). Blood was assayed for hematological parameters and iron metabolism parameters, muscle overuse markers i.e. creatin kinase (CK), lactate dehydrogenase (LDH), aspartate aminotransferase (AST), and kidney function (creatinine, cystatin C, estimated Glomerular Filtration Rate eGFR). Saliva was assayed for steroid hormone profile: testosterone, cortisol, estradiol, Dehydroepiandrosterone (DHEA).

Results

Results are shown in Table 1. Leukocyte count and composition were unchanged. Erythrocytes, hematocrit, hemoglobin and mean corpuscular hemoglobin content slightly decreased; mean corpuscular volume and red cell distribution width increased (all $p<0.001$). Serum transferrin and ferritin decreased, while soluble transferrin receptor increased. Serum iron and transferrin saturation were unchanged, as was reticulocyte count. Cryo-stimulation helped muscular recovery (increased LDH ($p<0.001$) and stabile CK and AST activities). Creatinine was unaffected while cystatin C was increased ($p<0.05$). Creatinine/cystatin C-based eGFR slightly decreased ($p<0.05$); eGFR and muscular biomarkers were unrelated, suggesting a real recovery effect of WBC. In saliva cortisol and DHEA were reduced ($p<0.05$) already after the first 2 WBC sessions. After 7 days (14 WBC consecutive sessions) cortisol, DHEA ($p<0.001$) and estradiol ($p<0.05$) were decreased, while testosterone was increased ($p<0.01$) as did the testosterone-to-cortisol ratio.

		Pre-WBC	Post-WBC	P value
Hematology	Leu (10^9/L)	6.10±1.28	5.69±1.58	n.s.
	Neu%	48.41±9.32	47.50±5.09	n.s.
	Ly%	39.58±9.01	39.95±5.71	n.s.
	Mo%	8.49±1.81	8.69±1.72	n.s.
	Eo%	2.50 (1.60-5.74)	2.75 (1.60-7.29)	n.s.
	Ba%	0.35 (0.20-0.70)	0.25 (0.10-0.84)	n.s.
	Neu (10^9/L)	2.85 (1.93-4.64)	2.70 (2.10-3.82)	n.s.
	Ly (10^9/L)	2.38±0.71	2.30±0.46	n.s.
	Mo (10^9/L)	0.50 (0.40-0.77)	0.50 (0.30-0.70)	n.s.
	Eo (10^9/L)	0.20 (0.10-0.37)	0.20 (0.10-0.37)	n.s.
	Ba (10^9/L)	0.020 (0.010-0.040)	0.020 (0.003-0.074)	n.s.
	RBC (10^{12}/L)	5.11±0.33	4.98±0.27	<0.001
	Hb (g/L)	150.6±8.4	147.0±6.2	<0.001
	Ht%	45.79±2.41	45.20±1.89	<0.01
	MCV (fL)	89.78±3.38	90.83±3.10	<0.001
	MCH (pg)	29.52±0.97	29.52±0.90	n.s.
	MCHC (g/dL)	32.9 (32.1-33.8)	32.5 (23.1-33.2)	<0.001
	RDW-CV%	13.09±0.44	13.39±0.42	<0.001
	Plt (10^9/L)	207±37	209±39	n.s.
	MPV (fL)	11.15 (10.23-12.07)	11.40 (10.04-12.08)	n.s.
Martial Status	Iron (mg/dL)	98.74 ± 21.72	92.22 + 23.45	n.s.
	Transferrin (mg/dL)	245.33 ± 27.44	239.74 + 22.97	<0.05
	Ferritin (µg/L)	159.64 ± 74.61	147.71 + 75.28	<0.05
	Transferrin saturation (%)	28 (19.1-40.9)	27 (17.1-37.8)	n.s.
	sTfR (mg/L)	1.12 (0.98-1.59)	1.21 (1.01-1.59)	n.s.

Muscle Overuse Markers	CK (U/L)	178.00 (88.40-910.60)	152.00 (84.20-739.40)	n.s.
	LDH (U/L)	172.0 (136.2-214.0)	190.0 (152.2-236.0)	<0.001
	AST (U/L)	25.00 (16.40-44.60)	28.00 (17.00-51.60)	n.s.
Kidney Function	Creatinine (mg/dL)	1.02 (0.90-1.23)	1.03 (0.89-1.27)	n.s.
	Cystatin C (mg/L)	0.73 (0.64-0.84)	0.75 (0.66-0.90)	<0.05
	eGFR-CKD-EPI (mL/min)	113.00 (97.40-126.50)	106.46 (88.40-131.10)	<0.05
Salivary Hormones	DHEA (pg/mL)	236.0 (16.0-1128.0)	57.10 (9.0-202.0)	<0.001
	17β-Estradiol (pg/mL)	2.265 (0.170-27.700)	1.665 (0.760-15.400)	<0.05
	Testosterone (pg/mL)	46.73 (25.67-188.9)	74.56 (25.05-151.80)	<0.01
	Cortisol (ng/mL)	2.425 (1.100-6.600)	1.380 (0.200-3.180)	<0.001

Table 1. Hematological and salivary parameters before (Pre) and after (Post) Whole Body Cryotherapy (WBC). Values are expressed as mean±SD or median (5th-95th percentile) depending on data distribution

Conclusions

In this sample of professional rugby players, cryo-stimulation modified the hematological profile, with a reduction in erythrocyte count and hemoglobinization paralleled by a change in martial status markers. The muscular recovery was stimulated by RBC, while kidney function was substantially unaffected. The modification in steroid hormone profile (particularly, increased testosterone and decreased cortisol) support the recovery and indicates an overall improvement of the psychophysical status.

References

1. Banfi G, Lombardi G, Colombini A, Lippi G. Whole body cryotherapy in athletes. Sports Med 2010; 40: 509-517
2. Bettoni L, Bonomi FG, Zani V, Manisco L, Indelicato A, Lanteri P, Banfi G, Lombardi G. Effects of 15 consecutive cryotherapy sessions on the clinical output of fibromyalgic patients. Clin Rheumatol 2013; 32: 1337-1345
3. Lubkowska A, Dolegowska B, Szygula Z. Whole-body cryostimulation-potential beneficial treatment for improving antioxidant capacity in healthy men-significance of the number of sessions. PLoS One. 2012; 7(10): e46352

THE EFFECT OF A RETURN TO PLAY CIRCUIT ON BICEPS FEMORIS ACTIVATION IN ELITE HOCKEY PLAYERS

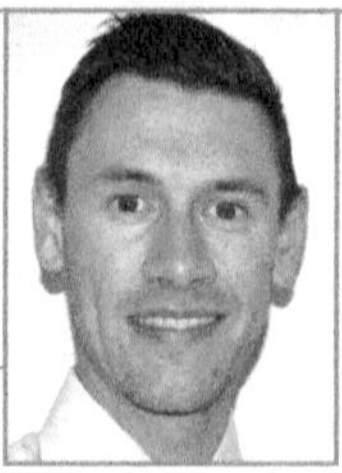

Andrews CJ[1], Neill MC[1], Tejani SR[1], Manolas L[1], Graus KSC[1], Appleby B[2], Rosalie SM[3], Netto KJ[1]

[1]School of Physiotherapy and Exercise Science, Curtin University, Perth, Australia; [2]Australian Institute of Sport, Perth, Australia; [3]University of Florence, Florence, Italy

Introduction

Judging return to sport following injury can involve a multitude of tests, one proposed method is a Return-To-Play Circuit (RTPC).
Assessing the recovery of a muscular injury is difficult, with a number of factors able to influence timeframes. It has previously been shown that the ability of an athlete to load an injured muscle can only be determined by sports-specific field testing (1). The use of a RTPC may therefore aid the clinician in judging a player's return to sport as it integrates movement patterns which mimic on-field demands.
It is not known what effect such circuits have on muscle activation patterns of the lower limb.
The purpose of this study was to investigate the muscle activation patterns of the Biceps Femoris (BF) during a RTPC as used by elite sports players. A secondary aim was to assess these patterns with modifications to the circuit. A RTPC used by hockey in Australia was tested in this study (Figure 1).

Methods

Nine professional, international level, field hockey players (mean±SD: age 24.4±3.8 years; height 1.79±0.05 m; weight 77.7±6.1 kg; international caps 91±77) who were all deemed fit to play by the team's medical staff were recruited following an information session.
Wireless, surface Electromyograph (EMG) sensors (Trigno wireless system, Delsys Inc, MA, USA) were taped to the left BF. Maximal isometric voluntary contractions were used for calibration.
The circuit consists of 10 sections including walking, jogging, zig-zags, sprinting and multi-directional components (Figure 1).
Two sections of the circuit were modified on subsequent runs to assess the effect on the BF in comparison to the original circuit (elongated sprint section of 10 m to 20 m; enlarged diamond shuttle of 6 m to 12 m). The circuit was run a total of eight times and included clockwise and anti-clockwise approaches. Players were rested for 5 minutes before and between the modified runs.
A customised software package allowed analysis of the EMG data in correlation with video recordings of the runs and thus delineated the separate sections of the circuit for statistical comparison. Both peak and mean muscle activation was analysed for each circuit section.

Results

The overall results from a repeated measures ANOVA revealed significant differences in both the peak and mean activation of the BF when comparing the different sections of the un-modified circuit. Higher activation patterns were seen when running at higher speed and in tasks involving a rapid change of direction (Table 1).
In the modified sections significant differences were seen in both peak and mean muscle activation patterns when compared to the corresponding sections of the original circuit. Peak activation in the modified sprint section was 131% of the un-modified (p=0.033); mean activation of 113% (p=0.042); peak activation in the modified diamond shuttle was 123% (p=0.043) and mean activation was 106% (p=0.026).

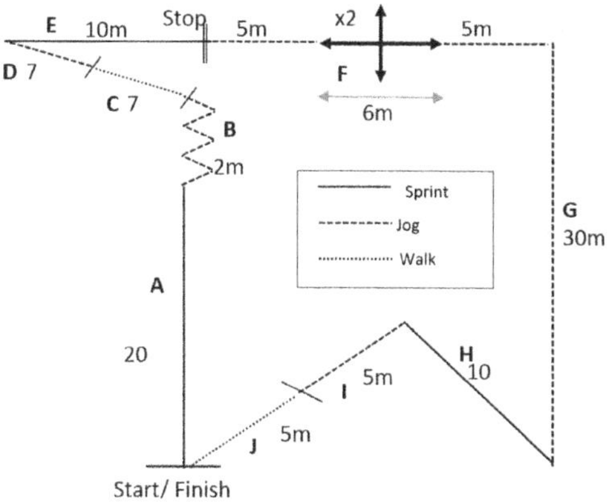

Sections A – J = 10 circuit components. Section E (sprint to stop) increased to 20m; Section F (reaction diamond) increased to 12m diameter in modified runs.

Figure 1. The return To Play Circuit (RTPC).

Section of the circuit	Peak	Mean
A	92.63±57.22	40.06±25.53
B	51.93±31.47	22.26±12.17
C	28.36±23.28	10.22±9.82
D	38.33±32.17	16.13±13.59
E	78.58±40.27	32.58±18.15
F	61.29±36.37	16.32±9.06
G	55.39±48.76	19.63±16.89
H	84.40±51.66	36.71±23.57
I	43.02±35.43	17.65±14.20
J	25.78±25.60	8.24±9.60

Table 1. Mean±SD values of EMG (Peak and Mean) of original circuit as % of Maximal Voluntary Isometric Contraction (MVIC).

Conclusions

Differences were seen between the higher-velocity components of the circuit, namely the sprint sections, zig-zags and diamond shuttle, suggesting that an effective RTPC needs a variety of components rather than simple straight-line tasks to assess the BF. The results show significant variations between the components and in the modified sections. Enabling the BF to be tested at varied levels of intensity and through selective omission, can enable a clinician to graduate BF load and thus return to play. The circuit assessed in this study was originally used for other sporting codes, namely Australian Rules football and Rugby Union; in addition, the physical demands of a hockey player are comparable to that of a footballer and thus the results of this study would have merit in football.

References

1. Tol JL, Hamilton B, Eirale C, Muxart P, Jacobsen P, Whiteley R. At return to play following hamstring injury the majority of professional football players have residual isokinetic deficits. Br J Sports Med 2014; 48: 1364-1369

Sunday, 10th April, 2016
POSTER AREA

FREE POSTER PRESENTATIONS

TRAINING & RE-TRAINING

Chairs

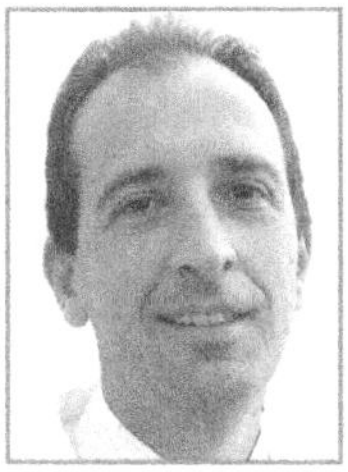

Luca Tomaello
(Turin, Italy)

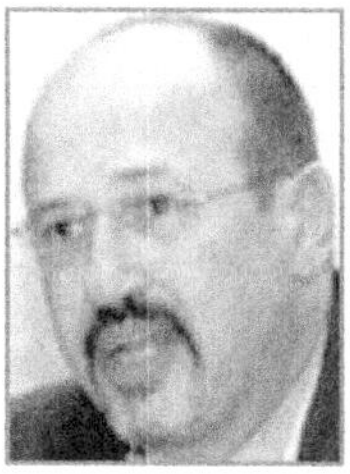

Nikos Tsouroudis
(Athens, Greece)

PH01 Neuromuscular performance of lower limbs six months after anterior cruciate ligament reconstruction **Roth R, Donath L, Mauch M, Weisskopf L, Faude O (Basel, Switzerland)**

PH02 Focal muscle vibration reverses quadriceps hypotrophy improving muscle fibres recruitment
Benedetti MG, Zati A, Cavazzuti L, Rainoldi A, Casale R (Bologna, Turin and Bergamo, Italy)

PH03 The effect of two different training approaches on physical performance in young soccer players **Perri E, Iaia F, Alberti G (Milan, Italy)**

PH04 Three stretching training methods to increase hamstrings flexibility in professional soccer players **D'Onofrio R, Tamburrino P, Manzi V, Bovenzi A, Mazzoni S, Tavana R, Tamburrino G (Milan, Italy)**

PH05 Effects of three different training programmes on instep kick in pre-adoloscent football players
Rossi A, Formenti D, Alberti G (Milan, Italy)

1

NEUROMUSCULAR PERFORMANCE OF LOWER LIMBS SIX MONTHS AFTER ANTERIOR CRUCIATE LIGAMENT RECONSTRUCTION

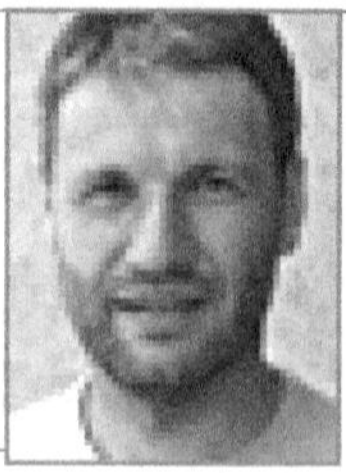

Roth R[1], Donath L[1], Mauch M[2], Weisskopf L[2], Faude O[1]

[1]Department of Sport, Exercise and Health, Basel; [2]Rennbahnklinik, Basel, Switzerland

Introduction

Injuries to the Anterior Cruciate Ligament (ACL) are a major concern in team sports, particularly in football. Players aim for a fast return to play after ACL surgery (2).
Although no consensus statements on return to play are available (2), the assessment of various clinical and performance parameters may support a successful return to play. Strength asymmetry is considered to notably affect biomechanical variables and injury risk at return to play (3). As athletic demands of playing football are challenging and comprise the risk of (re-)injury, athletes should be able to tolerate high biomechanical loads. The present study aimed to assess asymmetries of neuromuscular performance of the lower limbs six month after ACL surgery.

Methods

Ten patients (3 women, 7 men; age: 24.4±3.0 SD yrs; height: 174± (11) cm; weight: 74±15 kg) were compared to 10 healthy controls (29.4±6.1 yrs; 175±8 cm; 73±13 kg) who were pair-matched according to sex, height and weight.
Six months after ACL surgery (Hamstring autografts) both groups (64% were football players) performed a test battery consisting of isokinetic strength testing at a speed of 60°/s (Humac Norm, CSMi, Stoughton, USA) for knee flexion and extension, gait analysis on a treadmill (FDM-T, Zebris Medical, Isny, Germany), drop-jumps (DJ, drop height 20 cm) on a force plate (MLD, SPSport, Trins, Austria), unilateral dynamic postural assessment (ProKin, TechnoBody, Dalmine, Italy), the Y-balance and 6 m-timed-hop-test (1).
Muscle activity of four muscles (rectus femoris, vastus medialis, biceps femoris and medial gastrocnemius) was recorded at both legs via surface electromyography (Myon 320, Myon AG, Schwarzenberg, Switzerland). Muscle activation was calculated relative to maximal voluntary isokinetic contraction (MVIC). Absolute (Δ) and standardized mean differences (SMD) between the injured and uninjured limb in patients as well as between the injured limb in patients and the corresponding limb in controls were calculated with 90% confidence intervals.

Results

In patients differences between the injured and uninjured leg were observed with better results in the uninjured leg for leg extension strength (Δ=-18 Nm, [-14;-21], SMD=0.41), dynamic postural assessment (Δ=-146 mm, [-66;-227], SMD=0.35) and 6-m-timed-hop-test (Δ=0.23 s, [-0.09;0.36], SMD=0.51).
During drop-jumps muscle pre-activation between legs differed in all muscles (0.64<SMD<1.06) with a particularly higher pre-activation in Rectus and Biceps Femoris in the injured leg.

Large differences between patients and controls were observed for drop jump height (controls higher; Δ=-4.6 cm, [-5.7;-3.4], SMD=1.02) and contact time (patients shorter; Δ=-39 msec, [-9;-68], SMD=0.63). Moderate between-group differences occurred with poorer performance in patients for leg extension strength, stride length, unilateral standing balance and Y-balance performance (0.49≤SMD≤0.68). Moderate to large between-group differences in muscle pre-activation during the drop-jumps were measured for all muscles (0.64<ES<1.45). Patients had higher pre-activation in all muscles except for Biceps Femoris, with healthy controls showing a higher pre-activation.

	ACL patients (n= 10)		Matched controls (n= 10)	
	Injured leg	Uninjured leg	Corresponding to injured leg	Corresponding to uninjured leg
Maximal leg extension (Nm)	144±40	162±45	145±35	142±39
Maximal leg flexion (Nm)	104±30	107±21	109±22	104±21
Dynamic postural sway of the CoP (mm)	1077 ±341	1223±496	941±237	984±294
Y-Balance-Score	316 ±22	317±22	319±15	324±15
6-m-timed-hop-test (s)	2.56 ±0.56	2.33±0.31	2.44±0.30	2.37±0.30
Drop jump (cm)	25.6±5.9		34.0±4.9	
Contact time (s)	0.227±0.034		0.266±0.090	
PRE Rectus Femoris (%MVC)	28±18	16±14	35±19	40±18
PRE Biceps Femoris (%MVC)	34±18	31±9	41±33	64±20
PRE Vastus Medialis (%MVC)	26±12	38±18	59±18	55±31
PRE Gastrocnemius (%MVC)	140±71	144±70	180±94	162±104

Table 1. Results of the tests. CoP: center of pressure. PRE: Pre-activation during drop jumping, 0.150 s before initital contact (n=7).

Conclusions

The results of this pilot study showed that patients six months after ACL reconstruction exhibit different performance and muscle activation patterns in a battery of strength, gait, balance und jump tests. Differences in drop jump performance might be attributed to the altered recruitment patterns of the muscles. Neuromuscular performance tests together with muscle activation assessment may support return-to-sport decisions 6 months after ACL reconstruction.

References

1. Logerstedt D, Grindem H, Lynch A, Eitzen I, Engebretsen L, Risberg MA, Axe MJ, Snyder-Mackler L. Single-Legged hop tests as predictors of self-reported knee function after anterior cruciate ligament reconstruction the delaware-oslo ACL cohort study. Am J Sports Med 2012; 40: 2348-2356
2. Petersen W, Taheri P, Forkel P, Zantop T. Return to play following ACL reconstruction: a systematic review about strength deficits. Arch Orthop Trauma Surg 2014; 134: 1417-1428
3. Schmitt LC, Paterno MV, Ford KR, Myer GD, Hewett TE. Strength Asymmetry and Landing Mechanics at Return to Sport after Anterior Cruciate Ligament Reconstruction. Med Sci Sports Exerc 2015; 47: 1426-1434

FOCAL MUSCLE VIBRATION REVERSES QUADRICEPS HYPOTROPHY IMPROVING MUSCLE FIBRES RECRUITMENT

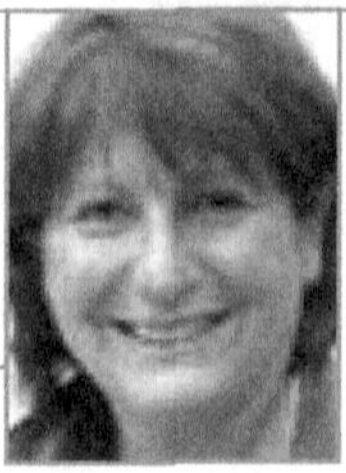

Benedetti MG[1], Zati A[1], Cavazzuti L[1], Rainoldi A[1], Casale R[2]

[1]Physical Medicine and Rehabilitation Unit, Istituto Ortopedico Rizzoli, Bologna;
[2]Habilita Care & Research Rehabilitation Unit, Zingonia, Bergamo, Italy

Introduction

The use of vibration has been used with a wide range of frequencies in different rehabilitation settings. Two wide categories of vibrating devices are actually used: the Whole-Body Vibration (WBV) and mechano-acoustic vibration locally applied on a single muscle (Local Vibration: LV).
LV has been used as a tool to improve muscle force (2), due to its neurophysiological effects both on muscle and on the central nervous system (1). These responses are characterized by an improvement in neuromuscular recruitment. This effect is thought to be particularly important in patients with knee diseases who experience a decline in quadriceps strength, generally associated with an overall reduction in muscle mass and decrease in proprioception. In these patients usually Neuro-Muscular Electrical Stimulations (NMES) are considered an efficient technique for quadriceps strengthening (3). The results of a randomized, controlled, single-blind trial are presented, which had as its primary goal the evaluation of the effects of LV on patients with documented hypotrophy and weakness of quadriceps muscle, in order to ascertain, through clinical and electrophysiological measures, weather LV is more effective that NMES in increasing the strength and improving the tropism of quadriceps muscle.

Methods

Thirty patients with painful knee Osteo-Arthritis (OA) were recruited for the present study, diagnosed as follows: first knee OA symptoms detected at least 6 months before study entry; radiographic evidence of knee femoro-tibial OA for the studied knee defined by the Kellgren and Lawrence grade 1-4; pain and functional limitation during physical activities. They were 14 males and 16 females, mean age 59±8 years, BMI 26.1±3.1 kg/m^2, moderately active.
Participants were randomly assigned into two groups: a study group, which was treated with LV (150 Hz, specifically set for muscle strengthening) by means of a commercial device VIBRA (e-Circle, San Pietro in Casale, Bologna, Italy), and a control group of patients treated with NMES (Compex Medical SA, Ecublens, Switzerland) 85 Hz and 4 Hz alternated frequency. All patients were treated in outpatients' regime for 10 days, 30 minutes per day.
Clinical measures taken pre and post treatment were WOMAC (Western Ontario and McMaster Universities Arthritis Index), Visual Analogue Scale (VAS), thigh circumference measured at 50% of the ASIS-superior patellar pole distance, Test Up and Go (TUG) and Stair climbing test. In addition, a subgroup of 20 patients (mean age 57±9 years, 8 females, 12 males, BMI 25.9±3.1 kg/m^2) were studied through the use of an isometric brace equipped with two torque transducers and surface Electromyogram (EMG) during isometric contraction (30% e 60% e 80% MVC) of quadriceps to indirectly asses changes in the muscle fiber composition and in the so called fatigue plot before and after treatment (1).

Results

At the end of treatment the Mann Whitney test evidenced a significant increase in thigh circumference for patients treated with LV ($p=0.026$), a reduction of TUG score ($p<0.0001$), Stair Climbing Test ($p= 0.022$), Womac ($p=0.002$) and VAS score for pain ($p=0.011$). This improvement was not significant in patients treated with NMES. sEMG analysis showed a changes in muscle fiber composition toward fiber II and a better muscle fiber recruitment leading to an increase in muscle force output in the group treated with LV.

Groups	n	WOMAC	VAS	Circumference	TUG	Stair Climbing
		Delta Pre-Post	Delta Pre-Post	Delta Pre-Post	Delta Pre-Post	Delta Pre-Post
VIBRA	15	-8.7±6.9	-1.4±1.6	0.6±1.1	-1.1±1.0	-3.8±3.6
NMES	15	-1.3±6	-0.1±1.1	-0.2±0.7	0.1±0.7	-0.6±5.5

Table 1. Delta values of the tests performed before (Pre) and after (Post) the treatment.

Conclusions

The present study confirms the effectiveness of LV in quadriceps strengthening. Electrophysiological findings originally demonstrate the effect of LV in enhancing muscle recruitment, modifying the muscle fiber composition.

References

1. Casale R, Ring H, Rainoldi A. High frequency vibration conditioning stimulation centrally reduces myoelectrical manifestation of fatigue in healthy subjects. J Electromyogr Kinesiol 2009; 19: 998-1004
2. Pietrangelo T, Mancinelli R, Toniolo L, Cancellara L, Paoli A, Puglielli C, Iodice P, Doria C, Bosco G, D'Amelio L, di Tano G, Fulle S, Saggini R, Fanò G, Reggiani C. Effects of local vibrations on skeletal muscle trophism in elderly people: mechanical, cellular, and molecular events. Int J Mol Med 2009; 24: 503-512
3. Vaz MA, Baroni BM, Geremia JM, Lanferdini FJ, Mayer A, Arampatzis A, Herzog W. Neuromuscular electrical stimulation (NMES) reduces structural and functional losses of quadriceps muscle and improves health status in patients with knee osteoarthritis. J Orthop Res 2013; 31: 511-516

THE EFFECT OF TWO DIFFERENT TRAINING APPROACHES ON PHYSICAL PERFORMANCE IN YOUNG SOCCER PLAYERS

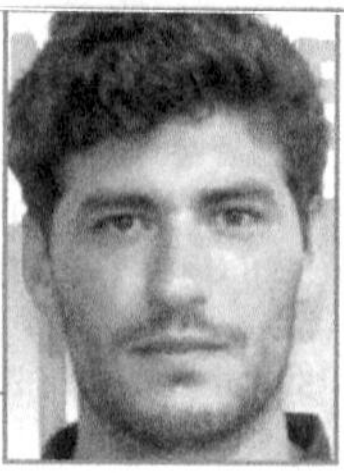

Perri E, Iaia F, Alberti G

Università degli Studi di Milano, Department of Biomedical Sciences for Health, Milan, Italy

Introduction

Via the triggering of different cellular signalling cascades, both, short-duration high-intensity and low-intensity high-volume training have been shown to upregulate several physiological mechanisms and therefore are important component of a training programme for enhancing work capacity (1, 2). However, no studies have directly compared these two divergent training approaches in soccer. Thus, the aim of the present investigation was to examine the effect of high-intensity vs endurance training on several football-related exercise performances in young soccer players.

Methods

During three weeks of the competitive season, nineteen young soccer players from Italian regional team (13.6±1.0 years; 169.5±6.9 cm; 56.8±10.2 kg), replaced their habitual fitness conditioning work with either Anaerobic/Speed-related training (AN n=9) or Aerobic-based training (AER n=10), three time per week. Anaerobic/Speed training consisted of attacking goal drills (8 x 15-30 s all-out, with 2-3 minutes of recovery-time) or small-sided games (7 x 60-90 s all-out, with 2.5-3.0 minutes of recovery time), whereas aerobic-based training was constituted by three, four sets of continuous drills lasting 6-8 minute each (85-90% of HRmax). Before and after the intervention, the players carried out the Yo-Yo intermittent recovery level 1(Yo-Yo IR1) and 2 (Yo-Yo IR2) test, a sprint test (20 m) and a Repeated Sprint Ability (RSA) (5 x 30 m, recovery 30 s).

Results

Significant improvements ($p<0.001$) were noticed between pre and post in the Yo-Yo IR1 (893±367 vs 1057±368 m; +15.5%, effect size (ES) 0.4) and Yo-Yo IR2 (246±64 vs 307±79 m; 19.9%, ES 0.9), whereas no interactions were detected between groups. No differences were observed in 20 m sprint (3.50±0.18 vs 3.47±0.17 s; $p>0.05$), RSA total time (26.15±1.30 vs 26.09±1.64 s; $p>0.05$) and RSA sprint decrement (2.29±1.19% vs 2.82±1.74%; $p>0.05$). No injured occurred during the intervention period.

Conclusions

In young male soccer players, three weeks of Anaerobic/ Speed-related training induced similar improvements in intermittent high-intensity exercise performance as aerobic-based training despite a 75% severe reduction in training volume. This findings could have an enormous impact also on others population such as the joints-compromised subjects who may have limitation in performing prolonged exercise training.

References

1. Iaia FM, Bangsbo J. Speed endurance training is a powerful stimulus for physiological adaptations and performance improvements of athletes. Scand J Med Sci Sports 2010; 20 Suppl 2: 11-23
2. Laursen PB. Training for intense exercise performance: high-intensity or high-volume training? Scand J Med Sci Sports 2010; 20 Suppl 2: 1-10
3. Nielsen JJ, M Fernstrom, K. Sahlin, J Bangsbo. Four weeks of speed endurance training reduces energy expenditure during exercise and maintains muscle oxidative capacity despite a reduction in training volume. J Appl Physiol 2008; 106: 73-80

THREE STRETCHING TRAINING METHODS TO INCREASE HAMSTRINGS FLEXIBILITY IN PROFESSIONAL SOCCER PLAYERS

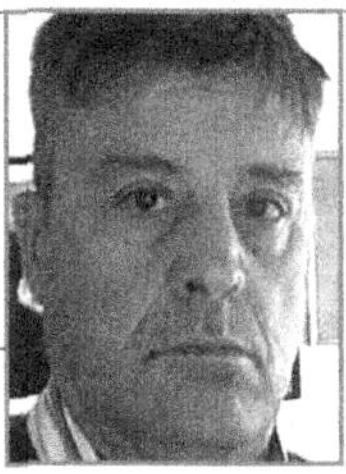

D'Onofrio R[1], Tamburrino P[2], Manzi V[3], Bovenzi A[3], Mazzoni S[3], Tavana R[3], Tamburrino G[2]

[1]Italian Scientific Society of Sport Rehabilitation and Posturology;
[2]Libera Associazione Medici del Calcio (LAMICA); [3]AC Milan, Milan, Italy

Introduction

There are many scientific articles in the international literature on the effects of static stretching, but only few studies have compared the different techniques of muscular stretching between them. The aim of this study is to analyse the differences between three methods of passive and active stretching and which of these has the most impact on increasing hamstrings flexibility.

Methods

The study involved 24 professional soccer players (average±SD age: 25.1±2.7; height: 1.90±0.07 m) participating in the First Division Italian Championship (Serie A). The players performed a Straight Leg Raise Test (SLRT) to assess the flexibility mainly related to the hamstrings and to establish the individual reference values before training (T1). The training protocol consisted in three sessions per week, for four weeks, of stretching exercises performed by the players previously divided into three groups:

- Group A (n=6) practiced a global postural stretching for the posterior chain, out of bench-stretch (6 x 20 seconds).
- Group B (n=6) practiced muscle stretching on the Nemes whole body vibrating platform (Nemes, Bosco System) in position Standing Pike Stretch (vibration at 20 Hz applied for 6 x 20 seconds).
- Group C (n=6) practised static analytical stretching (Anderson technique) 6 x 20 seconds.

All the players observed a rest of 10 seconds between stretches and performed the same technical soccer training. SLRT was repeated after the training (T2) and 14 days after the end of the training (T3).

Results

Results are shown in table 1.

	T1	T2	T3
Group A Right	74.5±11.5*#	91.3±9.1*§	88.8±9.3#§
Group A Left	73.8±10.0*#	93,6±8.0*§	91.0±8.2#§
Group B Right	80.8±4.5*#	91.0±5.6*	90.2±5.4#
Group B Left	80.9±4.6*#	92.6±6.6*	91.1±6.8#
Group C Right	77.6±9.7*#	86.1±6.6*§	81.4±7.7#§
Group C Left	77.6±8.1*#	87.6±6.9*§	83.5±6.6#§

Table 1. Results of the Straight Leg Raise Test (SLRT) performed to assess the flexibility in the three groups of professional players. T1: before training; T2: after four weeks of training; T3: 14 days from the end of the training. *P<0.05 T1 vs T2; # P<0.05 T1 vs T3; §P<0.05 T2 vs T3.

Conclusions

After training, significant improvements (P<0.05) of the performance in the SLRT were observed in the three studied groups of players. Among the studied no protocols of stretching, seems to be the more effective in order to improve hamstring flexibility (P>0.05). After 14 days from the end of the trainings we observed a decrease of the performances in the SLRT for two groups (Group A and C, P<0.05). Indeed the Group B (stretching during whole body vibration) showed a smaller but not significant decrease (P>0.05).

5

EFFECTS OF THREE DIFFERENT TRAINING PROGRAMMES ON INSTEP KICK IN PREADOLOSCENT FOOTBALL PLAYERS

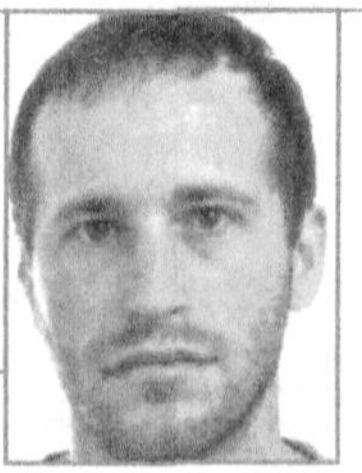

Rossi A, Formenti D, Alberti G

School of Exercise Sciences, Department of Biomedical Sciences for Health, Università degli Studi di Milano, Milan, Italy

Introduction

The Instep Kick (IK) is a basic element of a soccer game. It is a multi-joint activity affected by numerous factors, such as strength and power of the muscles involved in the kick (2), movement timing and stretch-shortening cycle among segments that contribute in the kick (3), and approach of the player to the ball (3).
The purpose of this study was to investigate the effects of specific (instep kick), non-specific (i.e., small side game and condition training) training on the speed of the ball in an IK on dominant and non-dominant legs in preadolescent Italian football players.

Methods

Eighteen male football players (age: 11 y, height: 1.45±0.09 m, weight: 36.9±6.0 kg) were recruited from an amateur Italian football team. Participants followed 6-weeks of specific training, in addition of their baseline football training and were randomly divided into three groups: 1) Instep Kick Group (IKG, n=6); 2) Conditional Group (CG, n=6) and 3) Small Side Games Group (SSG, n=6).
In all the training sessions (twice per week), IKG performed 20 IK (using maximum force) into the goal with dominant and non-dominant legs; CG performed four different conditional football exercises (i.e., 10 sets of the T-drill, 10 sets of 4 consecutives alternate bipodalic lateral jumps, 8 series of 5 consecutive bipodalic frontal jumps, 10 series of the stop-and-start drill); and SSG performed 20 minutes of 3 vs 3 small side game.
The football players were tested pre and post training periods on the speed of the ball in an IK on dominant and non-dominant legs. In each day test, participants performed four kicks with the left and the right leg and the speed of the ball was recorded using a speed radar gun (model#10-1925, Bushnell Outdoor Products, Overland Park, KS, USA). Among the 4 kicks, the higher speed recorded was used in the statistical analysis.
Two-way analysis of variance with repeated measures on one factor was used in order to detect differences among the three groups and between pre and post training period, in the dominant and non-dominant legs separately. Least Significant Difference test (LSD) was used as post-hoc analysis.

Results

Significant improvement in IK of about 5.7% was found in each group between pre and post training periods in dominant leg (Within-subjects difference: $F_{(1,15)}=21.805$, $p<0.001$) (Table 1).

Group	Dominant leg		Non dominant leg	
	Pre	Post	Pre	Post
IKG (n=6)	62.5±5.8	66.5±4.2	51.5±6.6	56.8±4.6
CG (n=6)	64.0±4.2	67.2±5.9	52.8±3.6	54.0±4.5
SSG (n=6)	60.5±7.2	62.8±5.9	54.8±6.7	55.7±6.9

Table 1. Results of the Instep Kick test (km/h) in the three groups of players. IKG: Instep Kick Group; CG: Conditional Group; SSG: Small Side Games group. Pre: before training; Post: after six weeks of training. Data are shown as mean±SD.

Significant interaction was found in non-dominant leg (Interaction: $F(2,15)=21.805$, $p=0.001$). The LSD post-hoc test showed statistical improvement only in IKG of 10.3% between pre and post training period ($p=0.002$).

Conclusions

The three different trainings produced the same improvement on the speed of the ball in an IK on dominant leg. Conversely, on non-dominant leg it was found different effects between training methods. In particular, the IKG obtained larger improvement than the CG and SSG on non-dominant leg.

The young football players often use the dominant leg to manipulate the ball (1), and for this reasons the dominant leg did not require any specific training to improve the speed of the ball in an IK. For the same reason, the 11 years old football players obtained larger improvement on non-dominant leg, probably because trained to repeat the IK numerous times.

References

1. Bjelica D, Popovic S, Petkovic J. Comparison of instep kicking between preferred and non-preferred leg in young football players. Montcn J Sports Sci Med 2013; 2: 5-10
2. Dörge HC, Andersen T B, Sørensen H, Simonsen EB, Aagaard H, Dyhre-Poulsen P, Klausen K. EMG activity of the iliopsoas muscle and leg kinetics during the soccer place kick. Scand J Med Sci Sports 1999; 9: 195-200
3. Kapidžić A, Huremović T, Biberovic A. Kinematic analysis of the instep kick in youth soccer players. J Hum Kinet 2014; 42: 81-90

Sunday 10th April, 2016 (morning)
MOUNTBATTEN ROOM

FREE ORAL PRESENTATIONS
CONTEST - FINALS - PART 1

BEST CLINICAL CASE HISTORY AWARD

Chairs

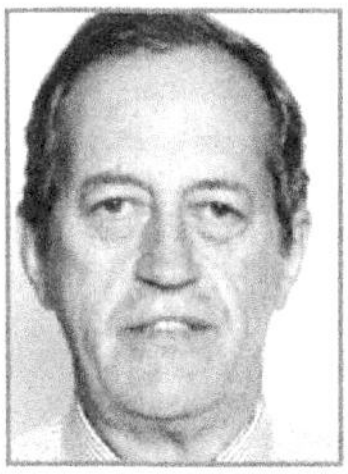

Peter Brukner
(Melbourne, Australia)

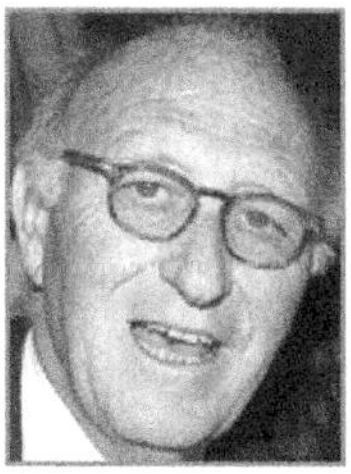

Antonio Delcogliano
(Rome, Italy)

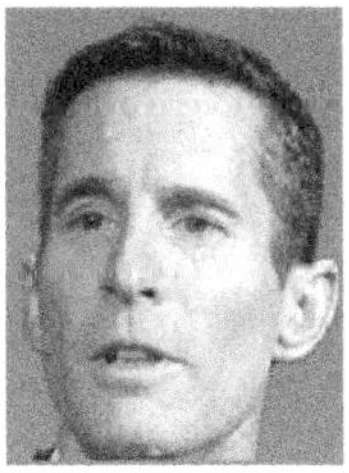

Bill Knowles
(Philadelpia, USA)

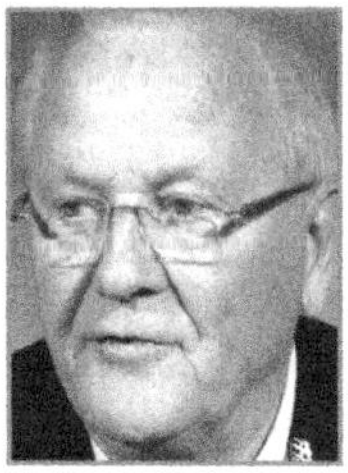

Lars Peterson
(Gothenburg, Sweden)

9:30 Performance optimised return to play following concussion in tournament football **Williams M, Iga J, Spencer SM (Burton-Upon-Trent, United Kingdom)**

9:42 Non-operative management and return to play soccer after second ACL injury **Arundale A, Snyder-Mackler L (Newark, USA)**

9:54 Rehabilitation after femoroacetabular impingement arthroscopy. When all is not enough **Vivo-Fernández I, Sanchez-Heredia MA, Jimeno-Serrano FJ (Murcia, Spain)**

10:06 A case of 12th rib costochondral fracture in an elite youth soccer goalkeeper **Robertson D, Materne O (Doha, Qatar)**

10:18 Return to pre- injury level football following multi-ligament reconstruction
Cady K (Cheltenham, United Kingdom)

10:30 Return to professional football following a third ACL reconstruction
Buckthorpe M, Zanobbi M, Batty P (London, United Kingdom)

10:42 Post-concussion syndrome and psychosocial issues in a professional academy footballer **Robinson TM, Forsdyke D (York, United Kingdom)**

10:54 End of the session

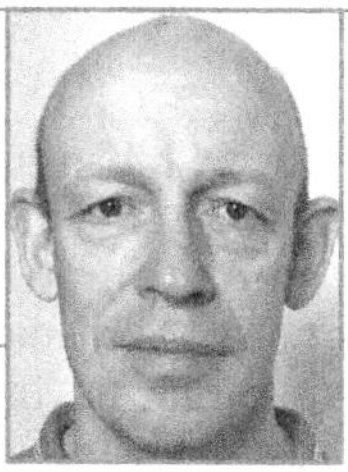

PERFORMANCE OPTIMISED RETURN TO PLAY FOLLOWING CONCUSSION IN TOURNAMENT FOOTBALL

Williams M, Iga J, Spencer SM

England U21 Medical Performance Dept, St George's Park, Burton-Upon-Trent, United Kingdom

Publication of the Zurich Consensus Statement of 2012 (1) offers common ground in the definition, diagnosis and management of concussed athletes, proposing a Graduated Return To Play (GRTP) protocol as the cornerstone for recovery. To permit multi-sport application, the GRTP protocol is broad in principle but lacks sport specificity.

We describe the management of concussion in a 21-year-old male professional footballer on the eve of a European U21 International Tournament, reflecting the need to maintain match preparedness and physical fitness within recognised GRTP guidelines amidst an intense tournament scenario.

Two days prior to the first group game a defender sustained a head injury in a collision with a team mate in a set-piece training routine. Pitch side management was in accordance with Advanced Resuscitation and Emergency Aid principles. Neurological assessment and profiling with the Sport Concussion Assessment Tool 3rd Edition revealed a significant increase in symptoms and symptom severity scores compared to his normal baseline.

Assessment the next morning revealed further deterioration in symptoms, symptom severity, concentration and balance scores. A 24-hour period of absolute rest was prescribed.

By day two post-injury all symptoms, concentration and balance scores had returned to their respective baselines. In accordance with the GRTP Stage 2, the player was taken for a supervised light aerobic session on a static bike. The session lasted 20 minutes in duration with a subjective Rating of Perceived Exertion (RPE) of 3 reported; his average Heart Rate (HR) was 126 bpm, with no time recorded at intensities greater than 85% of estimated HR max (3) (HR>85% Ext max).

Subsequent daily assessments revealed no adverse neurological reaction to increased training load.

To satisfy a return to sport specific exercise (GRTP Stage 3), the player was prescribed a modified Hoff Circuit consisting of an interval-based dribbling activity (4 minutes) intervened with a period of active recovery (3 minutes). He reported an RPE of 3 and covered a total of 4,195 metres in distance, with no high speed running (distance covered at speeds > 5.5 m/s) or sprinting (speed above 5.5 m/s and maintained for at least 1 s) exposure; his average HR was 141 bpm, with 17 minutes spent at intensities greater than HR>85% Ext max.

Progressing to more complex non-contact training drills (GRTP Stage 4) and reflecting the physical demands of his defensive role, drills were organised to replicate the typical movement patterns of his playing position. Within this session the player covered 3,329 meters: 242 meters at high speed, sprints 15, average HR 158 bpm, 25 minutes of HR>85% Ext max).

Day 5 post-injury was the second group fixture. Unable to assess response to full contact training (GRTP Stage 5), the player remained ineligible for selection. To align with tournament tempo, he was given a gym based session with no significant cardiovascular workout. This adjustment in training load permitted him to undertake full contact training the next day (duration 58 minutes, distance covered 3,843 meters, high speed running 185 meters, sprints 14, average HR 137 bpm, 44 minutes of HR>85% Ext max).

The implication of a concussion diagnosis for players, coaches and clinicians should not be underestimated. GRTP protocols in the Zurich Statement are broadly defined and open to interpretation by clinicians, their mandated timescales are an additional pressure within a tournament setting.

Squad replacement rules, emotional labiality of the player, self-declared fitness and retrospective admission of symptom severity, were all decision modifiers (2) in this scenario.
We believe this return to play protocol was specific to the challenges of an intensive international tournament. Progressive drills reflected the recommended physiological boundaries of the post-concussion GRTP protocols, while session content remained relevant to the defensive position of the player. Alignment of training load allowed the player to make a full return to competitive play for the final group game (Day 8 post-injury).
For future tournaments we propose medical performance staff consider position specific training drills within post-concussion guidelines to maximise return to fitness at the required tournament tempo. Furthermore, the priority should always remain the assessment and subsequent management of risk tolerance, regardless of the impact on collective performance aims.

References

1.McCrory P, Meeuwisse WH, Aubry M, Cantu B, Dvorak J, Echemendia RJ, Engebretsen L, Johnston K, Kutcher JS, Raftery M, Sills A, Benson BW, Davis GA, Ellenbogen RG, Guskiewicz K, Herring SA, Iverson GL, Jordan BD, Kissick J, McCrea M, McIntosh AS, Maddocks D, Makdissi M, Purcell L, Putukian M, Schneider K, Tator CH, Turner M. Consensus statement on concussion in sport: the 4th International Conference on Concussion in Sport held in Zurich, November 2012. Br J Sports Med 2013; 47: 250-258
2.Shrier I. Strategic Assessment of Risk and Risk Tolerance (StARRT) framework for return-to-play decision-making. Br J Sports Med 2015; 49: 1311-1315
3.Tanaka H, Monahan KD, Seals DR. Age-Predicted Maximal Heart Rate Revisited. J Am Coll Cardiol 2012; 37: 4-7

NON-OPERATIVE MANAGEMENT AND RETURN TO PLAY SOCCER AFTER SECOND ACL INJURY

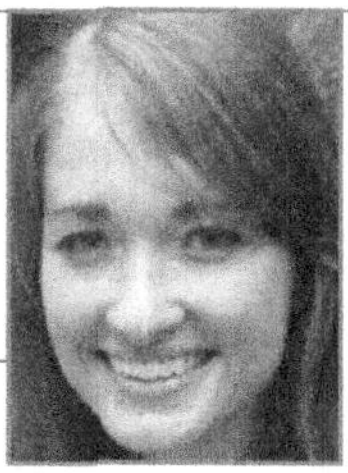

Arundale A, Snyder-Mackler L

The University of Delaware, Newark, USA

Introduction

Compared to primary Anterior Cruciate Ligament Reconstructions (ACLR), Anterior Cruciate Ligament (ACL) revisions have lower patient-reported outcomes and higher rates of subsequent knee operations. Non-operative management of primary ACL injuries has been studied, however there is little literature on non-operative management of second ACL injuries.

Case report

The athlete was a collegiate and professional central mid-fielder up to age 23, at which point he transitioned to playing amateur soccer three times a week. At age 30, he had a non-contact right ACL injury while playing soccer and an ACLR using allograft tissue. He returned to his pre-injury level and frequency of soccer and one year after ACLR scored 100% on the Knee Outcomes Survey- Activities of Daily Living (KOS), Global Rating of Perceived Knee Function (GR), and International Knee Documentation Committee 2000 Subjective Knee Form (IKDC). He had a non-contact re-injury to his right knee while playing soccer, planting his foot and cutting, five days shy of two years after his ACLR.

Examination (Day 1): Examination (Table 1) found right quadriceps inhibition and a 5° quadriceps lag with a straight leg raise. He had decreased stance time and Range Of Motion (ROM) on his right during gait, but no episodes of giving way. He also had limited patellar mobility, and reported 5/10 pain at worst.

Diagnosis: Magnetic Resonance Imaging (MRI) confirmed a full thickness graft rupture and revealed lateral bone bruising, but no concomitant meniscal or ligamentous injuries.

Intervention: Therapy initially focused on the athlete's effusion, ROM, gait, and quadriceps deficits. By the athlete's 4th visit (Day 10) he had 1+ effusion, 144° of knee flexion, 3/10 pain at worst, no gait or patellar mobility impairments, no quadriceps lag, and a quadriceps strength index of 84%. The athlete had KOS and GR scores of 84% and 85%, respectively, and continued to have no episodes of giving way. The athlete decided to pursue non-operative management as he wanted to return to sport but was moving in six weeks. Perturbation training (3) was initiated at the fifth visit after the athlete achieved trace effusion and full ROM. Progression of all exercises was determined by effusion and soreness rules (1). When the athlete could maintain stability and balance, perturbation training was progressed to include a soccer ball, and when the athlete could maintain trace or no effusion and no soreness between sessions a running progression was initiated (10th visit, Day 42) and subsequently the Interval Kicking Progression (11th visit, Day 49).

Outcomes: At the athlete's final visit before moving (12th visit, Day 51) he had a quadriceps strength index of 90%, 0/10 pain at worst, and scored 97% on KOS and 90% on the GR. He was given a detailed home exercise program which involved gradual initiation of agility exercises, advised to complete the interval kicking progression1 and given a return to sport plan which involved gradual introduction of field sessions (2). Six months after the athlete's second ACL injury he reported that he had returned to his pre-injury level of soccer again, and scored 100% on the KOS score and GR, and 95.4% on the IKDC.

Discussion

This case demonstrates the ability of an athlete to return to his pre-injury level of sport after non-operative management of an ipsilateral second ACL injury; applying the literature on non-operative management of primary ACL injuries successfully to second ACL injury rehabilitation.
Non-operative management may not be suitable for all athletes, but this athlete had no episodes of giving way, good quadriceps strength and self-report measures, and quickly resolved his initial impairments making him a good candidate (3). Objective criteria (e.g. soreness and effusion rules) and progressive programs (e.g. the Interval Kicking Progression) were integral to safely progressing and returning this athlete to sport. The outcomes of this case demonstrate that non-operative management of second ACL injuries can be successful and that more research is needed.

Anthropometrics		
Ethnicity	African-American	
Height	1.8 m	
Weight	81.2 kg	
Initial Evaluation Findings	**Left**	**Right**
Modified Stroke Test	0	3+
Active Knee Extension ROM	Hyper 8	Hyper 8
Active Knee Flexion ROM	147°	110°
Instrumented Laxity Measurement	7mm	9mm
Lachman's Test	-	+
Varus Stress Test	-	-
Valgus Stress Test	-	-
Posterior Drawer Test	-	-
Quadriceps Strength Index (KinCom, Chatanooga, TN, USA)	77%	

Table 1. Initial Evaluation. Instrumented Laxity Measurement performed with KT-1000, (MEDmetric Corporation, San Diego, California, USA).

References

1. Arundale A, Silvers H, Logerstedt D, Rojas J, Snyder-Mackler L. An interval kicking progression for return to soccer following lower extremity injury. Int J Sports Phys Ther 2015; 10: 114-127
2. Della Villa S, Boldrini L, Ricci M, Danelon F, Snyder-Mackler L, Nanni G, Roi GS. Clinical outcomes and return-to-sports participation of 50 soccer players after anterior cruciate ligament reconstruction through a sport-specific rehabilitation protocol. Sports Health 2012; 4: 17-24
3. Fitzgerald GK, Axe MJ, Snyder-Mackler L. Proposed practice guidelines for nonoperative anterior cruciate ligament rehabilitation of physically active individuals. J Orthop Sports Phys. 2000; 30: 194-203

REHABILITATION AFTER FEMOROACETABULAR IMPINGEMENT ARTHROSCOPY. WHEN ALL IS NOT ENOUGH

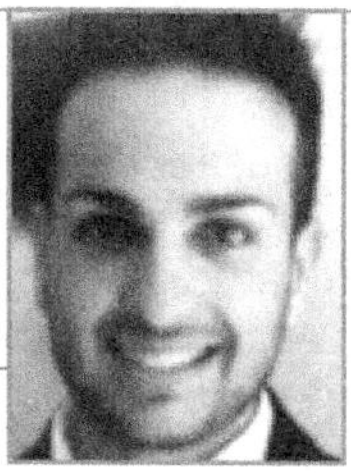

Vivo-Fernández I[2,3], Sanchez-Heredia MA[1], Jimeno-Serrano FJ[1,2]

[1]Innova, Health and Sport Institute, Murcia;
[2]Department of Physiotherapy, University of Murcia;
[3]Research Centre of Murcia Soccer Federation, Murcia, Spain

The purpose of this case report is to show the outcomes of rehabilitation of arthroscopic management of Femoro-Acetabular Impingement (FAI) in an elite male soccer player with 30 years old, 184 cm and 76 kg. He played at Spanish LaLiga first division as right defender since 2003 (19 years old), and he participated in almost 300 professional elite matches along these years (including Spanish U-21 National Team, UEFA Europe League and Champions League matches).
Left hip FAI diagnosis was made after several months of clinical hip pain and functional disability. After a few weeks of conservative treatment by team physiotherapy staff, finally FAI was treated by hip arthroscopy, labral debridement and acetabular cartilage repair (micro-fractures technique). After successful surgery, the player began rehabilitation with the team medical staff.
Two months after the hip surgery, the season finished and the player contract expired, so the rehab with the team medical staff was finished.
Hence, the player started a new rehabilitation program with our work team. In order to establish our rehab goals, at first, we assessed the hip Range Of Motion (ROM) with a universal goniometer, hip strength using a pressure biofeedback, and the footballer report us about the pain and functionality of the hip with the Copenhagen Hip and Groin Outcome Score (HAGOS). In addition we visually examined his movement patterns looking for motion patterns that led the hip to FAI, with the purpose of correct them. Results of first assessment are shown in Table 1.

	First assessment		**Final assessment**	
	Right	Left	Right	Left
Hip Internal Rotation (°)	30	10	40	40
Hip External Rotation (°)	50	25	50	45
Bent Knee Fallout Test	16	21	16	17
Thomas Test	0	0	0	0
Impingement Fadir Test	-	+	-	-
Impingement Faber Test	-	-	-	-

Table 1. Results of the first and of the final assessment (five months later).

Squeeze tests at 0°, 45° and 90° recorded 80 mmHg, 70 mmHg and 103 mmHg respectively.
HAGOS scores were 65 (pain), 55 (symptoms), 70 (activity daily living), 25 (sport/recreation), 20 (participation) and 32 (quality of life).
According to these results, we started with the objectives of reduce hip pain, improve range of motion and hip function.
First the player made functional combined exercises at the pool and the rehabilitation gym, increase the exercises goals according to the assessment by the physicals therapist team. Firstly we propose a program of hip ROM exercises, and low strength program in the pool combined with gym ROM exercises and correction of aberrant motion patterns by video-feedback, mirror exercises and spoken corrections. Low intensity stationary bicycle was used to warm up before gym sessions, and manual therapy was done at the end of each session. Every month, the hip surgeon checked the advances and every second month, hip Magnetic Resonance Imaging (MRI) was made for detect any change.
Along the following weeks, our player gained ROM, strength, motor control and the pain practically disappeared, so we integrate more strength and proprioceptive working like elastic bands, Total Resistance eXercise (TRX), functional strength exercises and low football skills exercises, like driving and passing the ball. On his own, our player increased his bike activity, developing an unexpected liking for the mountain bike. After five months, everything was better, and it was the moment to make a decision: our footballer met with the surgeon, a hip surgery expert and his agent to decide if he was ready to return to elite football. Results at that moment are shown in Table 1.
Squeeze tests at 0°, 45° and 90° recorded 100 mmHg, 95 mmHg and 120 mmHg respectively.
HAGOS scores were 90 (pain), 80 (symptoms), 90 (activity daily living), 65 (sport/recreation), 75 (participation) and 90 (quality of life).
Despite of a surgery and a rehab process that invited optimism, both surgeon and specialist advised our footballer not to return to elite football. Although he was better and better along the rehab, the cartilage had suffered a lot during the football career of the players, and the hip mixed pincer and cam deformity of the player did not predict a good future and involved a great risk for his health, with a subsequent risk of early hip osteoarthritis and even requirement of arthroplasty. Hopelessly, in one hand, we were sad because of the prohibition from part of surgery staff, but in the other hand, the hip of our player was notably improved on ROM, strength, functionality and pain; and despite all, our footballer was happiest than ever, he could not return to elite-football, but we gave him back a hip state better than he could imagine, and subsequently a quality of life that he didn't enjoy since this problem started.
Currently, he is able to do every daily activity without any pain, and although he did not return to play, he achieved return to sports, and now he transfers his old football passion and enthusiasm to mountain bike, riding large routes and sharing trainings with elite regional bikers.

Conclusions

Common sense and avoiding health risks for our athletes have to prevail before the desire of return to play.
Sometimes, achieving the rehab goals does not mean return to play.
Sometimes, not to be able to return to play does not mean not to be able to return to sport.

A CASE OF 12TH RIB COSTOCHONDRAL FRACTURE IN AN ELITE YOUTH SOCCER GOALKEEPER

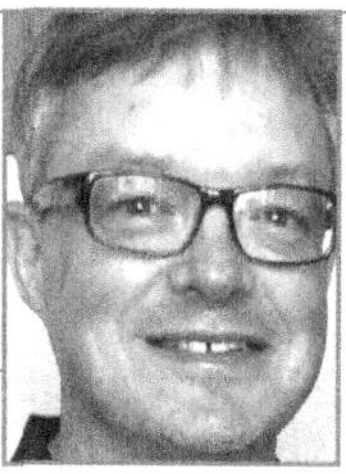

Robertson D[1], Materne O[2]

[1]Qatar Football Association, Qatar Football Association, Doha;
[2]Aspire Academy, Health Centre, NSMP, Doha, Qatar

Introduction

Acute impact-type chest wall injury is common in sports involving deliberate heavy contact, such as boxing and rugby (2). In soccer, chest injury is typically less severe and infrequent. Indeed, one 10-season study of youth soccer reports trunk and abdominal injury rates ≤0.5% (1). However, there is also evidence that goalkeepers are up to five times more likely to suffer injury to the trunk, compared to outfield players (3), and 30% more likely to suffer a training injury (1). Fracture of the floating ribs is a rare sports injury (2), and has not previously been reported in soccer. In this study we describe for the first time a 12th rib costochondral fracture (with associated internal oblique muscle enthesial injury) and the Return To Play (RTP) pathway. Awareness of youth and player-position factors was a crucial part of the overall medical management plan, which included safe collaboration with the goalkeeper coach.

Case report

An 18 years old goalkeeper was part of the squad in an international tournament (Age: 18.2 yrs; height: 185 cm; body mass: 67.7 kg; BMI: 19.8 kg/m^2; skinfolds: 49.0 mm). The injury mechanism was a, diving, saving movement, with a late sudden twisting, and change of direction, to save a close, low, hard shot. This resulted in a sudden violent muscle contraction in the trunk rotators.
The player completed the session but reported discomfort later. Visual Analogue Scale (VAS) on day 1 was 2/10, with apprehension, but no specific signs and no formal diagnosis. The player had physical therapies and trained next day. Despite careful follow-up, on day 4 the level of symptoms increased (VAS 5/10). Examination revealed focal chest wall signs around the 12th rib tip.
Sonography was positive (hypo-echoic) for injury to both the 12th costochondral joint and the adjacent internal oblique muscle enthesis (Figure 1 A-B). Magnetic Resonance Imaging scan confirmed the diagnosis, and excluded underlying intra-abdominal injury (Figure 1 C-D). X-ray was normal.

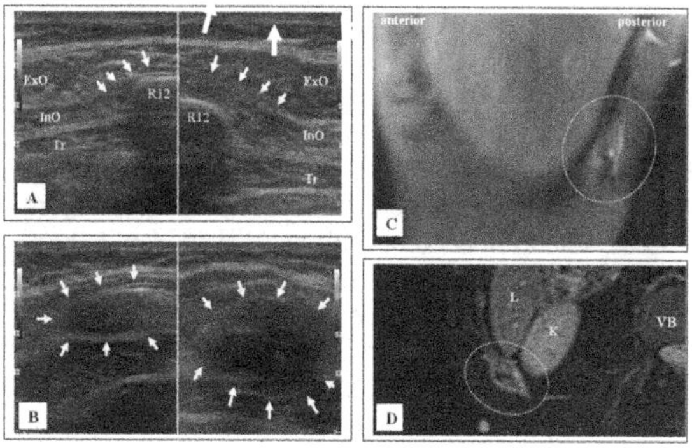

Figure 1. Show long (A) and short axis (B) comparative ultrasound scans (left, normal/right, injured). The arrows (A) show the internal oblique muscle attachments to the 12th rib; arrows (B) indicate the costochondral joint. Sagittal (C) and axial (D) MRI scan images reveal the swollen costochondral fracture and adjacent muscle injury (R12 = 12th rib; ExO = external oblique; InO = internal oblique; Tr = transversalis; K = kidney; L = liver. VB = vertebral body).

Therapeutic intervention

Management consisted of the following 5 steps (Table 1). 1) Therapeutic and analgesic modalities for first 4 days of minor non-specific symptoms; 2) 4 days of rest including therapeutic analgesic modalities and Ultrasound bone growth stimulator (Osteotron IV, Tokyo, Japan); 3) Progressive pain-free passive and active functional exercises including isometric, eccentric and concentric strengthening; 4) Higher threshold rehabilitation started at day 14, incorporating graduated functional progressions, co-contraction and position-specific movements; 5) RTP on day 20.

		Phase 1	Phase 2	Phase 3	Phase 4	Phase 5
		In tournament	Tissue recovery	Rehabilitation	Return to train	Return to play
		Day 1 to 4	Day 5 to 8	Day 9 to 13	Day 14 to 19	Day 20
Subjective	VAS (Range)	Moderate (2-5/10)	Moderate (1-4/10)	Minor (0-1/10)	Pain free (0/10)	Pain free (0/10)
	Apprehension	**High**	**Moderate**	**Low**	**Low**	**None**
Objective clinical assessment (VAS)	Internal Oblique	Moderate (2-4/10)	Minor (1-3/10)	Minor (0-1/10)	Pain free	Pain free
	Latissimus dorsi	Moderate (2-4/10)	Moderate (2-4/10)	Minor (0-2/10)	Minor (0-1/10)	Pain free
	Quadratus lumborum	Pain free	Pain free	Pain free	Pain free	Pain free
Palpation (VAS)	12th Rib	Moderate (2-3/10)	Moderate (2-3/10)	Minor (1-2/10)	Minimal (0-1/10)	Minimal (0-1/10)
Range of motion (Mean VAS)	Active lateral trunk flex	Limited (3/10)	No Limited (1/10)	No Limited (0-1/10)		
	Active trunk rotation	No Limited (1/10)	No Limited and pain free	No Limited and pain free	Full ROM and pain free	Full ROM, pain free, no recurrent sympt.
Treatment	Medicine	Ibuprofen 400 mg TDS	None	None	None	
	Manual therapy & soft tissue techniques	Once a day	Once a day	Once a day	Prior rehab / training	
	Cryotherapy	2 to 3 times a day	1 to 2 times a day	1 to 2 times a day	Post rehab/ train.	None
	TENS analgesic	once a day	once a day	None	None	
	Bone stimulator	None	Twice daily (2x20')	Twice daily (2x20')	Once daily (1x20')	
Rehabilitation	Cardiovascular		Bike	Bike	Rowing	
	Stretching	None	None	Progressively pain free	Normal	
	Range of motion		None	Active limited	Full	None
	Strengthening		None	Pain free Isom & Ecc	All + plyometrics	
	Co-contraction exerc		None	PFM	Goalkeeper specific	
Goalkeeper activity	Ball handling				No restriction	
	Over-head (drills - catching)	Full function in-competition manag.	Stopped	Stopped	Progressive	Normal goalkeeper training demands
	Throwing (short - long)				Progressive	
	Goal-kicking				Progressive	
	Diving				Progressive	

Table 1. Summary of medical management, including goalkeeper coach collaboration. Isom.: isometrics; Ecc: eccentric; PFM: Progressive Functional Movements.

Discussion

The peculiarities of the goalkeeping role carry increased risk of injury to head, trunk and hands (3). Key challenges in this particular case were both the timing of the injury (international tournament), as well as the injury's impact on goalkeeper-specific movements. Where chest wall injury symptoms persist or worsen, imaging is indicated. Musculoskeletal ultrasound is an ideal first line imaging tool, and is accurate, cheap and comparative. MRI is also a good investigation, and can exclude underlying visceral injury (2). X-rays do not usually pick up costal cartilage fractures (2). Computed Tomography scan gives more detail on the fracture, but means radiation exposure (2). Effective analgesia at the outset helped minimize sleep disturbance, aiding recovery. The period of rest was also important, as was the need for patience before commencing functional rehabilitation. Furthermore, recruitment of the goalkeeping coach's skills has been mooted already (3), and his involvement in targeted technical field drills was seen as beneficial for an efficient return to play. Moreover, the possibility of using an image-guided injection intervention to help symptom-control was discussed, but not employed.

Conclusions

This case offers the first description of a successful return to play for this unusual chest injury. The overall treatment and rehabilitation programme was 15 days (including 9 days rest from all football activities). This strategy resulted in an efficient, safe recovery, with no residual apprehension or recurrence. Finally, the functional progressions were position-specific, and at no stage was follow-up imaging felt necessary.

References

1. Le Gall F, Carling C, Reilly T, Vandewalle H, Church J, Rochcongar P. Incidence of injuries in elite French youth soccer players. A 10-season study. Am J Sports Med 2006; 34: 928-938
2. Lopez V, Ma R, Li, X, Steele J, Allen A. Costal cartilage fractures and disruptions in a rugby football player. Clin J Sport Med 2013; 23: 232-234
3. Ostojic S. Comparing sports injuries in soccer: influence of a positional role. Res Sports Med 2003; 11: 203-208

RETURN TO PRE- INJURY LEVEL FOOTBALL FOLLOWING MULTI-LIGAMENT RECONSTRUCTION

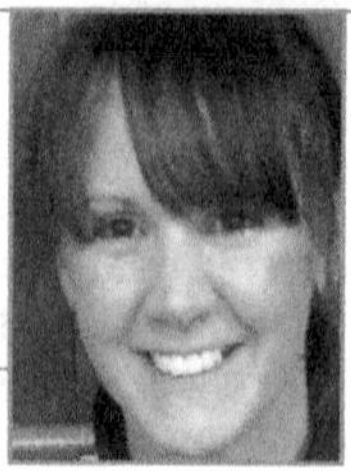

Cady K

The University of Gloucestershire, Cheltenham, United Kingdom

A 27 year old male semi-professional (ex-professional) midfield player (Stature 157 cm, Body Mass 72 kg) presented four months following a traumatic tibio-femoral dislocation of his right knee. This injury was sustained from a two footed tackle whilst participating in a league game.

He was immediately referred to A&E and a complete rupture of the Anterior Cruciate ligament (ACL), Posterior Cruciate Ligament (PCL), Lateral Collateral Ligament (LCL) and Bicep Femoris (BF) was diagnosed. He underwent an open postero-lateral corner reconstruction which included a reconstruction of his LCL by allograft and reattachment of his BF. Unfortunately the player experienced a postoperative infection and a manipulation under anaesthetic was carried out in order to regain his range of movement. He underwent a second operation two months later to reconstruct his ACL and PCL. The ACL was repaired using a hamstring graft and the PCL was repaired by allograft. The player was prescribed a Jack Brace which limited extension to 10 degrees for the first three months post ACL/PCL reconstruction. He was receiving weekly NHS physiotherapy post injury that consisted of hydrotherapy and mobility exercises. On presentation the player was still wearing the Jack Brace. This was to be removed in three weeks. On examination the player had 20 degrees active flexion and 10 degrees active extension which had not been improved with regular physiotherapy sessions. The Patello-femoral joint was restricted with no movement in all ranges and the tibia had no medial or lateral rotation. In addition, an arthrofibrosis was present. Due to the limited range of motion presented the consultant had stipulated a time frame of four weeks in order to gain 90 degrees flexion and terminal extension or he would perform another manipulation under anaesthetic. Patello-Femoral Joint (PFJ) mobility is key to regaining mobility of the Tibio-Femoral Joint (TFJ) but this joint had received no mobilisation after the surgery. Treatment in the first stage involved patellofemoral joint mobilisations, passive rotational mobilisation of the tibial femoral joint and soft tissue release to regain mobility and increase movement of the tibiofemoral joint. Isometrics were given to regain strength of the hamstrings and Vastus Medialis. As the mobility of the TFJ was improved this enabled strengthening to be achieved through the range and the player was able to progress to body weight squats at different ranges. The player continued with hydrotherapy strengthening and mobility exercises alongside cardiovascular maintenance and a lumbo-pelvic stability program. After four weeks of treatment, 90 degrees active flexion, 100 degrees passive flexion and full terminal extension were achieved. Full PFJ mobility had been achieved and the player had regained medial and lateral rotation of the TFJ. A fourth surgical procedure had been avoided as the treatment and rehabilitation program had addressed the joint mobility issues and this had been achieved within the fourth week period stipulated by the surgeon. Seven months post injury the player began jump landing retraining followed by the commencement of straight line running a month later. The player had maintained full terminal extension and had increased his flexion to 110 degrees. End of range flexion was restricted but pain free. Hamstring strengthening specifically targeting inner range and single leg work was increased. After sessions the player reported no swelling but some stiffness which reduced after stretching and mobilising on the foam roller. Ten months post injury the player was full paced running, turning and striking a ball with no pain or swelling. A strengthening program was maintained and the sports specific exercises were progressed into position specific drills such as running and changing direction with and without the ball and passing over different distances. These drills progressed to introduce the player to contact when receiving the ball, and tackling drills were also incorporated into the program. At twelve months the player returned to full unrestricted training at the same level of football and has been participating at this level ever since. After such a traumatic injury the player was not expecting to return to his pre injury level of sport and was pleased at being able to avoid a fourth operation.

RETURN TO PROFESSIONAL FOOTBALL FOLLOWING A THIRD ACL RECONSTRUCTION

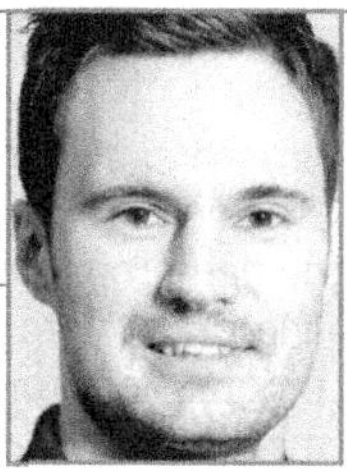

Buckthorpe M, Zanobbi M, Batty P

Isokinetic Medical Group, FIFA Medical Centre of Excellence, London, United Kingdom

Methods

This case report presents the successful rehabilitation and focused return to sport of a 28-year-old male professional footballer (midfielder) after his third Anterior Cruciate Ligament Reconstruction (ACLR) (second ipsilateral limb). The player was in the final year of his current playing contract at a Premier League Football Club (2014-2015). The surgical procedure involved arthroscopy partial medial meniscectomy, revision ACLR with hamstring and lateral tenodesis of the left knee.

Rehabilitation goals were to return the player back to professional football at the same level of performance with minimal risk of re-injury as quickly as possible.

A criterion based progression focused on function as opposed to time was adopted involving five phases of rehabilitation (1).

Phase 1: involved resolution of pain, inflammation and wound healing.

Phase 2: incorporated pool based rehabilitation and gym based physiotherapy to focus on restoration of swelling and range of motion, maintenance and restoration of basic movement patterns. Progression through this phase was severely delayed due to a rare occurrence of psued oaneurysm. The player underwent further surgery which involved aspiration, injection of PRP, exploration and excision of pseudo aneurysm and coagulation 46 days after his primary surgery.

Phase 3: focused on muscle strength and endurance, with an initial focus on isolated restoration of quadriceps, calf and posterior chain strength, with the second phase incorporating more global strengthening as well a focused approach on muscle imbalance correction and core/pelvic stability in order to create a well-balanced musculoskeletal profile on which to progress.

Phase 4: focused largely on neuromuscular training, incorporating a periodised progressive programme of neural training in addition to continued strengthening and aerobic re-conditioning. Aspects of this were incorporated into pool based rehabilitation to accelerate adaptations in neural function earlier in the programme. A progressive programme of agility based exercises to re-train movement control was undertaken alongside this neuromuscular training, which was specific to the functional recovery at that stage.

Phase 5: incorporated a greater focus on strength and conditioning alongside on-field rehabilitation in order to restore a football specific physiological profile, explosive neuromuscular performance and technical performance. Gradual transition from conscious to unconscious movement patterns and incorporation of more complex sport-specific skills was undertaken alongside increased training intensity and volume in order to prepare for the demands of actual training. Some final aspects of phase 5 were undertaken at the players' club and included reintegration into training and then return to competitive match play.

A focused approach on neuromuscular biomechanics, through the restoration of muscle imbalances and movement dysfunction and optimisation of neuromuscular function was incorporated throughout the programme.

Progression through the phases and ultimately back the team was guided through specific criteria. Isokinetic testing of maximal concentric knee extensor and flexor strength and muscle endurance guided progression through phase 3 to 4 (<25% deficit vs. contralateral limb) 4 to 5 (<15% deficit) and phase 5 to 6 (<10%). Our ACL specific movement analysis test was used as an indicator for progression from phase 4 to 5 (>80%) and then return to train (>90%). This involved analysis of movement capabilities and ACL risk factors with high speed cameras during sport specific movements; whilst running speed at lactate thresholds were used as a guide of aerobic fitness for return to train (2 and 4 mmol/L respectively, target: 11.5 and 13.5 km/h: final values upon return to the team were 12.3 and 14.0 km/h respectively).
The player returned to the team at six months following surgery. He completed the final two weeks of phase 5 at the club whilst being slowly reintegrated into full training with the team. The player completed in his first competitive match at seven months post-surgery and was able to sufficiently impress for the remainder of the season to secure a contract extension.
So far this season (2015-2016) the player has competed in 64% of his teams' competitive league fixtures.

References

1. Zanobbi M, Fazzini D, Marcheggiani GM. Rehabilitation in five phases. In: Roi GS, Della Villa S (Eds). Football medicine strategies for knee injuries. Calzetti Mariucci Editore, Torgiano, 2012, pp. 53-54

POST CONCUSSION SYNDROME AND PSYCHOSOCIAL ISSUES IN A PROFESSIONAL ACADEMY FOOTBALLER

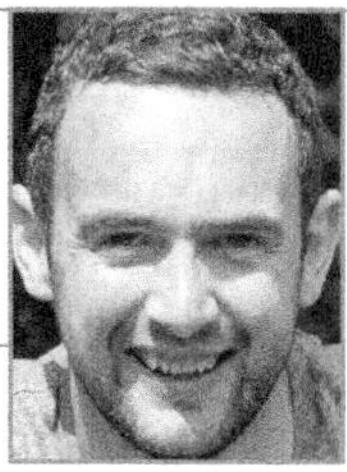

Robinson TM, Forsdyke D

York St John University, York, United Kingdom

A 17 year old, healthy male footballer (height 176.1 cm, weight 67.6 kg) whose only previous medical history was of regular migraines, playing as a forward at a professional football academy in England and also at U17 international level, sustained a concussion (Glasgow Coma Scale = 14, E4V4M6; E=Eye, V=Verbal, M=Motor) during training. He was referred to hospital for medical assessment at which point he recalled an earlier head injury two weeks prior, which had been previously unreported by the player, his diagnosis was two separate concussions in a two week period, during which time he had been playing competitively.
The player underwent Sport Concussion Assessment Tool (SCAT) 3 concussion testing and over the next four weeks, he underwent a further four SCAT 3 assessments (Table 1) and an Magnetic Resonance Imaging (MRI) scan, which reported no significant findings, in line with the majority of concussions (1). After assessment by the club's doctor four weeks post injury, a GRTP (Graduated Return to Play) was implemented which was to remain non-contact, this took place over the following two months.

SCAT 3 Test Date (post injury)	No. of symptoms	Symptom Severity Score
1 day	21	67
1 week	21	40
2 weeks	22	32
3 weeks	10	13
4 weeks	20	46
11 months (Follow Up)	22	82

Table 1. Sport Concussion Assessment Tool (SCAT) assessments.

Despite a resumption of moderate cardiovascular exercise the player continued to complain of symptoms (low concentration levels, poor memory, feeling of being in a "fog"); although these were not worsened with exercise. Due to the persistent symptoms, the player was referred to see a Consultant Neurosurgeon who confirmed the diagnosis of concussion and recommended a full GRTP over a period of three months up to full but non-contact training. The consultant noted no neurological deficits.
A successful GRTP over three months followed with technical coaches and medical staff noting excellent levels of training performance. The player however, complained of ongoing symptoms, although these were slightly improved. A referral from the Neurosurgeon to Neuropsychology followed to assess whether Neuropsychological issues were the cause of the symptoms of the player. One week later (seven months post injury), the player reported a significant worsening of symptoms and development of new symptoms (severe fatigue, headaches, stomach pains); he was unable to train or undertake any light exercise or engage in educational work.

Blood results indicated Hypothyroidism and referral to an Endocrinologist followed. Full endocrinology tests were undertaken and all results were within normal levels with the exception of thyroid function. Thyroxine was prescribed six weeks later and within a further six weeks, blood tests indicated thyroid function had returned to normal levels. During this time, the player was reporting severe symptoms of fogginess, lack of concentration and an inability to exercise due to extreme fatigue. These symptoms improved slightly with the medication and the return of his thyroid function to normal ranges.

At ten months post injury, with the recommendation from all medical practitioners involved in the care of the player, he was put on a GRTP. This successfully happened over a period of four weeks up to full training.

At eleven months post injury, the player returned to full training. He continues to report symptoms ("fogginess", poor concentration and memory) and is still undergoing Neuropsychological assessment to attempt to resolve some of these issues. His endocrine levels are regularly checked and are within normal levels.

Conclusions

The complex and sometimes vague symptoms of Post-Concussion Syndrome (PCS) can result in a complex differential diagnosis. In this case, with the added complexity of hypothyroidism, it proved very difficult to pinpoint any one cause of the PCS symptoms.

Research suggests a link between traumatic brain injury and dysfunction of thyroid and pituitary glands (2, 3), unfortunately there were no baseline blood test measures for the player, so whether the thyroid dysfunction was already underlying or not cannot be established. However, it would seem advisable for basic blood screening to form part of the assessment of the PCS patient.

With hindsight, it would appear that the majority of the symptoms experienced by the patient, both during the eleven months of injury and now the ongoing symptoms experienced while returned to play, have been caused by complex psychosocial issues. These issues should be considered during the rehabilitation of all concussion patients to hopefully avoid or reduce the length and severity of any PCS experienced.

References

1. Broshek DK, De Marco AP, Freeman JR. A review of post-concussion syndrome and psychological factors associated with concussion. Brain Injury 2015; 29: 228-237
2. Ives JC, Alderman M, Stred SE. Hypopituitarism after multiple concussions: a retrospective case study in an adolescent male. J Athletic Training 2007; 42: 431-439
3. Kimbler DE, Murphy M, Dhandapani KM. Concussion and the adolescent athlete. J Neurosci Nurs 2011; 43: 286-290

Sunday 10th April, 2016 (morning)
MOUNTBATTEN ROOM

FREE ORAL PRESENTATIONS CONTEST - FINALS - PART 2

BEST CLINICAL CASE HISTORY AWARD

Chairs

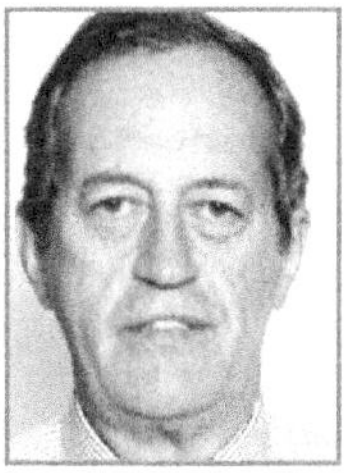

Peter Brukner
(Melbourne, Australia)

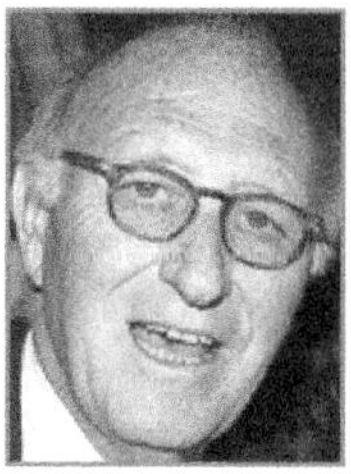

Antonio Delcogliano
(Rome, Italy)

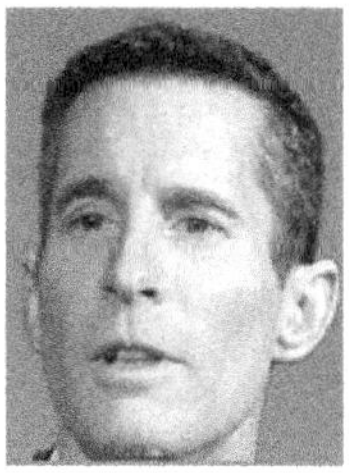

Bill Knowles
(Philadelpia, USA)

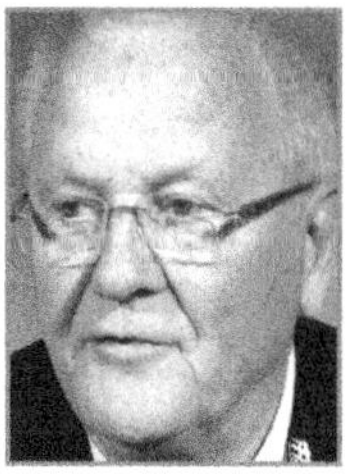

Lars Peterson
(Gothenburg, Sweden)

11:30	A team approach to anterior talo-fibular ligament rupture in an elite academy football player **Harris A, Rajeswaran G, Ahmad I (Enfield and London, United Kingdom)**
11:42	Return to play following hamstring tendinopathy and peripheral neuropathic pain **Battersby DB, Purdam C, Buchan C (Gold Coast, Australia)**
11:54	Exercise-induced bronchoconstriction: impact of therapy on health and performance **Jackson A, Hopker J, Dickinson J (Chatham, United Kingdom)**

12:06 The sky over New York: the backstage of Franco Baresi 1994 memorable World Cup final **Ferretti F, Ferretti A (Rome, Italy)**

12:18 Functional strength recovery in a professional female football player **Azzini M, Baroli M, Ventresca I (Verona, Italy)**

12:30 Rectus Femoris avulsion treated conservatively in a professional soccer player **Requena B, Aramberri M, Olmo J (Madrid, Spain)**

12:42 Successful return to play after conservative treatment of an Adductor Longus avulsion **Serner A, Chaabane M, Weir A (Doha, Qatar)**

12:54 End of the session

13:00 Award Ceremony for the best three clinical case reports

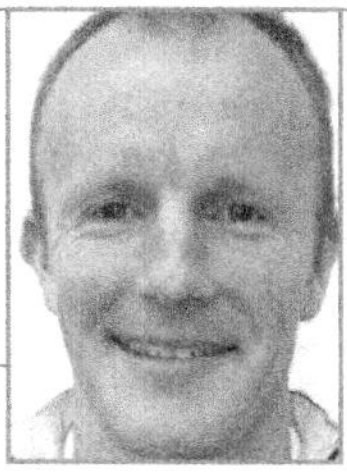

A TEAM APPROACH TO ANTERIOR TALO-FIBULAR LIGAMENT RUPTURE IN AN ELITE ACADEMY FOOTBALL PLAYER

Harris A[1], Rajeswaran G[2], Ahmad I[1]

[1]Department of Sport Medicine and Science, Tottenham Hotspur Football Club Training Centre, Enfield; [2]Department of Radiology, Chelsea and Westminster Hospital NHS Foundation Trust, London, United Kingdom

Case report

A 17-year-old right-footed male full back suffered a contact inversion right ankle injury causing inability to weight bear with tenderness and swelling over the lateral ankle. He was kept Non-Weight Bearing (NWB) and had an ultrasound scan by the Team Doctor which suggested a ruptured Anterior Talo-Fibular Ligament (ATFL). Magnetic Resonance Imaging (MRI) scan on day 4 and ultrasound by a Consultant Musculoskeletal (MSK) Radiologist at day 10 confirmed full thickness rupture of the ATFL.

Treatment

The player was empowered as being central to his rehabilitation and given responsibility for applying ice, self-compressions and regular elevation. He was offered prolotherapy, which is the injection of growth factor production stimulants to promote growth and repair of normal cells. Growth factors are most effective during the repair phase and therefore prolotherapy is ideally suited to treat disrupted collagen fibres in ligament tears (3). Although Prolotherapy has been used for ATFL strains, there is no published data to support its efficacy and no outcome data on its use in elite sport or on its use in full thickness ATFL injuries 2).

The player and family gave informed consent and were counselled regarding side effects of pain, stiffness, bruising, transient numbness and low risk of infection. Ultrasound guided prolotherapy was performed on day 10 with 2 mL 50% Dextrose in 1 mL 1% Lidocaine injected into the full thickness ATFL tear gap. No side effects were reported. Repeat ultrasound guided prolotherapy was performed on days 16 and 23 demonstrating a thickened, heterogeneous ATFL but no demonstrable fibre disruption, in keeping with a healing response.

Rehabilitation

Manual therapy such as Active Release Techniques (ART), Muscle Energy Techniques (MET) and joint mobilisations was used. From day 2 cardiovascular activities like Arm Crank Ergometry and seated boxing were used. Thoracic mobility, multi-planar planks and ankle, adductor, hamstring and gluteal strengthening exercises were increased in volume and progressed. Compex muscle stimulation was used for the calf complex. Pool walking and NWB deep water running were also commenced. Proprioceptive exercises were practised from day 13-17. From day 18 movement development drills, contact work in a closed chain gym setting and plyometric power sessions began. Alter Gravity running started at 60% body weight on day 20 until full body weight running at day 23.

Pitch-work was commenced on day 24 with straight line and slalom running. During the first 3 pitch sessions he ran pain-free at 81.0%, 87.5% and 97.0% respectively of his premorbid maximum speed. On day 25 the player completed a 31% match equivalent session, which compares different Global Positioning Systems (GPS) variables to what a player completes in a match. This gives us a more broad look at what the player is able to complete as part of their training or rehabilitation load, and allows safer progressions of acute to chronic load (1).
On day 28 pain-free shuttle runs and change of direction running was completed. Multi planar plyometric and power exercises were commenced in double leg stance before single leg. On day 30 he completed an intensive pitch session with a 57% match equivalent on GPS, on day 32 the player reached a new top speed on GPS while completing his extensive pitch session that had a 42% match equivalent.
In the week prior to Return To Training (RTT) he coped with a 30%, 40% and a 50% GPS match equivalent loading. He RTT at day 34 he returned to training after multiple staff clearance and played 45 minutes in a competitive match on day 45 (Figure 1).

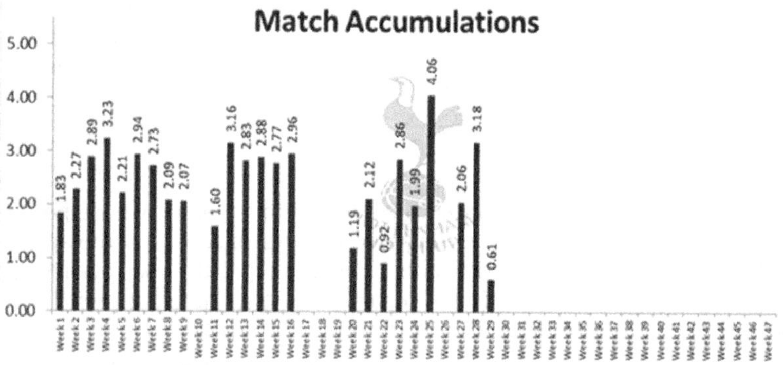

Figure 1. The injury occurred in Week 16, and the player was back in training in the latter part of Week 21.

Conclusions

This case report has shown how early diagnosis and multidisciplinary management can facilitate successful return to play. Empowering the player enabled him to return stronger with a low risk of recurrence. Rehabilitation should focus on physical, technical, mental and social aspects. He was reintegrated early to the team's off-pitch group injury prevention programme. This requires considerable staff communication, allowing the player to feel part of the group and happy with his rehabilitation: "When I returned from the injury I felt physically very good. I felt as fit as I did before I got injured. I have continued to work on my balance through doing different exercises in the gym. This allowed me to feel completely confident in my ankle during games and training".

References

1. Blanch P, Gabbett TJ. Has the athlete trained safely enough to return to play safely? The acute:chronic workload ratio permits clinicians to quantify a player's risk of subsequent injury. Br J Sports Med 2015; 2015 Dec 23. [Epub ahead of print]
2. Campbell RS, Dunn AJ. Radiological interventions for soft tissue injuries in sport. Br J Radiol 2012; 85: 1186-1193
3. Fullerton BD, Reeves KD Ultrasonography in regenerative injection (prolotherapy) using dextrose, platelet-rich plasma, and other injectants. Phys Med Rehabil Clin N Am 2010; 21: 585-605

RETURN TO PLAY FOLLOWING HAMSTRING TENDINOPATHY AND PERIPHERAL NEUROPATHIC PAIN

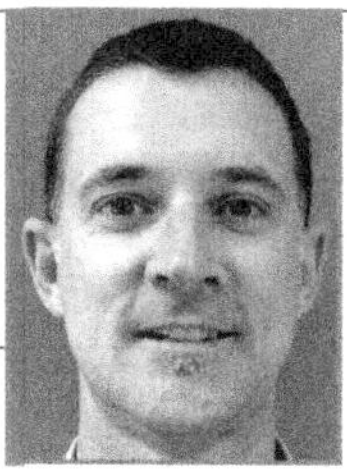

Battersby DB[1], Purdam C[2], Buchan C[3]

[1]Westfield Matildas, Physiologic, Gold Coast; [2]Australian Institute of Sport, Canberra; [3]Queensland Diagnostic Imaging, Gold Coast, Australia

This case relates to a 23 year old international female football player returning to play following a left proximal hamstring tendinopathy complicated by altered sciatic nerve neurodynamics. The player was a central midfielder, 53 kg and 158 cm tall, and was part of the Australian national team who had qualified for the 2015 FIFA Women's World Cup in June 2015.

In October 2014, during the domestic football season, the player complained of diffuse left groin, lateral hip, low back, ischial pain and paraesthesia in her posterior thigh and lateral shin. She had not experienced any episode of acute injury. Her key subjective findings included pain with driving, night pain, paraesthesia in her lateral lower leg, and pain sprinting (Table 1).

Key objective measures reproducing her symptoms were Straight Leg Raise (SLR) biased with hip adduction (Dr J. Rippstein, La Conversion, Switzerland), resisted prone knee bend at 30 degrees knee flexion (Microfet 2, HogganHealth Inc, USA) and single hamstring bridge (Table 1).

Magnetic Resonance Imaging (MRI) studies of her lumbar spine and pelvis showed no disc, joint or thecal pathology but a directed MRI of her proximal hamstring showed mild tendinopathy of her common hamstrings tendon origin and subtle signal alteration of the adjacent sciatic nerve. The diagnosis made, was proximal left hamstring origin tendinopathy and associated left sciatic nerve tethering causing peripheral neuropathic pain.

In early January 2015, with minimal improvement in her signs and symptoms, a review was conducted involving the team doctor, physiotherapists, the player and head coach.

A collaborative decision was made to rest the player from team training until April 2015, considered the latest time that she could return to training and be eligible for selection in the World Cup squad.

A decision was also made to perform a hydrodilatation and adhesiolysis of the sciatic nerve/hamstring tendon interface aiming to reduce the peripheral neuropathic component of her symptoms.

A specialist musculoskeletal radiologist experienced in the procedure conducted the hydrodilatation using ultrasound guidance. The SLR was assessed immediately before and after the procedure with significant improvement in both pain and range of motion. Three days post-procedure improvement was noted in all signs and symptoms (Table 1).

Assessment	Initial	Pre injection	Post injection 3 days	Return to play
Pain driving (minutes)	10	10	30	90
Night pain (VRS*)	6/10	5/10	2/10	0/10
Paraesthesia (VRS)	3/10	4/10	1/10	0/10
Sprinting pain (VRS)	6/10	Not sprinting	Not sprinting	0/10
SLR (angle in degrees)	Left p1** 60 // + hip adduction Right r2*** 84	Left p1 60 // + hip adduction Right r2 84	Left p1 74 // + hip add Right r2 84	Left r2 78 // hip adduction isq Right r2 84
Resisted prone knee bend at 30 degrees knee flexion (N)	Left p1 145 Right maximum 249	Left p1 158 Right maximum 246	Left p1 185 Right maximum 240	Left maximum 254 Right maximum 265
Single leg hamstring bridge (VRS, repetition maximum (RM))	Left 3/10, 1 RM Right 0/10, 20 RM	Left 3/10, 4 RM Right 0/10, 20 RM	Left 3/10, 10 RM Right 0/10, 20 RM	Left 0/10, 18 RM Right 0/10, 20 RM

Table 1. Subjective and Objective Measures. *Verbal rating scale; **onset of pain; ***end of range of motion.

The decrease in pain allowed a comprehensive tendon loading programme to commence, initially limiting hip flexion to reduce the compressive and tensile load on the tendon and sciatic nerve. The programme included combined concentric and eccentric knee flexion exercises with strength training progressing to increasing ranges of hip flexion and higher eccentric loads. In addition, specific running drills were introduced, initially at low intensity, frequency and volume. Neurodynamic techniques including sliders and SLR techniques were also included in her programme.

Leading up to her return to team training, the player completed football specific training every second day – building intensity and volume but controlling frequency of training sessions. Her training load was monitored through an electronic monitoring system (AMS) and was calculated on rate of perceived exertion and session time. Key subjective and objective signs were monitored with AMS and no progressions in training load were made if these measures deteriorated. The player returned to modified team training 13 weeks following injection and unrestricted return to play six weeks later, four weeks before the World Cup.

Conclusions

Proximal hamstring tendinopathy is often a recalcitrant presentation with significant participation and performance consequences. In the case presented, the interaction with the adjacent sciatic nerve complicated the condition, and addressing this allowed for more effective rehabilitation of the hamstring tendon. Collaborative team planning of the player's management and regular monitoring of the progression of training load, enabled the athlete to contribute to the team reaching the quarter finals of the FIFA Women's World Cup. She was satisfied with her performance at the tournament and continues to play at international level with no recurrence of her symptoms.

EXERCISE-INDUCED BRONCHOCONSTRICTION: IMPACT OF THERAPY ON HEALTH AND PERFORMANCE

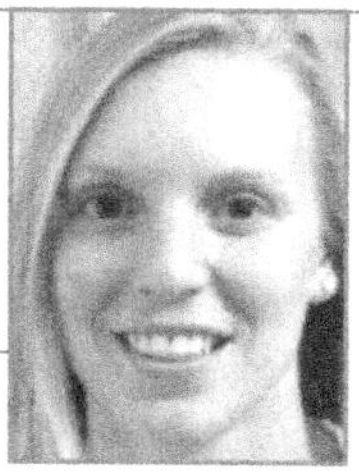

Jackson A, Hopker J, Dickinson J

School of Sport and Exercise Sciences, University of Kent, Chatham, United Kingdom

Many elite football players report respiratory symptoms during exercise. Using symptoms alone to diagnose asthma and Exercise Induced Bronchoconstriction (EIB) has resulted in 50% of professional football players receiving an inappropriate diagnosis (1). Furthermore, many players do not recognise or report exercise respiratory symptoms and therefore continue to play with no protection against asthma/EIB. This may lead to underperformance and has the potential to increase EIB severity through airway remodelling. Therefore, a diagnosis of asthma/EIB must be made with objective testing. When Premier League football players have been screened for asthma/EIB the prevalence has been reported to be 30% (2). This case study follows a player who was screened for EIB and treated appropriately. Over the course of 12 weeks' markers of airway function and exercise performance were assessed. The player was a male professional, championship level football centre back, age 30, height 188 cm, weight 90 kg. He had a previous symptom based diagnosis of asthma but reported symptoms only when pollen levels were high. He had a current prescription for Salbutamol. The player was initially screened for EIB as part of a club medical. The player underwent a respiratory assessment which comprised measurement of exhaled Nitric Oxide (FeNO) and a Eucapnic Voluntary Hyperpnoea (EVH) challenge. In the same week he also completed a submaximal Yo-Yo intermittent recovery test (YYIRsubmax). After 12 weeks the player repeated the EVH and YYIRsubmax tests. The player continued training and match play throughout. The player presented with a positive EVH challenge (a fall in Forced Expiratory Volume in 1 second (FEV1) of 40% post challenge). He was 1 of 10 players (48%) with a positive test out of 21 screened. The 40% fall in FEV1 indicates he has moderate to severe EIB. The team physician decided to alter medication in line with that recommend for moderate to severe EIB and the player was prescribed Seretide (long acting β_2 agonist and corticosteroid) and Salbutamol (β2 agonist) inhalers. After 12 weeks of taking the new treatment, the fall in FEV1 following the EVH challenge had reduced to 16%. The initial FeNO of the player was 181 ppb (parts per billion), classified as High (>50 ppb). After 12 weeks of medication this was reduced to 37 ppb, classified as Elevated (25-50), which indicates greatly reduced airway inflammation. Results from the YYIRsubmax show improved performance both in a reduction in player load of 13% (pre=108.2; post=93.61) and Heart Rate indices: maximum HR pre=205 bpm (beats per minute); post=197 bpm and mean HR pre=181 bpm, post=167 bpm, all indicating a reduced effort at the same workloads following the 12 weeks of using appropriate therapy. In conclusion a simple objective airway provocation challenge highlighted the player was under medicated for the severity of his EIB. The implementation of appropriate treatment resulted in reduced EIB severity, reduced airway inflammation and improved performance during the YYIRsubmax test. This case study demonstrates EIB is common in elite football players and the use of objective airway challenges can improve detection and treatment of EIB, which may result in improved aerobic performance.

References

1. Ansley L, Kippilen P, Dickinson J, Hull J. Misdiagnosis of exercise-induced bronchoconstriction in professional soccer players. Allergy 2012; 67: 390-395
2. Dickinson J, Drust B, Whyte G, Brukner P. Screening English Premier League football players for exercise induced bronchoconstriction. In: Numone, Hiroyuki, Drust, Barry, Dawson, Brian (Eds) Science and Football VII. Routledge, 2013: 341-346

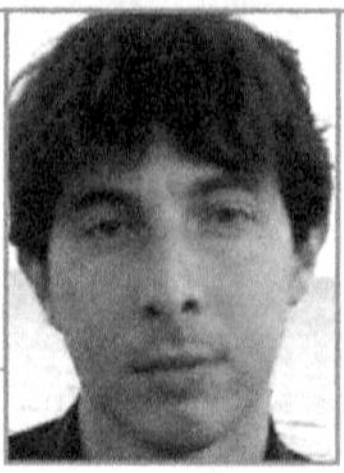

THE SKY OVER NEW YORK: THE BACKSTAGE OF FRANCO BARESI 1994 MEMORABLE WORLD CUP FINAL

Ferretti F, Ferretti A

Federazione Italiana Giuoco Calcio (FIGC) Medical Committee, Rome, Italy

As journalist and son of Dr. Ferretti, I will tell you this story speaking in the first person identifying myself with my father who told me this story.
I will never forget the blue sky over New York that Saturday at dawn, while Franco Baresi (34 y.o., 1.76 m, central defender) and I (Andrea Ferretti) were crossing the Big Apple from Lenox Hill Hospital, after a sleepless night following operation.
Everything began two days before, at Giants Stadium, where we had won a crucial match at the World Cup. But we couldn't be happy after Baresi's injury: bucket handle tear of medial meniscus. With no time to celebrate, coach Arrigo Sacchi called a meeting with the staff to set up a plan.
I proposed three options:
1) Flying Baresi back to Italy for treatment, as suggested by the physician of the club (AC Milan), Rodolfo Tavana).
2) Keeping Baresi in the USA, supporting him until the end of the World Cup (a poorly logical option due to pain and possible troubles to the locked joint).
3) Performing an immediate operation in NY (almost impossible to realize considering possible opposition by AC Milan football club).
About the last option, my colleague Paolo Zeppilli, a serial blabbermouth, said: "This is the best one because, if we go to the final, Baresi could play too!". That quite venturesome phrase unleashed the reaction of Vincenzo Pincolini, AC Milan athletic trainer "on loan" to the National team: "Please, don't talk nonsense", he said, creating a further embarrassing atmosphere.
But Arrigo Sacchi, got curious, asked me if Zeppilli's hypothesis was just fantasy. In a climate of tension, I answered that in theory if the operation could be performed no later than the next day and without any complications, the road to recovery for a possible final was feasible.
Coach Sacchi, who has always loved challenges, told me to consider operating. I had been entrusted with a huge responsibility.
I went to Baresi's room: he was in bed with a pillow under his knee. I explained that he had to be operated on to remove a meniscal fragment from the joint.
I asked if, where and when he would like to be operated on, but I kept silent about recovery time to avoid any pressure on him. He replied: "I want to be operated here, immediately". By phone Dr. Tavana insisted he wanted to come to attend the operation. I replied that in that case we would have had to wait until Monday, missing the most favorable moment. Later Dr. Tavana told me that we could proceed in his absence and that I had his and the whole of AC Milan's trust.
It was already nightime; I searched for Dr. Herschmann, Director of the local Medical Committee. He assured me that we could operate Baresi together the next day.
I wondered if I had chosen the best way; if I was really sure of the diagnosis; if it was really prudent to take all this responsibility without sharing it with the club, 6,000 km away.
When my colleague put the arthroscope inside the knee, a thought flashed through my head "Will he be able to do it"? After all, I just knew his scientific achievements, not his surgical skills! Although I didn't have a license to practice in the USA, in an emergency, I wouldn't have hesitated to pick up the tools and remove that damn piece of meniscus myself. Anyway, a few minutes later the meniscus flowed from the tiny incision: all done.

The following days were filled with trepidation for the fate of the team that, among the general skepticism, gradually acquired trust, despite heat, fatigue and other significant injuries. Meanwhile, slowly, quietly, Baresi recovered, helped by the limited quadriceps atrophy thanks to the short time elapsed from injury to surgery, even though no one could imagine the following developments. And so, from isometrics to isotonics and isokinetics, from the treadmill to the field, from the stands to the bench, after a couple of weeks Baresi was already alongside his team mates. When, in the semifinal, Alessandro Costacurta was issued with a yellow card and disqualified for the final, Baresi softly told me: "It's up to me, I'm ready" a shiver ran down my spine along with a lot of questions: "Will he be ready? Will his knee sustain such as stressful match as a final?" But I knew the course of events had already been determined.
The history of the final is well known. Italian defenders, led by Baresi, resisted 120 minutes assaults of two of the best forwards in the world, the Brazilians Romario and Bebeto.
The worldwide broadcasted tears of Baresi after the penalty kicks didn't hide the awareness that, thanks to a coordinated workteam of the club and National team medical staff, he could play one of the most important games in the history of Italian football.

5

FUNCTIONAL STRENGTH RECOVERY IN A PROFESSIONAL FEMALE FOOTBALL PLAYER

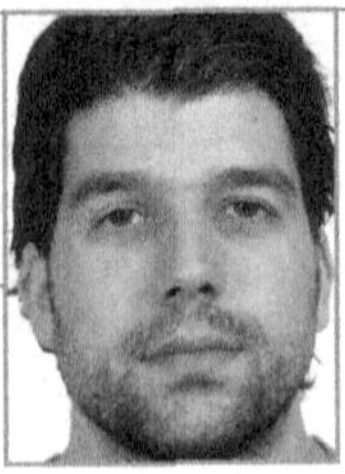

Azzini M, Baroli M, Ventresca I

Isokinetic Medical Group, FIFA Medical Centre of Excellence, Verona, Italy

Case report

A professional female football player (26 years old, height 168 cm, weight 60 kg), striker, playing in the Italian First League (Serie A) and in the National team, had an Anterior Cruciate Ligament (ACL) surgical reconstruction with Semi-Tendinosus-Gracilis (ST-GR) autologous tendons after right knee injury. She started rehabilitation in our Clinic seven days after surgery.

The Rehabilitation program was carried out in the following five phases: Phase 1, control of pain and swelling; Phase 2, recovery of the full Range of Motion (ROM); Phase 3, recovery of strength; Phase 4, recovery of coordination; Phase 5, Return To Play (RTP).

At the beginning of the protocol, work was dedicated to reducing pain and the swelling of the knee this was done with modalities (physical therapies), lymphatic massage and ice.

Once pain and swelling had been reduced the patient started working on her range of movement, firstly with knee extension and flexion until she managed to recuperate the full grades of Passive ROM (PROM). She did this by alternating passive movements including rope roller-skating, pendulum leg swinging and stretching exercises with ropes and wall bars, and active movements mainly using a recline bicycle.

The operated knee suffered a certain degree of articular stiffness that made the full recovery of PROM rather complex both in extension and flexion. Therefore the aquatic based rehabilitation was particularly important for improving articulation and reducing the oedema.

During this phase she did the threshold test to check her general physical condition and to plan her training according to results gained.

In order to recuperate the knee strength as soon as possible, she started with isometric exercises, with the help of electro-myo-stimulation (Compex, DJO International, Guildford, UK), and isotonic exercises performed with ankle-weights to strengthen knee extensors, and knee and hip flexors. She increased the workouts with closed kinetic chain exercises with Vector (Easytech, Florence, Italy) and leg press. At the same time, open kinetic chain exercises were applied with the Leg Extension machine and after approximately 60 days from surgery she added the exercises with the isokinetic machine (2). To monitor the maximum peak torque in all the rehabilitation sessions, at the beginning of the session an isokinetic test, consisting of 4 repetitions at 90°/s and 20 repetitions at 180°/s, was added.

During each session a minimum of 30 minutes of aerobic activity at an intensity corresponding to the aerobic threshold (assessed by an incremental running test) was carried out.

Later on we noticed a sudden halt in the progressive increase of strength (Table 2). We therefore decided to stop using the isokinetic training and substitute them with functional strength exercises (1). We used: squats, Bulgarian squats, lunges, proprioceptive courses in which the levels of difficulty were increased each time, step ups, bouncer and Bosu, all of which were integrated with the help of virtual reality with Nintendo Wii (Nintendo, Kyoto, Japan) and Microsoft Xbox (Microsoft, Redmond, USA) and the aid of specific generic programs or specific sports programs to recall the specific athletic movements.

With this method we saw a revival of the strength recovery right up to the evidence of a complete recovery in respect of the healthy limb. The patient has since been able to finish her personal recovery by passing on to the specific movement rehabilitation phase, on the field. In all the sessions the Heart Rate (HR) was monitored by HR Monitors (Polar Electro, Kempele, Finland).

	Phase 1	Phase 2	Phase 3	Phase 4	Phase 5
Under T2	80±11%	100±0%	89±1%	82±2%	31±13%
Between T2 and T4	13±18%	0±0%	10±8%	16±9%	80±11%
Over T4	7±29%	0±0%	1±9%	2±9%	80±11%

Table 1. Percent of the time spent at different metabolic intensities during the Five Phases of the Rehabilitation. T2: aerobic threshold (2 mmol/L of blood lactate); T4: anaerobic threshold (4 mmol/L of lactate).

	Knee Ext 90°/s		Knee Flex 90°/s		90°/s	Knee Ext 180°/s		Knee Flex 180°/s		180°/s
Session	**MPT**	**Increase**	**MPT**	**Increase**	**F/E**	**MPT**	**Increase**	**MPT**	**Increase**	**F/E**
1	109	--	64	--	59%	80	--	42	--	53%
2	113	4%	66	3%	58%	84	5%	47	12%	56%
3	116	3%	67	2%	58%	89	6%	49	4%	55%
4	118	2%	69	3%	58%	93	4%	55	12%	59%
5	115	-3%	64	-7%	56%	89	-4%	53	-4%	60%
6	104	-10%	63	-2%	61%	90	1%	55	4%	61%
7	104	0%	61	-3%	59%	90	0%	54	-2%	60%
8	105	1%	64	5%	61%	91	1%	57	6%	63%
9	115	10%	75	17%	65%	101	11%	67	18%	66%
10	129	12%	85	13%	66%	103	2%	70	4%	68%
11	134	4%	89	5%	66%	105	2%	73	4%	70%
12	136	1%	92	3%	68%	107	2%	75	3%	70%

Table 2. results of the isokinetic test performed before all the sessions of strength training. Ext: extension; Flex: flexion; MPT: maximal peak Torque (Nm); Increase: percentage increase between subsequent sessions; F/E: ration between Knee Flexors and Extensors Torques.

The athlete went back to play four months after surgery. However, she was psychologically fragile due to lack of faith in herself after the injury, on top of this she had a lot of pressure from both her team and the National team, as in June 2015 they were playing in the FIFA Women's World Cup in Canada, and she wanted to be fit enough to be called up to play. During the rehabilitation stage she had many difficult moments but in the end, thanks to her will power, dedication and hard work, she managed to go back to play in the last few matches in the Premier League and was also called up to play in the preliminary list for the FIFA Women's World Cup Canada 2015.

Conclusions

This case report point out the importance of three aspects: i) the psychological help to the injured player during the entire period of rehabilitation; ii) the functional strength exercises after ACL reconstruction, useful for strength recovery because they simultaneously involve multiple joints and muscles to improve strength, endurance, coordination, balance and agility; iii) HR monitoring during the entire recovery stage, allowing to give the desired amount of aerobic training useful to recovery the general fitness of the player.

References

1. Frank C, Kobesova A, Kolar P. Dynamic neuromuscolar stabilitation and sport rehabilitation. Int J Sport Phys Ther 2013; 8: 62-73
2. Knowles B. The difference between clinical rehabilitation and football reconditioning. In: Roi GS, Della Villa S (Eds). Football Medicine Strategies for Joint and Ligaments Injuries. Calzetti-Mariucci Editore, Torgiano, 2014: 162-163

RECTUS FEMORIS AVULSION TREATED CONSERVATIVELY IN A PROFESSIONAL SOCCER PLAYER

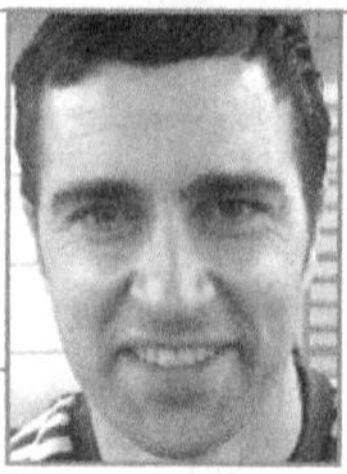

Requena B, Aramberri M, Olmo J

Real Madrid Club de Fútbol, Madrid, Spain

Introduction

Rectus Femoris (RF) proximal tendon avulsions are uncommon but severe football injuries (1). Controversy exists around their best treatment approach, either conservative or surgical (2, 3). We present a case report of this injury in an elite football player treated conservatively with one-year follow-up.

Methods

The patient is a 29 year old male elite midfielder, 1.75 cm height and 72.0 kg weight.
At the 25th minute of an international match the patient suffered a sudden pain in his left groin while kicking that repeated on the next sprint action, forcing him to leave the field.
A Magnetic Resonance Imaging (MRI) scan confirmed the diagnosis of left RF complete indirect and subtotal direct proximal tendon avulsion, with a bone-tendon gap of 11 mm.
A conservative treatment was chosen, combining a criteria-based, staged rehabilitation program with a Platelet-Rich Plasma (PRP) treatment as follows:

- Phase 1: Acute. Therapy: rest, compression, cryotherapy, RF relaxation. Plasma Rich in Growth Factors (PRGF; Endoret, BTI Biotechnology Institute, Colchester, UK) injection at the tendon gap on day 6th: 36 mL of peripheral blood were extracted by venipuncture directly into four extraction tubes containing 3.8% sodium citrate as anticoagulant, and centrifuged at 580 G for eight minutes at room temperature. 2 mL of PRP remaining above the red series and the buffy coat were separated, avoiding picking up the leukocytes. The four 2 mL fractions were put together in a single sterile tube and activated by adding 400 mg of calcium chloride right before infiltration of the total volume of 8 mL.
- Phase 2, day 8th: Biostimulation. Physiotherapy: Laser, ultrasound, diathermia, cryotherapy, hyperbaric chamber, draining massage, RF relaxation. Reconditioning: RF flexibility, RF activation and initial strength conditioning, initial general conditioning. PRP injection, day 16th, with the same procedure, but the volume injected was halved at 4 mL. After one day rest, Phase 2 was resumed.
- Phase 3, day 30th: Basic, low-energy functional rehabilitation. Criteria: formed scar in MRI, no pain, full RF length. Physiotherapy: former protocol plus tendon fibrolysis, gliding and mobility. Reconditioning: RF maximal strength, low-energy neuromuscular control and low-energy functional rehabilitation; conditioning: accumulation mesocycle (aerobic endurance, maximal strength).
- Phase 4, day 75th: Advanced, high-energy functional rehabilitation. Criteria: matured scar in MRI, >85% RF maximal strength, low-energy tasks accomplished. Physiotherapy as previous. Reconditioning: RF rapid strength & power, high-energy neuromuscular control and high-energy functional rehabilitation; conditioning: transformation mesocycle (anaerobic endurance, strength endurance)
- Phase 5: Return to Play (RTP). Criteria: high-signal scar in MRI, 100% RF maximal strength, high-energy tasks accomplished, maximal sprint and shot speeds recovered. Conditioning: realization mesocycle (speed, power, rapid strength). Return to Competition criteria: normalized training sessions General Positioning System (GPS)/Accelerometer data, and subjective confidence.

Injury control MRI scans were done at 1, 1.5, 2.5 and 3.5 months from the episode, showing the tendon healing progression.
Time to return to competition was 115 days. At that moment, functional testing showed a left RF eccentric isokinetic (Dinasystems BlackBox, Granada, Spain) functional strength of 480 N, and a left shot peak speed (Adidas Micoach Smart Ball, Düsseldorf, Germany) of 104 km/h, while GPS/accelerometer data registered a maximal sprint speed of 31 km/h, peak acceleration 4.5 m/s^2, and peak deceleration -4.9 m/s^2, all of these data coherent with his pre-injury scores.
Some residual discomfort was felt by the player for several months after the injury, but no more training sessions or games were missed.
At one year follow-up, the player was clinical and functionally asymptomatic, participating normally in training and games, and the MRI showed a stable tendon scar signal. Playing performance statistics were comparable to pre-injury levels.

Conclusions

This case report details the conservative treatment of a RF proximal tendon avulsion in an elite football player, which may be used as a clinical guide for similar injuries. The outcome show that it is possible to successfully treat this injury without surgery when a part of the direct portion remains attached and thus the tendon does not retract severely. In these cases, a return to competition in less than four months may be achieved.

References

1. Gamradt SC, Brophy RH, Barnes R, Warren RF, Thomas Byrd JW, Kelly BT. Nonoperative treatment for proximal avulsion of the rectus femoris in professional American football. Am J Sports Med 2009; 37: 1370-1374
2. Hsu JC, Fischer DA, Wright RW. Proximal rectus femoris avulsions in national football league kickers: a report of 2 cases. Am J Sports Med 2005; 33: 1085-1087
3. Ueblacker P, Müller-Wohlfahrt HW, Hinterwimmer S, Imhoff AB, Feucht MJ. Suture anchor repair of proximal rectus femoris avulsions in elite football players. Knee Surg Sports Traumatol Arthrosc 2015; 23: 2590-2594

SUCCESSFUL RETURN TO PLAY AFTER CONSERVATIVE TREATMENT OF AN ADDUCTOR LONGUS AVULSION

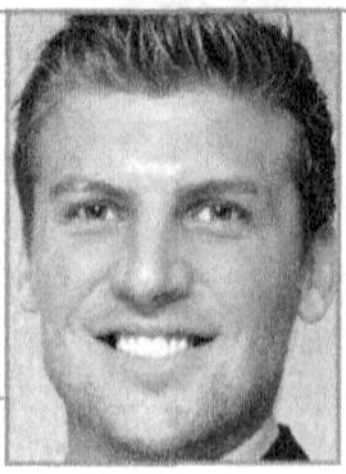

Serner A, Chaabane M, Weir A

Aspetar Orthopaedic and Sports Medicine Hospital, Doha, Qatar

A 24 year old (183 cm, 93 kg) male goalkeeper becomes the club's first choice as goalkeeper after his League club sells two goalkeepers, and the usual first goalkeeper encounters an Anterior Cruciate Ligament (ACL) injury during the pre-season.

During pre-season screening (2013) he had considerable right adductor-related groin pain with 7/10 pain during the Copenhagen Squeeze test, low squeeze test strength scores and inability to perform unilateral eccentric adduction strength test. With no other alternatives for the club, the player had to play while managing the groin pain. The player was pain free during the first game of the season; however, in the second game he was injured during an unremarkable save.

The player had severe pain, mainly in the adductor region with all adductor pain provocation positive, and palpation pain in the lower abdominal region and near the adductor longus insertion (8/10 pain). No palpable gap was present at the adductor insertion.

Magnetic Resonance Imaging (MRI) showed an adductor longus avulsion injury without considerable retraction and a connection of fibres anterior to the pubic bone.

Conservative treatment at the national sports medicine hospital was chosen, and the player followed a standardized criteria-based exercise treatment protocol consisting of five phases with specific progression criteria; initial focus on active flexibility, early activation, intensity progression, advanced strength and stability, and on pitch sports-specific training. The protocol includes an alternate day adductor focus progressing in intensity throughout the rehabilitation period and included; leg swings, hip circles, hip adduction and hip flexion with an elastic band, abdominal "woodchopper" exercise and a kicking exercise ("tension arc") with an elastic band, as well as the cross-country skiing exercise and the Copenhagen Adduction exercise.

After 61 days the player was clinically pain free (0/10) during the following criteria tests: palpation, maximal adductor stretch, maximal adductor contraction in full abduction, 10 RM hip adduction elastic exercise, 10 repetitions of the Copenhagen Adduction exercise, maximal straight sprinting, and maximal speed T-test.

After 66 days the player completed the sports-specific training, including long passes, goal kicks, standing and jump saves, Spider test and Illinois Agility test at 100% relative intensity, and was allowed return to team training in the club.

At discharge all clinical examination tests were pain free, there was fairly symmetric flexibility (side-lying hip abduction. Left(L): 45°; Right(R): 42°; Bent Knee Fall Out test: L 3.5 cm, R 3.5 cm). The player was pain free, but uncomfortable performing maximal eccentric adduction strength tests influencing the results, which showed a 29% lower eccentric adduction strength in the injured side; Side-lying Eccentric Adduction (L: 3.5 Nm/kg, R: 2.5 Nm/kg), and Supine Outer-range Eccentric Adduction (L: 2.7 Nm/kg, R: 1.9 Nm/kg), with a hand-held dynamometer (Commander Muscle Tester). Additionally, another MRI was performed showing considerable healing; however, with remaining oedema and detachment.

The player was advised to continue the training programme while progressively returning to full team training. The Copenhagen hip and groin outcome score (HAGOS) questionnaire including 6 subscales from 0-100 was also reported: Pain: 100; Symptoms: 89; Activity Daily Living (ADL): 100; function in sport and recreation (Sport/Rec): 100; participation in Physical Activities (PA): 100; Quality of Life (QOL): 95.
He returned to progressive team training on the 67th day after injury, and trained with no restrictions from day 80. As a new goalkeeper in the club had performed well, the injured goalkeeper was now the second choice, and there was no immediate pressure for an urgent return to matches. Additionally, due to a short break in the season, the goalkeeper played his first game (2nd team) after injury on day 105 despite being considered ready prior to this.
The player was followed up at two months after Return To Play (RTP), and at one year after injury with an extensive clinical examination and MRI at both time points. At both time points all clinical examination tests were pain free and the player reported no complaints from the injured area. HAGOS scores were: Pain: 98, Symptoms: 82, ADL: 95, Sport/Rec: 78, PA: 100, QOL: 90 at 2 months, and 100 on all subscales at 1 year.
Strength has considerably improved, but remained lower on the injured side at both time points; at 2 months: -9% in the side-lying eccentric adduction (L: 3.4 Nm/kg, R: 3.1 Nm/kg) and -25% in the outer-range eccentric adduction (L: 3.7 Nm/kg, R: 2.8 Nm/kg), and at 1 year: –15% in both the side-lying eccentric adduction (L: 3.3 Nm/kg, R: 2.8 Nm/kg) and supine outer-range eccentric adduction (L: 3.9 Nm/kg, R: 3.3 Nm/kg).
At 2 year post-injury the player still reports no complaints from the injury.
In conclusion, we have presented a successful RTP from an adductor longus avulsion injury in a professional goalkeeper managed with a criteria-based exercise treatment protocol.

Sunday 10th April, 2016 (afternoon)
POSTER AREA

FREE POSTER PRESENTATIONS CONTEST

BEST CLINICAL CASE HISTORY AWARD

Chairs

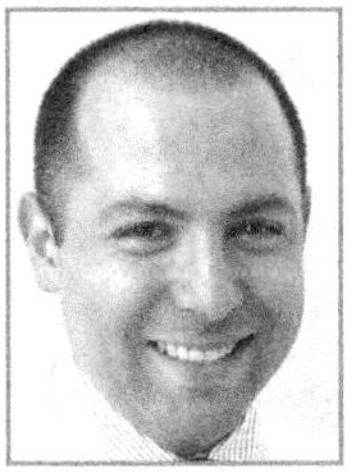

Giammaria d'Orsi
(Rome, Italy)

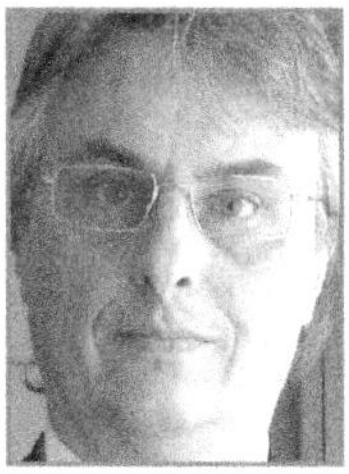

Davide Susta
(Dublin, Ireland)

PL01 Hamstring injury management and sprint mechanics in professional football
Setuain I, Lecumberri P, Izquierdo M (Pamplona, Spain)

PL02 Patellar tendon rupture after platelet rich plasma and steroid therapy for chronic tendinopathy
Nishio H, Kobayashi Y, Saita Y (Tokyo, Japan)

PL03 Partial avulsion of Adductor Longus fibrocartilage. not as innocent as it looks... **Dimitrakopoulou A, Schilders E (London and Leeds, United Kingdom)**

PL04 Return to play after hamstrings muscle injury: a safe, fast and effective case study of a professional football player **Loureiro N, Pereira R, Espregueira-Mendes J (Porto and Minho, Portugal)**

PL05 Traumatic miositis ossificans in a professional football player-when to return?
Ribeiro BV, Teixeira JFC, Noronha JC (Vila do Conde and Porto, Portugal)

PL06 Post-acute muscle injuries rehabilitation with radial extracorporeal shock wave therapy **Di Cosmo R (Genova, Italy)**

PL07 Shockwave treatment for hamstring injury in a youth level soccer player
Vincent KC, d'Agostino MC, Schaden W (Auckland, New Zealand; Milan, Italy; Vienna, Austria)

PL08 Return to play after hamstrings muscle injury
Furini F, Pagella F, Sandrelli L (Arquata Scrivia, Italy)

PL09 Differential diagnosis and conservative rehabilitation approach in hip impingement concerning footballers
Stergiou M, Stergiou E, Giannis C (Kozani, Greece)

PL10 Using level of specificity to monitor reconditioning load for a knee injury
Pajon D, Alvarez J, Colell D (Reus, Spain)

PL11 Pubic stress fracture and osteitis pubis in a 24 year old footballer
Chatterjee AD, Wilson J, Knight RR (Nottingham, United Kingdom)

HAMSTRING INJURY MANAGEMENT AND SPRINT MECHANICS IN PROFESSIONAL FOOTBALL

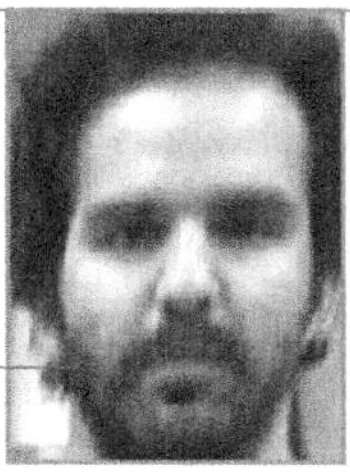

Setuain I[1,2], Lecumberri P[3], Izquierdo M[1]

[1]Public University of Navarra. Department of Health Sciences, Tudela;
[2]TDN, Orthopaedic Surgery and Advanced Rehabilitation, Pamplona;
[3]Movalsys Movement analysis solutions, Pamplona, Spain

Methods

A professional football player (age 19 years; height 177 cm; weight 70 kg; midfielder, Spanish 3rd Division) with a grade 1 Biceps Femoris long head injury was prospectively evaluated at the pre-season and post injury (the injury episode lasted 17 days).
The rehabilitation program consisted on a progressive range of motion both strength and neuromuscular training routines in order to archive maximal muscle function prior to attend to the sprint mechanics evaluation. Progression during the rehabilitation program was tracked by regular examinations targeting muscle force (i.e., Peak Torque and rate of torque development on an isokinetic device), core strength (through the use of hand held dynamometer), and passive and dynamic range of motion assessments.
Sprint mechanics was analyzed by the use of an inertial orientation tracker (MTw, 3D Human Orientation Tracker, Xsens Technologies BV, Enschede, The Netherlands) attached over the L3 region of the lumbar spine which provided kinematic variables at a sampling rate of 100 Hz. The IU combines nine individual MEMS (Micro-Electro-Mechanical Systems) sensors to provide a drift-free 3D orientation as well as other kinematic data: 3D acceleration, 3D rate of turn (rate gyro) and 3D earth-magnetic field. Moreover, its data fusion algorithm, based on the Xsens Kalman Filter for 3 degrees-of-freedom, computes statistically optimal high accuracy 3D orientation estimates with no drift from the 3D acceleration, rate of turn and earth magnetic field sensors. A customized software application was developed for data analyses and interpretation (Movalsys, Pamplona, Navarra, Spain).
The Horizontal component of the Ground Reaction Force, HGRF0 in (N); V0, in (m/s); steps Frequency (steps/s) and the rate of force application, in terms of the slope of the adjusted linear regression (SFV); were assessed on both legs during pre and post injury evaluation (1).

Results

The injured limb applied significantly greater Horizontal force during sprinting at the post-injury evaluation in comparison to baseline (HGRF0 1211.3±0.3 vs. 721.3±0.4 N for injured and unaffected limb respectively).
The coefficient of force application (SFV), however, demonstrated to be decreased in the injured limb in comparison to the contralateral healthy at post injury evaluation (SFV -1.45±0.3 vs. -2.51±0.1 for the healthy and injured limb respectively).
No further differences were found in the rest of the analyzed variables.

Conclusions

A unique result obtained with the novel inertial technology was that the force-application pattern during the sprint, seems to remain affected after a grade I hamstring strain injury in a professional football player.

The proposed inertial sensor based method for sprint mechanics analysis, seems to be a sensitive technology for team physicians and therapist to monitoring hamstring performance function during sprint mechanics when discharging player back to competition after a hamstring injury episode.

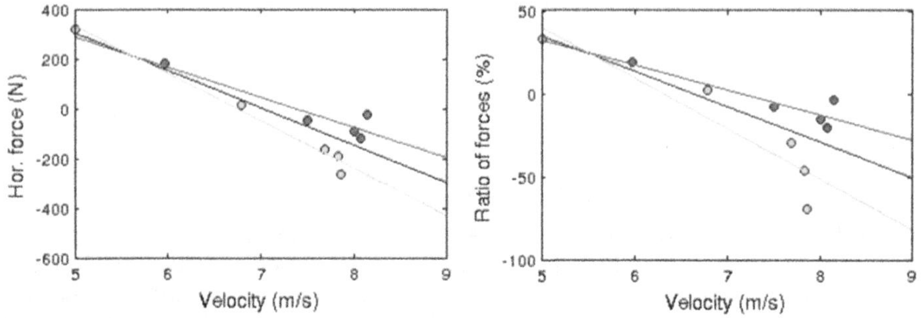

Figure 1. HGRF and velocity curve (right) and Ratio of HGRF vs. resultant GRF and velocity curve (left).

References

1. Samozino P, Rabita G, Dorel S, Slawinski J, Peyrot N, Saez de Villarreal E, Morin JB. A simple method for measuring power, force, velocity properties, and mechanical effectiveness in sprint running. Scand J Med and Sci Sports 2015 May [Epub ahead of print]. DOI: 10.1111/sms.12490
2. Setuain I, Martinikorena J, Gonzalez-Izal M, Martinez-Ramirez A, Gómez M, Alfaro-Adrián J, Izquierdo M. Vertical jumping biomechanical evaluation through the use of an inertial sensor-based technology. J Sports Sci 2015; 10: 1-9

2

PATELLAR TENDON RUPTURE AFTER PLATELET RICH PLASMA AND STEROID THERAPY FOR CHRONIC TENDINOPATHY

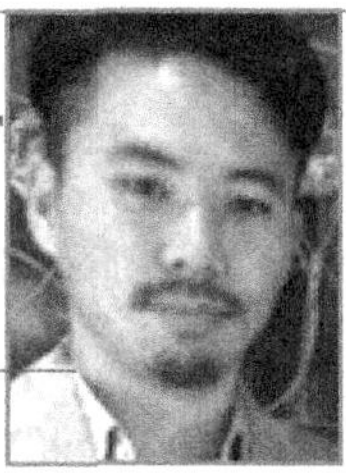

Nishio H, Kobayashi Y, Saita Y

Juntendo University, Tokyo, Japan

Introduction

There are various conservative treatments for chronic patellar tendinopathy such as local steroid injection, shock wave, and Platelet-Rich Plasma (PRP). However, the efficacy of these treatments remains to be controversial. Chronic patellar tendinopathy results in the denaturation of the tendon and rarely causes tendon rupture. We describe a case who sustained patellar tendon rupture after both steroid and PRP injections.

Case report

The case is a 22 years old Japanese male college football player (Tegner activity scale 7). His Body Mass Index (BMI) was 19.7 kg/m^2. He had been sustained patellar tendinopathy for 12 months before he visited our hospital. He had received three times of PRP therapy and corticosteroid injection. We prepared 2 mL of buffy-coat based leukocyte-poor PRP from 20 mL of peripheral blood using autologous preparation kit (Mycell, Kaylight Ltd, Israel; single centrifugation at 2000 g x 7 minutes; no activating agent was added), and mounted them multiply around the painful tender points. In this preparation method, platelet concentration is three times higher than whole blood and leukocyte is below the base line. We allowed him to walk and move his knee within the range he did not feel pain, and after 2-3 days, he returned to the same level of exercise before PRP therapy. Regarding steroid injection, 1 mL of Triamcinolone Acetonide was injected at the most painful point and he returned to play two days after injection. These treatments successfully relieved his symptoms, however, he did not undergo enough physiotherapy during this periods. Seven months after he underwent a local corticosteroid injection, he felt sudden pain with sound of "pop" when he braced his right leg against other player during kick motion. Radiographs indicated the presence of patella alta, and Magnetic Resonance Imaging (MRI) revealed a patellar tendon rupture. In the next day after the injury, he underwent surgery with primary suture plus augmentation using ipsilateral semitendinosus and gracilis tendons preserved their distal insertions on tibia (1). Since the quality of the tendon would be deteriorated due to persistent tendon inflammation, we added augmentation with intent to reduce the risk of re-injury after RTP soccer. Passive range of motion and isometric exercise of quadriceps and hamstrings were gradually initiated from the day after surgery. He started walking from the second day after surgery with knee extension brace and bracing continued for 4 weeks only when he walked. He started closed kinetic chain exercises from 6 weeks after the surgery and bracing had finished. He started jogging from 12 weeks after the surgery. Though there was no extensor lag at 6 months, his knee extension strength was only 58% compared with the left side. At 8 months, splinting and various training were permitted. Concerns regarding post-operative knee flexor weakness as both the gracilis and semitendinosus tendons were harvested, however, at 9 months, knee flexural muscular strength of the isokinetic concentric contraction recovered as strong as the left side. At 10 months, he gradually started soccer specific motions such as kicking and agility exercises with reaction movement. At 12 months, his knee extension strength reached to 86% as compared with the left side, and we could RTP soccer. He was able to return to full activity with no pain. At the follow up period of 18 months, he can play without any symptoms.

Conclusions

Although there are many case reports of a tendon rupture after corticosteroid injection, there are few reports after the PRP therapy. The corticosteroid can lead necrosis of tenocyte, whereas the PRP possess both anabolic and catabolic capacity. The effects of PRP differ from the cell compositions especially for leukocyte concentration. We used leukocyte-poor PRP in this case but it was not certain if PRP was involved in the cause of tendon rupture.
The most important message is that the physiotherapy is indispensable to cure the chronic patellar tendinopathy. The effect of desensitization of injection therapies is temporary and is not radical cure. We should note that too much intervention for desensitization can cause the neglect of player's efforts to collect their inappropriate motion that lead recurrence of sports injuries.

References

1. Takazawa Y, Ikeda H, Ishijima M, Kubota M, Saita Y, Kaneko H, Kobayashi Y, Sadatsuki R, Hada S, Kaneko K. Reconstruction of a ruptured patellar tendon using ipsilateral semitendinosus and gracilis tendons with preserved distal insertions: two case reports. BMC Research Notes 2013 Sep 8; 6: 361. doi: 10.1186/1756-0500-6-361

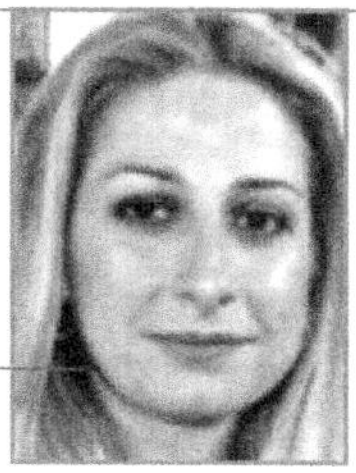

PARTIAL AVULSION OF ADDUCTOR LONGUS FIBROCARTILAGE. NOT AS INNOCENT AS IT LOOKS...

Dimitrakopoulou A, Schilders E

The London Hip Arthroscopy Centre at The Wellington Hospital, London; Fortius Clinic, London; Leeds Beckett University, Leeds, United Kingdom

Case Report

A 32-year-old male, professional footballer who played as goalkeeper at international level sustained a groin injury while performing a goal kick during a premiership football game. The mechanism was abduction in combination with extension of his right kicking leg. He felt a sharp pain in his right adductor area and was unable to continue playing. The patient had a history of adductor enthesopathy treated with a pubic cleft injection (2). Magnetic Resonance Imaging (MRI) revealed a partial avulsion of the right adductor longus fibrocartilage (25%, butterfly broken wing sign). The patient was treated non-operative with Rest Ice Compression Elevation (RICE) and progressively he regained about 85% of his normal level of activity but was not able to sprint flat out and do long goal kicks. During his training he reinjured himself and the MRI scan demonstrated further avulsion of his right adductor longus fibrocartilage (75%). The recurrent injury was further managed non-operatively but the patient was not able to return to his full activity. He sustained a third injury during training and the MRI showed a complete avulsion with displacement of the fibrocartilage. He was unable to play and clinical examination revealed pain during palpation on adductor area and resisted adduction. The footballer was treated surgically three months after his first injury. An incision was made over the adductor longus origin, the crural fascia was incised and the fibrocartilage was found avulsed and 3 cm displaced. The fibrocartilage footprint measured 1.5 x2.5 cm. Six non-absorbable anchors 2.4 mm (Mitek G2, De Puy) were positioned within the footprint of the fibrocartilage to reattach the enthesis. Excellent apposition was achieved. There were no immediate postoperative complications. A staged functional training programme of adductors was initiated consisting of close chain adductor strengthening followed by open chain and football specific adductor strengthening work. At eight weeks postoperatively, the patient had full range of movement without pain, with good strength of adductors/abductors (5/5). The patient had no limitations in his activities, returning to full training at 9 weeks and return to play at the same level at 11 weeks.

Conclusions

This case report highlights the progressive staged avulsion of the fibrocartilage of the adductor longus enthesis. Reviewing the MRI scans we can clearly demonstrate that the avulsion of the fibrocartilage occurs from lateral to medial as it is progressed from a partial to a complete avulsion. Patients with a partial avulsion of the fibrocartilage of adductor longus when they are not able to regain 100% of their pre-injury level of performance after non-operative management should be considered as candidates for surgical treatment. Selective partial adductor release (3) is the operation of choice and footballers return to play 4-6 weeks postoperatively. Further progression of this injury to a complete avulsion necessitates surgical reattachment of the fibrocartilage (1) and footballers return to play 10-12 weeks postoperatively. Therefore, the decision for surgical treatment is crucial for footballers to return to play promptly and at the same level.

References

1. Dimitrakopoulou A, Schilders E, Talbot JC, Bismil Q. Acute avulsion of the fibrocartilage origin of the adductor longus in professional soccer players: a report of two cases. Clin J Sport Med 2008; 18: 167-169
2. Schilders E, Bismil Q, Robinson P, O'Connor PJ, Gibbon WW, Talbot JC. Adductor-related groin pain in competitive athletes: role of adductor enthesis, magnetic resonance imaging, and entheseal pubic cleft injections. J Bone Joint Surg Am 2007; 89: 2173-2178
3. Schilders E, Dimitrakopoulou A, Cooke M, Bismil Q, Cooke C. Effectiveness of a selective partial adductor release for chronic adductor-related groin pain in professional athletes. Am J Sports Med. 2013; 41: 603-607

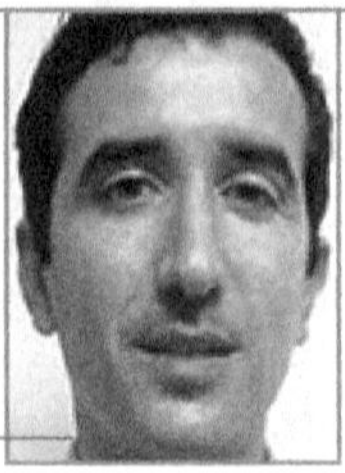

RETURN TO PLAY AFTER HAMSTRINGS MUSCLE INJURY: A SAFE, FAST AND EFFECTIVE CASE STUDY OF A PROFESSIONAL FOOTBALL PLAYER

Loureiro N[1,2], Pereira R[1,3,4], Espregueira-Mendes J[1,3,5,6]

[1]Clínica do Dragão, Espregueira-Mendes Sports Centre, FIFA Medical Centre of Excellence, Porto; [2]Paços de Ferreira FC, Paços de Ferreira; [3]Dom Henrique Research Centre, Porto; [4]Faculty of Health Sciences, University of Fernando Pessoa, Porto; [5]ICVS/3B's-PT Government Associate Laboratory, Braga/Guimarães; [6]Orthopaedics Department, Minho University, Minho, Portugal

Introduction

Hamstrings injuries are frequent in football, being the most common injury in the elite football player, with an approximate rate of 1/1,000 h (2). The median time to return to sport at the pre-injury level has been reported to be 31 weeks, ranging from 9 to 104 weeks (1).
One-third of the hamstrings lesions may recur, specially at the two first weeks of returning to play (3) reports in the literature suggest it is due to inadequate rehabilitation program or premature return to competition, but mainly due to incorrect physical loads of training.
This case report depicts the diagnosis, rehabilitation and return to play process of a first league football player. It will be presented a broad written record of the events as well as a video footage from the lesion moment to the celebration of the first goal (against a twice champions league winner) after the coming back.

Case report

We present a case report of a 28-year old male professional football player (82 kg, 1.86 m and 7.73% fat mass), playing as striker at the Portuguese First National League. During a game on September 6th 2015, at the 55th minute, the football player suffered a non-contact muscle injury to the distal third of the hamstrings muscles, on the right lower limb, during a sprint action.
The muscle injury was diagnosed trough clinical evaluation and ultrasound imaging. The diagnosis process revealed a muscle injury, which was classified as a type 2a lesion according British Athletics Muscle Injury Classification.
We report the rehabilitation process into three phases in order to clear up the whole process. These had different goals and objective criteria as requisite to evolve to the next phase, until returning to competition.
Acute phase. During the first 7 days of injury, the goal was to promote the analgesic process and accelerate the muscle healing. Thus, it was recommended relative rest. Moreover, it was applied physical modalities such as electrotherapy, thermotherapy and manual therapies (lymphatic drainage, myofascial release and brushing techniques) to reduce the pain and release adhesions. Additionally, there was a single eco-guided application (documented in video) of Platelet-Rich Plasma (PRP), 72 hours after the injury, aiming for better tissue healing. PRP was obtained from a sample of patients' venous blood drawn at the time of treatment. Freshly collected blood was centrifuged at 1,800 rotations/minute (rpm) (for 8 minutes). The preparation of PRP was accomplished inside a laminar flow hood. Additionally, the activation was made with calcium-chloride and 5 mL were delivered at the injurie site. The rehabilitation protocol was continued three days after these procedures were done.

- Functional recovery. After the first 7 days, we started the functional recovery phase, which aimed to reestablish the neuromuscular balance and recover the functional skills. The player underwent a strengthening program of the hamstrings, hip external rotators and extensors (these muscle groups were progressed under asymptomatic circumstances with more confidence -time frame of muscle tissue healing rationale- assisting the increasing in load after 12-15 days after injury, from active towards active resistive movement) and lumbo-pelvic motor control stabilization. Progressive agility training with specific football skills was also incorporated. In addition, proprioceptive training and single-leg landing exercises were performed by the players, with the physiotherapist supervision to correct the biomechanical and kinematics deficits.
- Progressive return to play. At the 20th day, the player returned to the field to start more football-specific exercises. The field training consisted in running, followed by agility and coordination training. The strengthening and flexibility training was also employed at this phase. The football-specific exercises were introduced progressively, in a controlled environment. On the 23rd day, the player integrated the team practice without any restrictions.

After 27 days from the injury, the football player stepped the grass once again to play in a professional game, showing full recovery from his injury coping with return to competition without symptoms or signs of impaired performance.

Conclusions

After following the good practices and evidence-based sports medicine recommendations we were able to help a professional football player to return in a safe and effective way after a 2nd muscle injury in 27 days. The follow-up is now reaching four months and there was not any sign of recurrence.

In spite of the positive results reported, we felt a lack of unequivocal criteria to progress in the rehabilitation process as well in decision process to decide on the return to play. Therefore, we rather based our intervention in scientific general guidelines, time frame of tissue healing and feedback from the athlete on intensity and complexity of the exercises experienced.

References

1. Askling CM, Tengvar M, Saartok T, Thorstensson A. Proximal hamstring strains of stretching type in different sports injury situations, clinical and magnetic resonance imaging characteristics, and return to sport. Am J Sports Med 2008; 36: 1799-1804
2. Ekstrand J, Hägglund M, Kristenson K, Magnusson H, Waldén M. Fewer ligament injuries but no preventive effect on muscle injuries and severe injuries: an 11-year follow-up of the UEFA Champions League injury study. Br J Sports Med 2013; 47: 732-737
3. Heiderscheit BC, Sherry MA, Silder A, Chumanov ES, Thelen DG. Hamstring strain injuries: recommendations for diagnosis, rehabilitation, and injury prevention. J Orthop Sports Phys Ther 2010; 40: 67-81

TRAUMATIC MIOSITE OSSIFICANS IN A PROFESSIONAL FOOTBALL PLAYER - WHEN TO RETURN?

Ribeiro BV[1], Teixeira JFC[2], Noronha JC[3]

[1]Rio Ave FC and National Beach Soccer Team, Vila do Conde;
[2]Rio Ave FC, Vila do Conde;
[3]Portuguese Federation of Football and Gestifute, Porto, Portugal

Case report

A high-level Portuguese first division midfield football player (male, 31 yrs old; 189 cm, 82 kg), right side dominant, sustained a contusion on his right quadriceps during a friendly match. Rest, ice, compression and paracetamol was advised. At 48 hours an ecography showed a haematoma in the vastus intermedius muscle. In the coming days the thigh was swollen, passive Range Of Motion (ROM) of the knee was 70° of flexion with the hip flexed at 90°. There was not change on the sensation of the lower limb. Palpation revealed a dull thigh, without any specific tenderness, consistent with the underling haematoma. Knee extension strength was graded 4+/5 and 5/5 with knee flexion. Three days later the thigh was painless. The pain-free physiotherapy included stretching and strengthening exercises, with and without electrostimulation, and pressotherapy. No local massage was done. On day 6 (d6), although the thigh was still swollen, and since he didn't have any pain and ROM around 100°, he was allowed to resume training with the team, but without kicking. Although the thigh was a bit swollen and the ROM was around 115°, his first game after injury was on d16, he performed quite well during the 90 minutes match. During the following week he could train quite well, feeling only light soreness. He played the 2nd game on d18, but on the following day he was clinically worse, the thigh was swollen, the knee flexion around 90°, with pain on the bent knee stretching. A Magnetic Resonance Imaging (MRI) was performed on d20 and it showed an hematoma (13.5 x 3.0 cm) in the Vastus Intermedius muscle. Drainage was attempted without success and a local injection of collagen was applied. He resumed the initial treatment. On d22 the knee flexion was 100° and on d23 it was 120°, with less volume and without any local pain. On d27 the ROM was normal, the volume of the thigh was much smaller and he started running painless with some physical training on the pitch, without kicking the ball. On d30 an ultrasound scan was performed by a radiologist in a private clinic and a heterogenic myositis ossificans in the vastus intermedius muscle was diagnosed (62.5 x 17.2 mm). Since the volume of the thigh was almost normal, he was painless and with full knee flexion, a decision had to be taken as far as return to play was concerned. After medical consultation with other doctors and a talk with the player and the coach, it was decided he could return to train with the team, but with a carbon fibre custom-made protection (20 x 15 cm), to protect the front thigh and to avoid any direct trauma. He could perform without any handicap related to the injury. The following weekly ultrasound scan showed regression of the size of the Myositis Ossificans (MO) and he progressively returned to his previous level of physical shape. On d39 it was his 1st official game without any further problem. On d80 the ultrasound scan still showed a residual injury (25.1 x 2.6 mm).

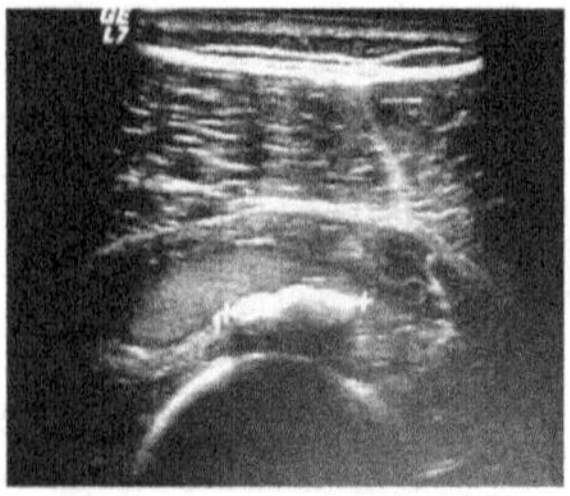

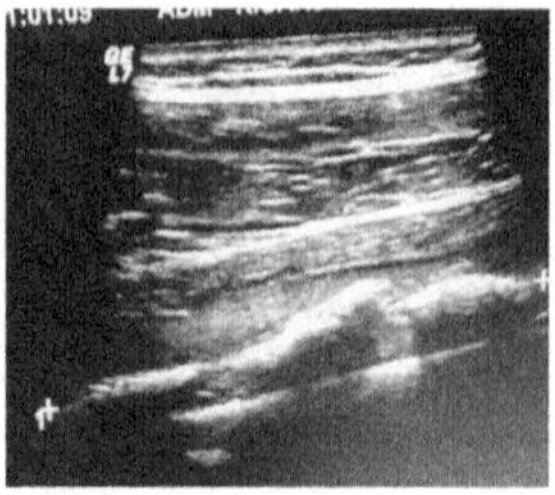

Figure 1. Ultrasound scan showing Myositis Ossificans.

Discussion

The posttraumatic MO is the proliferation of bone and cartilage within a muscle, as a complication in approximately 9-20% of large haematomas associated with muscle contusions and strains. There could be long lasting morbidity, with pain, limited ROM and stiffness (1, 2).
MO must be considered if the contusion becomes irresponsive to medical treatment, after 10 to 14 days of rest, with increasing pain and decreasing ROM (2). Our player had only a swollen thigh and limited ROM. A MRI was performed because it could also differentiate MO from a sarcomatous lesion (3).
The treatment performed was in accordance with the literature. The issue here was the timing of the return to train and to play. In the first moment the played was allowed to get back to the pitch when he was pain free and a ROM over 100°, although the existing o a small haematoma and that was a bad decision. Then, once the diagnosis of MO was done, 30 days later, the decision to let a very valuable, important and painless player, with a ROM of 120°, to get back to the pitch was questioned again. The decision to let him train, with local protection, turned to be right and wise. We conclude, no matter how important is the player, at least a period of four weeks must be respected for return to train and play in a case of a hematoma in the thigh and only if he is pain free and have a ROM over 120°. The ecography was a valuable tool for the follow-up on this injury.

References

1. Miller AE, Davis BA, Beckley OA. Bilateral and recurrent myositis ossificans in an athlete: a case report and review of treatment options. Arch Phys Med Rehab 2006; 87: 286-290
2. Torrance DA, Christopher deGraauw C. Treatment of post-traumatic myositis ossificans of the anterior thigh with extracorporeal shock wave therapy. J Can Chiropr Assoc 2011; 55: 240-246
3. Tyler P, Saifuddin A. The imaging of myositis ossificans. Seminars in musculoskeletal radiology. 2010; 14: 201-216

POSTACUTE MUSCLE INJURIES REHABILITATION WITH RADIAL EXTRACORPOREAL SHOCK WAVE THERAPY

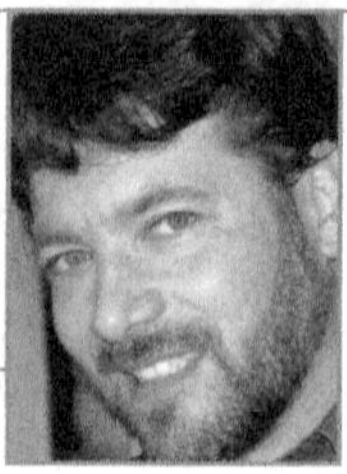

Di Cosmo R

Di Cosmo Phisiotherapy Clinic, Genova, Italy

Introduction

One of the most common muscle injuries in soccer affects the Rectus Femoris. The traditional therapeutic approach for partial lesions (i.e., rupture of the fibers of less than 50% of the muscle belly) relies on a variety of treatments that provide recovery times ranging from 25 to 35 days. After such an injury, residual muscular weakness may predispose to a re-injury or inadequate performance i.e., during running or shooting. Furtheremore the extensibility of the quadriceps can be affected and in some cases the deficit in Rectus Femoris flexibility after a second degree muscular injury by indirect mechanism, can be related to a large amount of fibrotic tissue or scar tissue, either on the whole muscle, already present before the injury. There are different modalities utilised in rehabilitation such as diathermy, Laser, continuous ultrasounds, and myo-electrical stimulation, but for this type of muscular injury the radial Extracorporeal Shock Wave Treatment (ESWT) is not so frequent.

Case report

A side back male semi-professional soccer player (age: 24 yrs; height: 170 cm; weight: 70 kg) usually involved in 3-4 sessions of training/week plus the match on Sunday, was affected by a muscular injury on the Rectus Femoris occurred by indirect mechanism during a sprint.
An Ultrasound scan performed 24 hours after the injury demonstrates a hypoechoic area of the right Rectus Femoris of 1.5 x 2.8 cm, still during contraction, 2.2 cm from the skin surface, referring to recent muscle injury of grade II, with extensive bruising around the wound and edema of adjacent soft tissues. The treatment started immediately with PRICE (Protection of the injured limb, Rest, Ice, Compression, Elevation) and ten diathermy treatments in two weeks, crutches for one week. After 58 days he had no pain during active movement, and during proprioceptive exercises, but the area of the lesion was hard, painful to acupressure and to passive analytic stretching. After warming up the pain was relieved, but could not carry out intense submaximal exercises, it does not respond positively to strengthening exercises, it had not improved quadriceps atrophy, the Range of Motion (ROM) in flexion of the knee with the thigh flexed to 90° was decreased by 50% compared to the contralateral. It was hypothesised that the Rectus Femoris was already fibrotic before the accident and what prevented it from healing. Three sessions of ESWT once a week were applied. The first session the machine was set at a pressure of 3 Bar, 15 Hz frequency and 8,000 shots on the Rectus Femoris and Vastus Lateralis with a plat pointer of 15 mm diameter. Massage and light analytical stretching to the entire quadriceps. In the second treatment ESWT was administered with a pressure of 4 bar, 8 Hz, 4,000 shots with 15 mm concave pointer on the Rectus Femoris, and 2 bar, 15 Hz, 500 shots with 7.5 mm in diameter plat pointer on the area of the lesion. Massage therapy and analytical stretching to the entire quadriceps. In the third treatment ESWT was administered with 3.5 bar, 10 Hz frequency, 5,000 shots with 15 mm in diameter plat pointer on all the quadriceps and adductors of the right thigh. The result was: no inflammation after all treatments, due to cavitation and wash-up of ESWT; increased blood microcirculation, rapid reactivation of tissue repair processes, disruption of fibrotic tissue. During the last 20 days of treatment the patient proceeded with rehabilitation training sessions on soccer pitch completely recovering the tropism of the quadriceps muscle and explosive strength. After 21 days from the starting treatment with ESWT the player was able to play his first game for 90 minutes, without problems and so for all the football matches. Based on the results achieved and more detailed studies, ESWT can be considered as successful modality to be included in the rehabilitation protocol after post-acute indirect muscle injury of the Rectus Femoris.

7

SHOCKWAVE TREATMENT FOR HAMSTRING INJURY IN A YOUTH LEVEL SOCCER PLAYER

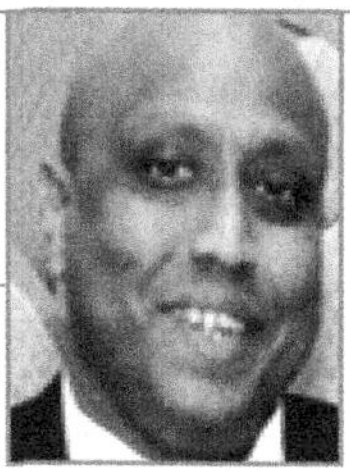

Vincent KC[1], d'Agostino MC[2], Schaden W[3]

[1]Kompass Health Associates, Auckland New Zealand;
[2]ESWT Centre, Rehabilitation Department, Humanitas Research Hospital, Milan, Italy;
[3]AUVA Trauma Centre, Vienna, Austria

This case study discusses the clinical outcomes of a 16 year old male (weigh: 76 kg; height: 180 cm) right footed centre-back, playing regional and national youth level soccer. The injury involved the strain of the right proximal hamstring reported as a sudden occurrence when sprinting during a game. The injury was initially managed by: rest, ice, pharmacogenics, eccentric stretching, and strapping which allowed the player to continue playing for some time. Over a 14 weeks (wk) period the condition progressed in severity and became indocile to this management strategy. The symptoms were most severe during sprinting and kicking, causing the player to be sidelined and unable to participate in team training. An ultrasound scan reported the presence of tendinosis occurring at the proximal hamstring region. This placed the player in a dilemma as his injury would cause him to miss the national U-17 selection to be held in five weeks. A cortisone injection was recommended but this was declined due to several concerns. We then recommended Extracorporeal Shock-Wave Treatment (ESWT), the rationale being its efficacy for a variety of chronic tendinopathies, safety, mechanics of action (1, 2), and systemic neutrality.

Clinical tests comprised of subjective reporting, palpation, limb size measurement, and Range Of Motion (ROM), collected at baseline, wk3, and wk24. Functional tests comprised of five sets of single leg jumps and single leg squats done in the fastest possible time to determine varus and valgus angles, and were assessed utilising wearable sensor technology (ViMove, Victoria, Australia), and was measured at baseline and wk24. ESWT was administered over 3 sessions at one week intervals utilising the electrohydraulic OrthoGold 100 (TRT/MTS Medical UG, Konstanz, Germany). 1,000 acoustic impulses at 0.19 mJ/mm^2 per session was aimed at the proximal hamstring origin region totalling 3,225 mJ/mm^2, while another 900 impulses was applied equally at 0.13 mJ/mm^2 over the proximal free, intramuscular hamstring tendon regions, and rectus femoris muscle, totalling 1,803 mJ/mm^2. All physiotherapy, strapping, and pharmacogenics were discontinued prior to commencement of ESWT. Concurrent rehabilitation protocol was recommended (Table 1) aimed at trunk stabilisation, neuromuscular control, endurance, joint motion, and overall strengthening, until return to play was achieved.

Rehabilitation Programme	Week 1	Week 2	Week 3	Week 4
Free style swimming	✓	✓	✓	✓
Aqua jogging	✓	✓	✓	✓
Core balance programme	✓	✓	✓	✓
Pain-free isometric stretch	✓	✓	✓	✓
Stationary cycling		✓	✓	✓
Low speed running			✓	✓
Indoor rowing		✓	✓	✓
Return to Soccer Training & Play				✓

Table 1. Return to play rehabilitation pathway.

The results of our case study showed a positive response to ESWT and the rehabilitation programme (Table 2) within a short timeframe. There was a significant reduction in pain symptoms, muscle hypertrophy, improvements to varus/valgus angles, and task capacity optimisation. The player also reported subjectively that he noted an increase in running speed, jump height, and balance, with less fatigue after recovery and return to play.

Clinical Assessments	Baseline	wk3	wk24
Subjective Pain (including palpation)	7.5	2.5	0.5
Mid-thigh circumference (R)	53.5 cm	56.9 cm	59.9 cm
Mid-thigh circumference (L)	58.7 cm	59.3 cm	60.3 cm
Hamstring ROM	52°	68°	84°
Funtional Assessment: Varus/Valgus angle range			
Single leg jump (L)	6°Var/7°Val	-	4°/4°Val
Single leg jump (R)	12°Var/7°Val++	-	3°Var/4°Val
Single leg squat (L)	4°Var/3°Val	-	2°Var/1°Val
Single leg squat (R)	11°Val++	-	1°Var/3°Val
Functional Assessment: Speed of completion			
Single leg jump (L)	16.47 s	-	14.03 s
Single leg jump (R)	UC*	-	14.02 s
Single leg squat (L)	26.09 s	-	23.26 s
Single leg squat (R)	UC*	-	23.33 s

Table 2. Comparison of baseline and post-ESWT scores at week 3 (wk3) and week 24 (w24). L: left; R: Right. Var: varus; Val: valgus. *UC: unable to complete task (5 repetitions); ++ Scores were taken from two of proposed five repetitions.

Hamstring injuries are commonly seen in soccer and remains a challenge to treat, and is often associated with slow healing process and high recurrence rate. From what has been elucidated to-date of the mechanics of action of ESWT is that, the mechanotransduction from the acoustic stimulus modulates a diverse homeostatic return on human tissue (i.e. microcirculation, cell proliferation, inflammatory modulation, collagen and protein synthesis etc.) (1, 2). The findings of this case study suggests that ESWT is an effective option which helped our soccer player recover from this challenging condition, enabling him to return to play within a short timeframe at optimal performance levels. There is a suggestive possibility that ESWT may be used to help prevent overuse syndromes via optimising tissue resilience to help cope with the stresses associated with soccer at all levels. This becomes an invaluable medical asset when considering actual playing time, career longevity, and investment protection for this great sport.

References

1. D'Agostino CM, Craig K, Tibalt E, Respizzi S. Shock wave as biological therapeutic tool: from mechanical stimulation to recovery and healing, through mechanotransduction. Int J Surg 2015; 24 (Pt B): 147-153
2. Sukubo NG, Tibalt E, Respizzi S, Locati M, d'Agostino CM. Effect of shock waves on macrophages: a possible role in tissue regeneration and remodeling. Int J Surg 2015; 24(Pt B): 124-130

RETURN TO PLAY AFTER HAMSTRINGS MUSCLE INJURY

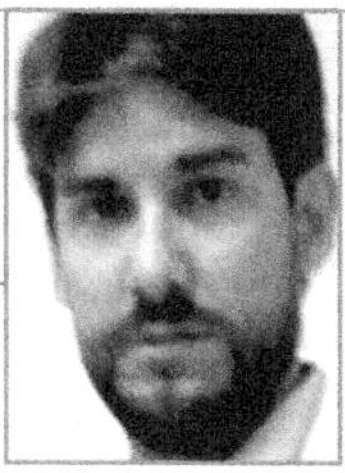

Furini F, Pagella F, Sandrelli L

Medical and Sports Rehabilitation Centre Argos Lab, Arquata Scrivia, Italy

On September the 18th 2015 a young 17 year-old male football player came to our Rehabilitation Centre after injury. He complained of pain (Visual Analogue Scale - VAS - 8/10) and functional impotence at the right hamstrings, arisen after a football training session. He played in the local team (Italian League D). He grew up with his team mates and his trainers, and now the concern of standing still because of the injury haunts him so much that he cannot even sleep at night. In the last year he changed his role from fullback to forward and in the new position he feels steady and determined.

During the medical consultation, he complained of pain due to the pressure of the middle-third and the proximal third of the muscle belly of the right Bicep Femoris. During the palpation, an oval area of tight elastic consistence is remarkable. An ultrasound scan was done in order to state the muscular damage: a II degree oval sprain of 25 mm x 10 mm at the proximal third of the right hamstrings. So, the RICE (Rest, Ice, Compression, Elevation) was suggested for two days and then a treatment with Tecartherapy (Human Tecar HCR701, Unibell, Lecco, Italy) was started with the device set in capacitive mode homeothermy for 15 minutes around the area of injury, with a draining course to the lymph nodes, followed by resistive mode in athermy on the area of the injury for 15 minutes. We performed 3 sessions on alternate days, obtaining a subjective pain reduction (VAS 4/10).

Eight days after the injury, respecting the pain threshold, some strength, endurance and balance exercises were carried out.

The functional assessment of strength was performed with the Isokinetic System Pro4 (Biodex, NY, USA) with 10 repetitions at 90°/s and 20 repetitions at 180°/s (Table 1).

Balance was measured with a postural stability test performed on Balance System SD (Biodex, NY, USA) (Table 1).

The rehabilitation process, which would have evolved according to the standard protocol but personalized depending on his response, was illustrated and agreed, after having reassured the patient on the possibility to full recovery and Return To Play (RTP). After having understood the duration and complexity of the treatment for a safe RTP, the patient decided to discuss about the case with his parents because his family couldn't afford the foreseen costs. Much to our surprise, the day after the patient came back to the centre in order to face the rehabilitative process thanks to the help of his grandfather and his Sports Society.

The rehabilitative protocol consisted in: Phase 1 (isometric exercises and stretching for 4 days); Phase 2 (eccentric then concentric exercises with elastic resistance and isokinetics for 4 days); Phase 3 (coordination exercises on instable balance board); Phase 4 (recovery of the technical gesture on the pitch).

In order to speed up the RTP, starting from the Phase 2, eight sessions of therapy with a selective mechanical-sound wave system (VIBRAplus, a-Circle, S. Pietro in Casale, Italy) were effected. The mechanical-sound vibrations on the muscle bellies of the anterior kinetic chain of the lower limbs (abductors, femoral rectum, anterior tibial) were applied at 300 Hz for 25 minutes and at 50 Hz for 5 minutes, 3 times a week.

Since the pain disappeared (VAS 0/10) and since the patient showed a good recovery of strength (1), endurance and balance, we proceeded with the application of the mechanical-sound vibrations also on the posterior kinetic chain (big gluteus, femoral bicep and sural tricep) at 150 Hz for 25 minutes and at 50 Hz for 5 minutes.

	First assessment	Last assessment
Days after the injury	8	20
Pain (VAS)	4/10	0/10
Knee Extensors Isokinetic 90°/s Peak torque (Nm)	167.9	177.0
Knee Flexors Isokinetic 90°/s Peak torque (Nm)	63.1	74.3
Knee Extensors Isokinetic 180°/s Peak torque (Nm)	97.2	136.5
Knee Flexors Isokinetic 180°/s Peak torque (Nm)	46.2	62.6
Balance (% of time in A zone)	50	100

Table 1. Functional strength and balance tests performed at the first and the last assessment 20 days after the start of the rehabilitation protocol.

After 20 days, the isokinetic test showed a complete strength recovery (Table 1) and our young football player was ready to face the last phase of the rehabilitative protocol on the pitch. This phase was overcome without any complication, so 25 days after the injury the athlete played his first match during a training (13 October 2015) and on the 18 October 2015 the first official match. After two months since our patient returned on the pitch, he did not show neither relapses nor other adverse events.

References

1. Zwolski C, Schmitt LC, Quatman-Yates C, Thomas S, Hewett TE, Paterno MV. The influence of qudriceps strength asimmetry on patient-reported function at time of return to sport after anterior cruciate ligament reconstruction. Am J Sports Med 2015; 43: 2242-2249

DIFFERENTIAL DIAGNOSIS AND CONSERVATIVE REHABILITATION APPROACH IN HIP IMPINGEMENT CONCERNING FOOTBALLERS

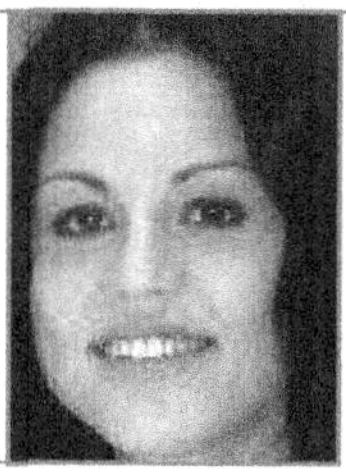

Stergiou M, Stergiou E, Giannis C

Ma.Ster Physio, Siatista, Kozani, Greece

Introduction

Femoro-Acetabular Impingement (FAI) is caused when the neck of the femur, due to limited internal rotation, contacts the pelvis biomechanically in an atypical manner. It is often misdiagnosed as a groin strain, knee or lumbar spine pathology, ovarian cysts, trochanteric bursitis, and/or abdominal region hernias (1).
Thus, the aim of this abstract is to highlight the importance of the differential diagnosis and conservative rehabilitation approach in case of FAI.

Case report

This case report deals with our personal experience of a 17 years old male football player (left back defender) with continuous complains in the hip area over the past two years. The footballer was recovering from a second degree Biceps Femoris strain (during a football match); he contacted our Clinic following a prescription by his physician. After having examined his history (family and clinical), we conducted clinical tests such as Range of Motion test, Fabers and Thomas test, and Trendelenburg sign test. The flexion, adduction and internal rotation test involved having the patient in a supine position on the examination table with the affected hip and knee flexed to 90 degrees. The hip which was then adducted and internally rotated provoked sudden and sharp pain to the athlete. Furthermore, hip flexion and internal rotation were measured and found to be 101°degrees and 9°degrees respectively. However, pain appeared with internal rotation. The footballer met specific criteria (<115° hip flexion, <15° internal rotation, or pain with internal rotation) and was exhibiting the clinical symptoms of FAI (2). In addition, given his multiple history of trauma, an examination of the lumbar spine and sacroiliac joint was conducted but both areas did not present any abnormality. Finally, an X-Ray confirmed the cam type FAI. Footprint and gait analysis tests (FootChecker 4.0, Loran Engeneering, Castel Maggiore, Italy) showed the following:

	Gait Static Analyses 60.3%		**Gait Static Analyses 54.6%**	
Foot	Average Pressure Pa(r)	Surface Contact cm^2	Average Pressure Pa(r)	Surface Contact cm^2
Left	50.8	84.0	45.4	62.8
Right	56.7	85.0	92.0	83.0

Table 1. Gait static analysis.

Steps	Duration (ms)	Average Pressure K Pa(r)
First Left	710	138.3
Second Right	680	133.7

Table 2. Gait Dynamic Analyses (Maximum Pressure).

The rehabilitation program aimed at a quick return to play and involved rehabilitation sessions of four times a week, with session being 70 to 100 minutes per day.
The program was divided into two phases. The first phase (5 sessions) aimed at decreasing pain by decompression of the hip area and included mobilization of the hip joint following orthopedic manual therapy principles (Grade IV mobilization of the anterior hip capsule, led to significant increase in gluteus maximum strength), stretching structures around hip complex, proprioception and effective weight transfer without compensatory movement patterns. Last but not least, in order to increase the neuromuscular coordination and function closed chain exercises were chosen.
The second phase (after 6 sessions)aimed at increasing the strength of the deep, intermediate and superficial hip muscles by allowing hip abductors and extensors to function in full range. It involved progressive exercises and more challenges to the lumbopelvic region. In addition, hip control (core stability) included stabilization of specific muscles such as the diaphragm, the Transversus Abdominis , the Obliquus Abdominis, the pelvic floor and multifidus contraction which provided segmental stability and led to a more explosive and efficient function of the hip abductors and adductors.
Simultaneously, we proceeded in stretching the tough muscles thus, improving hip muscle flexibility (from concentric to eccentric exercises) and joint mobility progressive proprioception to single one leg stand and balance. Finally, full rehabilitation involved cardiovascular activities such as running or cycling and simulated exercises in more functional positions.
In almost three weeks, the player returned back to play obtaining his joint position sense, proceeding from functional to dynamic and total control of his body through spinal stabilization and neuromuscular balance.
The initial feeling of the patient, which was intermittent pain aggravated by both physical activities and exercising in extreme football positions, was reduced to a minimum.

Conclusions

Our rehabilitation process and results suggest that orthopedic physical assessment and differential examination with early screenings, can lead to a more precise diagnosis on footballers with multiple trauma on the same anatomic area. Thus, tracing and identifying the cause of trauma will help physiotherapists provide a high quality rehabilitation programme that prevents further injuries, improves the existent trauma and reduces the recovery time needed to return back to play.

References

1. Philippon MJ, Maxwell RB, Johnston TL, Schenker M, Briggs KK. Clinical presentation femoacetablular impingement. Knee Surg Sports Traumatol Arthrosc 2007; 15: 1041-1047
2. Rothenfluh DA, Reedwisch D, Müller U, Ganz R, Tennant A, Leunig M. Construct validity of a 12-item WOMAC for assessment of femoro-acetabular impingement and osteoarthritis of the hip. Osteoarthritis Cartilage 2008; 16: 1032-1038

USING LEVEL OF SPECIFICITY TO MONITOR RECONDITIONING LOAD FOR A KNEE INJURY

Pajon D, Alvarez J, Colell D

Club de Futbol Reus Deportiu, Reus, Spain

Introduction

Exercise Level Of Specificity (LOS) is a method used as an intensity indicator to monitor training load in football periodization, the system is based in closeness of the task planned to the real match situation, the closer, the more intense the exercise is. The main goal of this case report was to adapt this system to a reconditioning program (it is already applied in the team periodization), and see if the workout done by the injured player, achieves a similar load level as the group and, object the progress in the level of specificity of the sessions; when the desired values are achieved we can take a return to play decision.

Case report

A 24 years old male professional football player, fullback, Spanish 2B league, (body mass 79.7 kg; height 184 cm) suffered a medial collateral ligament grade I injury in the left knee after a concussion during a match. The player underwent physiotherapeutic treatment during all the rehabilitation process. Day 1 and 2: injury evaluation by the doctor and Magnetic Resonance Imaging (MRI); the reconditioning program started on day 3. Day 10 was a rest day. In Table 1, we can see the 8 days reconditioning gym and on-field program, including day 12 (full training participation with the group), where every exercise has a time and a LOS value.

	EXERCISE	DAY 3	DAY 4	DAY 5	DAY 6	DAY 7	DAY 8	DAY 9	DAY 11	DAY 12
1	TIME (minutes)	15	15	15	20	20	20	20	15	18
	Level of Specificity	10	10	10	11	11	11	11	11	11
	Load	150	150	150	220	220	220	220	165	198
2	TIME (minutes)	25	30	30	23	27	30	30	40	21
	Level of Specificity	13,2	13,4	13,4	15	15	13,6	13,6	16	15
	Load	330	402	402	345	405	408	408	640	315
3	TIME (minutes)	10	10	10	20	26	23	10	15	34
	Level of Specificity	10	12	12,5	13,4	13,8	15	15	13,8	19
	Load	100	120	125	268	358,8	345	150	207	646
4	TIME (minutes)		15	10	15	15	10	14		
	Level of Specificity		10	13,8	11	11	10	14,4		
	Load		150	138	165	165	100	201,6		
5	TIME (minutes)			10	10			10		
	Level of Specificity			10	10			10		
	Load			100	100			100		
	TOTAL TIME (minutes)	50	70	75	88	88	83	84	70	73
	Average Specificity	11.07	11.35	11.94	12.08	12.70	12.40	12.80	13.60	15.00
	Session Load	580.0	822.0	915.0	1098.0	1148.8	1073.0	1079.6	1012.0	1159.0
	LAST 3 DAYS GROUP LOAD							1027.75	1041.0	

Table 1. Reconditioning program.

The description of the type of exercise referring to each LOS value can be found in Table 2. The time of the exercise multiplied by the LOS value gives us the exercise load; at the end of every session we can see the average LOS value and the total load of the session (sum of all exercises loads).
As we can see in the Table 1, there is a clear sessions progression of average specificity, that tendency shows that the situations that the player was exposed to in the reconditioning program, were more specific and intense as he was getting closer to join the group again.
The load results show the progression during the first days of rehabilitation and the adaptation of the reconditioning loads to the group values. This way, we make sure that the player returns to full participation with no accumulated fatigue and a minimum load achieved.
The player performed a 93 minutes match on the day 15; he did not experience unusual fatigue or soreness.
Taking this into account we can say that this is a simple and useful tool for professionals that cannot use latest technology to monitor training load, and gives us information to take a return to play decision.

Level of Specificity	Exercise Characteristics
10.0	Core Training + Mobility
11.0	General or Group Warm Up/ Propioception Injured Limb
12.0	Group Match Recovery Running / Bycicle Aerobic Z1
12.5	Running Aerobic Z1
13.0	Group Muscular Endurance Training
13.2	Muscular Endurance Training - Upper Body
13.4	Muscular Endurance Training - Injured Limb
13.6	Strength Training (Hipertrophy) - Injured Limb
13.8	Coordination Training
	Strength Training (Maximal / Eccentric) - Injured Limb
14.0	Group Tactical Positioning Work/ Combinative Actions
14.4	Basic Habilities with the Ball
14.8	Advanced Habilities with the Ball
15.0	Group 'Rondos'/ General Endurance Training
	Running Aerobic Z2
16.0	Group Explosive Strength Training / Plyometric Training
	Competitive Habilities/ Match Actions with or Without Opponent
17.0	Group Speed Training / 'Macro System' Situations
18.0	Aerobic Z3/ Group 'Meso-System' Situations
19.0	Group ' Micro- System' Situations / Training Match Situation
20.0	Competition Match

Table 2. Exercise Level of Specificity description.

PUBIC STRESS FRACTURE AND OSTEITIS PUBIS IN A 24 YEAR OLD FOOTBALLER

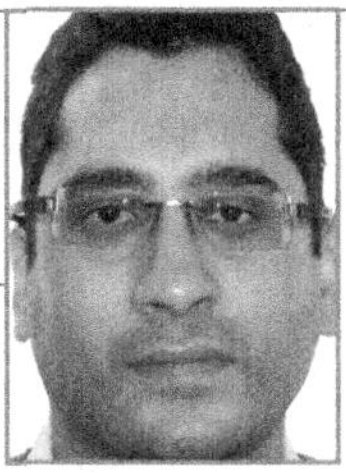

Chatterjee AD, Wilson J, Knight RR

Notts County Football Club, Nottingham, United Kingdom

Introduction

This case report presents a 24 year old male professional footballer diagnosed with a left pubic stress fracture and osteitis pubis. The patient plays in the first team at a League Two professional football club in England as a striker. He is 1.70 m tall, weighs 69.8 kg and is a right foot dominant player. The player initially presented with a 2-3 week history of left adductor related pain. He subjectively presented with pain when sprinting, changing direction and kicking. Magnetic Resonance Imaging (MRI) scans and plain radiograph confirmed a combination of a left side pubic stress fracture and osteitis pubis. It was decided that a conservative approach to this injury was warranted. This involved an offload period of 21 days. The player returned to running at 218 days and completed his first training session 244 days post diagnosis. This was a very challenging case due to the paucity of research relating to pelvic stress fracture rehabilitation in football. In order to provide the player with best possible outcome, advice was sort from a variety of other sports. The success of this case also relied on the player being able to understand the nature of his injury and being compliant with rehabilitation program despite its lengthy process. It is the opinion of these authors that medical teams may have sort to intervene surgically in order to accelerate the rehabilitation process.

Methods

The rehabilitation followed a criterion-based model, with 9 key stages of rehabilitation: 1. Acute management; 2. Static Core Stability; 3. Dynamic Core Stability; 4. Progressive Loading Phase; 5. Performance Phase; 6. Plyometric Phase; 7. Return to Running; 8. Return to Training (Sport Specific); 9. Return to Play. The player was required to meet specific criteria to progress through the phases of rehabilitation.

Phase	Criteria Examples
1. Acute management	Numerical Pain Rating Scale (NPRS) 0/10 on activities of daily living
2. Static Core Stability	Plank Matrix x 3 minutes NPRS 0/10 Adductor isometric squeeze 10 x 10 seconds
3. Dynamic Core Stability	Sport Specific Plank Test >2 minutes NPRS 0/10 Adductor Bridge 10 x 10 seconds
4. Progressive Loading Phase	Single leg elevated bridge and Single leg calf raises: maximal body weight test 30+ on each leg. Left and right within 5 repetitions Step Up, Sumo Squat, Lunge, Split Squat 3 x 8 x 25 kg Standing Long lever Adductor cable resistance 3 x 20 x 13 kg
5. Performance Phase	Back Squat: 2 x Body Weight x 5 repetitions Single leg press 2 x Body Weight x 10 repetitions
6. Plyometric Phase	Plyometric Matrix (Squat Jumps, Split Squat Jumps, Adductor Jacks, Fast calf raises, broncos, mountain climbers) 3 x 40 seconds
7. Return to Running	Alter-G x 30 minutes 80% Body Weight at 12.0 km/h Alter-G 10 x 1minute Interval Run (18 - 20 km/h) at 50% Body Weight Multidirectional Running 3 x 8 minutes at 60% heart rate max x 3 sessions
8.Return to Training (Sport Specific)	Complete position specific whole pitch modified Hoff circuit (1) in line with GPS (Catapult GPS, Melbourne, Australia) demands of training x 12 sessions including all ball work Complete 1 x 10 x 20 m x 20 kg sled sprints x 4 sessions Complete 2 x 8 x 100 m sprints with no adverse effect x 4 session
9. Return to Play	Complete squad predictable and unpredictable passing, shooting and crossing drills x 6 sessions Complete possession drills and small sided games x 6 sessions

Table 1. Phases of the rehabilitation.

Results

The player was absent from training for a total period of 244 days. During this he missed 113 training days and 44 matches. The player progressed through each of the phases in the time detailed in table 2. The player has since completed 53 training days (4350 minutes) and 12 games (500 minutes) with no relapse in symptoms.

Phase	Days in Phase	Exited Phase (days)
Acute management	21	21
Static Core Stability	7	28
Dynamic Core Stability	21	49
Progressive Loading Phase	57	106
Performance Strength	49	155
Plyometrics	11	166
Return to Running	52	218
Return to training (Sport Specific)	26	244
Return to Play	15	259

Table 2. Time spent in each phase.

Conclusions

Whilst pelvic stress fractures are a rarity in male footballers, this case highlights the importance of recognising their potential. The methods and results highlight how conservative management requires a stepwise progressive loading approach to minimise relapse and ensure optimal outcome.

References

1. Hoff J, Wisløff U, Engen LC, Kemi OJ, Helgerud J. Soccer specific aerobic endurance training. Br J Sports Med 2002; 36: 218-221

Sunday 10th April, 2016 (afternoon)
POSTER AREA

FREE POSTER PRESENTATIONS CONTEST

BEST CLINICAL CASE HISTORY AWARD

Chairs

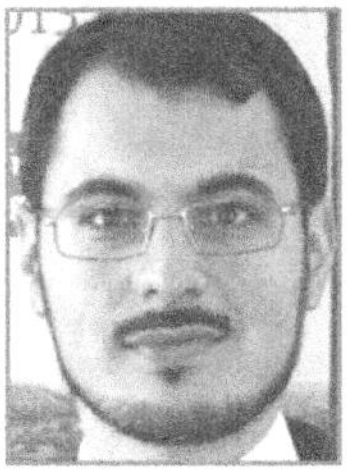

Giuseppe Filardo
(Bologna, Italy)

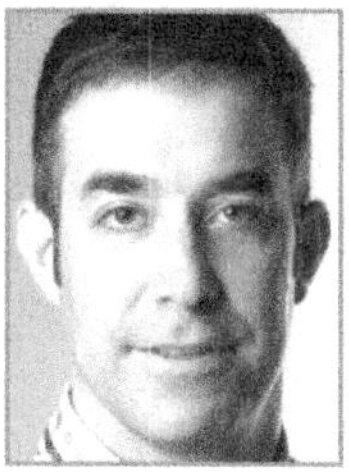

Gérgely Panics
(Budapest, Hungary)

PM01 Injury or disease flare with known seronegative arthritis
Janse van Rensburg DC, McCord J, Martin C (Pretoria, South Africa)

PM02 Return of a low adherence to treatment goalkeeper with osteochondritis in Brazil **Dorilêo CGLF, Pedrinelli A, Youssef M (São Paulo, Brazil)**

PM03 A case of chondrosarcoma of rib in a professional football player
Fukui T, Fujita I, Harada T (Kakogawa and Akashi, Japan)

PM04 Lisfranc injury repair with the tightrope and the Charlotte targeting device
Drampalos E, Clough TM (Wigan, United Kingdom)

PM05 A 22 year's old national team football player with increasing atraumatic ankle pain **Shimakawa T, D'Hooghe P (Doha, Qatar)**

PM06 Extraordinary cause of hip joint pain in a professional football player
Tzoanos G, Tsavalas N, Manidakis N, Chardaloumbas D, Kalliakmanis A (Heraklion, Crete; Athens, Greece)

PM07 Rehabilitation and return to play of a professional footballer following conservative management of lumbar spine disc herniation
Toolan AM (New York, USA)

PM08 Iliac crest avulsion fracture in immature elite soccer player: a stochastic return to play **Materne O, Robertson D (Doha, Qatar)**

PM09 Return to play of a professional female football player after eighty rehabilitation days
Angius M, Volpi P, Pinna M (Sassari and Milan, Italy)

PM10 Monitoring of an anterior cruciate ligament injury through infrared thermography **Fernández-Cuevas I, Arnáiz-Lastras J, Sillero-Quintana M (Madrid, Spain)**

PM11 A case of shortening the preoperative period before anterior cruciate ligament reconstruction **Kinugasa T, Ikeda K (Tsukuba-shi, Japan)**

1

INJURY OR DISEASE FLARE WITH KNOWN SERONEGATIVE ARTHRITIS

Janse van Rensburg DC[1], McCord J[2], Martin C[2]

[1]Sports Medicine University of Pretoria, Pretoria;
[2]McCord & Repton Physiotherapy, Pretoria, South Africa

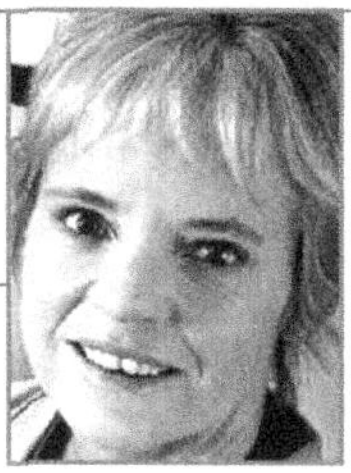

History

A 22 year old male midfield player (height 1.7 m, weight 70 kg) was diagnosed with seronegative arthritis in April 2013. He responded well to disease modifying treatment and was able to continue play for his Premier Soccer League team. Regular follow-up visits to monitor disease control and possible side-effects from medication were unremarkable. In September 2014 his team doctor arranged an emergency visit due to "uncontrolled" disease. On further enquiry and clinical examination it seemed more like a lateral meniscus problem of the left knee rather than a disease flare. Magnetic resonance imaging revealed a bucket handle tear of the lateral meniscus without florid synovitis. Inflammatory blood markers (C-reactive protein and erythrocyte sedimentation rate) were normal.

Treatment

His arthritis medication was maintained as previously and he was referred to an Orthopaedic Surgeon. An arthroscopic debridement including excision of the torn part of the meniscus and hypertrophic synovium in the lateral gutter was performed. His rehabilitation programme commenced pre-operatively. Emphasis was placed on the myofascial release of the posterior and spiral lines (2). The pre- and post-operative rehabilitation programmes were based on the Sport Science Lab principles (1).

Pre-operative rehabilitation included dynamic, functional core and pelvic stability exercises on a ball, balance and proprioceptive training on slant boards and pipes, non-weight bearing (open chain) eccentric strengthening of gluteus medius and hamstrings. Manual and electrotherapy techniques comprised soft tissue massage and gentle joint mobilisation, and ultra-sound respectively. Kinesiology taping (drainage technique) was used to decrease pre-operative swelling. Interval stationary cycling, to maintain cardio respiratory fitness was included in the programme.

Post-operatively, days 1 and 2 entailed soft tissue techniques to manage swelling, gait re-education (full weight bearing without crutches), and accessory and physiological patella-femoral and tibio-femoral joint mobilisation techniques to aid in restoring knee flexion and extension range.

Days 2-7, miniature bilateral balance boards for balance and proprioceptive re-education, eccentric strength training of hamstring and gluteal muscles in functional movement patterns, and stationary cycling for cardio-respiratory fitness training was introduced.

During week 2 of his post-operative rehabilitation he could start jogging on grass with running shoes while interval training was continued on a stationary bike. Strength training of core, pelvis, hamstrings and gluteus maximus were adapted and progressed to continuously challenge different strengths and endurance. Rhythmic drills using ladders to progress the foot programme, and simple foot-eye coordination drills commenced.

On day 10 the sutures were removed and wounds had healed. A pool strengthening programme was started with plyometric jumps and advanced to a leg-press machine doing 'throw-offs'. A progressive linear sprinting programme was started while continuing with the progressive strengthening programme.

Day 14 introduced multi-directional running drills, plyometric drills on the floor and general agility drills on a step machine and on the field.
At week 3 football specific drills were added to the programme, as well as progressive plyometric drills.
By week 4 he was cleared for full training with his team. Return to play approval was based on a combination of pre-season screening measurements compared to advanced football specific drills. He was able to commence play after five weeks.
He successfully continued play, but unfortunately in July 2015 had an injury to the right knee which proved to be a root attachment tear of the posterior horn of the medial meniscus.

Lessons learnt

1. In a patient diagnosed with an inflammatory disease, not all symptoms and signs attributes to the chronic disease.
2. The response to rehabilitation for a player with controlled disease is the same as for a player with no disease.
3. Contrary to popular belief, patients suffering from seronegative arthritis can participate in high level sport if the disease is well controlled.

References

1. MacMillan G. Sport Science Lab. Internet: c2016. Available from: http://www.sportsciencelab.com/training-programs
2. Myers TW. Anatomy trains: myofascial meridians for manual and movement therapists. Elsevier, Philadelphia, 2014

RETURN OF A LOW ADHERENCE TO TREATMENT GOALKEEPER WITH OSTEOCHONDRITIS IN BRAZIL

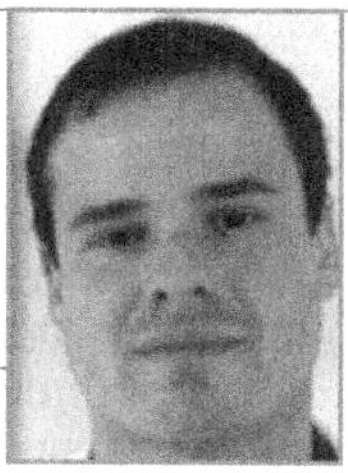

Dorilêo CGLF, Pedrinelli A, Youssef M

Hospital das Clínicas, University of São Paulo, São Paulo, Brazil

Methods

In September of 2014, a eleven years old Male Football Goalkeeper had his first consult in the sports medicine ambulatory because of a insidious pain in the medial side of the left knee, that lasts for two years, worsening in the last seven months, with functional limitation and decrease of sports performance (had to left a competition). The patient deny joint effusion, instability, trauma, fractures or previous injury in the left knee. His Physical Exam was: anthropometrical characteristics: aligned lower limbs, semi-flexion of the knees, bilateral shortening of the hamstrings, valgus of the Rearfoot; left knee: normal Range Of Motion (ROM) static and dynamic valgus, ligaments and meniscus tests negative, pain on palpation in the articular line and medial tibial plateau, absence of joint edema, Wilson Test and Wilson Sign positive (3), gait with external rotation of the affected limb. The patient had a RX of the left knee (showing only an Osteoma in Proximal Fibula) and a Computadorized Tomography, with a 15 mm fragment in the Medial Femoral Condile, suggestive of Osteochondritis Dissecans (OCD) in the most prevalent site (2). The first consult conduct: solicited limb scanometry, laboratory exams, RX exam for bone age determination and Magnetic Resonance Imaging (MRI) the patient was not cleared for any sports activity until the results of the exams, and it was said to the parents of the patient that if OCD would be confirmed, it was fundamental to success in the healing process a good adherence (1) to the conservative treatment (initial rest, with no weight bearing and physical therapy). After two weeks, the patient returned, with the results: normal scanometry and laboratory exams, bone age of 11 years old and on the sagittal scan of the MRI it was seen a fragment in the Medial Femoral Condile, diagnostic confirmed by the gold standard exam: OCD, it was decided that the treatment would be conservative.
Initially six weeks with no bearing and physical therapy with monthly reevaluation, it was explained that the duration of the conservative treatment is not cleared established, but, it should not last for more than six months, and it success is strongly associated with a good adherence (3). The physical therapy started in the facilities of the Medical Department of his Football team (three sessions of 1.5 hour weekly, analgesy with Transcutaneous Electrical Nerve Stimulator (TENS) and ice, stretching and isometric strengthening) and one session of 3 hours of swimming pool weekly (deep running, stretching and strengthening exercises, sportive gest, balance and proprioception exercises). Two weeks after that, the patient returned with good evolution, with no pain in the daily activities, and a new consult was scheduled in four weeks. Despite the return scheduled in the first week of November, because of force majeure, the goalkeeper just returned in our ambulatory after the summer, saying that after November it was not possible to do the physical therapy in his team facilities, and he did some physical therapy with his sister, who was a physiotherapist, in a public square form November until 10th of March (four months after the scheduled meeting, with a total time of five months of diagnostic), the day that the patient returned with a new MRI and solicited a consult, scheduled one week after that.

On 17th of march of 2015, the patient was totally asymptomatic, with the physical exam of left knee showing normal ROM, no pain in the articular line, Wilson test and sign negative. The MRI of February showed a healing process of the OCD. It was solicited RX in the tunnel view antero-posterior and lateral, which were normal. In this day, it was determined the return to play: training sessions (cardio respiratory exercises and specific exercises for goalkeeper) twice a week, with one game in the weekend (not cleared for more sports activities than that) and return in four weeks. Patient returned after one month totally asymptomatic, totally cleared for training sessions and competitive football in April of 2015 with seven months of conservative treatment. In may, another control RX of the left knee was made, because of the osteoma in Fibula, the patient remains in clinical segment in our sports medicine department.

References

1. Kessler JI, Nikizad H, Shea KG, Jacobs JC Jr, Bebchuk JD, Weiss JM. The demographics and epidemiology of osteochondritis dissecans of the knee in children and adolescents. Am J Sports Med 2014; 42: 320-326
2. Mestriner LA. Osteochondritis Dissecans of the knee: diagnostic and treatment. Rev Bras Ortop 2012; 47: 553-562
3. Wilson JN. A diagnostic sign in osteochondritis dissecans of the knee. J Bone Joint Surg Am 1967; 49: 477-480

3

A CASE OF CHONDROSARCOMA OF RIB IN A PROFESSIONAL FOOTBALL PLAYER

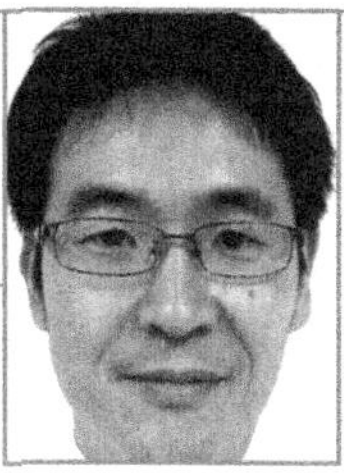

Fukui T[1], Fujita I[2], Harada T[1]

[1]Department of Orthopaedic Surgery, Hyogo Prefectural Kakogawa Medical Center, Kakogawa; [2]Department of Orthopaedic Surgery, Hyogo Prefectural Cancer Center, Akashi, Japan

Our department has been in charge of medical care of a professional football team in J1 League (top league of football in Japan). Medical checks are performed to survey general condition for all players every season and consist of blood examinations, a chest X-ray, an electrocardiography, and an echocardiography, the purpose of those is mainly to rule our heart diseases. We experienced a rare case of chondrosarcoma of rib found out by the medical check. The objective of this paper is to report the treatment and return to football about this case.
The patient was 31-year-old male and had no particular medical history. An abnormal shadow was indicated in his chest X-ray, therefore additional chest Computed Tomography (CT) was performed to show that the proximal part of right 8th rib was thin and roundly expanded measuring 5 cm diameter. Irregular calcification was noted inside the lesion. On Magnetic Resonance Imaging (MRI), the mass lesion showed iso-intensity on T1-weighted images and iso- to high-intensity on T2-weighted images, and was partially enhanced by gadolinium.
CT-guided core needle biopsy was performed and the tumor was diagnosed low grade chondrosarcoma. The patient underwent wide resection of the lesion with a proximal part of the right 8th rib and the right 7th and 8th intercostal nerve. The final histological diagnosis was chondrosarcoma grade 1.
The player started jogging two weeks after the surgery and returned to full training eigth weeks after the surgery. However, pain in his back was caused by a contact with another player few days later. After continuing rehabilitation, he returned to full training again at four months after the surgery and played in a League match at five months after the surgery.
Three years passed after the surgery and there was no evidence of recurrence or metastasis of the tumor in follow-up imaging examinations, and he keeps playing football as a professional player in domestic highest level.
We found two complications during the follow-up. One was weakness and decreased contraction of Rectus Abdominis and Oblicuus Abdominis muscles. This was supposed to be induced by resection of intercostal nerves which control those muscles. The other was a fatigue fracture of the right 7th rib. It was indicated after full return to play and treated by Low Intensity Pulsed Ultrasound (LIPUS) to complete union. This fracture could be speculated to occur with relating to increased load on adjacent rib of the resected 8th rib.
Intercostal nerve can be used as nerve graft in clinical setting of orthopaedic surgery, however it is unusual the patients complain about the weakness of abdominal muscles and it can be recognized as a particular complication to top athletes. Similarly, a fatigue fracture of rib is not common complication following rib resection and might have happened because the current case is a professional sports player.
Malignant tumor arising in a professional football player is an extremely rare case and it is difficult to get sufficient information about return time to play and whether return to play is possible or not, therefore the contents of this report would be meaningful.

LISFRANC INJURY REPAIR WITH THE TIGHTROPE AND THE CHARLOTTE TARGETING DEVICE

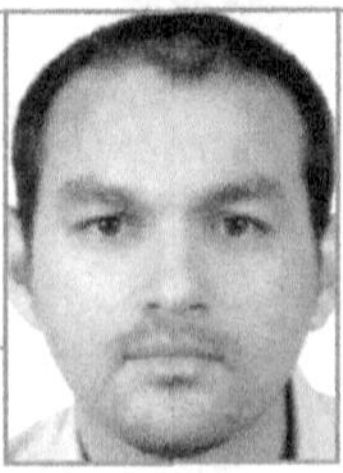

Drampalos E, Clough TM

Department of Orthopaedic Surgery, Wrightington Hospital, Wigan, United Kingdom

Introduction

Lisfranc injuries are rare, but can be catastrophic for the professional elite player, ending their career. They need accurate early diagnosis, anatomical reduction and robust stabilization.
Various surgical treatments exist, with stabilization using screws, bridging plates, wires and primary Lisfranc fusion. Screw stabilization has the drawback of a second operation to remove metalwork (1), potentially delaying return back to the game or risking slow progressive subsequent re-displacement. Dorsal bridging plate has the advantage of not breaching any joint with metalwork, but is bulky on top of the foot, in the area where most footballers strike the ball and can also cause extensor tendon tethering. Use of K-wires, has generally been abandoned. Primary fusion is reported, but return to play is limited with this technique.
Stabilization with a suture button (TightRope, Arthrex, Inc, Naples, Fl, USA) has only been previously reported in two case series but not in the elite football setting (2, 3). It offers advantages of a more physiologic, less rigid mode of fixation and the unlikely need for re-operation to remove metalwork (3). The use of the Tightrope device, with concomitant use of a Targeting guide, the Charlotte Lisfranc Reconstruction System (Targeting Device and Guide Wire, Wright Medical Group, Inc, Memphis, USA) has not been reported. The authors feel this technique offers more accurate positioning of the suture button avoiding multiple drilling or fracture. The purpose of our study was to confirm the advantages of the above technique in an elite football player.

Methods, Results

A 19 year old male professional (English Championship) football player (defender) sustained an axial load, hyper plantar flexion injury to the foot during a match. He suffered immediate pain and had to come off. He underwent RICE (Rest, Ice, Compression, Elevation) therapy, assessment and initial investigation with an Magnetic Resonance Imaging (MRI) scan, followed by Computed Tomography (CT) scan. This confirmed rupture of the Lisfranc ligament, widening and displacement across the Lisfranc zone. Surgery was recommended.
Under general anesthesia with a tourniquet, a dorsal incision over the Lisfranc zone was made, debris removed and the area anatomically reduced. The Targeting Device (Charlotte Lisfranc Reconstruction System) was applied, holding the reduction and allowing accurate placement of a guide wire, which was then over drilled under fluoroscopic control. The TightRope was pulled through the drill hole engaging the lateral wall of the second metatarsal base and the medial wall of the medial cuneiform. Dynamic assessment was performed to determine stability. In this case, there was additional instability through the intercuneiform joints and consequently a second Tightrope placed across medial to intermediate cuneiform, stabilizing them. Further dynamic checks confirmed full stability. Post operatively a backslab was applied and the patient mobilized on crutches non weight bearing for 2 weeks. Following wound review at two weeks, the foot was placed into a below knee removable boot. Physiotherapy was commenced, with active and passive range of movement exercises and light Theraband activities, but the patient was continued non weight bearing for a further

four weeks. Chemical thromboprophylaxis was maintained for six weeks. At six weeks, radiology confirmed a reduced Lisfranc joint. He was then allowed progressive weight bearing in the boot, but no weight bearing out of boot. At 10 weeks radiology again confirmed a reduced Lisfranc zone. Clinically there was no tenderness over the area. He was then allowed to discard the boot, commence a progressive, nonimpact graduated resistance programme (but including AlterG). As he hit target specific goals, running was introduced (13-14 weeks). By 15 weeks, he had progressed with running, had started cutting and twisting and was ready to commence ball work. The patient returned to full match play at 20 weeks.

Conclusions

The authors believe the TightRope device with the concomitant use of the Charlotte targeting device (which has not been reported), allows for accurate intra-operative positioning of the suture button avoiding multiple drilling, provides robust stabilization even in high demands of the professional football setting, and has the advantage of not requiring further surgery for removal, speeding up return to play.

References

1. Deol RS, Roche A, Calder JD. Return to training and plating after acute Lisfranc injuries in elite professional soccer and rugby players. Am J Sports Med 2016; 44: 166-170
2. Brin YS, Nyska M, Kish B. Lisfranc injury repair with the Tightrope device: a short-term case series. Foot Ankle Int 2010; 31: 624-627
3. Charlton T, Boe C, Thordarson DB. Suture button fixation treatment of chronic Lisfranc injury in professional dancers and high-level athletes. J Dance Med Sci 2015; 19: 135-139

A 22 YEAR'S OLD NATIONAL TEAM FOOTBALL PLAYER WITH INCREASING ATRAUMATIC ANKLE PAIN

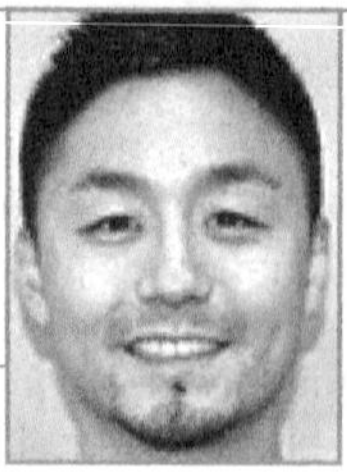

Shimakawa T, D'Hooghe P

Aspetar Hospital, Aspire Zone, Doha, Qatar

Case report

A 22 year-old professional and National Team football player presented with fierce anterior ankle pain.

He was unable to play and experienced complaints during normal daily activities. No recent trauma to the ankle had occurred that could have elicited the complaints.

The pain started suddenly during training and then gradually worsened until he was completely unable to play and even started limping. It took 2 weeks from the initial pain onset to the first clinical visit. No associated anomalies were present.

Physical examination revealed no anomalies: a (pain-) free Range Of Motion (ROM) as well as normal plantar- and dorsiflexion and negative drawer test.

Conventional radiography of the foot and ankle demonstrated no abnormalities. Due to a clinical mismatch towards standard radiology, a Computed Tomography (CT) scan was made revealing minor radiolucent abnormalities of the talar body suspicious for a minor talar body stress fracture. Hereafter a Magnetic Resonance Imaging (MRI) was made demonstrating the suspected stress fracture/bone infarctus of the talar body.

Based on the MRI the fracture was classified as stable without displacement.

Initially the player was treated conservatively in a short leg Non Weight Bearing (NWB) cast for 4 weeks followed by a walking cast for 4 weeks. 6 weeks after the first MRI was taken -because of worsening pain during the conventional treatment period, a new MRI was made.

Unfortunately, the MRI revealed progressive oedema in the fracture.

Consequently it was decided to perform an arthroscopic-assisted internal compression fixation of the fracture by means of a minimal invasive compression screw fixation (Figure 1).

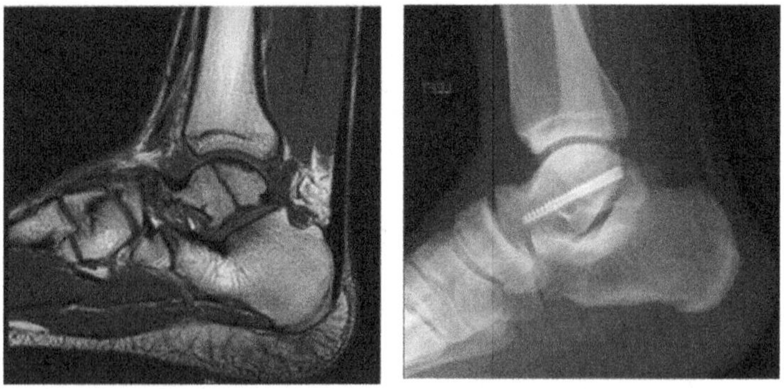

Figure 1. Left: MRI showing progressive oedema in the fracture. Right: fixation of the fracture by means of a minimal invasive compression screw fixation.

Post operatively the patient was placed in a NWB cast for 2 weeks and a Partial Weight Bearing (PWB) walker boot for 4 more weeks.
Physiotherapy was started after cast removal and full weight bearing was allowed starting from 6 weeks postoperatively. From the start of week 8 postoperatively, he started training individually with a progressive rehabilitation protocol for 4 more weeks. Three months post-surgery he returned to the pitch playing at his pre-injury level, he was pain free and showing a full range of ankle motion.

Discussion

Stress fractures are the most common overuse injuries in athletes, however talar body are rare (2, 3). In athletes, especially football player in case, significant pathogenic movements predisposing to a talar stress fracture can be identified in the repetitive restricted axial loading while sprinting, kicking the ball or landing after a heading attempt. The load that has to be absorbed during these actions created by the ground impact, the extremes in plantar- /dorsiflexion of the foot (kicking the ball) and other traumatic actions should be considered important pathogenic factors in repetitive ankle injuries. Stress fractures are known for their prolonged healing period (1). The described case can be classified as a Hawkins type 1 fracture. These fractures have a good prognosis as the risk of avascular necrosis is less than 15%. As shown in the presented case, proper positioning can be achieved by means of a relative non-invasive intervention, meaning an arthroscopic-assisted minimal invasive internal fixation with a compression screw. It is unknown why the oedema between the two talar particles progressed after the initial good alignment treated with cast immobilization. A possible explanation for the increased oedema may lie in the prolonged immobilization period as this is known to increase osteopenia. Also, movement of the foot in the cast or walking with the cast could be a cause of the oedema progression. In this case however the patient stated he did not walk while wearing the cast and he was found to be compliant by his team staff. A case report of a player with secondary progression of such a fracture is presented.

Conclusions

This is a report of a stress fracture/bone infarctus of the talar body with secondary progression after initial conservative treatment. It is important to keep it in mind in case of a primarily undisplaced fracture which is treated conservatively, as apparently secondary progression, even in an immobilized patient, may occur.
If a high demand athlete presents with a talar body stress fracture, an immediate operative fixation is indicated. The return to play time is considered crucial in this player's profile and no initial wait and see.
The importance of this case is to alert the team physicians that talar body stress fractures/bone infarctus in an elite football player, with a visible fracture line on T1 images, need immediate operative fixation in order to achieve a perfectly feasible and appropriate return to elite play.

References

1. Kaeding CC, Yu JR, Wright R, Amendola A, Spindler KP. Management and return to play of stress fractures. Clin J Sport Med 2005; 15: 442-447
2. Motto SG. Stress fracture of the talar body. Clin J Sport Med 1996; 6: 278-279
3. Rossi F, Dragoni S. Talar body fatigue stress fractures: three cases observed in elite female gymnasts. Skeletal Radiol 2005; 34: 389-394

EXTRAORDINARY CAUSE OF HIP JOINT PAIN IN A PROFESSIONAL FOOTBALL PLAYER

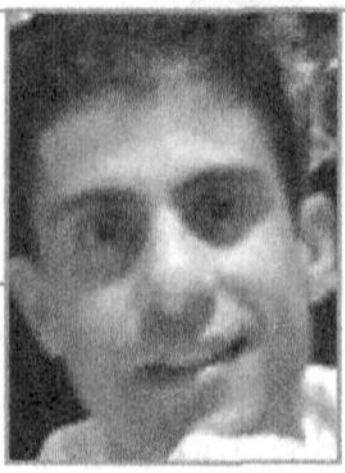

Tzoanos G[1], Tsavalas N[1], Manidakis N[1], Chardaloumbas D[1], Kalliakmanis A[2]

[1]Tzoanos Sports Clinic, Heraklion, Crete; [2]Athens Medical Center, Athens, Greece

Introduction

Hip pain in athletes is a common entity. Associated symptoms frequently can be attributed to hip labral tears, adductor strain, pubic osteitis or sports hernia. Magnetic Resonance Imaging (MRI) is indicated to differentiate the pathology. Although rare, osteoid osteoma should be included in the differential diagnosis of hip pain in football players. We present a case of a professional football player with a benign bone tumour (osteoid osteoma) in the hip.

Case report

A 24-year-old male, professional football player, suffered from right hip pain for approximately three months before consulting our sports clinic. He had persistent pain while playing and pain at night. There was no history of trauma, surgery or previous right hip problems, and no mechanical symptoms were reported. The pain located at the lateral aspect of the hip and groin and described as sharp and constant. Sporting activities including playing worsened the pain. Physiotherapy and Diclofenac failed to offer relief and his pain had progressed during the past three months, resulting in referral to our sports clinic.

On examination, his right hip showed reduced passive internal rotation due to pain. Provocative tests for labral hip tears, adductor strain, pubic osteitis and sports hernia, conditions were negative. Examination of the spine and knee was unremarkable.

A Computer Tomography (CT) and Magnetic Resonance Imaging (MRI) reformatted views showing the cortical lytic lesion, the mineralized central nidus (white arrow) and the surrounding sclerosis (Figure 1).

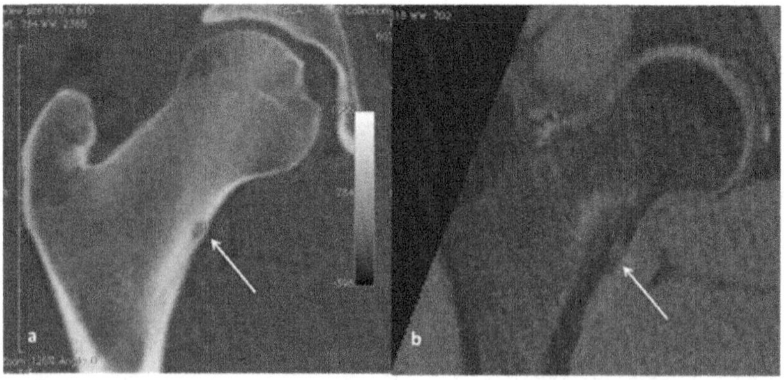

Figure 1. Computed Tomography (a) and Magnetic Resonance Imaging (b) reformatted views showing the cortical lytic lesion, the mineralized central nidus (white arrow) and the surrounding sclerosis

There are various modalities for available for the treatment of osteoid osteoma ranging from oral Nonsteroidal Anti-Inflammatory Drugs (NSAIDs), radiofrequency ablation to surgical excision. The results of treatment vary between reports. Our choice of our treatment option was CT-guided radiofrequency ablation due to the availability of the treatment, reported efficacy and minimal complications associated with the procedure.
The procedure was performed without any complications. The player was allowed to return to football training within 3 weeks after the CT-guided radiofrequency ablation. His training scheme was initially reduced in intensity, full intensity training was progressively introduced over the following three weeks. He was able to fully participate in training and play matches without limitations after six weeks.

Conclusions

Osteoid osteoma is a benign bone tumour in the hip, often seen in an adolescence male, but rare in football players. A classic symptom is night pain relieved by Aspirin. Radiographic appearance of nidus surrounded by thick sclerotic margin is diagnostic. Localising the lesion key in the management of this condition. MRI and CT are the gold standard diagnostic tools.
Full symptomatic and functional recovery within six weeks after CT-radiofrequency ablation of osteoid osteoma of the hip can be expected.

REHABILITATION AND RETURN TO PLAY OF A PROFESSIONAL FOOTBALLER FOLLOWING CONSERVATIVE MANAGEMENT OF LUMBAR SPINE DISC HERNIATION

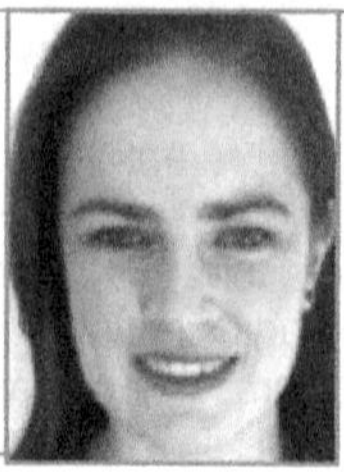

Toolan AM [1,2,3]

[1]Hospital for Special Surgery, FIFA Center of Medical Excellence, New York;
[2]New York City Football Club, New York; [3]United States Soccer Federation, USA

The patient was a 30 year old professional male soccer player, who is 1.93 m tall and a member of the Greek National team. He presented after six months of acute-on-chronic low back pain, due to lumbar disc herniations at the L4/L5 and L5/S1 levels. Prior to undergoing conservative management at our institution, Hospital for Special Surgery, he had two epidural injections and several courses of physical therapy, which were unsuccessful in resolving his low back and posterior thigh pain symptoms.

A physical therapy evaluation was performed three days following epidural steroid injection at the L5 and S1 nerve root levels. Of note on initial evaluation, the athlete had a general fear of movement, especially lumbar flexion, and was severely limited in all lumbar and thoracic spine movements. His Fear Avoidance Beliefs Questionnaire (FABQ) and Oswestry Disability Index (ODI) scores were high at 52/66 and 82% respectively. He demonstrated a +Straight Leg Raise (SLR) and +Slump tests for dural tension. He had significant para-spinal muscle guarding, a flattened lumbar lordosis with an associated posterior pelvic tilt, +Thomas test for hip flexor and quadriceps tightness, decreased hamstrings flexiblity, poor deep abdominal strength, measured at Level 1b on the Sahrmann stabilization scale. He had mild myotonal weakness (4-/5) of the L4, L5 and S1 innervated muscle groups.

Treatment strategies employed following initial evaluation were the McKenzie mechanical diagnosis and treatment technique, involving repeated and prolonged lumbar spine extension for symptom reduction. Thoracic and lumbar spine mobilization and manipulation techniques were applied, as well as active release therapy and Graston technique to address soft tissue restrictions. Pelvic floor and deep abdominal stabilization training was commenced, as well as isolated strengthening to address his proximal hip weakness. When lower extremity strength was 5/5 on manual muscle testing, underwater and anti-gravity treadmill training were commenced.

At four weeks post-injection, he demonstrated a 20° improvement in his lumbar spine flexion, as measured by spinal inclinometer, a 10° improvement in thoracic rotation bilaterally. His SLR test was (-) for dural tension and through education and positive reinforcement of movements and activities he has previously feared, his FABQ score was reduced dramatically to 29/66.

At 8 weeks post-injection, his lumbar and thoracic spine ranges of motion were within normal limits. He could squat symmetrically without pain, and his lower extremity flexiblity was grealty improved. His deep abdominal strength measured at Sahrmann Level IIIb. He underwent a gradual return to soccer-specific activities, in a program which specifically targeted ever-increasingly complex spine movements and loading.

13 weeks into his rehabilitation program, this player demonstrated full Active Range of Motion (AROM) of his lumbar and thoracic spine, 5/5 LE strength including hip abduction and extension, excellent deep abdominal core strength and endurance, and a greatly reduced fear of re-injury (FABQ 12/66; ODI 8%). A single leg hop test for power revealed his leg strength of the initially weaker left leg was 94% of his uninvolved side. At this time-point, he was able to participate fully in training, without any recurrence of low back or leg pain symptoms, with a professional club team in New York with the goal of earning a new contract. He was discharged from the care of this physical therapist with a spinal mobility and core strength maintenance program.

Conclusions

1. Understand the necessity of identifying fear avoidance behaviors and kinesiophobia in footballers with chronic pain, and treatment strategies for this troubling phenomenon.
2. Principles involved in conservative management and rehabilitation of an athlete following lumbar disc herniation (1, 2, 3).
3. Highlighting the importance of addressing the entire kinetic chain in a footballer with low back pain.
4. Recognize the dynamic demands of the game of soccer on the core and spine, and therefore be able to replicate the required movements as part of a progressive rehabilitation program.

References

1. Reiman MP, Sylvain J, Loudon JK, Goode A. Return to sport after open and microdiscectomy surgery versus conservative treatment for lumbar disc herniation: a systematic review with meta-analysis. Br J Sports Med Br J Sports Med. 2016; 50: 221-230
2. Watkins RG. Great rehabilitation and great physical bodies allow professional athletes undergoing lumbar discectomy to return to sport at a high rate. Spine J 2011; 11: 187-189
3. Wellington KH, McCarthy KJ, Savage JW, Roberts DW, Roc GC, Micev AJ, Terry MA, Gryzlo SM, Schafer MF. The professional athlete spine initiative: outcomes after lumbar disc herniation in 342 elite professional athletes. Spine J 2011; 11: 180-186

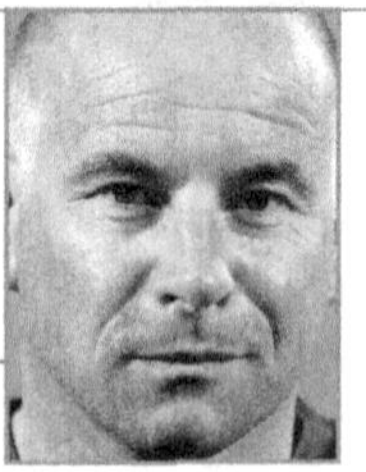

ILIAC CREST AVULSION FRACTURE IN IMMATURE ELITE SOCCER PLAYER: A STOCHASTIC RETURN TO PLAY

Materne O[1], Robertson D[2]

[1]Aspire Academy, Health Centre, NSMP, Doha; [2]Qatar Football Association, Doha, Qatar

Introduction

Avulsion fractures are a common injury in skeletally immature elite athletes. Iliac crest avulsion fracture is recognized to be an unusual pelvis pathology, and there is a lack of published studies describing a comprehensive rehabilitation process (2). In youth elite soccer development, a variety of different parameters need to be take into account when considering optimal rehabilitation and return to play; these include clinical and functional progressions. In addition, maturation, motor-learning (3), player profile, soccer and match characteristics (1) are also key considerations. This case study describes a Return To Play (RTP), through conservative management of an iliac crest avulsion fracture in an elite adolescent soccer player, in a differential learning model.

Case report

A 16 year old male centre-back soccer player, early maturer (age at injury: 16.4 yrs.; Peak Height Velocity, PHV, onset: +2.46 yrs; bone age: 17.6 yrs; height: 174.9 cm; trunk height: 92.8 cm; leg length: 82.1 cm, arm span: 183.5 cm, body mass: 70.1kg; BMI: 22.9 kg/m^2; skinfolds: 43.9 mm). The injury occurred while playing soccer, a sudden sharp and severe pain onset at the left lateral pelvic (standing leg) at the moment of executing a long cross of the ball to the left, with his right leg. There was immediate inability to full weight-bear. At the emergency hospital, X-ray (Figure 1) revealed an avulsion fracture (7 mm laterally displaced) of the whole anterior portion of the left iliac crest. The Magnetic Resonance Imaging (MRI) confirmed the extent of the iliac crest damage, located at the growth plate.

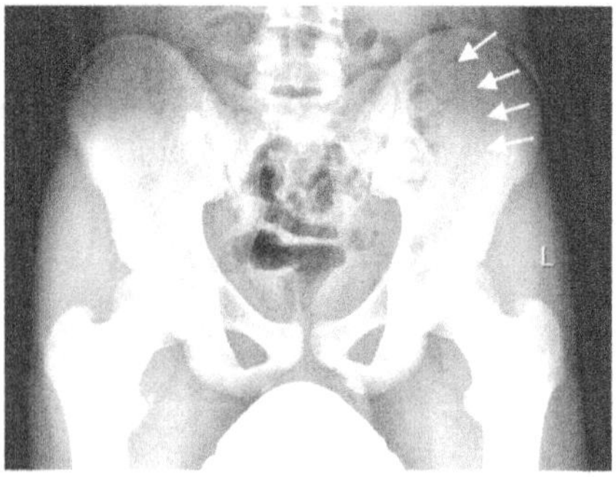

Figure 1. X-Ray frontal view of the pelvis showing the avulsion fracture of the left (L) iliac crest.

Therapeutic intervention

The rehabilitation design has been a five stages plan (Table 1). A lumbosacral molded bracing orthosis, wrapping around both iliac crest, has been custom-made and was worn for four weeks by the player. This consisted of three weeks in Partial Weight Bearing (PWB) on crutches, and one week (pain-free) in Full Weight Bearing (FWB). Physical therapy started at stage 2, with postural synergy exercises at a low-threshold, between the Involved Muscles (IM) associated with the iliac crest (Transversus Abdominis, External and Internal Oblique, Quadratus Lumborum, Gluteus Medius, Tensor Fasciae Latae, Sartorius, Iliacus).

STAGES	1	2	3	4	5
Weeks	1 to 2	3-4	5-8	9 to 10	11 to 16
Main Objectives	Healing stage	Introduction to passive, dynamic and synergy postural work	Functional rehabilitation	Return to train	Return to play and follow-up
Lumbosacral brace	Yes	Yes	No	No	No
Weight Bearing	Crutches (NWB to PWB)	Crutches (week 3) (PWB to FWB)	FWB	FWB	FWB
Number of sessions	0	6	26	16	28
Sessions per week	0	3+3	5+6+7+8	8+8	0+10+8+6
Total hours	0	7	26	18	27
Hours per week	0	2.5+4.5	5.0+6.0+7.5 +7.5	8+10	0+12+10+5
Rehabilitation aim	Full rest, regular review and monitoring	LT postural control, synergy of involved muscles (no rotation)	HT postural control, synergy of involved muscles (resistance and rotation)	Recover sports specific movements. Field rehabilitation	Field rehabilitation Progressive re-insertion to the team
Rehabilitation objectives	-	ROM and stretching	ROM, stretching Functional Movement Strength	Coordination, speed, agility, re-introduce ball and soccer tasks	Team involvement and position specific demand
Type of muscles contraction (IM)	-	Postural isometric and eccentric (Vs. gravity)	Isometric, eccentric and concentric (Vs. external load)	Multi contraction in all motion	High energy specific multi contraction
Differential learning	-	Introduction to differential model	Low level of variability and CONT INT	High level of variability in low CONT INT	High level of variability and CONT INT
Cardio	-	NWB (e.g. bike)	Biking, Aqua-jogging Running	Running	Running
Game & playing position characteristics	-	-	Low intensity < 13.0 km/h) High-intensity 13.1 to 16 km/h	Very high-intensity 16.1 to 19 km/h Sprinting > 19.1 km/h Biomechanics constraint	All different intensity and characteristics.
Aqua therapy (hours)	-	1.5 hours	6 hours	3 hours	-

Table 1. Synopsis of the 5 stages rehabilitation and return to play progression. NWB: No Weight Bearing; PWB: Partial Weight Bearing; FWB: Full Weight Bearing; LT: Low Threshold; HT: High Threshold; ROM: Range of Motion; IM: Involved Muscles; Differential learning: movement constraint imposed during rehabilitation & field rehab; CONT INT: Contextual interference: the effect on learning of the degree of functional interference found in a practice situation when several tasks must be learned and are practiced together.

Stage 3 initiated more functional progress with isometric, eccentric and concentric strengthening of the IM, including external load and rotation. Match performance characteristics (total game distance, different intensity of running, biomechanics constraint) helped optimise the rehabilitation process. Player profile data was used as well (maximal aerobic speed, position-specific demand). All was integrated into a differential learning model, involving acyclic, random variability of constrains, and decision making.
A conservative approach was chosen, as the literature suggests surgery only when the displacement of the fragment is ≥2 cm (2). Youth soccer development is a unique environment, with ongoing skill acquisitions, in which young players are improving their physical abilities throughout growth and maturation. Moreover, match running performance characteristics have been shown to be affected by age and playing position (1). Indeed, the rehabilitation team should acknowledge that the playing level of the team which the injured player is rejoining, is likely to be higher than the pre-injury standard. Lastly, stochastic perturbation (training with larger movement variations) produced a greater performance in two football tasks; this produced higher retention than the traditional model, which uses more monotonous repetitions of movements (3).

Conclusions

In this case the growth plate was not yet completely fused, and the MRI still showed signs of apophysitis. Nevertheless, the player recovered fully, and participated again at international level 3.5 months later without pain or recurrence after 6 months. Implementation of a differential learning model that takes into account match and individual characteristics in rehabilitation, may enhance the RTP and support clinical decision making, in youth elite soccer.

References

1. Buchheit M, Mendez-Villanueva A, Simpson B, Bourdon P. Match Running Performance and Fitness in Youth Soccer. Int J Sports Med 2010; 31: 818-825.
2. Porr J, Lucaciu C, Birkett S. Avulsion fractures of the pelvis – a qualitative systematic review of the literature. J Can Chiropr Assoc 2011; 55: 247-252
3. SchÖllhorn W, Hegen P, Davids K. The nonlinear nature of learning. A differential learning approach. Open Sports Sciences J 2012; 5 (Suppl 1-M11): 100-112

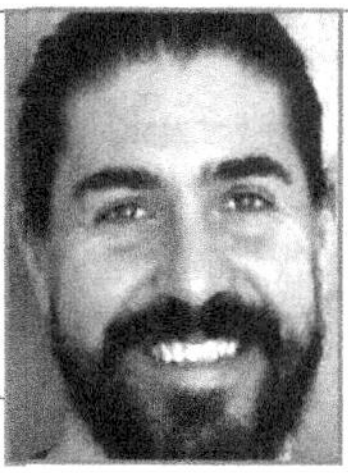

RETURN TO PLAY OF A PROFESSIONAL FEMALE FOOTBALL PLAYER AFTER EIGHTY REHABILITATION DAYS

Angius M[1], Volpi P[2], Pinna M[1]

[1]Kiness Physiotherapy Center, Sassari;
[2]Istituto Clinico Humanitas, Rozzano (Milan), Italy

Introduction

The Anterior Cruciate Ligament (ACL) injury is one of the most common, devas¬tating and serious knee injuries in athletes, in particular in the Pro-soccer female players (1).
Recent reports have provided new information understanding ACL injury and the prevention and rehabilitation of the injury. Anterior translation of the tibia is the primary mechanism of the injury. The kind of differences in movement patterns are likely due to differences in training and skill levels. Rehabilitation of the reconstructed knee is critical for the successful return to risky cutting and jumping activities. New rehabilitation and prevention programs need to be developed to improve compliance to prevention programs. Movement patterns may need to be evaluated in actual football game conditions (2).
Return to full athletic activity after Anterior Cruciate Ligament (ACL) reconstruction is the goal for patients and for rehabilitation staff. The decision on when and if patients can return to competition is based on different tests and criteria (1).
Athlete homecoming to play is often dictated by graft stability (anterior posterior tibiofemoral motion), patient confidence, post surgical timeline, and subjective medical team opinion. At the time more conservative therapeutic approaches may limit progression to later stages of rehabilitation and possibly delay successful return to sport.

Case report

The aim of this Case Report was to show how an elite female professional soccer player can return in the Major Italian Football League eighty days after ACL reconstruction by Semitendinosus Tendon (ST). At the time of operation she was a midfield player of the Italian National Team soccer. The anthropometrical characteristics of this Caucasian player were: height 160 cm and weight 53 kg, and she was 28 years old. She had the characteristics of power athletes. After surgery, the patient started the rehabilitation program with a home based exercises program for core stability. Five days after surgery she started with an early weight-bearing without braces and closed kinetic chain exercises. After 10 days she started with a swimming pool conditioning program and continued with closed kinetic chain exercises and metabolic conditioning on the rehabilitation gym.
The first run was played on a treadmill after 45 days. The first official match was after 80 days. The football player suitability was determinated after less than 80 days after surgery. We based the rehabilitation program on functional criteria from a systematic review of ACL literature (1, 2, 3): continuous passive motion, rehabilitative bracing, neuromuscular electrical stimulation, early weight-bearing, home versus supervised physical therapy, open versus closed chain kinetic exercise programs, accelerated rehabilitation and a variety of miscellaneous tools. We worked in a multilateral functional approach starting from the analysis of the faulty movement patterns that probably had generated the injury (2, 3).
After two years the patient play in the Major Italian Football Leagues without any laxity or ligament or muscles injuries.

Conclusion

This rehabilitation program based on literature evidence and functional goals by a variety of miscellaneous tools, permitted to a professional female soccer player the return to play after 80 days with no complication or muscle or ligament injuries at the two years follow up.

References

1. Alyson F, Byrnes R, Paterno MV, Myer GD, Hewett TE. Neuromuscular training improves performance on the star excursion balance test in young female athletes. J Orthop Sports Phys Ther 2010; 40: 551-558
2. McClure. Accelerated versus non accelerated rehabilitation after anterior cruciate ligament reconstruction. A prospective, randomized, double-blind investigation evaluating knee joint laxity using roentgen stereophotogrammetric analysis. Am J Sports Med 2011; 39: 2536-2548
3. Myer GD, Paterno MV, Ford KR, Quatman CE, Hewett TE. Rehabilitation after anterior cruciate ligament reconstruction: criteria-based progression through the return-to-sport phase. J Orthop Sports Phys Ther 2006; 36: 385-402

MONITORING OF AN ANTERIOR CRUCIATE LIGAMENT INJURY THROUGH INFRARED THERMOGRAPHY

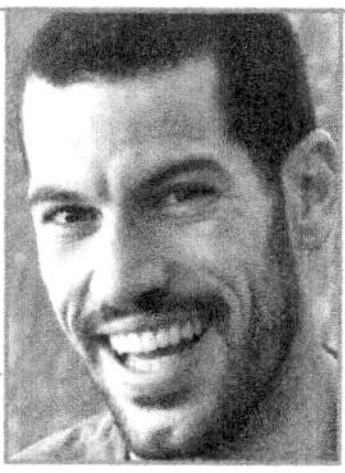

Fernández-Cuevas I, Arnáiz-Lastras J, Sillero-Quintana M

Sports Department, Faculty of Sciences for Physical Activity and Sport (INEF), Technical University of Madrid, Spain

Introduction

Despite the improvement of technology, injuries are still a huge problem for professional football teams, regardless of their budget or reputation. Moreover, injuries are not just a health matter, but also an economic problem for the team, and obviously a factor influencing the individual and team performance. In this work, we present a singular and unique case study about the Anterior Cruciate Ligament (ACL) injury evolution on a football player: from the day before of the injury until the return to play. What makes unique this case study is that during the whole process, the football player was monitored by Infrared Thermography (IRT). IRT is a safe, non-invasive and low-cost technique that allows for the rapid recording of radiating energy that is released from the body. IRT measures this radiation, directly related to skin temperature (Tsk) and has been widely used since the early 1960s in different areas. Recent technical advances in infrared cameras have enhanced new and old applications of IRT on humans (beyond diagnostic techniques). Among others, the prevention and monitoring of injuries has been showed as one of the most interesting and useful applications of this technique.

Case report

The male subject was 22.03 years old, 161.6 cm height and 64.6 kg weight at the time of the injury. He played as midfielder in a third division football team in Spain, training four times a week. The subject was monitored during eight months at least once a week.

Thermal pictures were taken following the directions of most standard protocols (3). For this, the subject remained in an isolated room for at least 10 minutes of acclimation at a temperature average of 20.1±1.31°C and a humidity of 43.8±7.5% recorded by a BAR-908-HG weather station (Oregon Scientific, Portland, USA). All measures were taken in the morning (between 7:20 am and 8:00 a.m.) with a T335 infrared camera (FLIR Systems, Täby, Sweden) and were automatically analysed with ThermoHuman software, extracting the skin temperature asymmetry (ΔT_{sk}) from right and left front knee. Pain perception was measured using a CR10 Borg scale.

The subject suffered a contact fault during a training session on the 24th October 2011 (day 0). Everyone on the field heard a distinctive "crack" coming from his right knee. The team doctor diagnosed an ACL injury Grade 2 that was confirmed the day after in the hospital. At that time, the subject was taking part on a data collection for a PhD study with IRT. The day after the injury, the subject and the authors decided to use IRT to monitor the whole injury evolution.

Before the surgery (from day 12 to 94), the subject followed a progressive programme five days a week with isometric and concentric exercises to prepare the limb muscles and to maintain the physical condition. After the surgery (from day 111 to 242), the rehabilitation programme consisted on a progressive adaptation to gain range of motion, to reduce the inflammation, to strengthen the muscles, to gain ability and confidence. The results can be divided into 3 phases (Figure 1).

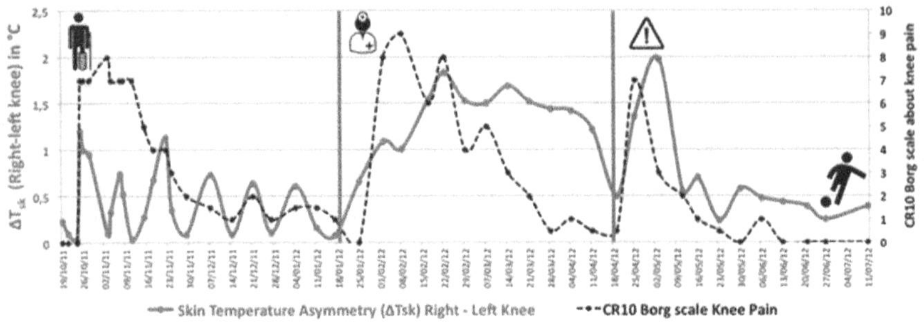

Figure 1. Skin temperature asymmetry (ΔTsk; left side scale) and Pain (CR10; right side scale) evolution after the ACL injury.

Firstly, from the injury to the surgery, we saw a decrease on pain perception and regular ΔT_{sk} variations, from the biggest (+1.20°C on day 1) to the smallest difference (+0.08°C on day 82). Secondly, from the surgery (day 95), we found a similar decrease evolution of pain but a different ΔT_{sk} behaviour, which is maintained during the first weeks of the rehabilitation due to the exercises performed (2). The third phase started some weeks before the return to play (day 175), when the subject felt again a "crack" on his right knee during his first game in a training session. ΔT_{sk} (+1.36°C) and pain increased but fortunately, ACL was not torn again. We restart the rehabilitation, which ended on the 27th June 2012 (day 242) with his first game, and the last one of the season for the team.
As conclusion, IRT results were especially useful regarding the return to play: since Tsk is directly related to the inflammation and muscle activity, it helped both the medical and technical staff to adapt and optimize the rehabilitation process. In addition, the subject described us how IRT helped him to visualize their evolution, and somehow motivated him to move forward despite the relapse (Figure 2).

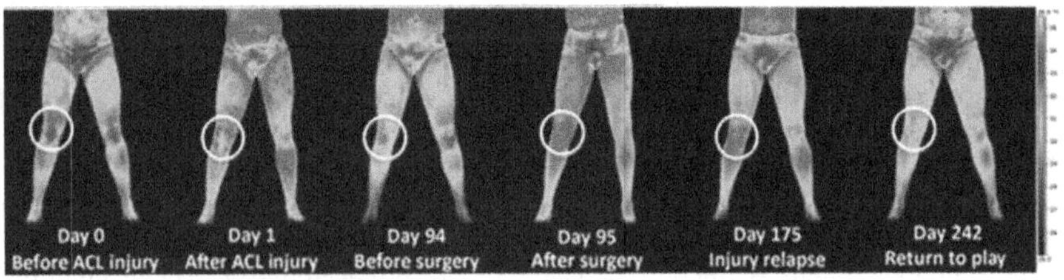

Figure 2. Infrared images of the subject in specific moments from the day before the injury (day 0) to the return to play (day 242).

References

1. Costello J, Stewart IB, Selfe J, Karki AI, Donnelly A. Use of thermal imaging in sports medicine research: a short report. Int Sportmed J 2013; 14: 94-98
2. Piñonosa S, Sillero-Quintana M, Milanović L, Coterón J, Sampedro J. Thermal evolution of lower limbs during a rehabilitation process after anterior cruciate ligament surgery. Kinesiology 2013; 45: 121-129
3. Ring EFJ, Ammer K. The technique of infra-red imaging in medicine. Thermology International 2000; 10: 7-14

A CASE OF SHORTENING THE PREOPERATIVE PERIOD BEFORE ANTERIOR CRUCIATE LIGAMENT RECONSTRUCTION

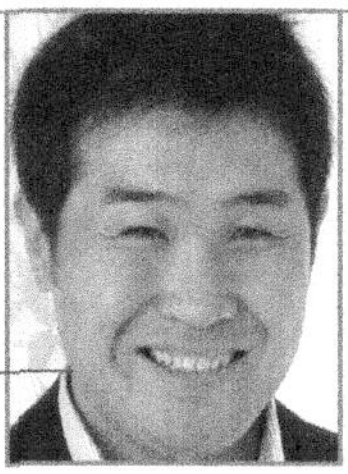

Kinugasa T, Ikeda K

Ichihara Hospital, Tsukuba-shi, Japan

Anterior Cruciate Ligament (ACL) rupture is a common injury, often requiring a significant amount of time (more than six months) for recovery in order to Return To Play (RTP). After one's injury, physicians in Japan often delay immediate treatment in order to prevent arthrofibrosis. Shelbourne reported patients who had an ACL reconstruction operation within seven days of injury had a significant increase in arthrofibrosis compared to those who had surgery after 21 days (1). Several cytokines, such as the platelet-derived growth factor-beta and the transforming growth factor-beta, might be associated with the fibrotic events (2). It is thought that the reduction of inflammation and hemorrhage allows for early operation of ACL reconstruction. To eliminate the risk of an excessively stiff knee, there is the implementation of this early procedure for the ACL rupture cases without any other ligament injuries or complications such as Medial Collateral Ligament (MCL) detected by Magnetic Resonance Imaging (MRI). A 21-year old male midfielder (weight 60 kg, height 163 cm) and member of the university football team, recognized a popping sound in his right knee when performing a cutting maneuver while decelerating. The team trainer performed the RICE (Rest Ice Compression Elevation) procedure on him immediately and informed the hospital physicians of his current physical condition. The next day he had a medical examination in our hospital. The anterior drawer test, the pivot shift test and the Lachman test all came back positive. The KT-1000 was used to measure anterior tibial displacement and differentiation against naive side was 10 mm. We confirmed the ACL rupture and lateral meniscus tear in his knee by MRI. The other ligaments in his leg, including MCL, were intact. He was given Nonsteroidal Anti-Inflammatory Drugs (NSAID) and a cryotherapy unit. Three days after his injury, we performed anatomical outside-in ACL reconstruction with semitendinosus alone. Skin incisions were two 5 mm portal for the arthroscopic procedure, one 5 mm incision for the outside-in procedure and one 3 cm oblique incision to harvest the semitendinosus and make the tibial bone tunnel. A ZipLoop with ToggleLoc (Biomet, Warsaw, USA) and a Double Spiked Plate Tibial Fixation system (Smith & Nephew, Andover, USA) were used for fixation. Tiny flap tear occurred around the posterior horn of lateral meniscus and partial meniscectomy was performed. A tourniquet was not used and total operation time (by two operators) was 84 minutes. After the operation, his knee was fixed with a brace. Seven days later, a hinged ACL brace was attached and a Range Of Motion (ROM) exercise regime was put into place. We allowed 1/2 Partial Weight Bearing (PWB) from postoperative two days and full Weight Bearing (FWB) at 21days. He obtained a full ROM and started jogging after two months, non-contact football practice at Post-Operative Month (POM) five. He returned to the game at POM six. At POM 24, we found his knee fully stabilized and the differentiation of KT-1000 was null. For reduced inflammation and reduced hemorrhage, team trainer's proper implementation of first aid on the fields is necessary. Arrangement for examinations, hospitalization and operation are crucial at an early stage. Effective communication between doctors and trainers saves time in the long run. All members involved should make an effort to bridging any gaps in communication along the way. In our hospital, special devices for knee ligament injury are always on hand, ready to be used to repair or reconstruct ligaments. Hospital staff communication (keeping all members, i.e. orthopedic surgeons, anesthesiologists, radiologists, nurses, etc..., involved and informed at all times) and having the right devices on standby are important for efficient RTP management.

References

1. Shelbourne KD Wilcken JH Mollabashy A DeCarlo M. Arthrofibrosis in acute anterior cruciate ligament reconstruction. The effect of timing of reconstruction and rehabilitation. Am J Sports Med 1991; 19: 332-226
2. Watson RS, Gouze E, Levings PP, Bush ML, Kay JD, Jorgensen MS, Dacanay EA, Reith JW, Wright TW, Ghivizzani SC. Gene delivery of TGF-β1 induces arthrofibrosis and chondrometaplasia of synovium in vivo. Lab Invest 2010; 90: 1615-1627

Sunday 10th April, 2016 (afternoon)
FLEMING ROOM

INVITED SPEAKERS

FUNCTIONAL EXERCISES AND RETURN TO PLAY

Chairs

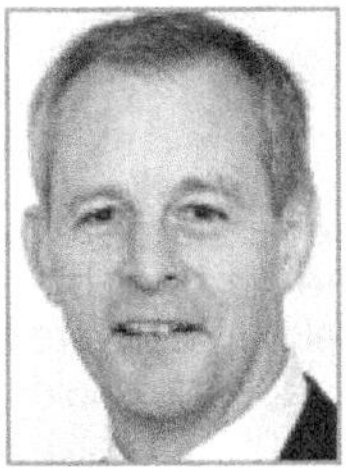

Tim Spalding
(Coventry,
United Kingdom)

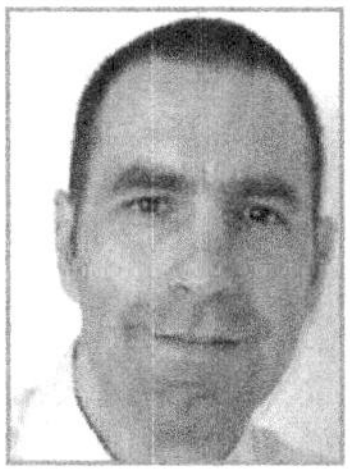

Marco Zanobbi
(London, United Kingdom)

14:30	The foundation of return to play: no pain, no swelling, full ROM **Helen Millson (Ipswich, United Kingdom)**
14:45	The progressive load concept in return to play process **Simone Rivaroli (Milan, Italy)**
15:00	Neuromuscular training in return to play **Tim Hewett (Rochester, USA)**
15:15	Manual therapies and exercise in return to play process **Alessandro Diquigiovanni (Bologna, Italy)**
15:30	Functional training approach: progression from the beginning to return to play **David Clancy (London, United Kingdom)**
15:45	Discussion
16:00	End of the session

THE PROGRESSIVE LOAD CONCEPT IN RETURN TO PLAY PROCESS

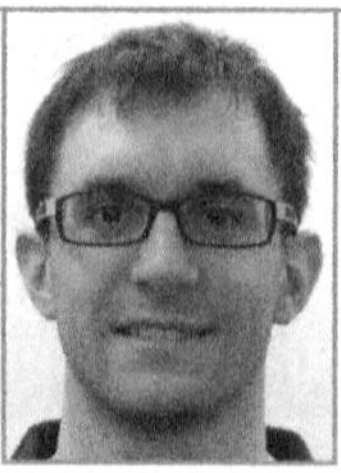

Rivaroli S

Isokinetic Medical Group, FIFA Medical Centre of Excellence, Milan, Italy

We define the load as all the functional, physical, technical, tactical and psychological solicitations that the athlete is subjected to during the process of re-conditioning or training. The progressiveness is one of the main principles to take into consideration for the proper planning of the load.
To better describe the concept of load, it is necessary to analyze the concept of external load (the objective quantification of the tools used during the training) and internal load (the amount of all the stresses and inputs that the body receives when exposed to external load, is strictly subjective) (1).
The study of progressive load in the area of Return To Play (RTP) stems from the necessity to adapt the daily practice to the patient, with the aim of obtaining the needed physical shape to go back to the field. In order to estimate the proper progression of the load in RTP, it is necessary to consider each part constituting the load through the monitoring of every single stimulus (combination of components of the load) and the correct administration of the combination of all stimuli.
In literature have been identified the following constituents of the external load:

- Intensity: amount administered
- Density: ratio between the span of training and the span of recovery.
- Frequency: number of administrations in the timeframe.
- Volume: number of series for repetitions.
- Duration: total of time span of training and time span of recovery.

It is necessary to monitor and quantify the way the athlete reacts to stimuli (monitoring of the internal load). According to the literature, this is possible through objective assessments of the internal loads, such as the monitoring of the heart rate in telemetry, the accumulation of lactate in relation to the increase in the intensity of the exercise (that which is calculated in the threshold test) and the value of oxygen that is consumed in the unit time for muscle contraction ($V'O_{2max}$). The subjective component of the internal load can be monitored, on the other hand, thanks to the scales of perception of effort, such as the Borg scale. With regard to the more rehabilitative approach to the progressiveness of loads, the literature tends to stress the importance of safety criteria that can be divided into two wider categories: the first security category is based on the recovery time necessary between one working session and the following one. This management of loads has to be estimated on the basis of a precise scheduling of the return to sport of the athlete, that which takes into consideration periods of training and recovery with regard to the subject's responses. The second category is represented by the progression through the five phases of rehabilitation. To proceed to the subsequent stages, it is necessary to monitor the proper achievement of the previous ones, so to avoid overloads (2). In conclusion, if the load is administrated appropriately in terms of progressiveness, intensity and specificity also in relation to safe recovery time, it is presumable to obtain long term adaptations and consequently the achievement, maintaining and even improvement of the performance for the return to play of the athlete.

References

1. Impellizzeri FM, Rampinini E, Marcora S. Physiological assessment of aerobic training in soccer. J Sports Sci 2005; 23: 583-592
2. Mithoefer K, Hambly K, Logerstedt D, Ricci M, Silvers H, Della Villa S. Current concepts for rehabilitation and return to sport after knee articular cartilage repair in the athlete. J Orthop Sports Phys Ther 2012; 42: 254-273

EVIDENCE BASED STRATEGIES FOR EFFECTIVE RETURN TO SPORT AFTER ACL RECONSTRUCTION

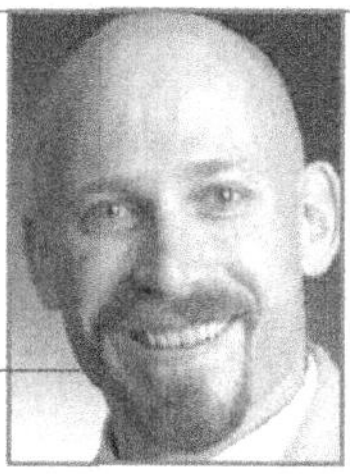

Hewett TE

Mayo Clinic Biomechanics Laboratories, Sports Medicine and Orthopedic Surgery

Reconstruction is the standard of care for athletes who suffer Anterior Cruciate Ligament (ACL) rupture. Most ACL Reconstruction (ACLR) surgery restores mechanical stability of the knee, but post-surgical outcomes vary.

Less than 50% of ACLR athletes return to sport (RTS) within the first year after ACLR, and about 30% of young, active ACLR athletes will go on to a second ACL injury.

The outcomes after a second ACL injury and surgery are significantly worse than outcomes after primary injuries.

As advances in graft reconstruction and fixation techniques improve to restore passive joint stability to the pre-injury level, successful RTS after ACLR is predicated on numerous post-surgical factors. Second ACL injury is strongly correlated to *modifiable* post-surgical risk factors. Biomechanical abnormalities and neuromuscular asymmetries are prevalent in this cohort, can persist despite high function levels, and represent control deficits and imbalances that are associated with second injury.

Decreased neuromuscular control and high risk movement biomechanics, which are heavily influenced by abnormal trunk and lower extremity movement, predict both first and second ACL injury risk.

These findings indicate that abnormal movement biomechanics and neuromuscular control profiles are likely both residual to, and exacerbated by, the initial injury. Evidence Based strategies are necessary to develop effective interventions targeted to these impairments in order to optimize safe return to high-risk activity.

MANUAL THERAPIES AND EXERCISE IN RETURN TO PLAY PROCESS

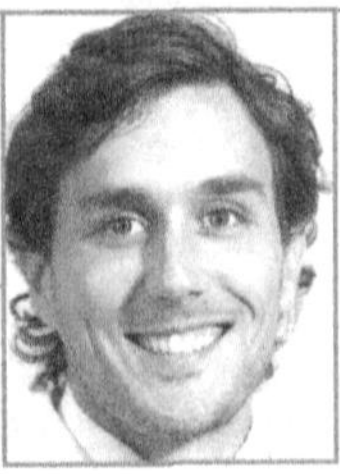

Diquigiovanni A

Isokinetic Medical Group, FIFA Medical Centre of Excellence, Bologna, Italy

There is a growing body of evidence that shows how manual therapies such as chiropractic and osteopathy play a major role in helping professional and amateur football players in the Return to Play (RTP) process. Manual adjustment of an axial or peripheral joint represents a well-documented neuromuscular input. The science behind how such input affects segmental and global neuro-mechanics is certainly more consistent than ever before. On top of that there is an important anecdotal and empirical knowledge that is documented by the many spinal specialists that work alongside medical doctors, physical therapists and fitness coaches in many football teams. High velocity low amplitude thrust to spinal or axial joints is most commonly used to alleviate the algic phase of many common pain syndromes like non-specific low back pain or cervicogenic pain and headaches. In addition to pain relief and improving mechanics and healthy affrentation to the brain, manipulative therapy can greatly contribute in minimising Muscular Inhibition (MI) by acting on its causes. Recognised research trials (2) have shown a correlation between sacroiliac joint manipulation and a 7.5% average reduction of MI in anterior-knee pain patients. The study followed twenty-eight patients with anterior knee pain randomly assigned to either a treatment or a control group. Following a functional spinal assessment the treatment group underwent chiropractic spinal manipulation aimed at correcting Sacro-Iliac (SI) joint dysfunction. The control group received no manipulation. Prior to and after the manipulation and/or the lower back functional assessment, knee-extensor moments, MI and muscle activation during full effort isometric knee extensions were measured. Although the study had a relatively small patient pool, it supports what many professional athletes experience daily when they seek chiropractic or osteopathic treatment to maximise their athletic performances. Appendicular manipulation may also play an important role in the RTP process. Research shows that ankle sprain patients present a reduced ipsilateral hip abductor strength, when compared with the contralateral side. The altered biomechanics of the ankle may represent a significant ascending component that needs to be addressed in recovering strength. A complete rehabilitation protocol for an ankle sprain should also include manipulation to restore appropriate joint motion and affrentation. From a spinal standpoint, research as well as experience tells spinal specialists that altered biomechanical relations within the spine, invariably lead to muscle spasm. We know in fact that spinal movement deviating from the norm does stimulate receptors in spinal and paraspinal tissues, activating neural reflex centres within the spinal cord or higher centres (1). Spinal Manipulative Therapy (SMT) is able to interrupt this loop to normalise spinal motion and favour appropriate affrentation (1). Recent research has shown that patients who responded to SMT displayed statistically significant decrease in spinal stiffness and an increase in multifidus thickness ratio. This was sustained for more than seven days, which was not the case in control groups that did not receive SMT in this particular study (3). Beyond providing a neuro-mechanical input, the spinal specialist can play an important role by aiding the rehab specialist in tailoring exercises in the RTP process of the injured player. Functional exercises significantly help spinal manipulation to "hold" in time by reinforcing correct neuro-motor patterns.

References

1. Haldeman S. Spinal manipulative therapy in sports medicine. Clin Sports Med. 1986; 5: 277-293
2. Suter E, McMorland G, Herzog W, Bray R. Conservative lower back treatment reduces inhibition in knee-extensor muscles: a randomized controlled trial. J Manipulative Physiol Ther 2000; 23: 76-80
3. Wong AY, Parent EC, Dhillon SS, Prasad N, Kawchuk GN. Do participants with low back pain who respond to spinal manipulative therapy differ biomechanically from non-responders, untreated controls or asymptomatic controls? Spine 2015; 40: 1329-1337

FUNCTIONAL TRAINING APPROACH: PROGRESSION FROM THE BEGINNING TO RETURN TO PLAY

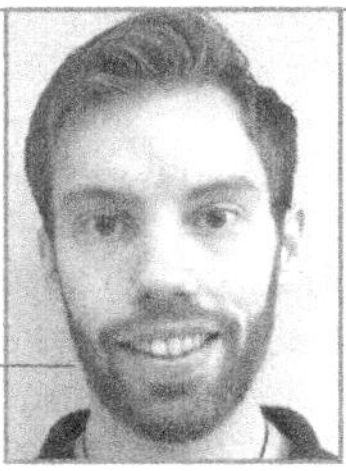

Clancy D, Zanobbi M, Marconato A, McGowan T, Pirotti E, Shanks-Weston H, Buckthorpe M

Isokinetic Medical Group, FIFA Medical Centre of Excellence, London, United Kingdom

Introduction

The functional training approach refers to the rehabilitation (rehab) science of training the body to meet the specific demands of life and sport. It is the action of training the function, thereby preparing the body for a specific role for which it was designed and built. It is an important part of the 5-phase rehab process (2), evolving from the early stages all the way to its completion at the point of Return To Play (RTP).

Discussion

Functional exercises are multi-planar, multi-articular, involve strength and endurance along with coordination and balance. They are advantageous as they stimulate the neuro-muscular and cardio-vascular systems, increase movement confidence and are helpful in injury prevention strategies.

The goal of training using functional exercise is to improve upper and lower extremity coordination and conditional skills, and increase lumbo-pelvic strength, endurance and proprioception. This contributes to improved movement quality and activation patterns. An ideal programme should improve not only muscular stability but also functional stability (1).

The functional training approach progressing from the beginning to RTP can be clearly seen with the functional pyramid paradigm (figure 1).

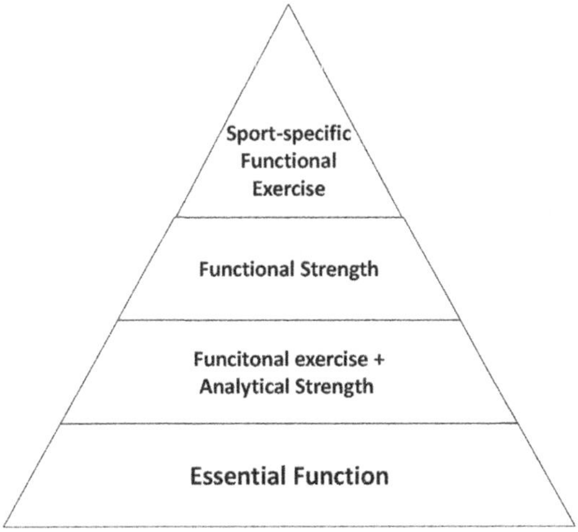

Figure 1. The functional pyramid paradigm.

In the initial phases of recovery, in the absence of adequately sufficient pure strength, conscious function needs to be trained to facilitate automation of activities of daily living. Functional training, or training essential function is key in order to restore essential movement patterns. Restoring normal gait in the pool is a great way to make progress in these early stages of the rehab process, coupled with gym-based rehab.
The ensuing stage involves restoring normal strength parameters; this further helps improve functional capability. Functional strength exercises refer to a specific type of exercise that is geared to increased maximum strength and endurance, using different muscle groups and joints simultaneously, in actions requiring balance and coordination.
One of the most significant factors that can influence movement quality and function is strength. When we are training strength it should be with the aim to enhance the ability to produce force in movement and develop the strength to re-stabilise joints to prevent injury. Single joint maximal strength is a form of strength, providing a marker of potential capacity to produce force in movement. It does not actually tell us about force expression in function. When interpreting strength it is important to recognise the form of strength required in function.
Isolated or machine-based strength is the capacity of a muscle to produce force, whereas in functional situations, movement is influenced by other factors, thus functional strength is the ability to produce force in postures specific to sporting or functional situations. This can be referred to as strength capability, the ability to produce force in a desired situation. Training both is imperative. Initially restoring strength capacity, then training the capability to express this strength in movement is of paramount importance to graduate towards end-stage RTP elements.
In the later phases of end-stage rehab, functional training is a significant component of the RTP paradigm. It is about building on the success of the gym and focusing principally on movement coordination, with the sole purpose to train the neuromuscular system to achieve a sound movement profile. Sports-specific exercise evolves naturally from progressive functional exercises and these are critical to adequately prepare a person/athlete for their respective field of play.

Conclusions

Functional training is at the very core of rehab from early post-operative treatment right through to field-based technical execution preceding a healthy RTP. This is because effective rehab is centered upon optimally restoring function capability from start-to-finish. Functional exercises, contrary to popular belief can be used at the earliest stages of the rehab process, and not solely when there is symmetrical limb muscle strength.
This can be seen clearly in the functional training pyramid. At the start of the rehab process essential function must be restored. Mid-way through rehab pure strength must be increased to facilitate more optimal functional recovery; following this functional strength exercises form an integral part of rehab. Finally, technically advanced sports-specific exercise contributes to creating the right musculoskeletal profile and movement pattern prior to RTP.

References

1. Yildiz Y, Aydin T, Sekir U, Cetin C, Ors F, Kalyon TA. Relation between isokinetic muscle strength and functional capacity in recreational athletes with chondromalacia patellae. Br J Sports Med 2003; 37: 475- 479
2. Zanobbi M, Fazzini D, Marcheggiani GM. Rehabilitation in five phases. In: Roi GS, Della Villa S (Eds). Football medicine strategies for knee injuries. Calzetti Mariucci Editore, Torgiano, 2012, pp. 53-54

Sunday 10th April, 2016 (afternoon)
CHURCHILL AUDITORIUM

INVITED SPEAKERS

MONITORING RETURN TO PLAY PROCESS

Chairs

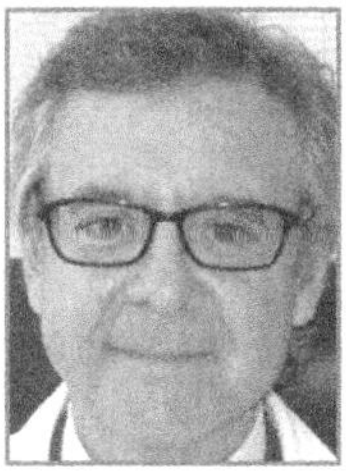

Gianluca Melegati
(Milan, Italy)

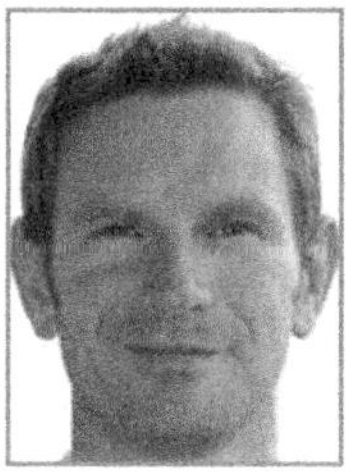

Barry Drust
(Liverpool, United Kingdom)

14:30 The value of pre-season testing and screening for return to play
Peter Ueblaker (Münich, Germany)

14:45 Imaging's role in the return to play process?
Justin Lee (London, United Kingdom)

15:00 Hop testing as an indicator for return to play
Eanna Falvey (Dublin, Ireland)

15:15 Blood and laboratory test options
Giuseppe Banfi (Milan, Italy)

15:30 Role of patient reporting in return to play outcomes
James Irrgang (Pittsburgh, USA)

15:45 Discussion

16:00 End of the session

THE VALUE OF PRE-SEASON TESTING AND SCREENING FOR RETURN TO PLAY

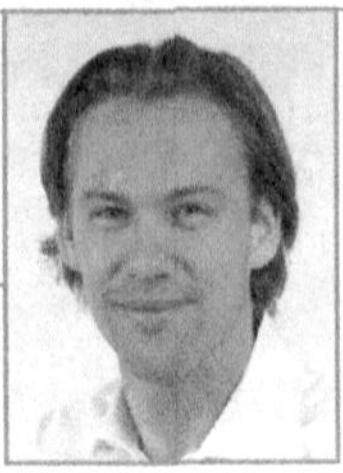

Ueblacker P, Mueller-Wohlfahrt HW

MW Center for Orthopedics and Sports Medicine, Munich, Germany

Numerous tests are available to assess the fitness and the medical condition of football players. Testing procedures differ from club to club, at least at elite level.

Fitness testing must be differentiated from medical testing; general medical, from cardiac and musculoskeletal tests.

Testing and screening need to be clinically reasoned, it should be considered that there is a treatment or prevention strategy available as a consequence of abnormal data.

Preseason testing and screening can help to obtain base line data to assess physical changes over time and to proof the effectiveness of rehabilitation before Return To Play (RTP) (e.g., fitness parameter, strength of thigh muscles, Range Of Motion of joints, etc...).

They can further help to implement individual prevention strategies through a better understanding of individual risk factors for injuries like previous injury, poor lower limb power, reduced balance, deficits in the lumbo-pelvic muscles, etc...

However, there is no recent study on the value of pre-season testing and screening in relation to RTP and there is much debate about the significance of various risk factors and the success of prevention programmes.

Optimal rehabilitation should aim for identification and compensation of individual (fitness and musculoskeletal) deficits that affect performance, rehabilitation should serve to reduce the risk of preventable injuries, to optimize performance, improve fitness and to bring the athlete to safe RTP with minimal risk of re-injury.

Since pre-season testing and screening examinations are usually only a snapshot of the athletes condition at one time point, regular check-ups should be performed during an entire rehabilitation process.

IMAGING'S ROLE IN THE RETURN TO PLAY PROCESS?

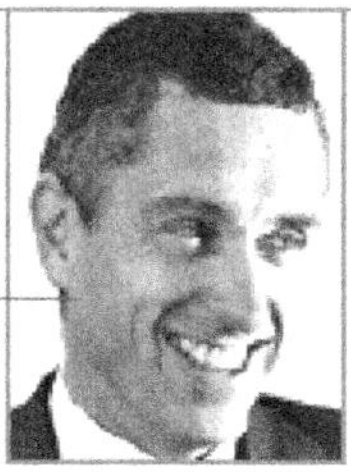

Lee J

Fortius Clinic, London; Chelsea and Westminster Hospital, London, United Kingdom

Introduction

With the development of sports medicine as a specialist clinical area, the role of imaging in management of football-related injuries is slowly transitioning from diagnosis to prognosis. Although there is conflicting evidence of the value of imaging in this group, it is widely accepted that imaging plays a vital role in determining injury pattern and therefore predicting time out. However, there are some controversies in the imaging literature and sometimes it is difficult for the sports physician to determine whether imaging is necessary or not in the management of his or her players following acute injury.

Magnetic Resonance Imaging

Various Magnetic Resonance Imaging (MRI) grading systems are now in use to describe muscle injuries in athletes. The UEFA Champions League Study Group published the largest series of hamstring injuries to date and concluded that MRI accurately correlates with time out from play (1). The identification of intramuscular tendon involvement has been recognised as a major predictor of injury recovery time (2).

Ligament injuries of the knee and ankle are a major cause of loss of playing time in footballers. MRI is essential in making accurate diagnosis of the grade and pattern of injuries in these players to ensure that the player is optimally managed. Unexpected cruciate ligament injuries are not uncommon and if missed, will have devastating consequences both for player and club.

Cartilage injuries involving the knee, hip and ankle require imaging, or direct visualisation by arthroscopy or open surgery. Accurate detection of injuries to hyaline cartilage or intra-articular fibrocartilage such as to the menisci or labrum of the hip cannot be made clinically. High grade acute cartilage injuries in footballers are potential causes of protracted loss of playing time and frequently require surgical intervention which in itself induces a further loss of playing time.

Bony injuries in footballers occur either as a result of direct trauma or overuse and subsequent development of stress injury. The stress injury spectrum ranges from simple periostitis to complete displaced stress fracture. Imaging classification systems for bone stress are widely used and help determine prognosis in this injury.

Conclusions

Imaging plays a vital role in accurately determining injury pattern and severity in elite footballers and allows the medical team and club to plan for loss of playing time in that individual.

The role of MRI in predicting return to play has gained interest in the published literature recently and its role will continue to develop over time with the recognition of which are the most important determining factors at time of original injury.

References

1. 1.Ekstrand J, Healy JC, Waldén M, Lee JC, English B, Hägglund M. Hamstring muscle injuries in professional football: the correlation of MRI findings with return to play. Br J Sports Med 2012; 46: 112-117
2. Pollock N, James, SL, Lee JC, Chakraverty R. British Athletics muscle injury classification: a new grading system. Br J Sports Med 2014; 48: 1347-1351

HOP TESTING AS A PREDICTOR OF RETURN TO PLAY

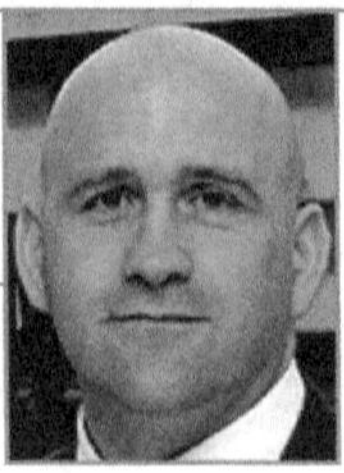

Falvey ÉC

Sports Medicine Department, Sports Surgery Clinic, Dublin;
Department of Medicine, University College Cork, Cork;
Irish Rugby Football Union, Dublin, Ireland

Return To Play (RTP) decisions are a vital conclusion to complete rehabilitation in an athletic population. While strength and speed may be objectively measured reliably and reasonably cost-effectively, multi-directional stability proves more difficult. Particularly in the office or clinical rooms setting. Functional movement screening often utilises the single leg squat for this purpose. The controlled, planned nature of this movement fails to account for significant hip and torso movements, both significant factors in changing centre of mass and muscular activation rates around the hip and knee. Three dimensional analysis of the single leg squat provided a moderate insight into knee control while landing, it did not however provide a meaningful insight into hip and pelvis control or loading during sporting movements (2).
A number of double- and single-leg sagittal plane hop tests are described as Physical Performance Tests (PPT) particularly for the knee. The one leg hop for distance is the most often studied PPT. Other testing includes 6 m timed hop, crossover hop for distance, one-leg hop for distance: triple hop, single leg vertical jump, single leg squat, triple jump. The ease of utilization and reproducibility explains the frequent use of such tests in pre-season testing and in RTP decisions. They are understandably well represented in the literature.
There is, however, conflicting evidence regarding the validity of the hop test. A recent review of the hop test outlined methodological issues around published data and when combined with the quality of the measurement properties, the level of evidence was generally limited or conflicting. There was moderate evidence that the hop test is responsive to changes during rehabilitation (1).
The lateral single leg hurdle hop is a novel biomechanical screening exercise proposed as part of a testing battery for athletic groin pain patients. Both single-leg consecutive hopping, and nonconsecutive hops have been used as measures of stiffness, and function in rehabilitation (3).
Unlike stationary or forward hopping however, the lateral hurdle hop is a more effective means of stressing frontal plane control patterns typical of field-based sports. In addition the non-consecutive nature of the testing may also have greater ecological validity to sporting actions in comparison to consecutive hoping.

References

1. Hegedus EJ, McDonough S, Bleakley C, Cook CE, Baxter GD. Clinician-friendly lower extremity physical performance measures in athletes: a systematic review of measurement properties and correlation with injury, part 1. The tests for knee function including the hop tests. Br J Sports Med 2015; 49: 642-648
2. Marshall BM, Franklyn-Miller AD, Moran KA, King EA, Strike SC, Falvey ÉC. Can a single-legged squat provide insight into movement control and loading during dynamic sporting actions in athletic groin pain patients? J Sport Rehabil 2015 May 6. [Epub ahead of print]
3. Myer GD, Paterno M V, Ford KR, Quatman CE, Hewett TE. Rehabilitation after anterior cruciate ligament reconstruction: criteria-based progression through the return-to-sport phase. J Orthop Sports Phys Ther 2006; 36: 385-402

LABORATORY TESTS TO DEFINE RECOVERY IN FOOTBALL PLAYERS

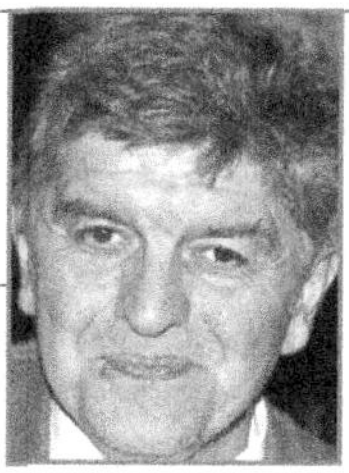

Banfi G[1], Lombardi G[1], Locatelli M[2]

[1]IRCCS Galeazzi, Milan
[2]Laboratorio Analisi, IRCCS San Raffaele, Milano, Italy

The role of laboratory is crucial to define the health status and complete recovery of a football player after traumas, surgery, overuse/overtraining and/or rehabilitation.
Traumas and surgery should be followed by haematological evaluations, due to possible blood loss and/or erythrocyte destruction. The complete recovery of haemoglobin and, consequently, regular number and morphological characteristics of erythrocytes are fundamental findings for assuring complete fitness and return of potential performances typical of the athlete. The stability of haemoglobin during the season characterizes football players, whereas the parameter is deeply influenced and modified by competitions in different sports disciplines. Thus, the control and monitoring of haemoglobin, through the evaluation of critical difference and not only the reference range, is important to define the real and effective recovery of the athlete.
The haematological evaluation is important also for evaluating possible modifications of immune systems response, particularly when the athlete is suffering from viral and/or bacterial infectious diseases. The analyses of lymphocytes are important for defining immunological deficiencies. Allergy analyses could be added to the classical leukocytes studies of immunological response.
Hormones are usually analysed for evaluating the health status and possible performance and for avoiding possible overreaching, but are more important to evaluate the recovery from traumas, immobilization, and incomplete training. Steroids are commonly measured, but some different stress hormones, and metabolism ones (thyroid and parathyroid molecules, for example) could be analysed. These analyses could be used also for evaluating the combined effects of training restraint or decrease and frequent travels and modification of regular chronological biorhythms.
Vitamins and amminoacids are defining the correct nutritional status, which could modified by the detraining and immobilization.
Bone markers, especially some molecules recently proposed for studying the interrelationship between bone and metabolism, are precious to define the restart of the regular bone actions, not only biomechanical, but also metabolic.

Sunday 10th April, 2016 (afternoon)
PICKWICK ROOM

FREE ORAL PRESENTATIONS

MUSCLE AND TENDON INJURIES

Chairs

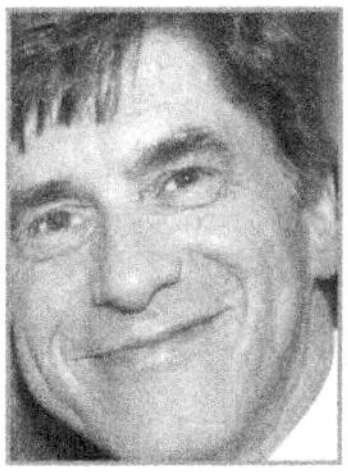

Gianni Nanni
(Bologna, Italy)

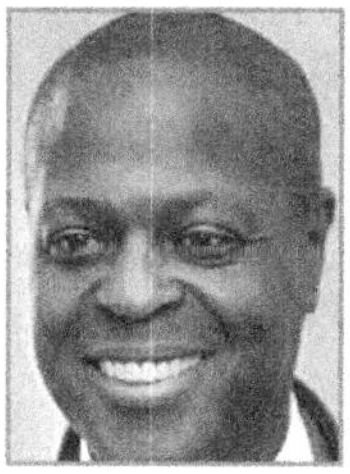

Ralph Rogers
(London, United Kingdom)

14:30 Targeting the low back improves return to play in athletes with functional hamstring disorders **Kakavas G, Colloca CJ, Hegazy Afifi M, Malliaropoulos N (Athens, Greece; Chandler and Moscow, USA)**

14:40 Groin problems are common at all levels of play in Norwegian male football **Harøy J, Clarsen B, Thorborg K, Hölmich P, Bahr R, Andersen TE (Oslo, Norway; Copenhagen, Denmark)**

14:50 Acute groin injuries in athletes; reliability of MRI assessment **Roemer F, Serner A, Hölmich P, Thorborg K, Niu J, Weir A, Tol JL, Guermazi A (Doha, Qatar; Erlangen, Germany; Boston, USA; Amager-Hvidovre, Denmark)**

15:00 Clinical predictability of MRI findings in athletes with acute groin pain **Serner A, Weir A, Tol JL, Thorborg K, Roemer F, Guermazi A, Hölmich P (Doha, Qatar; Amager-Hvidovre, Denmark; Erlangen, Germany; Boston, USA)**

15:10 Which is the optimal day for magnetic resonance imaging after acute hamstring injuries? **Wangensteen A, Bahr R, Almusa E, van Linschoten R, Whiteley R, Witvrouw E, Tol JL (Doha, Qatar; Oslo, Norway; Ghent, Belgium; Amsterdam, The Netherlands)**

15:20 Running exposure and hamstring injury risk in elite Australian footballers
Ruddy J, Timmins R, Pollard C, Opar D (Melbourne, Australia)

15:30 Hamstring strength in soccer players with and without previous hamstring injuries
Lee JWY, Tso KW, Yung PSH, Chan KM (Hong Kong, China)

15:40 Effectiveness of Nordic hamstring to improve injury risk factor on futsal players
Boroh Z, Sudarsono NC, Ilyas EI (Jakarta, Indonesia)

15:50 Above and beyond Bicep Femoris
Blandford L, Pedersen C, Mottram S (Bristol, United Kingdom; Helsingborg, Sweden)

16:00 New eccentric exercise mode for rehabilitation after muscle injury
Landkammer Y, Sassmann R, Herfert J, Wicker A (Salzburg, Austria)

16:10 A biochemical analysis of muscle injuries in football during rehabilitation
Tymvios C (Nicosia, Cyprus)

16:20 Discussion

16:30 End of the session

1

TARGETING THE LOW BACK IMPROVES RETURN TO PLAY IN ATHLETES WITH FUNCTIONAL HAMSTRING DISORDERS

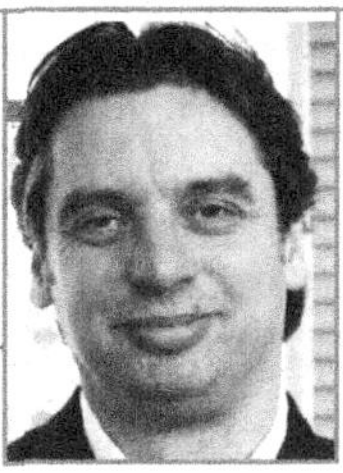

Kakavas G, Colloca CJ, Hegazy Afifi M, Malliaropoulos N

Fysiotek Spine and Sports Laboratory, Athens, Greece; International Spine Research Foundation, Chandler, Arizona, USA; Department of Movement Sciences, University of Idaho, Moscow, USA

Introduction

Hamstring Muscle Injuries (HMI) are among the most common time-loss sports injuries and the most common sports injury in football (1). Clinical presentation of athletes with (HMI) include pain, weakness, and increased fatigability locally as well as loss of motor control in the lumbopelvic region (2). However, treatment targeting the lumbo-pelvic region among athletes with HMI is not often implemented.

The objective of the current study was to compare two rehabilitative treatment programs, one including targeting treatment to the lumbo-pelvic region on clinical findings and return to play among elite football players. A second aim was to analyze clinical predictors of return to play.

Methods

Sixteen consecutive athletes in the Greek Super Football League (ages 21-32 years) diagnosed with acute HMI and Functional Muscle Disorder (FMD) within five days of injury were randomly assigned in to 1 of 2 rehabilitation groups. Inclusion criteria for all participants consisted of the presence of HMI with no Magnetic Resonance Imaging signs of structural hamstring strain, a positive slump test, <3 kg/cm Pain Pressure Threshold (PPT) upon digital algometry (Digital Algometer, CLA, Bethany Beach, Delaware, USA) to the involved Biceps Femoris (BF) muscle belly, ipsilateral Sacro-Iliac Joint (SIJ) and L5 and L4 spinous processes, and positive isometric hamstring digital muscle strength testing (Digital Muscle Tester, MicroFET2, Hoggan Scientific, Salt Lake City, Utah, USA). These variables were again re-assessed at the conclusion of treatment and used as outcome measures for group comparisons and predictor variables in this randomized clinical trial.

Eight athletes received standard supervised HMI rehabilitative treatment consisting of passive interventions of therapeutic ultrasound, hamstring massage and Nordic progressive hamstring exercises (Standard Treatment group: ST). The other eight athletes were assigned to a program of impulsive mechanical manipulation and manual therapy delivered to targets in the lumbar spine, sacroiliac joint and the involved BF with the Impulse iQ (Neuromechanical Innovations, Chandler, Arizona, USA) and core lumbar stability exercises (Mechanical Manual Therapy group: MMT). Both groups received treatments three times a week for three weeks prior to re-evaluation.

A series of mixed design 2x2 ANOVA's were conducted with time (pre-post) as the within-subjects factor and treatment group (ST vs. MMT) as the between-subjects factor with Bonferroni correction. Days to return to play were compared among groups using an independent t-test, and linear regression analyses were conducted to predict days to return to play from the objective clinical outcome variables. Significance was set at $p<0.05$ for all analyses.

Results

For the two treatment regimens, return to play was nearly two-fold significantly shorter in the MMT group (mean±SD: 14.6±1.4 days) compared with the ST group (25.4±6.1 days) ($p=0.001$).
At re-examination, all athletes in the MMT group were observed to have a negative slump test, whereas a positive slump test remained in 50% of the STG group.
Comparing pre-post mean hamstring muscle strength, significant improvement was observed in both groups ($p=0.002$) with improvement favored in the MMT group (+9.8±2.2 kg) compared to the ST group (5.8±4.2 kg ($p=0.001$).
Within group analyses demonstrated significant improvements in pre-post PPT in both groups for examinations of the SIJ, L5, L4, and the BF ($p<0.015$). Significantly greater improvement in PPT was found however for the MMT group for the SIJ, L5, BF (Table 1).
Linear regression models predicted a moderate correlation between return to play and improvement in PPT at the SIJ (R2=0.578; $p=0.001$), and L5 ($R^2=0.366$; $p=0.013$). No other significant predictors of return to play were observed for the other clinical outcomes evaluated.

Level	MMT group (kg/cm²)	ST group (kg/cm²)	p
SIJ	4.33±0.87	0.75±0.62	0.014*
L5	4.01±1.19	1.58±1.15	0.002*
L4	2.88±0.82	1.75±1.16	0.092
BF	3.95±1.34	1.59±1.27	0.004*

Table 1. Mean±SD of pre-post improvements in Pain Pressure Threshold (PPT) for clinical assessments made at the Sacro-Iliac Joint (SIJ), L5 and L4 spinous processes, and the Biceps Femoris muscle (BF) among the Manual Mechanical Therapy (MMT) and the Standard Treatment (ST) groups. *Significant differences between groups.

Conclusions

In this randomized clinical trial MMT targeting both the HMI and lumbo-pelvic spine was shown to be more effective than a standard HMI rehabilitation program for improvement in objective measures of FMD and HMI, and returning elite football players to sport participation.
These results, combined with the findings that L5 and SIJ PPT improvement predict return to play among athletes in the current study suggest that treatment targeting the lumbo-pelvic spine is an important consideration in HMI rehabilitation among athletes.
Further studies are needed to verify the lasting benefit of treatment on HMI and the possible role of applying MMT protocols for FHD rehabilitation to reduce the commonly high rate of re-injury of this type of injury.

References

1. Ekstrand J, Hagglund M, Walden M. Epidemiology of muscle injuries in professional football (soccer). Am J Sports Med 2011; 39: 1226-1232
2. Silder A, Sherry MA, Sanfilippo J, Tuite MJ, Hetzel SJ, Heiderscheit BC. Clinical and morphological changes following two rehabilitation programs for acute hamstring strain injuries: a randomized clinical trial. J Orthop Sports Phys Ther 2013; 43: 284-299

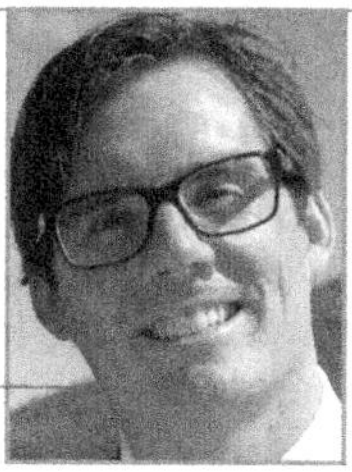

GROIN PROBLEMS ARE COMMON AT ALL LEVELS OF PLAY IN NORWEGIAN MALE FOOTBALL

Harøy J[1], Clarsen B[1], Thorborg K[2], Hölmich P[2], Bahr R[1], Andersen TE[1]

[1]Oslo Sports Trauma Research Center, Department of Sports Medicine, Norwegian School of Sport Sciences, Oslo, Norway; [2]Department of Orthopaedic Surgery, Sports Orthopedic Research Center-Copenhagen (SORC-C), Amager-Hvidovre Hospital, Faculty of Health Sciences, University of Copenhagen, Copenhagen, Denmark

Introduction

The majority of surveillance studies in football use a time loss injury definition (2). However, many groin injuries result from overuse, leading to gradually increasing pain and/or reduced performance without necessarily causing an absence from football training or match play. Thus, the true extent of groin injuries in female and male football is likely underestimated when traditional injury surveillance methods are used. Purpose: To investigate the prevalence of groin problems among football players of both genders and at different levels of play using a new surveillance method developed to register both acute and overuse problems.

Purpose

To investigate the prevalence of groin problems among football players of both genders and at different levels of play using a new surveillance method developed to register both acute and overuse problems.

Methods

We registered groin problems during a 6-week period of match congestion using the Oslo Sports Trauma Research Center (OSTRC) Overuse Injury Questionnaire (1).
A total of 240 players from 15 teams across different levels were included and responded weekly to the questionnaire using a mobile application (Spartanova, Spartanova NV, Gent, Belgium).
We calculated the weekly prevalence of all groin problems and substantial groin problems, defined as problems leading to at least moderate or severe reductions in training volume or sporting performance, or a total inability to participate.

Results

Among the 240 participants, the overall response rate to the six weekly questionnaires was 94-98% across different levels and for both genders.
Over the six weeks, 112 male players (59%) and 20 female players (45%) reported at least one episode with groin problems. The average weekly prevalence of all groin problems (±95% confidence interval) was 32% for elite male (±5%), 31% for sub-elite male (±9%), 29% for amateur male (±7%), 23% for U19 male (±9%) and 14% for female elite players (±4%).
Elite male players had an increased risk of reporting groin problems (odds ratio: 3.1; 95% confidence interval: 1.5 to 6.4; p=0.03) compared to elite female players. There was, however, no difference between the different levels of play for senior male players.
The average weekly prevalence of substantial groin problems (±95% confidence interval) was 13% for elite males (±2%), 7% for sub-elite males (±2%), 12% for amateur males (±2%), 7% for U19 males (±4%) and 4% for female elite players (±0%). There was no difference in the risk of reporting substantial groin problems between elite male and elite female players or across different levels of play for senior male players.

Conclusions

We found a high prevalence of groin problems among male Norwegian footballers during a period with match congestion.
Elite male players had three times higher risk of reporting groin problems compared to elite female players, while playing level did not influence the risk of reporting groin problems.

References

1. Clarsen B, Myklebust G, Bahr R. Development and validation of a new method for the registration of overuse injuries in sports injury epidemiology: the Oslo Sports Trauma Research Centre (OSTRC) overuse injury questionnaire. Br J Sports Med 2013; 47: 495-502
2. Waldén M, Hagglund M, Ekstrand J. The epidemiology of groin injury in senior football: a systematic review of prospective studies. Br J Sports Med 2015; 49: 792-797

ACUTE GROIN INJURIES IN ATHLETES; RELIABILITY OF MRI ASSESSMENT

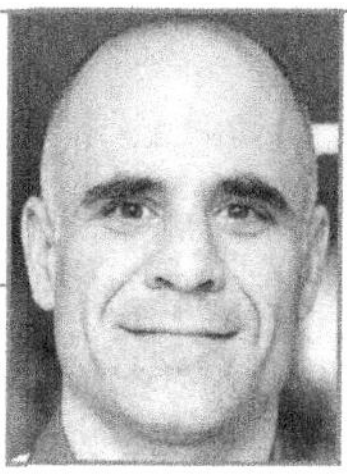

Roemer F[1,2,3], Serner A[1,4], Hölmich P[1,4], Thorborg K[4], Niu J[5], Weir A[1], Tol JL[1], Guermazi A[1,3]

[1]Aspetar, Orthopaedic and Sports Medicine Hospital, Doha, Qatar; [2]Department of Radiology, University of Erlangen-Nuremberg, Erlangen, Germany; [3]Quantitative Imaging Center (QIC), Department of Radiology, Boston University School of Medicine, Boston, MA, USA; [4]Sports Orthopaedic Research Center–Copenhagen (SORC-C), Department of Orthopedic Surgery, Copenhagen University Hospital, Amager-Hvidovre, Denmark; [5]Clinical Epidemiology and Training Unit, Department of Medicine, Boston University School of Medicine, Boston, MA, USA

Introduction

Groin injuries are common in football and most published literature on groin pain in athletes, including imaging, focuses on long-standing symptoms, for which a reliable Magnetic Resonance Imaging (MRI) protocol has already been developed (1). An imaging assessment system for acute injuries is still lacking, and only two studies have evaluated the role of imaging in the assessment of acute groin pain.

A prospective study from 1999 using both clinical examination and ultrasound found that only 1 out of 13 injuries, which were clinically diagnosed as muscle or tendon injuries could be confirmed using ultrasound (2).

Another more recent prospective study reporting on 110 athletes with acute groin injuries, using clinical, ultrasound and MRI examination, provided a general overview of injury locations (3). In that study MRI evaluation was coded with a simple dichotomization of acute lesion presence or absence, and no data on the reproducibility of the radiological assessment was provided.

To date it is unknown whether MRI data on acute groin injuries may be assessed in an elaborate fashion taking into account anatomical location, severity and extent of injury, and associated imaging findings in the groin region with adequate reproducibility including ordinal grading and continuous measurements.

The purpose of this study was therefore to develop a multi-dimensional MRI assessment instrument with a focus on acute musculo-tendinous groin lesions, and evaluate the scoring reproducibility.

Methods

Male athletes (18-40 y) who participated in competitive sports and who presented within seven days of an acute onset of sports-related groin pain were included.

All athletes underwent MRI according to a standardized groin-centered protocol. After several calibration sessions, a system was developed assessing location, grade, and extent of muscle strains, peri-lesional hematoma, as well as other non-acute findings commonly associated with long-standing groin pain. Kappa ($\mathcal{K}$) statistics and intraclass correlation coefficients (ICCs) were used to examine intra- and inter-rater reproducibility.

Results

The 75 randomly selected male athletes were on average 26.6±4.4 years (range: 18-37 yrs).
Sports played were football (76%), basketball (9%), handball (9%), and 5% were athletes from other sports.
85 different acute muscular lesions and 19 different non-acute lesions were scored.
The most commonly affected muscle was the Adductor Longus (43%), followed by the Rectus Femoris (16%).
The most common non-acute finding was pubic bone marrow oedema, which was present in at least one side in 55% of the athletes.
Further common pathologies were central disc protrusions/superior osteophytes and peri-symhyseal sclerosis.
Almost perfect intra- and inter-rater agreement ($\mathcal{K}$=0.81-1.00) was found for lesion presence/absence, number of acute lesions per athlete, muscle location, as well as lesion grading and oedema location in the axial plane, whereas oedema location in the coronal plane had substantial agreement ($\mathcal{K}$=0.70-0.85). The measures of the extent of oedema were also almost perfect with ICCs between 0.89-0.99 for both acute lesions and non-acute lesions. Similarly, the measures of the extent of the partial tears and complete tears/avulsions showed almost perfect reproducibility (ICC = 0.83-0.99).

Conclusions

Standardized MRI scoring of acute groin injuries using a multi-dimensional MRI assessment instrument is feasible with good reproducibility. This provides a stronger foundation for further research to determine the clinical significance of specific features, and their potential prognostic value in return to play estimations.

References

1. Branci S, Thorborg K, Bech BH, Boesen M, Magnussen E, Court-Payen M, Nielsen MB, Hölmich P. The Copenhagen Standardised MRI protocol to assess the pubic symphysis and adductor regions of athletes: outline and intratester and intertester reliability. Br J Sports Med 2015; 49: 692-699
2. Ekstrand J, Hilding J. The incidence and differential diagnosis of acute groin injuries in male soccer players. Scand J Med Sci Sports 1999; 9: 98-103
3. Serner A, Tol JL, Jomaah N, Weir A, Whiteley R, Thorborg K, Robinson M, Hölmich P. Diagnosis of acute groin injuries: a prospective study of 110 athletes. Am J Sports Med 2015; 43: 1857-1864

CLINICAL PREDICTABILITY OF MRI FINDINGS IN ATHLETES WITH ACUTE GROIN PAIN

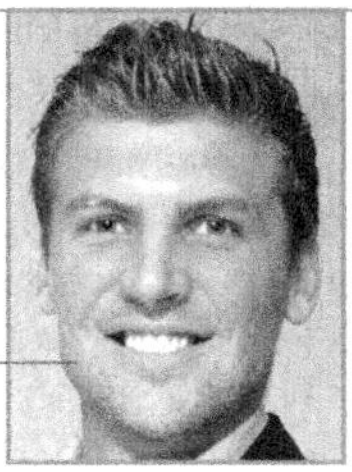

Serner A[1,2], Weir A[1], Tol JL[1], Thorborg K[2], Roemer F[1,3,4], Guermazi A[1,4], Hölmich P[1,2]

[1]Aspetar Orthopaedic and Sports Medicine Hospital, Doha, Qatar;
[2]Sports Orthopaedic Research Center-Copenhagen (SORC-C), Arthroscopic Center Amager, Department of Orthopaedic Surgery, Copenhagen University Hospital, Amager-Hvidovre, Denmark;
[3]Department of Radiology, University of Erlangen-Nuremberg, Erlangen, Germany;
[4]Quantitative Imaging Center (QIC), Department of Radiology, Boston University School of Medicine, Boston, MA, USA

Introduction

Acute groin injuries are common in sports, but little is known about the value of clinical examination or imaging. Diagnosing acute groin injuries can be challenging and discrepancies between clinical and radiological findings have been found (1).

As Magnetic Resonance Imaging is not readily available for many clinicians, the primary aim of this study was to investigate whether clinical examination tests can predict a positive or negative MRI (MRI+/-) in athletes with acute groin injuries. The secondary aim was to assess the accuracy of determining the location of injuries in MRI+ cases only.

Methods

81 male athletes (age 25.8±4.4 yrs) with an acute groin injury during sports were consecutively included.

The athletes were mainly football players (57% soccer and 20% futsal), 9% basketball players, 6% handball players, 5% volleyball players, and 2% from other sports.

A standardized clinical examination using pain provocation test for the adductors, hip flexors, and abdominal muscles, as well as an MRI investigation, was performed within seven days of injury.

Sensitivity (SN), Specificity (SP), positive and negative likelihood ratios (LR+/-) and predictive values (PPV and NPV) were calculated, and Receiver Operating Characteristic (ROC) statistics and the Area Under the Curve (AUC) was used to describe the discriminative value.

Results

There were 17 (21%) athletes with a negative MRI. In MRI positive cases 85 different muscle and/or tendon injuries were found in 64 athletes. In 46 (57%) athletes there was an MRI+ adductor injury, in 18 (22%) a MRI+ hip flexor injury was reported with 8 Iliopsoas, 8 Rectus Femoris and 2 Sartorius injuries. Only one abdominal injury was found on the MRI, therefore further analysis was not performed for abdominal tests. Fair to good discriminative values for an MRI+/- injury for most individual adductor and hip flexor examination tests (AUC >0.70) were found. Of the individual examination tests palpation showed the highest probability of ruling out an MRI+ injury with an NPV of 0.91 (95%CI 0.69, 0.98) and 0.96 (95%CI 0.85, 0.99) for adductor and hip flexor palpation respectively. Highest predictability of a MRI+ injury was found with all specific tests positive: PPV 0.83 (95%CI 0.58, 0.96) and 0.86 (95%CI 0.42, 0.99) for adductor and hip flexor tests, respectively.

No improvements of discriminative values were found from the ROC analysis.
Adductor palpation, resisted outer-range adduction and the squeeze test in hip neutral position were best at accurately determining an MRI adductor injury (all AUC 0.87; PPV 0.92-0.97).
Hip flexor tests were generally poor at predicting an accurate injury location.
For both Iliopsoas and Rectus Femoris injuries palpation provided the most accurate result (AUC 0.93 (95%CI 0.87, 0.99) and 0.96 (95%CI 0.91, 1.00), respectively), the PPV of an accurate injury location was however only 0.50 (95%CI 0.26, 0.74) and 0.62 (95%CI 0.32, 0.85).

Conclusions

We found higher probability of predicting a negative MRI than a positive MRI.
Palpation was the best test to rule out a positive MRI.
Individual adductor pain provocation tests (adductor palpation, resisted outer-range adduction, adductor stretch, and the squeeze test in hip neutral position) provided approximately 80% probability of predicting a positive MRI in the adductors.
Positive adductor examination tests were more accurate than hip flexor tests, and also provided high confidence in an accurate injury location.
Individual hip flexor pain provocation tests had poor probability of predicting a positive MRI, and appear insufficient to differentiate between a MRI+ iliopsoas and rectus femoris injury in the initial examination of acute groin injuries.

References

1. Serner A, Tol JL, Jomaah N, Weir A, Whiteley R, Thorborg K, Robinson M, Hölmich P. Diagnosis of acute groin injuries: a prospective study of 110 athletes. Am J Sports Med 2015; 43: 1857-1864

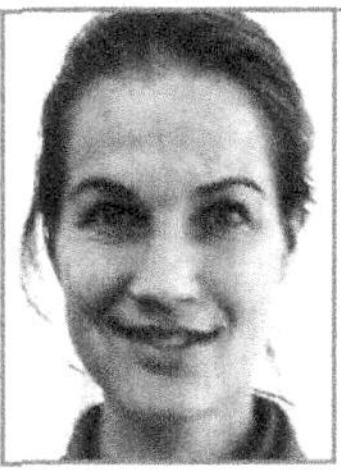

WHICH IS THE OPTIMAL DAY FOR MAGNETIC RESONANCE IMAGING AFTER ACUTE HAMSTRING INJURIES?

Wangensteen A[1,2], Bahr R[1,2], Almusa E[1], van Linschoten R[1], Whiteley R[1], Witvrouw E[1,3], Tol JL[1,4]

[1]Aspetar, Orthopaedic and Sports Medicine Hospital, Doha, Qatar; [2]Oslo Sports Trauma Research Center, Department of Sports Medicine, Norwegian School of Sport Sciences, Oslo, Norway; [3]Department Rehabilitation Science and Physiotherapy, Faculty of Medicine and Health Sciences, Ghent University, Belgium; [4]Amsterdam Center for Evidence Based Medicine, Academic Medical Center, Amsterdam, The Netherlands

Introduction

The Return To Play (RTP) process after acute hamstring injury, the most common non-contact muscle injury in professional football with increasing injury rates (1), begins at the day of injury occurence. There is currently no evidence that Magnetic Resonance Imaging (MRI) can predict RTP accurately (3). However, the prognostic studies are based on a single MRI scan obtained at different time points following injury and the evolution of MRI appearance after a muscle strain during the acute stage is not known. Furthermore single MRI scanning is widely used to support or refute the clinical diagnosis. Thus, the optimal timing of MRI imaging for correct diagnosis and to potentially provide a more precise RTP prognosis remains unknown.
Purpose: To investigate the time course of MRI changes and the optimal timing of MRI imaging after acute hamstring muscle injuries.

Methods

In this descriptive study, a standardised MRI examination was completed ≤1 day after injury in professional or recreational athletes presenting with a clinical diagnosis of acute hamstring injury assessed for eligibility at a sports medicine hospital.
If the initial MRI revealed positive signs of injury (increased signal intensity on fluid sensitive sequences), consecutive MRIs were obtained daily throughout the subsequent week. MRI parameters of the daily MRI images from day 1 through day 7 were scored by a single radiologist using a standardised scoring form (2). The changes in the length (cm), volume (cm3) and cross-sectional area (cm^2) of the oedema and the longitudinal extent of the tear (cm) were assessed with descriptive statistics and repeated measures analysis of variance (ANOVA). The overall main effect and pairwise comparisons with Sidak adjustments were reported with a significance level set at $p<0.05$.

Results

Out of 132 males athletes assessed for eligibility between January 2014 and December 2015, 13 were included in the study, of which 7 were professional athletes playing football or other sports and 5 were recreational athletes.

After imaging on day 1, all had positive MRIs.

One patient dropped out after the first MRI, while 12 (median age 31 years, range 20-49) completed the study (11 completed all 7 days of imaging, and 1 completed 5 days). On day 1, the mean (95% CI) for the length of the oedema was 13.0 cm (8.5-17.5), the volume of oedema was 57.4 cm^3 (13.0-101.9), the cross-sectional area was 4.9 cm^2 (1.8-7.9) and the length of the tear was 2.4 cm (0.2-1.4). A minor trend towards a decrease from day 1 to day 7 was seen. After repeated measurements, there was an overall time effect (ANOVA, p-values $\leq$0.005), but after Sidak adjustments for multiple pairwise comparisons, there were no significant differences between any of the days for either the length of oedema (p-values ranging from 0.26 to 1.00), volume of oedema (p-values ranging from 0.52 to 1.0) or cross-sectional area (p-values ranging from 0.14 to 1.0). The length of the tear, present in 5 of the athletes, showed only minimal changes during the 7 days of imaging and was detectable from day 1 (as fluid collection).

Conclusions

The changes in the extent of oedema (length, volume and cross-sectional area) after an acute hamstring injury were minimal, with a minor decreasing trend from day 1 throughout day 7.

The longitudinal extent of tear was virtually constant and dectectable from the first day after injury. The day-to-day changes of the MRI features within the subjects were considerably smaller than the larger variability between subjects. These findings support that the radiological diagnosis can be obtained correctly from day 1 to 7 and that the limited predictive value of MRI for RTP is probably not explained by the variation in timing of the MRI after the acute hamstring injury.

References

1. Ekstrand J, Waldén M, Hägglund M. Hamstring injuries have increased by 4% annually in men's professional football, since 2001: a 13-year longitudinal analysis of the UEFA Elite Club injury study. Br J Sports Med. 2016 Jan 8; doi:10.1136/bjsports-2015-095359
2. Hamilton B, Whiteley R, Almusa E, Roger B, Geertsema C, Tol JL. Excellent reliability for MRI grading and prognostic parameters in acute hamstring injuries. Br J Sports Med. 2013 Sep 13; doi:10.1136/bjsports-2013-092564
3. Reurink G, Brilman EG, de Vos R-J, Maas M, Moen MH, Weir A, Goudswaard GJ, Tol JL. Magnetic resonance imaging in acute hamstring injury: can we provide a return to play prognosis? Sports Med 2015; 45: 133-146

RUNNING EXPOSURE AND HAMSTRING INJURY RISK IN ELITE AUSTRALIAN FOOTBALLERS

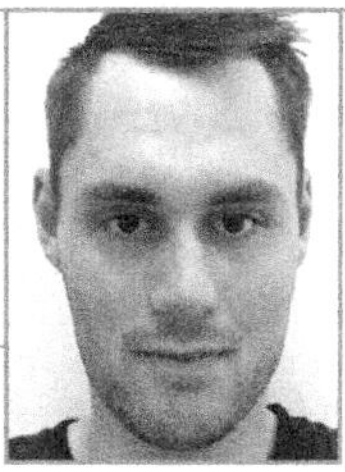

Ruddy J, Timmins R, Pollard C, Opar D

Australian Catholic University, Melbourne, Australia

Introduction

Hamstring Strain Injuries (HSIs) are the most common injury in elite Australian football. A number of modifiable risk factors have been previously examined, however despite thorough scientific investigation, the incidence, and particularly the recurrence, of HSI in Australian football has not declined.
The purpose of the current study was to investigate the association between running exposure derived from Global Positioning Systems (GPS), and future HSI risk in Australian footballers.

Methods

Two-hundred and twenty elite male Australian footballers (age: 23.4±3.5 years; height: 188.0±7.5 cm; mass: 87.2±8.5 kg; years of playing experience: 4.7±3.5) provided GPS data (OptimEye S5, Catapult Sports, Melbourne, Australia) from every training session and match for an eight month period.
Injury history, demographic data and prospective HSI reports, including magnetic resonance imaging confirmation, were also collected.
Univariate Relative Risk (RR) of subsequent HSI was determined for 36 running exposure variables. Variables which resulted in significant increases in RR of subsequent HSI were entered into logistic regression models, and the probability of subsequent HSI was estimated.

Results

Twenty-eight HSIs occurred.
Distance covered in the previous week at speed above 20 km/h (≥2461 m, RR=2.6, p=0.018), and above 24 km/h (≥594 m, RR=3.1, p=0.005) and week-to-week change in distance above 10 km/h (≥2865 m, RR=2.4, p=0.034), above 20 km/h (≥514 m, RR=2.4, p=0.034) and above 24 km/h (≥ 140 m, RR=4.3, p=0.001) significantly increased RR for subsequent HSI.
The number of efforts performed in the previous week above 10 km/h (≥587, RR=3.1, p=0.005), above 20 km/h (≥114, RR=3.8, p=0.018) and above 24 km/h (≥31, RR=3.8, p=0.018) and week-to-week change in the number of efforts performed above 10 km/h (≥125, RR=3.5, p=0.001), above 20 km/h (≥26, RR=3.5, p=0.001), and above 24 km/h (≥8, RR=3.5, p=0.001) significantly increased RR for subsequent HSI.
Logistic regression identified the largest increase in the probability of sustaining a HSI in the following week based on running exposure variables was never greater than 5%.

Conclusions

Greater running exposure in the previous week, as well as a greater week-to-week change in running exposure in the previous week, increased the risk of sustaining a HSI in the subsequent week. The use of GPS technology to monitor an athlete's running exposure following return to play may assist with preventing the recurrence of HSI.

HAMSTRING STRENGTH IN SOCCER PLAYERS WITH AND WITHOUT PREVIOUS HAMSTRING INJURIES

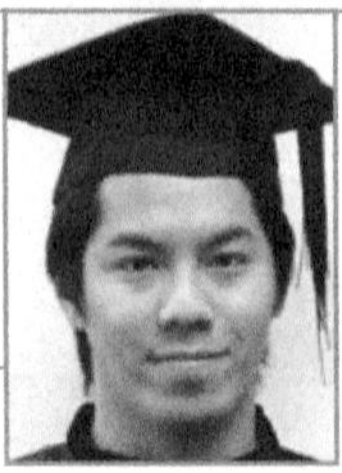

Lee JWY, Tso KW, Yung PSH, Chan KM

Department of Orthopaedics and Traumatology, Prince of Wales Hospital, Faculty of Medicine, The Chinese University of Hong Kong, Hong Kong, China

Introduction

Hamstring Strains Injuries (HSI) are the most prevalent injuries in professional football which accounted for 12% of the total injuries (2). To date, isokinetic dynamometry is considered the gold standard for evaluating knee flexor strength and had been widely adopted by previous prospective cohort studies investigating knee flexor strength as a risk factor of future HSI (1). However, this method is limited by various factors, including time, cost, and lack of portability of the device.
The aim of this retrospective study is to examine hamstring strength for football players with and without previous injury by a novel hamstring strength test.

Methods

Thirty-six elite and sub-elite male football players (8 unilateral hamstring injured, and 28 uninjured) from five clubs playing in the Hong Kong first, second, third division were recruited.
The mean (±SD) age was 24.0±5.6 years, height 176.4±8.1 cm, and weight 69.1±10.1 kg.
Each player was invited to attend one session of the novel hamstring strength test. The novel test has a good reliability and concurrent validity (ICC (2.1) =0.82; r=0.90). It is based on Nordic hamstring exercise.
Subjects were instructed to lower the upper body from a kneeling position as slow as possible until he reached a breaking point where the participant could no longer withstand the fall.
The forward tilting of trunk angle were recorded by a smartphone (iPhone 6s, Apple Inc., California, USA), that attached at the lower back. Hamstring strength and fatigue resistance of participants were tested by the Chinese University of Hong Kong (CUHK) hamstring strength test (3) during the 2014-15 season. After retrieving the maximum tolerable angle, the eccentric peak torque of player was calculated with an equation developed from our previous study.
Data were analysed by independent t-tests to determine for any significant difference between the means of dependent variables of hamstring injured group and uninjured group.

Results

Among the hamstring injured players, 75% of players strained hamstring in a competitive match situation, 6 out of 8 players injured their medial side of the dominant leg. Sprinting is the most common mechanism of HSI in this study which accounted for 75% of total injuries.
Players with previous hamstring injury showed strength deficit in the novel CUHK hamstring strength test (hamstring injured: 153.7±67.4 Nm; uninjured: 198.1±48.0 Nm; $p<0.05$).

Conclusions

The novel hamstring strength test demonstrated its ability to detect hamstring strength difference between players with and without a history of hamstring strain injuries within 12 months. This strength measure can provide a quick and convenient alternative for evaluations of hamstring strength throughout the rehabilitation period.

References

1. Croisier JL, Forthomme B, Namurois MH, Vanderthommen M, Crielaard JM. Hamstring muscle strain recurrence and strength performance disorders. Am J Sports Med 2002; 30: 199-203
2. Ekstrand J, Hagglund M, Waldén M. Injury incidence and injury patterns in professional football: the UEFA injury study. Br J Sports Med 2011; 45: 553-558
3. Lee JWY, Yung PSH, Li C, Chan HCK, Chan KM. Reliability and validity of a novel field based hamstring strength test for association football. In: Roi GS, Della Villa S (Eds). Football Medicine Strategies for Muscle and Tendon Injuries. Calzetti Mariucci Editori, Torgiano, 2013, pp. 215-216

EFFECTIVENESS OF NORDIC HAMSTRING TO IMPROVE INJURY RISK FACTOR ON FUTSAL PLAYERS

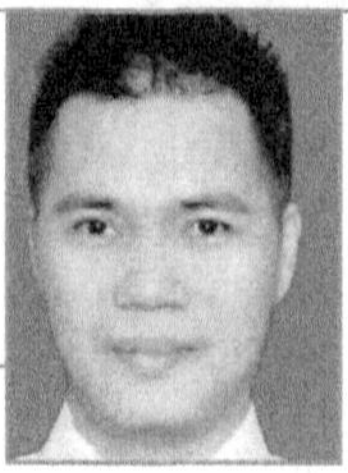

Boroh Z[1], Sudarsono NC[1], Ilyas EI[2]

[1]Sports Medicine Division, Community Medicine Department, and [2]Department of Medical Physiology, Faculty of Medicine, Universitas Indonesia, Jakarta, Indonesia

Introduction

Football has the highest injury incidence rate compared to any other sports (1).
Hamstring muscle injury is the most frequent injury in football. Researched by Wood et al. in professional football found that hamstring muscle injury incidence in football is 12% (3). Hamstring strain is mostly found on running, jumping and ball kicking exercises.
Futsal is multi sprint with higher intensity compared football. That is why the probability of hamstring muscle injury in futsal is higher than in football, as confirmed by Junge et al. who have found an incidence of 191/1,000 playing hour on futsal compared to 92/1,000 playing hour on football (2).
In Nordic Hamstring exercises the eccentric contractions performed during every movement is aimed to improve the eccentric strength of hamstring muscles, reducing the risk of muscular injuries.
The purpose of this research was to establish if the Nordic Hamstring exercise is effective as adjunct exercise to improve the strength of Knee Extensors.

Methods

Thirty one semi-professional collegiate student male futsal players (age ranges between 18 and 21 years) in Jakarta, Indonesia, were participated in this research.
They were divided into two groups: the first group consisted of 16 players (Treatment Group) and the second one consisted of 15 players (Control Group). Mean of Body Mass Index (BMI) of treatment group is 21.86±2.31 kg/m^2 and 21.90±3.21 kg/m^2 for control group.
Treatment Group performed routine exercise and Nordic Hamstring exercise for four weeks Table 1). Type of exercise of Nordic hamstring is isotonic eccentric.

Week	Sessions /week	Sets / Repetitions
1	2	2 / 5
2	2	2 / 6
3	3	3 / 6
4	3	3 / 8

Table 1. Protocol of Nordic Hamstring exercise.

Control group performed only routine exercises, consisting 3 part of exercises: warming up, stretching (static and dynamic stretching), exercises for endurance, strength, speed, technical drills and cooling down. Both groups performed routine exercises 5 sessions/week.
The Knee Extensor and Flexor muscular strengths were measured before and after treatment on both groups by using an isotonic dynamometer (Hur leg curl, Ab Hur Oy, Kokkola, Finland). The Protocol of measurement is the player sitting down on the isotonic dynamometer, the position of limbs places both the hip angle and knee angle at approximately 90°. Players flex and extend their knee. Each movement was performed three times, the best one was taken as result.
The differences of the results in both group before and after treatment were assessed by using paired t-test ($p<0.05$).

Results

The results (Table 2) showed that Players of the Treatment Group improved their Hamstring (i.e., Knee Flexors) strength in both limbs (Right: p=0.029; Left: p=0.007), and also improved the balance between Left and Right Knee Flexors strength (p=0.016), but there were no improvements on Knee Flexors/Extensors strength ratios. On the control group, there were no improvement of the Knee Flexors strength, no balance improvement, and no improvement on Knee Flexors/Extensors strength ratio.

Group	Limbs	Knee Flex		Diff %	Knee Ext		Diff %	KF/KE	
		Before	After		Before	After		Before	After
Treatment	R	67.31±26.08	81.12±17.37	20.5	163.75±25.85	160.31±22.88	- 1.49	0.411	0.506
	L	74.00±19.82	83.31±15.22	12.6	163.81±27.85	161.44±28.77	- 2.13	0.452	0.516
Control	R	69.80±24.77	73.20±18.98	4.87	168.80±36.33	168.07±35.62	- 0.44	0.413	0.435
	L	67.33±19.59	69.00±16.60	2.47	160.33±39.06	161.73±36.06	0.87	0.420	0.427

Table 2. Results of the strength tests performed before and after training in both groups of players. Strength data (N) are shown as mean±SD. Knee Ext: knee extensors (quadriceps); Knee Flex: knee flexors (hamstrings); R: right limb; L: left limb; Diff: difference in %.

Conclusions

Nordic Hamstring training carried out with a four weeks protocol, as adjunctive exercise, was effective to improve Knee Flexors (i.e., hamstring) muscle strength, and also the balance between Left and Right Knee Flexors strength on collegiate student futsal players.

This result probably helps in preventing hamstring muscle injuries, but this hypothesis needs further epidemiological studies.

References

1. De Loes M. Epidemiology of sports injuries in the Swiss organization "Youth and Sports" 1987-1989: Injuries,exposure and risks of main diagnoses. Int J Sports Med 1995; 16: 134-138
2. Junge A, Dvorak J, Graff-Baumann T, Peterson L. Football injuries during FIFA tournaments and the Olympic Games, 1998-2001. Development and implementation of an injury-reporting system. Am J Sports Med 2004; 32: 80-89
3. Woods C, Hawkins RD, Maltby S, Hulse M, Thomas A, Hodson A. The football association medical research programme: an audit of injuries in professional football - analysis of hamstring injuries. Br J Sports Med 2004; 38: 36-41

ABOVE AND BEYOND BICEP FEMORIS

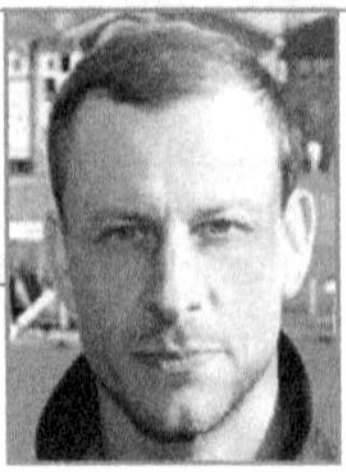

Blandford L[1], Pedersen C[2], Mottram S[1]

[1]Movement Performance Solutions, Bristol, United Kingdom;
[2]Arena Fysio, Helsingborg, Sweden

Introduction

The most commonly injured hamstring, Bicep Femoris (BF) receives the greatest focus within return to play strategies. Yet, assessment and subsequent training of its synergists, located in regions above, below and within the hamstring group itself, questions standard protocol. This case study considers how multi-joint movement assessment, informing on synergistic interactions related to BF, can support return to play interventions.

Methods

Whilst BF remains a principle cause of hamstring related time loss, 'silent partner', synergistic musculature deserve attention during return to play. In line with this premise, one week following a grade II, BF strain, an academy level player, based at a professional club (age: 16 yrs; height: 183 cm; mass: 68 kg) was assessed using a multi-joint, multi-intensity movement analysis tool, The Performance Matrix (TPM). Testing cognitive movement control, reliability literature for this tool has recently been published (2). Informing on relative contribution of multiple synergists, TPM reports the site, direction and recruitment threshold of related movement deficits, in addition to returning a score; a score of 0 out of 50 is deemed optimal. Additionally, hip flexion range of motion was assessed; straight leg raise to 70° and hip extension with a Thomas test.
Based on the findings of week 1, a training plan focussed on enhancing the movement control deficits associated with BF synergists, was delivered. Testing was repeated 6 weeks post injury.

Results

Table 1 shows movement analysis results for lumbo-pelvic and hip region performed at week 1 and week 6. Testing score fell from 28 to 19 out of 50. A
dditionally, positive tests of bilateral restrictions of Rectus Femoris and hamstrings, present in week 1, were negative by week 6.

Site, direction & threshold of uncontrolled movement	Week 1	Week 6
Hip flexion, low threshold	Uncontrolled	Controlled
Lumbar extension, high threshold	Uncontrolled	Controlled

Table 1. Results of most relevance to BF injury.

Discussion

Six weeks post injury, the player was available for selection. Whilst achieving the principle aim of any return to play strategy, the targeting of synergists highlighted as inefficient during testing, was seen to be followed by successful resolution of hamstring and Rectus Femoris restrictions, and the control issues of both lumbar extension and hip flexion. These factors have been associated with an Anterior Pelvic Tilt (APT) alignment, a marker related to both hamstring injury, and poor recruitment efficiency of BF synergists, the gluteals (3). If gluteal recruitment proves ineffective in managing eccentric challenges elicited by APT moments, such as hip flexion and lumbar extension, BF may substitute for this deficit.

APT is also associated with lack of extensibility of hip flexor musculature; hip flexor restriction is also seen to impact gluteal recruitment. A lack of hip extension range in footballers, accompanied by 60% deficit in Electromyographic (EMG) activity of gluteus maximus but a 15% increase in BF during squatting has been seen (1).

Conclusions

Assessment of synergistic contribution, may inform training strategies during the return to play phase. If conducted regions interacting with BF, interventions may address issues existent between BF and its synergists. If a return to play focus only adheres to predictable length or strength deficits within BF, synergistic interactions, associated to this outcome, may remain unresolved. Multi-regional assessment, draws focus to 'silent partner synergists', rather than just the overt outcome of deficits.

References

1. Mills M, Frank B, Goto S, Blackburn T, Cates S, Clark M, Aguilar A, Fava N, Padua D. Effect of restricted hip flexor muscle length on hip extensor muscle activity and lower extremity biomechanics in college-aged female soccer players. Int J Sports Phys Ther 2015; 10: 946 954
2. Mischiati C, Comerford M, Gosford E, Swart J, Ewings S, Botha N, Stokes M, Mottram SL. Intra and Inter-Rater Reliability of Screening for Movement Impairments: Movement Control Tests from The Foundation Matrix. J Sports Sci Med 2015; 14: 427-440
3. Oh JS, Cynn HS, Won JH, Kwon OY, Yi CH. Effects of performing an abdominal drawing-in manoeuver during prone hip extension exercises on hip and back extensor muscle activity and amount of anterior pelvic tilt. J Orthop Sports Phys Ther 2007; 37: 320-324

NEW ECCENTRIC EXERCISE MODE FOR REHABILITATION AFTER MUSCLE INJURY

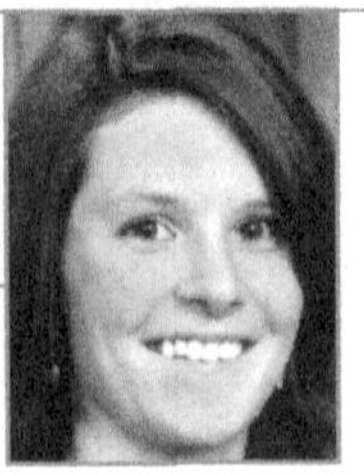

Landkammer Y, Sassmann R, Herfert J, Wicker A

Institute of Physical Medicine and Rehabilitation,
Paracelsus Medical University, Salzburg,

Introduction

The important role of eccentric muscular force development prior to a power activity maybe the most substantial during high-power sport activities (e.g. running, sprinting, jumping). The whole muscle-tendon unit participates in dissipating, or temporarily storing the energy, while forces within a muscle are used to decelerate a limb or body segment. If the muscle-tendon unit is too weak to handle the decelerating forces, injury to the muscle, myotendinous junction, the tendon itself, and the osteotendinous insertion may occur (1). Hence the need for implementing eccentric exercise in the rehabilitation phases is given. Therefore a new eccentric training device, Eccentron (BTE, Denver, USA), is used in our case report.

Case report

A 14 year old male football player (forward, youth league, height 1.78 m, weight 58 kg) ruptured the bony detachment of his right Rectus Femoris, confirmed by Magnetic Resonance Imaging (MRI) and X-ray.

40 days after the injury, upon completion of the early rehabilitation phase, we initiated an isokinetic concentric training (Biodex System 4 Pro, New York, USA) in the open kinetic chain.

In the isokinetic test performed in the 6th rehabilitation session (55 days after the injury) we measured Peak Torque (PT) at 60, 180, 240°/s angular speeds. Results showed no significant deficit in the knee extensors but a significant deficit in the knee flexors, as well as a higher agonist/antagonist ratio on the left side (74- 90.7%) compared to the right side (69.1- 75.4%) (Table 1).

	Ext 60°/s	Flex 60°/s	Flex/Ext 60°/s	Ext 180°/s	Flex 180°/s	Flex/Ext 180°/s	Ext 240°/s	Flex 240°/s	Flex/Ext 240°/s
Injured (R)	192.8	133.2	69.1%	141.5	99.5	70.3%	134.9	101.6	75.4%
Uninjured (L)	195.8	145.1	74.1%	145.3	131.8	90.7%	132.7	116.2	87.5%
Deficit Uninj/Inj (L/R)	1.5%	8.2%	--	2.6%	24.5%	--	-1.6%	12.5%	--

Table 1. First assessment 55 days after injury and on the sixth session of isokinetic training. Peak Torques (PT) in Nm at three different angular speeds, and % differences between Left-Uninjured (L) and Right-Injured (R) legs and between knee Flexors (Flex) and Extensors (Ext).

After the first test the patient performed an isokinetic training in eccentric mode once a week for four weeks. The protocol alternately included three sets of 10 repetitions of knee extension and flexion in eccentric mode at 90°/s and two sets of 15 repetitions at 120°/s, with 60 seconds of rest between sets. This protocol leads to the results showed in Table 2, assessed by a second isokinetic test, performed 88 days after injury.

	Ext 60°/s	Flex 60°/s	Flex/Ext 60°/s	Ext 180°/s	Flex 180°/s	Flex/Ext 180°/s	Ext 240°/s	Flex 240°/s	Flex/Ext 240°/s
Injured (R)	216.9	118.2	54.5%	141.2	97.4	69.0%	127.1	93.7	73.7%
Uninjured (L)	202.8	158.4	78.1%	140.0	125.7	89.7%	143.4	72.9	50.9%
Uninj/Inj (L/R)	-6.9%	25.3%	--	-0.8%	22.5%	--	11.3%	-28.4%	--

Table 2. Second assessment 88 days after injury. Peak Torques (PT) in Nm at three different angular speeds, and % differences between Left-Uninjured (L) and Right-Injured (R) legs and between knee Flexors (Flex) and Extensors (Ext).

After the second test, the patient started with training sessions on the new recumbent stepper-ergometer Eccentron with visual feedback, where the patient resists the alternately moving pedals at an individual force capacity. The training protocol was: three sets of 4 minutes, load of 600-800 N, pedal frequency of 12-20 repetitions per minute. After one minute of warming up with 50% of maximum resistance, the resistance was increased up to ±20% of the maximal resistance, followed by one minute of cooling down with again 50% of maximum resistance.
After four training sessions with the Eccentron, the isokinetic test performed 123 days after the injury showed a further increase of PT, and deficits always lower than 10% (Table 3).

	Ext 60°/s	Flex 60°/s	Flex/Ext 60°/s	Ext 180°/s	Flex 180°/s	Flex/Ext 180°/s	Ext 240°/s	Flex 240°/s	Flex/Ext 240°/s
Injured (R)	220.5	147.8	67.0%	153.9	123.5	80.3%	143.4	120.1	83.7%
Uninjured (L)	226.4	151.2	66.8%	147.9	135.8	91.8%	143.5	131.0	91.3%
Uninj/Inj (L/R)	2.6%	2.3%	--	-4.0%	9.0%	--	0.0%	8.4%	--

Table 3. Third assessment 123 days after surgery. Peak Torques (PT) in Nm at three different angular speeds, and % differences between Left-Uninjured (L) and Right-Injured (R) legs and between knee Flexors (Flex) and Extensors (Ext).

Conclusions

According to the literature (1), eccentric muscle training is an important part of functional recovery especially in sports with high muscular demands and challenging tasks, like football.
Eccentric training, also with new eccentric machines (i.e., Eccentron) can be successfully included into rehabilitation and training.

References

1. LaStayo PC, Woolf JM, Lewek MD, Snyder-Mackler L, Reich T, Lindstedt SL. Eccentric muscle contractions. Their contribution to injury, prevention, rehabilitation, and sport. J Orthop Sports Phys Ther 2003; 33: 557-571

A BIOCHEMICAL ANALYSIS OF MUSCLE INJURIES IN FOOTBALL DURING REHABILITATION

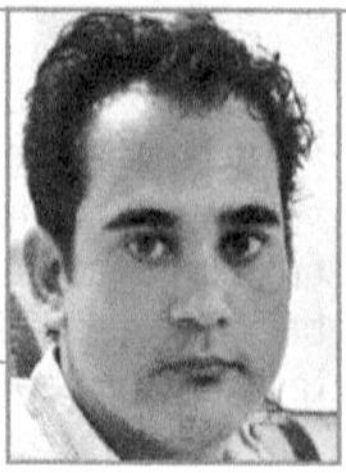

Tymvios C

Omonoia FC; BHS Diagnostics, Nicosia, Cyprus

Introduction

This study was conducted in Cyprus, on football players of League A and B, in order to study the assumption that biochemical evaluation could be used to treat and/or prevent muscle injuries on football players. The study lasted 5 years (2010-2015).

Methods

223 healthy and injured male football players (age 17-37yrs) were biochemically assessed during the season (June 2010 - May 2015). Muscle strain injury was defined as any grade 2 or 3 strain injury resulting from over-extension of the flexors muscles of the lower limb. Minor injuries resulting from hard kicks and other stretched muscles in other areas of the body were excluded from the study.

The study, therefore, mainly focused on injuries of the Biceps Femoris muscle. Diagnosis and progress of the injury were assessed with ultrasound and Magnetic Resonance Imaging (MRI).

The subjects were assessed in the following occasions: a) beginning of the season, b) every 2 months during the season (2 days after a game) and c) during the injury period (weekly).

Blood samples were collected from the antecubital vein.

The biochemical markers analyzed were: Full Blood Count (FBC), magnesium (in red blood cells), zing, phosphorus, calcium, progesterone, estradiol, testosterone, free testosterone, SHBG, albumin, cortisol, DHEA-S, CRP, IL-6, TNF-α, IgA, Super Oxide Dismutase (SOD), Glutathione Peroxidase (GPX), Glutathione (G), Vitamins B3, B6, B12, D3, DPD, Creatine Phosphokinase (CPK) and pH (in saliva and urine).

Fully accredited clinical laboratory with external (ISO 15189:2012 and RIQAS) and internal controls and biochemical analyzers (Cobas 311 and Cobas 411, Roche, Mannheim, Germany) were used in order to perform the tests.

Results

31 football players felled into the definition of injury during the course of the study (2010-2011: 8 injuries; 2011-2012: 9 injuries; 2012-2013: 7 injuries; 2013-2014: 3 injuries; 2014-2015: 4 injuries). CPK increases radically (4-10 fold) upon the event of a muscular injury however it could not be used as secure marker of muscle injury due to its high sensitivity in tissue damage.

Inflammation markers TNF-α and IL-6 increase by 4-6 fold, 2-4 weeks before injury. Further to this there is a significant decrease during the course of rehabilitation, period in which they return to normal levels.

Change in oxidative stress markers SOD (increase 65±12%), GPX (increase 120±23%) and G (decrease 55±14%) in combination with high levels of inflammation markers TNF-α, IL-6, low body pH (<5), low magnesium levels (<1.8 mg/dL), IgA (<100 mg/dL) and phosphorus (<2.4 mg/dL) were associated with increase chance of injury by approximately nine fold.

In rehabilitation period, footballers with higher levels of magnesium, zing and urine and saliva pH had faster recovery time from footballers with low values. Low values of Vitamins B1 (<2.5 μg/dL), B6 (<3 ng/mL) and B12 (<200 pg/mL) in blood stream where associated with slow progress during rehabilitation.

Laboratory Test	Before Injury	After Injury	After RTP	Normal Reference Values
Hemoglobin* (g/dL)	13.9±2.13	14.2±2.35	15.8±2.02	13.0-18.0
Magnesium⁺ (mg/dL)	1.84±0.3	2.13±0.45	2.03±0.33	1.7-2.55
Zing (μg/dL)	68±10.1	110±15.3	103±12.1	73-127
Phosphorus (mg/dL)	2.2±0.8	2.8±0.7	3.5±0.6	2.5-5.0
Calcium (mg/dL)	9.3±1.3	9.6±0.8	9.5±0.8	8.4-10.2
Progesterone (ng/mL)	0.9±0.1	0.98±0.08	0.96±0.07	0.2-1.4
Estradiol (pg/mL)	33.4±4.8	28.4±3.2	29.6±3.8	7.63-42.6
Testosterone (ng/mL)	3.2±0.4	4.6±1.3	5.8±2.9	2.8-8.0
Free Testosterone (pg/mL)	9.2±0.8	13.1±2.8	13.6±3.8	8.8-27.0
SHBG (nmol/L)	43.3±5.8	28.5±3.3	32.6±3.2	0.350-200
Albumin (g/dL)	4.5±1.2	4.4±1.4	4.4±1.4	4.2-5.3
Cortisol (nmol/L)	680±117	530±180	390±110	171-536
DHEA-S (μg/dL)	260.0±22.8	373.0±33.3	365.0±30.6	160-449
IL-6 (pg/mL)	5.6±0.8	2.8±1.2	<1.5	< 1.5
TNF-α (pg/mL)	435±52	185±26	78±8	42-203
IgA (mg/dL)	78±12	125±15	240±18	70-400
SOD (U/g Hb)	23000±1700	18500±1400	14900±1350	5000-16000
GPX (U/g Hb)	215.0±15.3	190.0±19.8	98.0±11.8	81-109
G (uM/L)	467±55	450±65	830±48	>669
Vitamin B1 (μg/dL)	2.6±0.8	2.3±0.8	12.3±2.4	2.5-7.5
Vitamin B6 (ng/mL)	2.6±0.6	2.8±0.7	18.8±2.2	3-17
Vitamin B12 (pg/mL)	425±65	430±67	1203±95	200-950
Vitamin D3 (ng/mL)	28.5±4.8	28.8±4.8	33.3±4.5	>50
DPD (ngDPD/mg)	14.4±1.5	12.7±1.7	15.5±1.8	8.4-19.7
CPK# (U/L)	280±180	1400±444	150±74	80-500
pH&	4.6±0.9	4.1±0.6	6.8±1.8	5.5

Table 1. Biochemical results of injured (31) players Before Injury, three days After Injury and two days after Return To Play (RTP). The average injury period was 6 weeks. Note that some results may be altered due to extensive supplementation during rehabilitation period. *Football players with any type of anemia where excluded from the average of hemoglobin measurements. +Magnesium was measured in red blood cells (not serum). #Extremely high values of CPK before injury (i.e. values above 2200 U/L) were excluded from the study. &In order to measure the pH accurately we asked the subjects no to eat or drink before the samples were taken. The following equation was used: (2 x saliva pH + urine pH) / 3 = Average pH).

No evidence suggested that levels of Vitamin D3 and calcium affect muscle strain injuries or rehabilitation; nonetheless normal DPD (bone density) was found to be strongly related with faster recovery. Finally altered ratios between DHEA:Testosterone:Cortisol and Testosterone:Free Testosterone:Estrogen were clearly altered before the course of a muscle strain injury but failed to show any significant benefits during rehabilitation period.

Conclusions

Muscle injury can be successfully monitored biochemically with accuracy and precision. In this study we show that extensive study of biochemical markers during the season could be a valuable tool for the medical team and fitness coach in order to treat (and prevent) muscle strain injuries in football and secure a faster and accurate return to play period.

References

1. Mueller-Wohlfahrt HW, Ueblacker P. Muscle Injuries in Sports. Thieme, Stuttgart/New York, 2013, pp. 267-292

Sunday 10th April, 2016 (afternoon)
FLEMING ROOM

INVITED SPEAKERS

FOOTBALL RECONDITIONING AND RETURN TO PLAY

Chairs

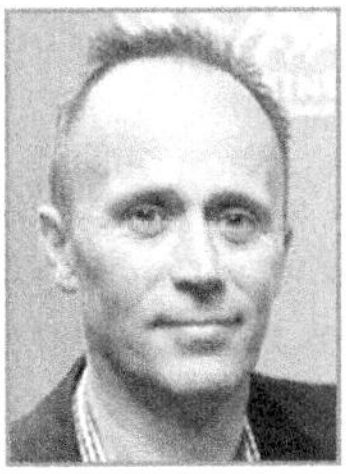

Bryan English
(London, United Kingdom)

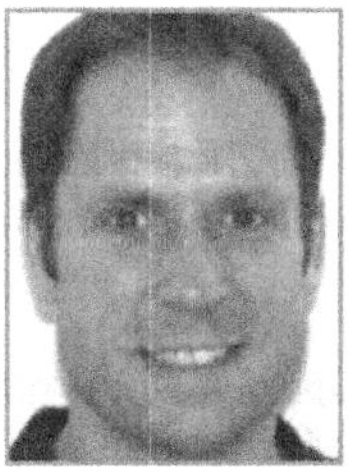

Chris Neville
(Blackburn, United Kingdom)

16:30	Science of football reconditioning and return to play **Gregory Dupont (Lille, France)**
16:45	Use of the pool in football reconditioning **Pierre-Louis Puig (Capbréton, France)**
17:00	The use of pitch in football reconditioning **Shad Forsythe (London, United Kingdom)**
17:15	Planned performance reconditioning-the bridge for a return to team training **Bill Knowles (Philadelphia, USA)**
17:30	From football reconditioning to the first competitive match **Mo Gimpel (Southampton, United Kingdom)**
17:45	Discussion
18:00	End of the session

SCIENCE OF FOOTBALL RECONDITIONING AND RETURN TO PLAY

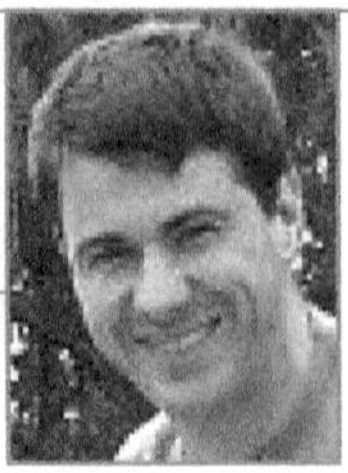

Dupont GM

Faculty of Health, Life and Social Sciences, Research Department for Sports and Exercise Science, Edinburgh Napier University, Edinburgh, United Kingdom

Introduction

Following an injury, a rehabilitation process is implemented by the medical team, with the aim to return the player to training and matches as soon as possible. During the rehabilitation period, players can lose the training-induced adaptations if they cease training or only perform reduced amounts. In soccer, such a lack of activity is associated with large decrements in maximal oxygen consumption, moderate to very large impairments in intermittent-running performance, small to moderate negative changes in body composition, a moderate decline in sprint performance and small to moderate decrements in muscle power (2). However, this period could be also considered as a window of opportunity to improve some specific qualities and at least to maintain the other ones. This process includes implementing strategies targeted at psychology of the player specific nutritional programmes, and increasing/maintaining some physical qualities. This role generally conducted by the conditioner requires carefully quantifying the workload as the spike in the acute: chronic workload ratio is associated with higher risk of injury (1). The reconditioning stage during the rehabilitation period could have a significant influence on the risk of re-injury. As little is known about the reconditioning process used by professional football teams, it would be interesting to survey this practice. Therefore, the purpose of this study is to analyse the current practice and perceptions in professional football clubs concerning the conditioners role during the return to play process after hamstring injuries, which are the most common muscle injury in football.

Methods

A survey was administered to 25 English premier and French premier league football clubs. The survey included 17 questions on conditioning during the rehabilitation period from the injury through to the criteria to validate return to play.

Results

Nineteen medical and sport science teams responded (76%).

During the first phase after injury, conditioning program is mainly focused on maintaining a level of aerobic fitness and upper strength through mainly hand bike (50% of the responses) at a moderate intensity (60%) and upper body strength (83%) at a moderate intensity (93%).

During the second phase, the physical program includes mainly bike (100%) at a moderate intensity (65%) to high-intensity (35%), upper body strength (94%) at a moderate intensity (65%) to high-intensity (35%), lower body strength (78%) at a low intensity (31%) to moderate intensity (69%).

During these 2 phases, a specific nutrition plan was provided by 68% of the teams with the main objective to avoid fat-mass increase (54%).

During the functional phase, 83% of the teams prescribe a progressive return to full team training. Four full training sessions (83%) are recommended before a return to match-play.
The training load was mainly monitored with rating of perceived exertion scale (77%), heart rate (71%), and duration (59%). Global Positioning Systems were used by only 35% of the teams during this period and were mainly focused on high-speed distance (100% of the responses).
The tests before returning to play are used by 72% of the teams and include sprints (71%), maximal strength (57%) and strength imbalance (57%). Psychological states were tested by only 29% of the teams.
The threshold set as criteria for return to play in these tests were above 90% of the initial values previously tested for sprints speed (90%), maximal strength (88%) and strength imbalance (89%).

Conclusions

This survey reports the most common practices and perceptions of premier league football medical and sport science departments regarding the conditioning role during the rehabilitation period. It would be worthwhile to determine the level of scientific evidence for these practices in order to analyse the gap between practice and research.

References

1. Blanch P, Gabbett TJ. Has the athlete trained enough to return to play safely? The acute:chronic workload ratio permits clinicians to quantify a player's risk of subsequent injury. Br J Sports Med 2015 Dec 23. pii: bjsports-2015-095445. [Epub ahead of print]
2. Silva JR, Brito J, Akenhead R, Nassis GP. The transition period in soccer: a window of opportunity. Sports Med 2015 Nov 3. [Epub ahead of print]

USE OF THE POOL IN FOOTBALL RECONDITIONING

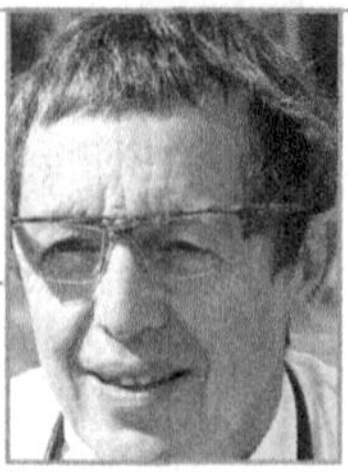

Puig PL

Centre Européen de Rééducation du Sportif (CERS), Capbreton, France

Increasing interest in aquatic physical therapy in football reconditioning can be attributed to a greater variety of exercises in a low-stress physical environment where axial and compressive forces are reduced with a heavy volume of aerobic training. Running in water, specifically Deep-Water Running (DWR) is a great tool for preventing overuse injuries and water resistance is the main force to be won during locomotion in water and it requires a high energy cost that does not exist in traditional running-based training. Using the water to regain lost mobility, to strengthen weakened muscles and to restore the neuromuscular control is often implemented with the aim of optimizing performance, preventing injury, or providing news sports skills.

Physical properties of water

Buoyancy and viscosity are key elements in designing effective exercises for treating athletic injuries. The buoyant force of water decreases the effective weight of an individual in proportion to the degree of immersion. The ability to control joint compression forces by varying degrees of immersion is of primary benefit in the design and prescription of therapeutic exercises. The advantage of viscosity of water is indirect: when the person moves through the water, resistance is felt. Thus, a relatively simple method of reducing impact forces and eccentric loading while still providing sufficient stimulus for physiological and sports-related improvements would be to perform plyometric training in a swimming pool.

Muscle strengthening using the viscosity of water

Water acts as an accommodating resistance. The advantage of accommodating resistance is that it matches the patient's applied force or effort. Because the resistance of the water equals the force exerted, the likelihood of exacerbation or re-injury is reduced dramatically. Water acts as a variable resistance. The term variable refers to being able to change the speed or velocity of the movement. Unlike isokinetic strength-training apparatus, which limit exercises to a preset velocity, it is possible to change limb speeds during each repetition in the water. Because most human motion is variable in nature, functional gains are more likely to be made.

Cooperative movements of lower extremities

An advantage of aquatic physical therapy is the extensive range of exercises that require alternating or symmetric movements of the limbs and associated joints. These movements encourage increased involvement of the affected limbs by inducing the injured side to match the effort and range of motion of the uninjured side. The propulsive movement patterns of formal swimming strokes require arm and leg actions that combine symmetric or alternating patterns of motion.

Cooperative movements of lower extremities

An advantage of aquatic physical therapy is the extensive range of exercises that require alternating or symmetric movements of the limbs and associated joints. These movements encourage increased involvement of the affected limbs by inducing the injured side to match the effort and range of motion of the uninjured side. The propulsive movement patterns of formal swimming strokes require arm and leg actions that combine symmetric or alternating patterns of motion.

Aquatic stretching

The therapeutic advantages of early restoration of joint mobility are well documented. The inactive injured athlete is predisposed to muscle atrophy, soft tissue weakness, decreased joint mobility, and possible increases in pain. Also, functional deficits may be addressed sooner with early mobilization. Aquatic stretching is a series of stretching exercises done in varying depths of water to quickly restore flexibility, produces muscle relaxation and decrease muscle soreness following intense workouts.

Neuromuscular training

Inadequate neuromuscular control of the body's trunk or core may compromise dynamic stability of the lower extremity and result in increased abduction torque at the knee, which may increase strain on the knee ligaments and lead to injury. Injuries occurring in football players that used neuromuscular training tended to be less severe. There is a specific preventive effect on knee injuries as well as ankle injuries. Most studies placed a special emphasis on core stability and proper knee alignment. The aims are to improve neuromuscular control during static and dynamic movements and to produce less strain to the joint. Because the effects of gravity are minimized with immersion, the proprioceptive input from the force of gravity is negated. Thus, the pool is an ideal medium to retrain this sense. Multi-intervention exercises can be performed in a variety of combinations of balance training, agility, stretching, plyometrics, running exercises, cutting and jumping/landing technique. Core body stability and strength training is critical to transfer kinetic energy from the upper to the lower extremity via the trunk musculature. Because any upper or lower extremity exercise must be stabilized by the trunk in the pool, most of these exercises also train the core. Core muscle activity precedes lower extremity muscle activity in the temporal sequence of many athletic tasks.

Cardiorespiratory fitness

DWR has been shown to compare favorably with land-based exercise. Maximum heart rate values for aquatic running ranged from 89% to 95% of values measured on land. Because of the physiologic changes occurring with immersion, the athlete should train at a heart rate 17 to 20 beats per minute lower than on land. The rate of perceived exertion is often unreliable due to the effects of skill and comfort on perceived exertion. As with any exercise session, an appropriate warm-up and cool down are essential. Optimally performed DWR requires minimal range of motion at the shoulders and a large range of hip and knee motion. Flotation vests may be used when teaching the athlete a deep-water technique. If weight bearing is allowed, the athlete can exercise in shoulder-deep water. Ankle floats, and fins increase the lever arm and resistance. Vertical kicking can be performed with or without fins and should be initiated with a small flutter kick. The program should be as sport specific as possible.

Aquatic plyometric training

Benefits from this type of training include improved measures of muscular strength, power and vertical jump, joint function and stability, reduced incidence of serious knee injuries and running economy. Performance of aquatic plyometric training could lead to similar benefits, but with reduced risks due to the buoyancy of water. Although buoyancy reduces the stretch reflex and amount of eccentric loading during aquatic plyometric exercise, athletes encounter greater than normal resistance during concentric movements because of the viscosity of water. The aquatic plyometric training exercises included power skips, spike approaches, single- and double-leg bounding, continuous jumping for height, squat jumps with blocking form, and depth jumps. The subjects were encouraged to perform all exercises in an explosive manner, and to apply their maximal effort on all maneuvers. Depth jumps were performed involving submerged boxes. The subjects began by squat jumping from the pool floor onto the submerged box, then squat jumping without hesitation as high as possible and landing on the floor at which point they immediately squat jumped as high as possible.

Football sport skills

The ability to control the ball is the key to many other skills, and juggling is also a very good way to practice ball control. Therefore, a player can only master the technique of controlling the ball if he coordinates the various parts of his/her body.

Sport-specific activities can be duplicated using aquatic equipment. Resistance can be added via buoyant or surface. Moreover, because the athlete is free floating and not stabilized on the pool's bottom, exercises require a great deal of trunk stabilization. Stabilization exercises can be performed in both open-chain and closed-chain positions. A variety of resistive and stabilization activities can be performed in provocative positions.

USE OF THE PITCH IN FOOTBALL RECONDITIONING

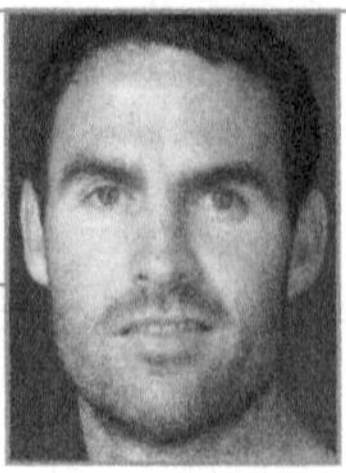

Forsythe S

Arsenal Football Club, London, United Kingdom

London Based Arsenal Football Club competes primarily in the English Premier League and while the Premier League is Arsenal's Primary competition, the club has enjoyed Champions League Football since the 1998-99 season and often competes simultaneously in the FA Cup and League Cup. The psycho-physical demands placed on our squad, competing in as many as four different competitions each season is extremely high, and understandably injuries of varying types and severity will occur. Arsenal's three full-time Fitness/Strength & Conditioning staff work closely with our medical team to capture relative pre-testing data and screening on our players to assist us in planning their training and recovery strategies, periodize their load, and bring them back to full training and match fitness as quick as possible.

At Arsenal Football Club we look at determining our Return to Play in a Progressive way.

1. Determining, Ready to Run: knowing that each injury has a different set of priorities Arsenal's Performance Team (Medical and Fitness teams) utilizes our pre-season testing and in-season monitoring of strength loads and biomechanical performance to gauge when our player is ready to start running. When these markers are achieved the athlete can progress to run.
2. Ready to Train: Arsenal's Performance Team utilizes our pre-season testing, in-season monitoring, and previous match/training data to set bench marks for starting and progressing through our running progression while mixing in football skill activities as tolerated. We try when possible and as tolerated to make the process sport and position specific. When these markers are achieved the athlete can progress to training
3. Ready to Play: Arsenal's Medical and Fitness utilize our prior in-season training monitoring and match data to determine a set of benchmarks our player must reach in order to available for match selection.

As Arsenal's Performance Team our primary goal during the 'Return to Play' process is to challenge our players when ready by placing them in an appropriate position/progression to succeed before taking the next step. We do realize that we work in highly competitive professional football environment and at times appropriate progression and the needs of the team do not always match up. At these times risk to the individual player and team need to be addressed collectively as a staff.

Sunday 10th April, 2016 (afternoon)
CHURCHILL AUDITORIUM

INVITED SPEAKERS

OBJECTIVE EVALUATION IN RETURN TO PLAY DECISION

Chairs

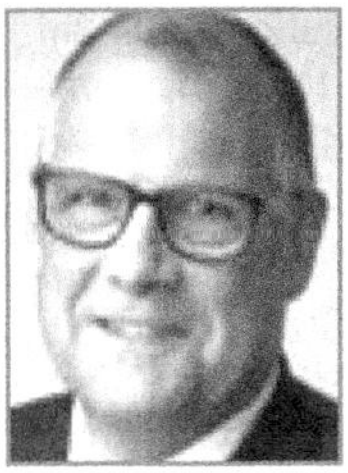

Paul Jackson
(Bath, United Kingdom)

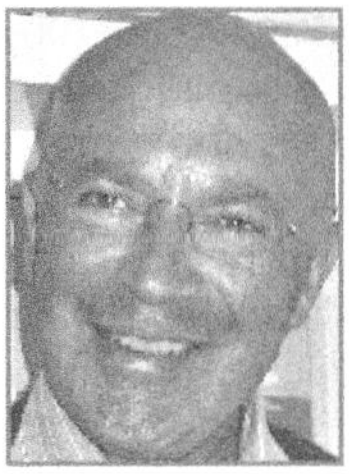

Donato Rosa
(Neaples, Italy)

16:30 Movement analysis for return to play decision making
Andy Franklyn-Miller (Dublin, Ireland)

16:45 The role of isokinetic testing in return to play decision making
Jesús Olmo (Madrid, Spain)

17:00 The aerobic and anaerobic threshold test
Davide Fazzini (Bologna, Italy)

17:15 Laxity measurement tools
Stefano Zaffagnini (Bologna, Italy)

17:30 Football specific field testing
Gary Lewin (London, United Kingdom)

17:45 Discussion

18:00 End of the session

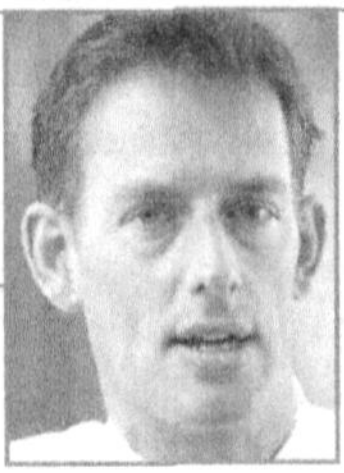

MOVEMENT ANALYSIS FOR RETURN TO PLAY DECISION MAKING

Franklyn-Miller A

Sports Surgery Clinic, Dublin, Ireland and Centre for Health, Exercise and Sports Medicine, University of Melbourne, Australia

Introduction

Although fitness to return to play is often described as the ability to execute sport specific tasks with a normal Range Of Motion (ROM) and with no pain (1), we all appreciate that this is not absolute, players can often compromise movement coordination or optimal execution to achieve a score or complete a task. In football, there are currently no return to play tests (2), which examine change of direction or agility abilities despite the predominance of this movement as part of the game. Currently we see clinical examination, ROM, strength and power tests and then a timeline of injury as the most common tool used as return to training.
There is existing literature in Anterior Cruciate Ligament (ACL) rehabilitation with more complex tasks including single leg hop for distance, counter movement jump and drop landing which assess movement competence alongside strength ratios in Isokinetic dynamometry (3).
As part of original work in the investigation of rehabilitation post ACL injury and athletic groin pain we examined a side hurdle hop, a planned 110° cut and a unplanned 45-90°cut in the 3D laboratory assessing kinematics and kinetics of the movement coordination and reproducibility in both an injured and un-injured population.
After examining the literature on agility and change of direction tests in an uninjured population, we devised a multi directional challenge test which incorporated a anaerobic, change of direction, agility, linear, curvilinear and prone components not only using time as an outcome but the movement competence of key movements. The objective was to first test the reliability of the test, then the movement variability of the execution of the biomechanics components and then the variability of in season performance changes prior to adopting a field version utilising inertial sensors.

Methods

Sixteen multidirectional field sport athletes (mass: 76.4±5.5 (SD) kg, height 177.6±4.7 cm, age 25.5±6.0 years) were recruited and tested during the 2015 season. Participants were selected from a variety of soccer, rugby, hurling and Gaelic football teams and they were all amateurs of varying competitive levels. All participants completed informed consent. The study was approved by the Sport Surgery Clinic Hospital Ethics Committee
The proposed test, named VU, is made up of three components, the first part tests acceleration, deceleration, change of direction and single leg power production (Figure 1). From the initial part, the athlete continues into the U run (curvilinear load). As the athlete comes to the end of the second U, they then continue into the straight line sprint for 20 m. The straight line run performed at this stage of the test will assess the athlete's ability to reach maximum velocity while under fatigue over a prolonged distance. At the end of the 20 m sprint a defender will direct a left or right cut at 45° in an unplanned direction.

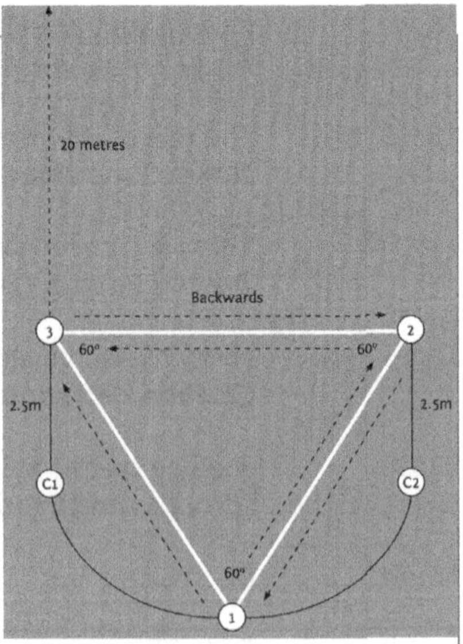

Figure 1. The VU test.

Participants undertook the VU test on two different test days exactly one week a part. The test was undertaken in very similar conditions, with the same grass football pitch surface and dry weather conditions on both testing occasions. Each athlete was quasi-randomised to determine which side they would start the test on. Participants undertook the test on test day 1 and 2 in the same order. Athletes were asked not to undertake any vigorous exercise on the day prior to testing. Testing procedure was exactly the same on both occasions. Participants undertook two practice trials of each movement (submaximal practice trials for the cutting maneuvers) before capture.
Time to completion of the VU test was measured using timing gates (Smart Speed, Fusion Sport, Sumner Park, Australia) placed at the start and end point of the VU test. The test began by breaking the first timing gate with a hurdle hop. In order to examine the test retest reliability of the VU test, we first analysed the normality in the distribution of the data using a Shapiro-Wilks W test. We then proceeded to examine the test retest reliability between both testing days in both the dominant leg and non-dominant legs. A Student's t-test was used to detect significant differences between tests. Each participant acted as his or her own control, reducing variability and increasing statistical power. The significance level was set at $P<0.05$.
Intraclass Correlation Coefficients (ICC) were calculated with a 95% Confidence Interval (CI) and Coefficient of Variation (CV) were used. Analysis of variance was with ANOVA and post hoc Tukey test with Bonferoni correction were undertaken to detect differences between tests.

Results

Test-retest reliability displayed excellent reliability as shown in Table 1.

	Test 1	**Test 2**	**Test 1**	**Test 2**
Mean±SD	21.23±1.81	21.01±2.01	20.81±1.65	21.15±1.85
CI (low - high)	20.26 - 22.19	19.93 - 22.08	19.93 - 21.69	20.17 - 22.14
CV	0.09	0.10	0.08	0.09
ICC	0.96		0.93	
ICC (low - high)	0.90 - 0.99		0.81 - 0.98	
CV of variation	0.49		0.68	
P	0.226		0.120	

Table 1. test-retest reliability.

Conclusions

The VU test has been demonstrated to be a highly reliable field based test. The test can identify deficits in performance. The role of this test in specifically identifying issues related to lower limb injury such as hamstring injury needs to be investigated further, and the biomechanical variability of testing and in season perfromance variability of those measures need confiming prior to examination of field based inertial measures.

References

1. Creighton DW, Shrier I, Shultz R, Meeuwisse WH, Matheson GO. Return-to-play in sport: a decision-based model. Clin J Sport Med 2010; 20: 379-385
2. Paul DJ, Gabbett TJ, Nassis GP. Agility in Team Sports: Testing, Training and Factors Affecting Performance. Sports Med 2015 Sports Med. 2015 Dec 15. [Epub ahead of print]
3. Undheim MB, Cosgrave C, King E, Strike S, Marshall B, Falvey É, Franklyn-Miller A. Isokinetic muscle strength and readiness to return to sport following anterior cruciate ligament reconstruction: is there an association? A systematic review and a protocol recommendation. Br J Sports Med 2015; 49: 1305-1310

THE ROLE OF ISOKINETIC TESTING IN RETURN TO PLAY DECISION MAKING

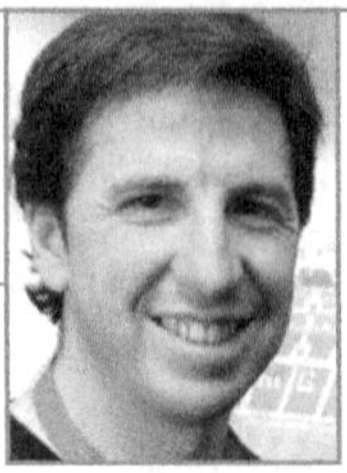

Olmo J

Real Madrid CF, Madrid, Spain

Return to Play Decision Making should consist in a multifactorial analysis, namely:
- Clinical Data: Physical examination, Imaging, Time.
- Functional Data: Analytical physical data - range of motion, strength, proprioception- and integrated functional data - functional motion, functional strength, functional control.
- Athletic condition.
- Football-specific playing adaptation.

From these data, doctors can estimate a percentage or readiness and a re-injury risk for Return To Play (RTP). Classic isokinetic machines has been directed to test muscular strength in standard, non-functional exercises aimed to isolate the tested muscle group as much as possible. From this setup, normative agonist/antagonist and bilateral ratios can be obtained for isolated muscles, both in concentric and eccentric modes. This kind of approach allows for a good information of the strength of one muscle group, but only limited information about its performance in functional, football-specific situations. As an advantage, there is plenty of information about the normative data to follow for evaluating the strength status of a determined muscle group against its contralateral one, its antagonist, or a population sample. Particularly in football, muscle strength levels around the knee and hip are of interest, inasmuch as they are involved in common football injuries, and can be compared with normative data in footballers. This kind of classic isokinetic equipment, in isotonic mode, also allows for training and testing of muscle contraction control in controlled setups, again mostly in non-functional motions. Recently, a new generation of isokinetic devices is emerging. Our work group are involved in the development of one such machine (1), and are accumulating growing data from its use in football players. This new generation has several key features that are oriented to a more functional, sport-specific actions strength testing, including:
- Pulley, cable-driven, non-guided, free kinematics resistance, which allows for infinite functional muscular exercises.
- Linear motion with force testing expressed in Newtons (N), as opposed to classic isokinetic angular motion torque testing in Newton * meters (Nm)
- Not only Isokinetic, but also 'Pleokinetic' modes, in which we can variate the velocity of the pulley along the range of motion in a linear fashion as will, allowing for acceleration and deceleration in an independent manner for concentric and eccentric phases.

This way, this new device is more functional in a double sense: enables more functional exercises, and the motion can be switch to more natural, non-isokinetic contraction modes. For applying this new equipment to rehabilitation and RTP evaluation, firstly we develop exercises that reproduce the injury mechanism, by positioning the player in the concrete functional gesture, and applying the pulley traction to mimic the injury-causing vector; and secondly, we adjust the velocity of the device in a deceleration eccentric mode to provide a very specific kinetic resistance to the eccentric contraction. This way, we can train and evaluate the specific deceleration muscle strength that opposes to the harmful injury vector. We hope that this new generation isokinetic devices will bring a more efficient strength training for injury rehabilitation and prevention, and a more specific strength testing for return to play decision making.

References

1. Olmo J. The Haefni HHE 1.0 system. A new isokinetic and pleokinetic device. In: Roi GS, Della Villa S. (Eds) Football medicine strategies for muscle and tendon injuries. Calzetti Mariucci Editore, Torgiano, 2013, pag. 89-90

THE AEROBIC AND ANAEROBIC THRESHOLD TEST

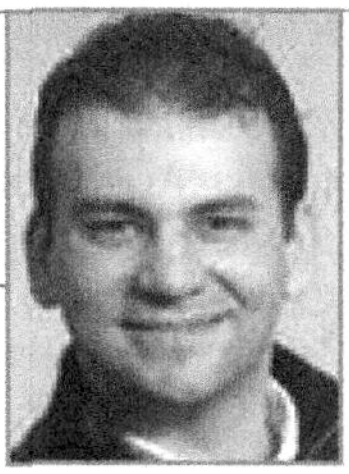

Fazzini D[1], Roi GS[1,2]

[1]Isokinetic Medical Group, FIFA Medical Centre of Excellence, Bologna;
[2]Department of Neurological, Biomedical and Movement Sciences, University of Verona, Verona, Italy

During a 90-minute football match, elite-level players run about 10 km at an average intensity close to the anaerobic threshold (i.e., 80-90% of maximal Heart Rate, HRmax) (3). However, the stop and go pattern of play lead players to repeated high intensity bouts which must be supported by a high rate of energy mainly coming from the anaerobic glycolytic sources, with average heart rate above 90% of HRmax also in recreational footballers (2). Moreover, during recovery between bouts the aerobic metabolism become mainly involved as well as for covering the energy requirements of playing at submaximal intensity.

There is a wide agreement that the aerobic and anaerobic characteristics (among others) can be considered important for a football player, and several protocols of functional assessment have been proposed. In our Clinics we utilize an incremental treadmill test to assess the aerobic and anaerobic thresholds of injured as well as healthy players.

The aerobic threshold can be defined as the intensity of exercise at which anaerobic glycolytic energy pathways start to be a significant part of energy production. This intensity conventionally corresponds to a blood lactate concentration of 2 mM. The anaerobic threshold can be defined as the intensity of exercise at which lactate builds up in the blood faster than it can be cleared away. This intensity conventionally corresponds to a blood lactate concentration of 4 mM. The incremental protocol of the threshold test is performed running on a treadmill, starting at 7 km/h with speed increments of 2 km/h every three minutes until the anaerobic threshold is reached (Bosquet L, Léger L, Legros P. Methods to determine aerobic endurance. Sports Med 2002; 32: 675-700). At the end of every three minutes step, measurements of the Heart Rate (HR) (Heart Rate Monitors, Polar Electro, Kempele, Finland), and blood lactate concentration (Lactate Analyzer YSI 1500 Sport, Yellow Spring Corp., Yellow Spring, USA) from capillary samples from an ear lobe are taken. Aerobic and anaerobic thresholds (conventionally at 2 and 4 mmol/L of lactate, respectively) are then calculated in terms of speed (km/h) and HR (bpm) from the relationships between speed and lactate and between speed and HR; these thresholds are used to individualize the intensity of the training sessions in healthy players.

Players	N	Age yrs	HR T2 bpm	HR T2 % HRmax	T2 Speed km/h	HR T4 bpm	HR T4 % HRmax	T4 Speed km/h
Professional male footballers	72	26±4	164±10	84±5	11.7±1.7	185±10	92±4	14.3±1.4
Professional male futsal players	14	25±4	157±12	80±6	12.7±1.5	174±9	89±5	15.3±1.4
Professional female footballers	22	23±6	169±9	86±3	9.9±1.2	181±8	92±3	12.0±1.2
Recreational male footballers	19	23±4	161±15	82±7	10.9±1.2	176±12	89±6	13.7±0.7
Injured male footballers*	50	23±6	158±12	80±6	8.9±1.6	180±11	91±3	11.4±1.6

Table 1. Reference values of threshold test for professional male, professional female, recreational male football players, professional futsal players and injured male football players participating in the Italian Championships. HR: heart rate; T2: threshold at 2 mmol/L of lactate; T4: threshold at 4 mmol/L of lactate. *First threshold test performed 93±37 days after ACL reconstruction (Della Villa S, Boldrini L, Ricci M, Danelon F, Snyder-Mackler L, Nanni G, Roi GS. Clinical outcomes and return-to-sports participation of 50 soccer players after anterior cruciate ligament reconstruction through a sport-specific rehabilitation protocol. Sports Health 2012; 4: 17-24).

It is well known that the resting period imposed by an injury primarily affects the cardiorespiratory fitness. In football players the aerobic threshold speed frequently decreases up to around 8 km/h when the player become able to return to running after three months of rest (i.e., after Anterior Cruciate Ligament Reconstruction; Table 1).
In injured players the cardiorespiratory fitness (together with body composition, muscular strength and endurance, and flexibility) should be considered one of the five specific components of the health-related physical fitness, (1). So, from a metabolic point of view, the first aim of the functional recovery after injury is to restore the physical fitness of the player with specific re-training and adequate lifestyle. This can be attained starting from the early phases of the rehabilitation where the aerobic work is performed through low impact activities, e.g. in the pool, or in the gym with stationary cycling, elliptical machines exercises or arm cranking, checking the suitable and personalized intensity from the % of the maximum theoretical HR.
After the solution of the first phase (inflammation and swelling), and after recovery of both full range of motion (phase 2) and a sufficient level of strength (phase 3), the injured player can restart with running and in few sessions she/he becomes able to be involved in the threshold test.
The threshold test is crucial for injured players because it allows the rehabilitation team to plan a personalized re-training for the cardiorespiratory fitness, checking the intensity from the HR corresponding to the thresholds. For an injured football players this personalized re-training usually consists of three sessions/week of 30 minutes of aerobic work at intensity corresponding to 2 mM of lactate (aerobic threshold), and one session/week with 6+6 minutes of work at intensity corresponding to 4 mM of lactate (anaerobic threshold), with 3-5 minutes of rest in between. In this way it is possible to recover around 2 km/h of aerobic threshold speed in four weeks. As a consequence, checking tests for thresholds should be repeated after around 4-5 weeks of aerobic re-training.
The aim of recovery of cardiorespiratory fitness for professional male football players, is to attain a minimum speed of 11.5 km/h and 13.5 km/h for aerobic and anaerobic thresholds respectively or a reference threshold speed, as for example indicated in Table 1, also considering the playing roles (Table 2).

Players	N	Age yrs	HR T2 bpm	HR T2 % HRmax	T2 Speed km/h	HR T4 bpm	HR T4 % HRmax	T4 Speed km/h
Goalkeepers	7	28±5	157±7	83±4	9.9±1.7	181±12	94±5	13.7±2.1
Defenders	21	25±4	165±11	84±5	12.0±1.6	187±11	93±4	15.5±1.1
Midfielders	24	26±5	161±10	83±5	12.4±1.5	183±9	92±5	16.0±1.1
Forwards	20	25±4	168±10	86±4	11.8±1.4	187±10	93±4	15.0±1.5

Table 2. Reference values of threshold test for professional male football players participating in the Italian Championships, divided by roles. HR: heart rate; T2: threshold at 2 mmol/L of lactate; T4: threshold at 4 mmol/L of lactate (Roi GS, Perondi F, Venturati G, Nanni G, Palaia G, Farnedi D, Mandarino F, Rosa EM. Frequenza cardiaca ed allenamento nel gioco del calcio. SdS 2000; 49: 47-51).

References

1. American College of Sports Medicine. ACSM's health-related physical fitness assessment manual. Lippincott Williams & Wilkins, Philadelphia, 2013
2. Krustrup P, Aagaard P, Nybo L, Petersen J, Mohr M, Bangsbo J. Recreational football as a health promoting activity: a topical review. Scand J Med Sci Sports 2010; 20(S1): 1–13
3. Stølen T, Chamari K, Castagna C, Wisløff U. Physiology of soccer: an update. Sports Med 2005; 35(6): 501-536

LAXITY MEASUREMENT TOOLS

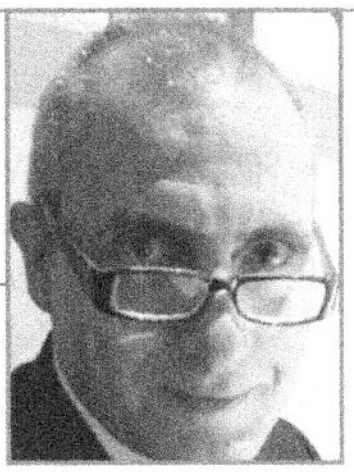

Zaffagnini S

Istituto Ortopedico Rizzoli, Bologna, Italy

Introduction

Anterior Cruciate Ligament (ACL) reconstruction is currently the seventh most common surgical procedure in the United States (2). Return to sport and especially to pre-injury level represents for the most sporting patients a crucial outcomes after the reconstructive surgery. A timely and precise diagnosis is certainly the first step to allow it. Even if a careful history, detailed preoperative Magnetic Resonance Imaging (MRI) and physical examination will always remain fundamental for a complete evaluation, the possibility to perform an instrumented objective and quantitative evaluation of joint dynamic laxity would represent a great decision support for orthopaedic surgeons dealing with ACL injuries.

Currently, the technology to measure knee joint laxity includes intraoperative navigational systems, portable devices such as accelerometers, gyroscopes and image analysis software, dynamic roentgen stereo-photogrammetric analysis, and full body motion analysis systems. These devices provide objective data regarding the kinematics of the knee following ACL injury and reconstruction under controlled testing environments.

Methods

For the purposes of navigational assessment of knee laxity, the clinical tests commonly analyzed are: Lachman and anterior drawer tests for anterior-posterior laxity assessment, internal/external rotation test at 30° and 90° of knee flexion, Varus/Valgus stress tests at 0° and 30° of flexion (VV30) and the Pivot-Shift test.

The analysis is performed with a high level of precision making the navigation systems considered the gold standard for laxity evaluation. In order to overcome the limit of invasiveness and high costs an innovative non-invasive systems for knee dynamic laxity evaluation, namely KiRA (Orthokey LLC, Delaware,USA), has been developed (1).

KiRA is a medical device based on accelerometer that analyses the severity of knee laxity, providing both real-time graphics and quantitative information about the Pivot-Shift and Lachman tests. The devices is connected wirelessly with a common tablet equipped with the free-available app. The sensor simply needs to be fixed on the tibial bone by the provided hypoallergenic strap.

Moreover, are now available Image analysis techniques that directly quantifying tibial translation along the lateral aspect of the knee joint during Pivot Shift test. Such systems use the laptop camera to record the video during the Pivot Shift test. In order to facilitate the quantification of movement stickers circular markers are attached to the skin over three bony landmarks which are: lateral epicondyle of the knee, Gerdy's tubercle and the fibular head.

The Roentgen Stereo-photogrammetric Analysis (RSA) has been developed to assess the stability of bone-prostheses interfaces. Initially, it was based on a procedure that required tantalum beads fixed into both the prosthesis and the bone. Recently, the application of the RSA has evolved to study not only the micro-movements and micro-adjustments of the bone-prosthesis interface, but also joint kinematics. It is now possible, using MRI models, to analyze joints kinematic in ACL deficient knees or after surgical reconstruction.

For all the technology that has been described to enhance the accuracy of ACL reconstruction, the fact remains that in order to limit the risk of re-injury the evaluation of both biomechanical and neuromuscular aspects of the athlete need to be considered during the postoperative phase.

A solution to overcome the issue may be the use of a motor analysis system to perform on-the-field data acquisition. Currently, there are multiple motion analysis systems available. Xsens system (Xsens Technologies, Enschede, The Netherlands) and Microsoft Kinect Sensor (Microsoft Corp, Redmond, USA) are the most technological advanced of their kind.

Conclusions

Quantitative measurements of joint laxity in the setting of ACL surgery offer the potential of maximizing surgical and rehabilitation outcomes offering an objective quantification of the deficit. These assessments can be done in the preoperative, intraoperative, and postoperative phases or during daily life activities.
In the future, these applications may lead to development of a standardized treatment algorithm for the ACL-injured patient with the goal of achieving maximum athletic potential while at the same time preventing post-traumatic Osteoarthritis for the patients.

References

1. Lopomo N, Zaffagnini S, Signorelli C, Bignozzi S, Giordano G, Marcheggiani Muccioli GM, Visani A. An original clinical methodology for non-invasive assessment of pivot-shift test. Comput Methods Biomech Biomed Engin 2012; 15: 1323-1328.
2. Moller E, Weidenhielm L, Werner S. Outcome and knee-related quality of life after anterior cruciate ligament reconstruction: a long-term follow-up. Knee Surg Sports Traumatol Arthrosc 2009; 17: 786-794

Sunday 10th April, 2016 (afternoon)
PICKWICK ROOM

FREE ORAL PRESENTATIONS

JOINT INJURIES

Chairs

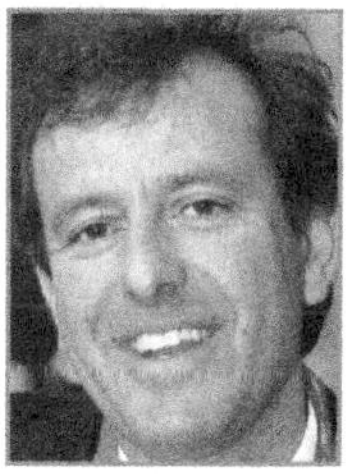

Furio Danelon
(Milan, Italy)

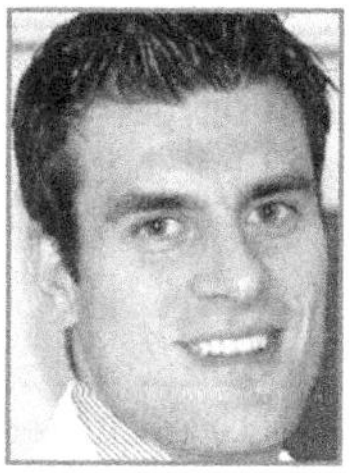

Kyriakos Tsapralis
(Bologna, Italy)

16:30 Maximum oxygen uptake in ACL-injured professional soccer players: preliminary results **de Almeida AM, Santos-Silva PR, Pedrinelli A, Hernandez AJ (São Paulo, Brazil)**

16:40 Quality of movement assessment in footballers six months following ACL reconstruction **Toolan A, de Mille P, Nguyen J, Selvaggio E, Do H, Chiaia T, Brown A (New York and New Brunswick, USA)**

16:50 Which and why neuromuscular significant deficits remain despite the return to sports? **Andrade R, Pereira M, Leite P, Vidal R, Pereira R, Espregueira-Mendes J (Porto and Gaia, Portugal)**

17:00 Real-time dynamic assessment for return to sport in ACL injury **Aginsky KD, Cale-Benzoor M (Tel Aviv, Haifa, and Netanya, Israel; Witwatersrand, South Africa)**

17:10 Patellar tendon healing after anterior cruciate ligament reconstruction in football players **Tzoanos G, Tsavalas N, Manidakis N, Chardaloumbas D, Kalliakmanis A (Heraklion, Crete; Athens, Greece)**

17:20 Non professional athletes return to play after acl reconstruction: a two years follow up **Ruggiero G, Re V, Falzone E, Mastio M, Respizzi S (Milan, Italy)**

17:30 Discussion

18:00 End of the session

MAXIMUM OXYGEN UPTAKE IN ACL-INJURED PROFESSIONAL SOCCER PLAYERS: PRELIMINARY RESULTS

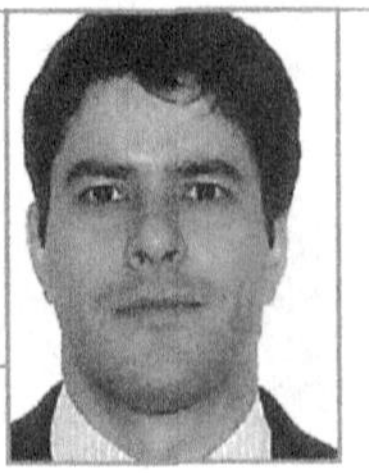

de Almeida AM, Santos-Silva PR, Pedrinelli A, Hernandez AJ

Department of Orthopedics and Traumatology, São Paulo University Medical School, FIFA Medical Centre of Excellence, São Paulo, Brazil

Introduction

The Anterior Cruciate Ligament (ACL) rupture is considered a major injury and may affect the career of professional soccer players. Surgical ACL reconstruction is often required to treat the resulting knee instability. Although ACL reconstruction is considered a successful procedure in restoring knee stability, literature shows that only 55% of the participants return to competitive sports participation after surgery (1). Soccer players need technical, tactical and physical skills to succeed, such as good knee function and aerobic capacity.

Our purpose is to evaluate maximum oxygen uptake ($V'O_{2max}$) in ACL-injured professional outfield soccer players and after a six-month period of post-operative rehabilitation, compared to a control group of healthy professional soccer players.

Methods

Thirty-six athletes with ACL injury were evaluated and underwent ACL reconstruction with hamstrings graft. The study is being carried, and until now 14 athletes completed the six-month post-op rehabilitation, and were compared to 16 healthy professional soccer players.

Maximum oxygen uptake was evaluated with a modified Heck protocol pre-op and post-op (after 6 months), and compared to the control group.

Knee function questionnaires (Lysholm and subjective IKDC), isokinetic testing (Biodex Medical Systems Inc, New York, USA) and body composition evaluation (InBody, Seoul, Korea) were also performed.

Statistical differences were assessed by Student's t-test (significance at $p<0.05$).

Results

Results are shown in Table 1.

	Pre-op	Post-op	Controls	Pre-op vs Post-op	Pre-op vs Controls	Post-op vs Controls
Age (yrs)	22.3±3.8	-	24.1±5.4	-	n.s.	-
$V'O2_{max}$ (mL/kg/min)	45.4±6.9	48.7±3.9	57.4±4.2	n.s.	<0.001	<0.001
Body fat (%)	15.9±4.9	13.0±3.9	13.3±4.2	n.s.	0.03	n.s.
Quadriceps deficit (%)	23.3±19.3	14.1±10.9	8.4±7.4	n.s.	<0.001	0.04
Lysholm	75.9±11.8	93.6±6.2	98.5±2.9	<0.001	<0.001	0.002
IKDC	57.1±17.9	84.0±13.3	98.1±3.4	<0.001	<0.001	<0.001

Table 1. Results as mean±SD assessed in control subjects and in ACL patients before (Pre-op) and 6 months after (Post-op) surgery. n.s.: non-significant difference

Mean time between injury and surgery was five months. Preoperative $V'O_{2max}$ was 45.4±6.9, post-operative 48.7±3.9 and controls 57.4±4.2. We found a statistically significant difference between controls and ACL-injured athletes, both pre-op and post-op ($p<0.001$).
No significant differences were found comparing ACL patients pre-op and post-op. ACL pre-op group body fat percentage was significantly higher than controls (Table 1).
Quadriceps peak torque deficit at 60°/s was significantly higher in ACL pre-op and post-op compared to controls.
Knee function questionnaires results improved significantly when comparing pre-op vs pos-op, but the results were lower compared to controls ($p<0.001$).

Conclusions

Although ACL reconstruction was successful in improving knee function and symptoms, we observed that maximum oxygen uptake was significant lower in the ACL group, even after six months of rehabilitation.
Desired levels of $V'O_{2max}$ in professional soccer players are about 60 mL/kg/min (3), and lower aerobic capacity is related to poorer performance (2).
We also showed that ACL-injured athletes had a higher body fat percentage compared to controls, and higher quadriceps strength deficit. Therefore, we conclude that, for optimal performance, professional soccer players rehabilitation should focus not only in knee function, but also in keeping body composition, muscle strength, and aerobic capacity.

References

1. Ardern CL, Taylor NF, Feller JA, Webster KE. Fifty-five per cent return to competitive sport following anterior cruciate ligament reconstruction surgery: an updated systematic review and meta-analysis including aspects of physical functioning and contextual factors. Br J Sports Med 2014; 48: 1543-1552
2. Helgerud J, Engen LC, Wisloff U, Hoff J. Aerobic endurance training improves soccer performance. Med Sci Sports Exerc 2001; 33: 1925-1931
3. Stølen T, Chamari K, Castagna C, Wisloff U. Physiology of soccer: an update. Sports Med 2005; 35: 501-536

QUALITY OF MOVEMENT ASSESSMENT IN FOOTBALLERS SIX MONTHS FOLLOWING ACL RECONSTRUCTION

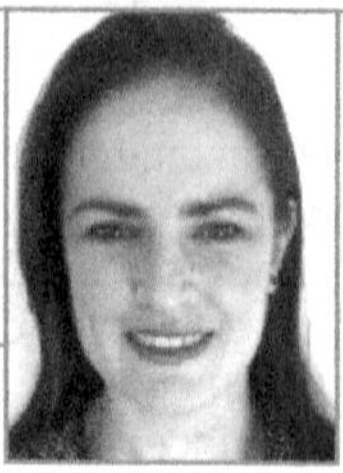

Toolan A[1,2], de Mille P[1], Nguyen J[1], Selvaggio E[1], Do H[1], Chiaia T[1], Brown A[3]

[1]Hospital for Special Surgery, FIFA Medical Center of Excellence, New York;
[2]New York City Football Club, New York, [3]Rutgers University, New Brunswick, USA

Introduction

Anterior Cruciate Ligament (ACL) injury prevention programs evaluate Quality of Movement (QM) to identify and correct high-risk movement patterns. However, Return To Play (RTP) decisions post-ACL Reconstruction (ACLR) are often based on non-football related quantitative measures such as isokinetic tests and/or time from surgery, with six months post-ACLR being a common expectation for RTP. Re-injury rates as high as 23% in the first 12-months (3), and 30% at 15-year follow up (2), have been reported in the literature. In a sample of 100 footballers, Brophy et al. (1) found a higher ACLR revision rate in female (20.0%) vs male (5.5%) footballers.

Purpose

To evaluate whether footballers are ready to RTP six months post ACLR using a QM Assessment (QMA).

Methods

A QMA, developed by the staff of the Sports Rehabilitation and Performance Center at Hospital for Special Surgery, including nine dynamic tasks (squat, single leg (SL) stance, step down, SL squat, jump in place, side to side jump, broad jump, hop to opposite, SL hop) progressing from double- to single-limb vertical and horizontal movements was administered to 50 footballers (age 19±5 years, 37 male, 13 female) six months post-ACLR.
The participation level of these footballers ranged from middle school to collegiate level. Tasks were viewed from the frontal and sagittal planes by a physical therapist and performance specialist. Movements were evaluated live for risk factors associated with ACL injury (strategy, depth, control, symmetry, and alignment). The proportion of patients exhibiting risky movement patterns for each task was calculated. Chi-square or Fisher's Exact test was used to determine if there were differences in movement patterns between males and females.

Results

The proportion of patients demonstrating risky movement patterns for a task ranged from 55% to 100%. All 50 footballers exhibited risky movement patterns for at least one task and 55% of patients displayed risky movement patterns in five or more of the nine tasks. In activities involving unilateral strength and control, 80% of footballers assessed demonstrated abnormal movement patterns. Rates of risky movement patterns were not different between males and females for all tasks ($P>0.1$ for all tasks).

Conclusions

Six months has been cited as a probable time for RTP post-ACLR; thus this is often the expectation of the athlete heading into surgery. Our data shows that footballers demonstrate multiple QM patterns associated with initial ACL injury, as well as 2nd injury six months post-operatively. Altered movement patterns evident in tasks as simple as a SL stance remained with the footballer through tasks of increasing difficulty. We recommend that therapists integrate QM screening into rehabilitation with a focus on movement retraining to address mechanical risk factors prior to RTP, to reduce the risk of second injury.

References

1. Brophy R, Schmitz L, Wright R, Dunn W, Parker R, Andrish J, McCarty E, Spindler K. Return to play and future ACL injury risk after ACL reconstruction in soccer athletes from the Multicenter Orthopaedic Outcomes Network (MOON) group. Am J Sports Med 2012; 40: 2517-2522
2. Hui C, Salmon L, Kok A, Maeno S, Linklater J, Pinczewski L. Fifteen-tear outcome of endoscopic anterior cruciate ligament reconstruction with patellar tendon autograft for "Isolated" anterior cruciate ligament tear. Am J Sports Med 2011; 39: 89-98
3. Paterno M, Schmitt L, Ford K, Mitchell R, Myer G, Huang B, Hewett T. Biomechanical measures during landing and postural stability predict second anterior cruciate ligament injury after anterior cruciate ligament reconstruction and return to sport. Am J Sports Med 2010; 38: 1968-1978

WHICH AND WHY NEUROMUSCULAR SIGNIFICANT DEFICITS REMAIN DESPITE THE RETURN TO SPORTS?

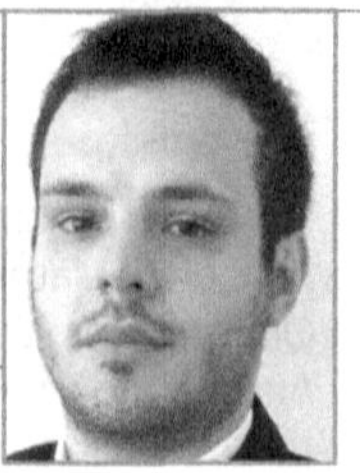

Andrade R[1], Pereira M[2], Leite P[2], Vidal R[1], Pereira R[1], Espregueira-Mendes J[1]

[1]Clínica do Dragão, Espregueira-Mendes Sports Centre, FIFA Medical Centre of Excellence, Porto; [2]Escola Superior de Saúde Jean Piaget, Gaia, Portugal

Introduction

The Return To Sport (RTS) criteria after Anterior Cruciate Ligament Reconstruction (ACLR) are still an important issue under debate concerning the safety and performance of the athlete. In this sense, it has been reported a RTS rate around the 75%, however only 43% return the pre-injury competitive level (1). Hence, accurate and reliable objective criteria is required (2). A lower limb asymmetry under 10% and a concentric Hamstrings/Quadriceps (H/Q) ratio between 0.5 and 0.8 has been suggested as one of the objective criteria for readiness to RTS (3).
Our study's objective was to assess the knee isokinetic muscular balance, at least, 1 year after the ACLR.

Methods

Twenty-five amateur athletes (23 male e 2 female; 24.0±4.5 yrs, range 18-35; 1.76±0.1 m; 74.7±14.2 kg) who underwent ACLR (12 with Bone-Patellar-Tendon-Bone (BPTB) and 13 with hamstrings) and have returned to competitive sports were recruited for this study. All the ACLR were performed elsewhere.
The dominant lower limb was injured in 16 players (40%) and the mechanism of injury was contact in 5 (20%) and noncontact in 20 (80%) athletes.
The isokinetic assessment protocol for the quadriceps and hamstrings muscles, was composed by 2 series of 6 and 8 concentric repetitions, and 60°/s and 180°/s, respectively (Doc Genu, Easytech, Florence, Italy).
A standard range of motion was applied and gravity correction procedures were assured for all athletes.

Results

The 25 athletes were involved in different sports: football (n=18); rugby (n=4); handball (n=2); indoor hockey (n=1).
There was significant differences between the injured and uninjured lower limbs regarding the quadriceps on Maximal Peak Torque (MPT) at the 60°/s and on the Total Work (TW) at 60°/s for both quadriceps and hamstrings ($p<0.05$).

	Quadriceps		Hamstrings	
	Injured	Uninjured	Injured	Uninjured
MPT 60°/s	222.5±40.4	230.6±42.5*	128.0±29.1	132.6±28.9
MPT 180°/s	135.4 ±30.9	137.1±30.4	84.3±17.5	84.9±16.8
TW 60°/s	914.9±220.4	993.9±235.3*	506.8±156.5	564.2±163.4*
TW 180°/s	873.5±233.1	877.6±217.4	491.3±147.5	498.0±145.6

Table 1. Mean±SD of Maximal Peak Torque (MPT) values (Nm) and of Total Work (TW) values (J) for both quadriceps and hamstrings muscles. *p<0.05.

	Injured	Uninjured	Range
60°/s	57.0±8.1	57.2±8.1	40-75
180°/s	62.9±10.7	62.4±10.2	45-85

Table 2. Mean±SD of the H/Q concentric ratio (%).

The individual analysis showed that 80% of the athletes had a bilateral deficit higher than 10%. Moreover, 36% of the athletes exhibited a H/Q concentric ratio bellow the recommended range. A more detailed analysis revealed that two thirds of these had hamstrings graft ACLR.
In addition, 9 athletes (44%) showed an atypical behavior, i.e., the ratio decreases with increasing velocity.

Conclusions

Overall, 80% percent of the athletes were playing without being aware of the significant bilateral asymmetry in isokinetic neuromuscular performance. Additionally, 36% of the athletes revealed an H/Q concentric ratio bellow the recommended range, being the majority identified within hamstrings graft ACLR subset. Furthermore, there were significant statistical differences in bilateral comparison of the total work, disfavoring the injured lower limb. These deficits may put the athlete in hazard for re-injury.
These results reflect the need for a more comprehensive full rehabilitation, a stricter assessment of the readiness for RTS and a regular monitoring of the motor skills and neuromuscular performance, even after the RTS.

References

1. Andriolo L, Filardo G, Kon E, Ricci M, Della Villa F, Della Villa S, Zaffagnini S, Marcacci M. Revision anterior cruciate ligament reconstruction: clinical outcome and evidence for return to sport. Knee Surg Sports Traumatol Arthrosc 2015; 23: 2825-2845
2. Espregueira-Mendes J, Pereira R, Monteiro A, Pereira H, Sevivas N, Varanda P. Sports and anterior cruciate lesions. Rev Chir Orthop Reparatrice Appar Mot 2011; 97: S472-S476
3. Undheim M, Cosgrave C, King E, Strike S, Marshall B, Falvey É, Franklyn-Miller A. Isokinetic muscle strength and readiness to return to sport following anterior cruciate ligament reconstruction: is there an association? A systematic review and a protocol recommendation. Br J Sports Med 2015; 49: 1305-1310

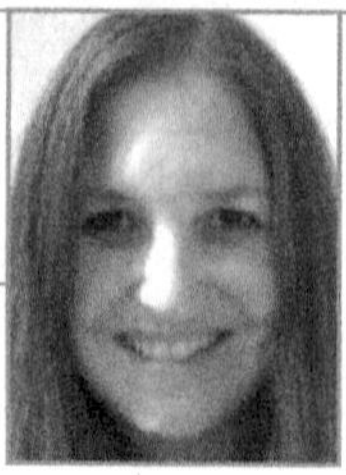

REAL-TIME DYNAMIC ASSESSMENT FOR RETURN TO SPORT IN ACL INJURY

Aginsky KD[1,2], Cale-Benzoor M[1,3,4]

[1]Physimax Technology, Tel Aviv, Israel; [2]Physiotherapy Department University of the Witwatersrand, South Africa; [3]Haifa University, Haifa, Israel; [4]Wingate Institute, Netanya, Israel

Introduction

There is a high occurrence of Anterior Cruciate Ligament (ACL) injuries in football players. Following injury neuromuscular control, strength, mobility and stability are compromised, thus it is important to objectively assess these during decision making for Return To Play (RTP). However, there is a distinct lack of kinematic-based criteria for RTP following ACL injury.
PhysiMax Technology (Tel Aviv, Israel) has developed 3D software for reliable, real-time, objective, functional assessment providing feedback on quality of movement (2). The software adds a new and important dimension to the rehabilitation process and the clinician's decision making in football RTP. In order to RTP, the footballer should display adequate stability, neuromuscular control, mobility and strength during a bilateral and unilateral landing and dynamic tasks. Real-time assessment of a drop jump task as measured by the Landing Error Scoring System (LESS) can be used to assess the biomechanical and neuromuscular parameters for potential risk of ACL re-injury for RTP (1). Dynamic unilateral tasks, such as the Single Leg Squat (SLS) should be used to assess unilateral deficits such as excessive knee valgus; increased medio-lateral displacement and adequate, symmetrical depth over ten repetitions following an ACL Reconstruction in football players (3).

Methods

This was a pilot study to assess the real-time dynamic assessment of the lower extremity in elite, male, football players. The following functional tasks were assessed using the 3D Physimax Technology (Tel Aviv, Israel): bilateral drop jump task scored using the reliable and valid Landing Error Scoring System (LESS) to determine landing symmetry, joint displacement during landing, neuromuscular control, mobility and stability; unsupported SLS to determine neuromuscular control, hip muscle dysfunction and knee stability; a supported SLS to determine the difference in maximal knee flexion between the supported and unsupported SLS assessing dynamic knee stability (deficit of 10 and 15% between the supported and unsupported SLS indicates moderate dynamic knee stability and above 20% indicates poor stability); a lunge test to determine the degree of ankle dorsiflexion; a repeated single leg vertical jump task to assess vertical jump height and landing accuracy.

Results

Twenty-five elite, male, football players (25.2±4.8 years; height: 180±7 cm and weight: 75.8±7.4 kg). Mean LESS 17 and 22 scores were good to moderate (5.4±2.0 and 6.6±2.2 respectively).
The LESS kinematics are shown in Table 1. The mean unsupported SLS scores were good and symmetrical (Dominant: 4.9±1.3; Non-dominant: 4.4±1.0).
Kinematic data for the SLS are shown in Table 2. Footballers had moderate dynamic knee stability (Dominant: 17.4±14.4%; Non-dominant: 10.5±14.7%. Mean ankle dorsiflexion on the dominant side was 23.7±6.1° and 25.1±7.1° on the non-dominant side. Mean unilateral vertical jump height was adequate and symmetrical (Dominant: 35.2±4.1 cm; Non-dominant: 36.6±4.8 cm).

Kinematic Parameter	Dominant	Non-Dominant
Medial knee position at initial contact (°)	-1.0±4.4	-1,8±4.4
Medial knee displacement (°)	5.1±12.2	3,6±9.8
Knee flexion at initial contact (°)	17.5±13.8	18,5±13.9
Knee flexion displacement (°)	62.0±26.1	61,4±25.7
Hip flexion at initial contact (°)	22.9±15.7	24,4±15.3
Hip flexion displacement (°)	42.3±27.7	41,9±28.0
Lateral trunk flexion at initial contact (°)	-0.2±2.1	
Trunk flexion at initial contact (°)	21.4±6.0	
Trunk flexion displacement (°)	1.8±9.9	

Table 1. Mean±SD of LESS kinematic results for the dominant and non-dominant sides in elite male football players (n=25). Negative medial knee position = knee varus; Negative lateral trunk flexion: to non-dominant side.

Kinematic Parameter	Dominant	Non-Dominant
Maximal knee valgus (°)	13.6±14.9	14.8±12.2
Maximal knee flexion (°)	81.5±18.1	78.5±16.3
Maximal hip Flexion (°)	75.7±18.2	73.9±18.1
Pelvic hike (°)	4.2±4.6	1.5±5.4
Lateral trunk flexion (°)	-1.1±4.3	1.8±5.0
Trunk rotation (°)	1.9±3.4	0.9±3.4

Table 2. Mean±SD of unsupported SLS kinematic results for the dominant and non-dominant sides in elite male football players (n=25). Negative lateral trunk flexion: to non-dominant side.

Conclusions

The introduction of this objective, real-time, dynamic movement assessment importantly enhances clinical decision making for return to play in football players following ACL injury.
Further research is required to develop football-specific, kinematic-based criteria for return to play.

References

1. Bizzini M, Hancock D, Impellizzeri F. Suggestions from the field for return to sports participation following anterior cruciate ligament reconstruction: soccer. J Orthop Sports Phys Ther 2012; 42: 304-312
2. Padua D, Boling M, DiStefano L, Onate J, Beutler A, Marshall S. Reliability of the Landing Error Scoring System- Real Time, a Clinical Assessment Tool of Jump- Landing Biomechanics. J Sport Rehab 2011; 20: 145-156
3. Waters E. Suggestions from the field for return to sports participation following anterior cruciate ligament reconstruction: basketball. J Orthop Sports Phys Ther 2012; 42: 326-336

PATELLAR TENDON HEALING AFTER ANTERIOR CRUCIATE LIGAMENT RECONSTRUCTION IN FOOTBALL PLAYERS

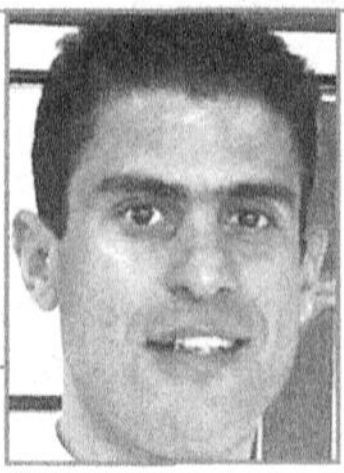

Tzoanos G[1], Tsavalas N[1], Manidakis N[1], Chardaloumbas D[1], Kalliakmanis A[2]

[1]Tzoanos Sports Clinic, Heraklion, Crete; [2]Athens Medical Center, Athens, Greece

Introduction

To investigate the healing process of the patellar tendon donor site at 12±2 and 24±2 months following Bone-Patellar-Bone (BTB) autograft Anterior Cruciate Ligament (ACL) reconstruction.

Methods

Twenty six male and four female amateur football players, with a mean age of 25 years (range: 20-32 years) were enrolled in our study. They had undergone BTB autograft ACL reconstruction, and were examined at 12±2 and 24±2 months postoperatively. Both donor and contralateral healthy tendons were evaluated with a high frequency (12 MHz) linear-array ultrasound transducer (Philips ATL HDI 5000 Sono CT, Philips, Eindhoven, The Nederlands). All patients returned to fully participation at 7±1 (range: 6-8) months after surgery, and exhibited no symptomatology at the time of the study. The Maximum Antero-Posterior (MAP) and Maximum Transverse (MT) diameters of the patellar tendon and associated defect at the site of the tendon incision were measured at its proximal, middle and distal thirds using electronic calipers. The presence of vascular flow was examined with color and power Doppler imaging. Echogenicity of the patellar tendon defect was graded as low, mixed or normal compared to the contralateral tendon.

Results

There was no statistically significant difference between the mean MAP and MT diameters of the donor tendons at 12±2 and 24±2 months postoperatively ($P>0.05$). The mean MAP and MT diameters of the patellar tendon defect at 24±2 months were significantly smaller compared to 12±2 months postoperatively ($P<0.01$). The mean MAP diameter of the harvested tendon was significantly greater at all measured sites in comparison to the contralateral tendon at 12±2 and 24±2 months postoperatively ($P<0.01$). There was no statistically significant difference between the mean MT diameters of the donor and healthy tendons at 12±2 and 24±2 months postoperatively ($P>0.05$). At 12±2 months postoperatively, the mean MAP diameter of the patellar tendon defect was 4.0±2.1 mm, 4.7±2.8 mm and 4.1±2.4 mm at the proximal, middle and distal third of the tendon respectively. Accordingly, the mean MT diameter of the defect was 3.3±2.2 mm (proximal third), 2.9±1.6 mm (middle third) and 2.1±0.9 mm (distal third). The vast majority (N=22) of tendon defects showed low echogenicity. Mixed echogenicity was found in 6 of them, while 2 patients demonstrated normal echogenicity of the harvested tendon. At 24±2 months postoperatively, the mean MAP diameter of the patellar tendon defect was 0.3±0.3 mm, 0.4±0.4 mm and 0.3±0.3 mm at the proximal, middle and distal third of the tendon respectively. Accordingly, the mean MT diameter of the defect was 0.3±0.3 mm (proximal third), 0.2±0.2 mm (middle third) and 0.2±0.2 mm (distal third). The vast majority (N=27) of patients demonstrated normal echogenicity of the harvested tendon. One tendon defect showed low echogenicity, while mixed echogenicity was found in two of them. No tendon exhibited any signs of neovascularization at 12±2 and 24±2 months postoperatively.

Conclusions

Patellar tendons after BTB ACL reconstruction in our group of football players were characterized by increased thickness at 12±2 and 24±2 months postoperatively. Signs of solid healing were evident in a minority of patients by 12±2 months and the vast majority of them by 24±2 months. No inflammatory changes were observed in our asymptomatic subject at 12±2 and 24±2 months postoperatively. Return to play did not seem to affect the normal reparative process of the patellar tendon.

NON PROFESSIONAL ATHLETES RETURN TO PLAY AFTER ACL RECONSTRUCTION: A TWO YEARS FOLLOW UP

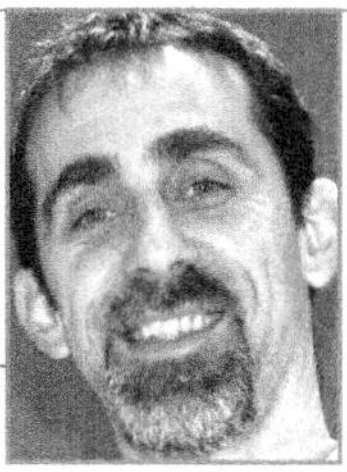

Ruggiero G[1], Re V[1], Falzone E[1], Mastio M[2], Respizzi S[1]

Humanitas Research Hospital, [1]Dipartimento di Riabilitazione e Recupero Funzionale and [2]Ortopedia Artroscopica e Ricostruttiva del Ginocchio, UO di Ortopedia V, Milan, Italy

Introduction

Despite many papers have been published about this topic, findings reported in the literature do not clarify definitely the predictability of the clinical and functional outcome after Anterior Cruciate Ligament (ACL) reconstruction.
Joint stability and return to performance are fundamental features in assessing the functional outcome but their correlation does not seem so clear.
Furthermore, daily clinical practice points out another matter of interest: do pre-operatory outcome expectations and perceived functional outcome meet different criteria in relation to different levels of participation in sport? And what if we focus on amateur athlete?
Our purpose was to assess clinical and functional outcomes, and their correlations with sport participation, in order to identify the real pattern of return to play after ACL reconstruction in amateur football player.

Methods

We selected 14 patients (males, mean age, at the time of follow-up, 35±10 yrs), mean follow-up of 22.4 months (range 16.1-30.6) after ACL reconstruction from the same surgical team and same standard technique with hamstring harvest, all practicing, pre operatively, football at non-professional level.
Revision surgery, peripherical lesions with associated procedures, meniscus suture repair and females were excluded. Patients underwent a telephone interview about their experience in return to sport and subsequently were enrolled for an assessment session which included clinical examination and functional testing. Assessment included: Pivot Shif testing using KiRA (Orthokey, Lewes DE, USA); Single Hop for Distance (3); Knee Bending 30s; Flexibility and Isokinetic Testing (PRIMA-ISO, Easytech, Borgo S. Lorenzo, Italy).
Patients were also asked to fill in four questionnaires (Lysholm, Oxford Knee score, ACLRSi, and Tampa Scale for Kinesiophobia).

Results

Eight patients (57%; RTS group) returned to sport at the same level.
Five patients (62.5%) returned to sport after not less than 6 months; 3 (37.5%) returned between 3 and 6 months. Four patients (50% of RTS group) returned to sport without any supervision or assistance on field.
Symptoms reported at the time of reprise mainly included: fear of re-injury, pain and feeling the knee different.
In three patients (37.5%), symptoms persisted at the time of follow-up.
Six patients (43%; NotRTS group) did not return to play: 4 (66.6%) have tried to, but did not succeed; 2 (33.3%) decided to abandon without trying.

Both groups showed a mean Oxford Knee Score (RTS=47.4; notRTS=42.3) corresponding to satisfactory knee function according to scale grading values (Murray DW, Fitzpatrick R, Rogers K, Pandit H, Beard DJ, Carr AJ, Dawson J. The use of the Oxford Hip and Knee Scores. J Bone Joint Surg [Br] 2007; 89-B: 1010-1014).
A better Lysholm Score always resulted in a better outcome. RTS group mean score (97.1±6.9) showed results corresponding to excellent; nRTS group mean score (88.3±6.2) showed results corresponding to good. All patients in RTS group had a better score than the nRTS one.
Total raw score in TSK was clearly better in RTS group and mean TSK value in Not-RTS group is higher than the cut-off value (2).
Pivot Shift with KiRA (Orthokey, Lewes DE, USA) showed a higher mean value in RTS group. In both groups the mean difference between operated and not-operated knee (RTS=0.5; notRTS=0.4) corresponded to a glide grade of Pivot-shift (1).
Agonist-antagonist ratio mean value (at 90°/s) was, in the operated knee, 61±14% in RTS group and 74±39% in NotRTS group. Despite the normal mean value in RTS group, 3 patients showed a knee Flexors/Extensors ratio higher than 66%.
In both groups 50% of patients had significant difference (>10%) in extensor muscles strength operated versus not operated knee.

Groups	n	KiRa	SHT	KB 30s	Flex	MPT E 90°/s	MPT F 90°/s	Lysholm	OKS	ACLRSi	Tampa
RTS	8	2.9±0.9	133.4±44.7	39.8±18.5	-1.0±10.1	127±9	78±17	97.1±6.9	47.3±1.4	57±5	18±1
NotRTS	6	2.2±0.4	117.0±34.2	32.9±18.5	4.7±6.3	123±6	77±33	88.3±6.2	42.3±6.2	73±9	29.3±0.3

Table 1. Results (mean±SD) of the study. KiRA: Pivot Shif test; SHT: Single Hop Test for distance (cm); KB 30s: Knee Bending for 30 s; Flex: Flexibility; MPT: maximal Peak Torque (Nm); E: knee extensors; F: knee flexors.

Conclusions

The amateur athlete deserves a peculiar attention in functional assessment before discharge from acute rehabilitation path in order to better evaluate clinical and functional features which can predict the patient's condition in order to return to play.
Specific functional questionnaires (Lysholm, TSK and ACLRSi) and functional tests (single hop for distance) seem to be effective in evaluating patient's functional capability related to return to play.
Isokinetic Test or quantitative measurement of Pivot Shift Test alone seems not to strictly correlate with functional outcome and performance.

References

1. Berruto M, Uboldi F, Gala L, Marelli B, Albisetti W. Is triaxal Accelerometer reliable in the evaluation and grading of knee pivot-shift phenomenon? Knee Surg Sports Traumatol Arthrosc 2013; 21: 981-985
2. Monticone M, Giorgi I, Baiardi P, Barbieri M, Rocca B, Bonezzi C. Development of the Italian version of the Tampa Scale of Kinesiophobia (TSK-I): cross-cultural adaptation, factor analysis, reliability, and validity. Spine 2010; 35: 1241-126
3. Myer GD, Schmitt LC, Brent JL, Ford KR, Barber Foss KD, Scherer BJ, Heidt RS Jr, Divine JG, Hewett TE. Utilization of modified NFL combine testing to identify functional deficits in athletes following ACL reconstruction. J Orthop Sports Phys Ther 2011; 41: 377-387

SYMPOSIA Saturday

Symposium ECOSEP (European College Of Sports and Exercise Physicians)
11+ and return to play
Saturday 9th April 11:30-13:00 – Mountbatten Room (sixth floor)

Symposium BPMpro
Helping medical staff to screen, assess and monitor players to return to play faster
Saturday 9th April 11:30-13:00 – Darwin Room (sixth floor)

Symposium International Federation of Sports Physical Therapy (ISFTP)
Return to play – Optimize load
Saturday 9th April 13:00-14:30 – Fleming Room (third floor)

Symposium ISEH (Institute of Sport Exercise & Health)
Concussion management and return to play
Saturday 9th April 13:00-14:30 – Churchill Auditorium (ground floor)

Symposium Sports Surgery Clinic
3D biomechanics in return to play decision making after ACL reconstruction
Saturday 9th April 13:00-14:30 – Mountbatten Room (sixth floor)

Symposium Soccer System Pro
Turn data into intelligence: how software can play a role in sports medicine
Saturday 9th April 13:00-14:30 – Darwin Room (sixth floor)

Symposium Cryoaction
Whole body cryotherapy in elite sports
Saturday 9th April 13:30-14:30 – Pickwick Suite (first floor)

Symposium FIDIA
IAHA tailor treatment for athletes with different needs
Saturday 9th April 14:30-16:00 – Mountbatten Room (sixth floor)

Symposium TRB Chemedica
Current treatments in elite sports for tendinopathies. Evidence and clinical experience
Saturday 9th April 14:30-16:00 – Darwin Room (sixth floor)

Symposium West African Sport Medicine Association
Saturday 9th April 16:30-18:00 – Mountbatten Room (sixth floor)

Symposium TMG
Tensomyography
Saturday 9th April 16:30-18:00 – Darwin Room (sixth floor)

SYMPOSIA Sunday

Symposium UTC Imaging
Novel approaches for the management of tendinopathy
Sunday 10th April 8:00-9:30 – Pickwick Suite (first floor)

Symposium DJO
Returning to play: reducing the risks of recurrent injury in sport
Sunday 10th April 8:00-9:30 – Darwin Room (sixth floor)

Symposium Indiba Activ
Stem cell proliferation by 448 kHz frequency
Sunday 10th April 9:30-11:00 – Darwin Room (sixth floor)

Symposium FC Barcelona - Muscletech Network
Muscletech technology and return to play
Sunday 10th April 13:00-14:30 – Fleming Room (third floor)

Symposium ISMuLT (Italian Society of Muscles, Ligaments & Tendons)
Evidence based medicine in muscles, ligaments and tendon disorders: ISMuLT guidelines
Sunday 10th April 13:00-14:30 – Churchill Auditorium (ground floor)

Symposium Myontech
Muscle activation data (EMG) from wearables in injury prevention and rehabilitation
Sunday 10th April 13:00-14:30 – Darwin Room (sixth floor)

Symposium Podactiva
Biomechanics and podiatry in elite football
Sunday 10th April 14:30-16:00 – Darwin Room (sixth floor)

Saturday, 9th April 2016 (morning)
MOUNTBATTEN ROOM (sixth floor)

SYMPOSIUM

11+ AND RETURN TO PLAY

Chairs

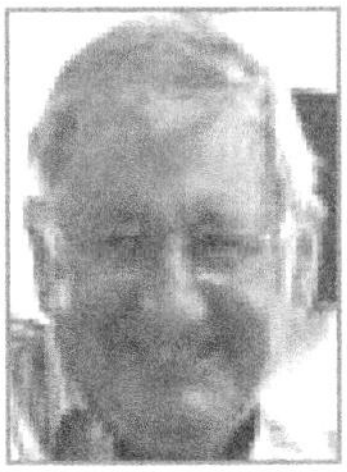

John King
(London, United Kingdom)

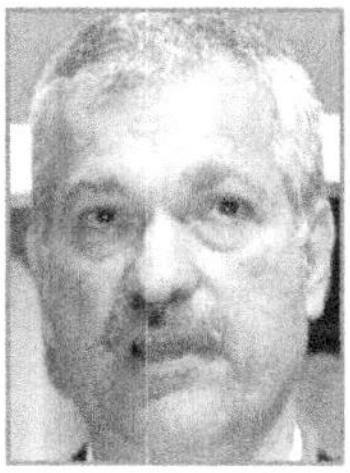

Nikos Malliaropoulos
(Thessaloniki, Greece)

11:30	11+ ways to prevent and Play **Mario Bizzini (Zurich, Switzerland)**
11:45	11+ Ways to educate and play **Kyriakos Tsapralis (Bologna, Italy), Asimenia Gioftsidou (Komotini, Greece)**
12:00	Team physician's view to return to play **Zafal Iqbal (London, United Kingdom)**
12:15	Imaging view to return to play **Otto Chan (London, United Kingdom)**
12:30	Nutrition view to return to play **Otto Chan (London, United Kingdom)**
12:45	Team environment in return to play **Xavier Valle (Barcelona, Spain)**
13:00	End of the workshop

FIFA 11+ APPLICATION EFFECTS ON LOWER LIMB BALANCE AND MUSCLE STRENGTH

Arsenis S[1], Gioftsidou A[1], Malliou P[1], Beneka A[1], Tsapralis K[2], Aggelousis N[1]

[1]Department of Physical Education and Sports Science, DUTH, Komotini, Greece;
[2]Isokinetic Medical Group, FIFA Medical Centre of Excellence, Bologna, Italy

Introduction

The benefits of warm-up are known for the preparation and the protection of the body of the athletes before participating in sports (2). FIFA 11+ is a complete warm-up package that can replace the typical football warm-up before the training (1). The main objective of this program is the training of neuromuscular control, proper posture and control of the body during the exercises. The purpose of this study was to evaluate the effect of the injury prevention program FIFA 11+ (level 2) application, on lower limb balance ability and knee flexors and extensors muscle strength, as an effective approach to reduce injury risk in Greek male football players.

Methods

Thirty-two male football players, participating in the young championship of the first Greek division, were randomly divided into two subject groups (n=16 each), one control group (C group) (aged 19.31±0.87 years), and one training group (F group) (aged 18.87±0.80 years). The F group followed the FIFA 11+ (level 2) injury prevention program 3 times per week for 8 weeks. Before the commencement of the study, the F group participated in a two days course (including a theoretical part and a practical part about FIFA 11+ exercises). Therefore, it decided to reach the second level of FIFA 11+ difficulty, because the players had a history of practicing the exercises of the level 1 in the past. The total duration was about 20-25 minutes. The C group continued the usual warm-up. The usual warm up involved a combination of running, stretching, technical exercises with the ball and small-sided games. The total duration was about 20-25 minutes.
Biodex Stability System was used to assess balance ability (deviations from the horizontal plane) in both groups at baseline (T0) and after completing the FIFA 11+ program (T8). Additional isokinetic knee joint moment measurements (concentric flexors/extensors and eccentric flexors) performed at two different angular velocities, first at 60°/s and then at 180° /s. For each angular velocity, muscle group and leg, the contraction with the highest peak moment value was considered for further analysis. One-way repeated measures ANOVA was used to test for differences between the measurements and between groups.

Results

Two main results were obtained, the FIFA 11+ program increased:
1) concentric flexors strength at 60°/s (for the dominant F (1,30= 5.66; $p<0.05$), and non-dominant leg F (1,30)= 9.61; $p<0.01$) and
2) total Stability Index (SI) (for the dominant F (1,30= 6.01; $p<0.05$), and non-dominant leg F (1,30) = 10.6; $p<0.01$) and Anterior-Posterior index (AP) (for the dominant F (1,30= 8.24; $p<0.01$), and non-dominant leg F (1,30)= 34.1 $p<0.001$).

Conclusions

Performing FIFA 11+ injury prevention program for 8 weeks can improve lower limb balance ability and hamstrings muscle strength, elements which are very important for prevention of hamstring muscle strains and lower limb ligament injuries in football.

References

1. Bizzini M, Impellizzeri F, Dvorak J, Bortolan L, Schena F, Modena R, Junge A. Physiological and performance responses to the "FIFA 11+" (part 1): is it an appropriate warm-up? J Sports Sci 2013; 31: 1481-1490
2. Subasi S, Gelecek N, Aksakoglu G. Effects of different warm-up periods on knee proprioception and balance in healthy young individuals. J Sports Rehab 2008; 17: 186-205

Saturday 9th April (morning)
DARWIN ROOM (sixth floor)

SYMPOSIUM

HELPING MEDICAL STAFF TO SCREEN, ASSESS AND MONITOR PLAYERS TO RETURN TO PLAY FASTER

Chairs

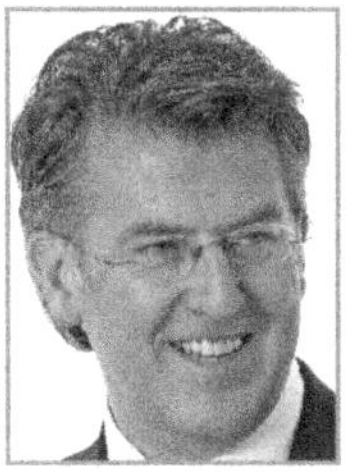

Martin Gossling
(Chilbolton, United Kingdom)

11:30	Welcome and introduction to BPMphysio **Martin Gossling (Chilbolton, United Kingdom)**
11:45	Screening from a clubs perspective **Craig Pead (Chilbolton, United Kingdom)**
12:00	Live demonstration of BPMphysio
12:30	BPMphysio from an orthopaedic surgeons point of view **Nick Birch (Chilbolton, United Kingdom)**
12:45	Discussion
13:00	End of the workshop

Saturday 9th April (afternoon)
FLEMING ROOM (third floor)

SYMPOSIUM

INTERNATIONAL FEDERATION OF SPORTS PHYSICAL THERAPY (ISFTP) RETURN TO PLAY - OPTIMIZE LOAD

Chairs

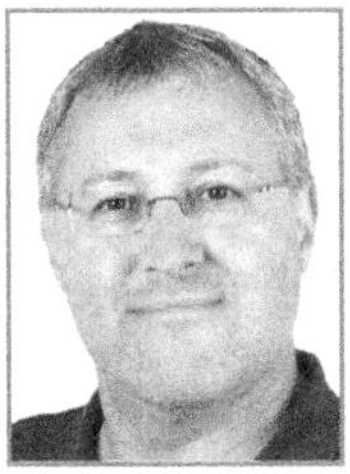

Mario Bizzini
(Zurich, Switzerland)

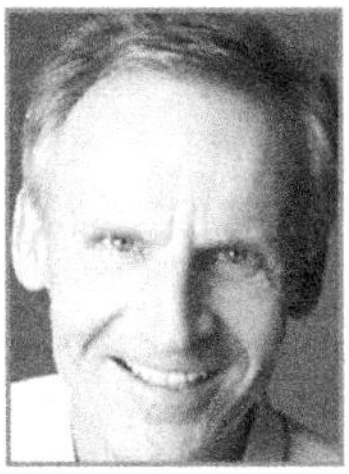

Karim Khan
(Doha, Qatar)

13:00 Introduction

13:10 Return to play: towards an international consensus
Clare Ardern (Doha, Qatar)

13:25 Optimizing load in return to play: is it feasible?
Phil Glasgow (United Kingdom)

13:40 Functional tests in return to play: where we're now?
Erik Witvrouw (Doha, Qatar)

13:55 Return to play in elite soccer: from the lab to the field
Holly Silvers (Santa Monica, USA)

14:15 Return to play in elite rugby: from the field to the field
Stephen Mutch (Edinburgh, United Kingdom)

14:30 End of the workshop

Saturday 9th April (afternoon)
CHURCHILL AUDITORIUM
(ground floor)

SYMPOSIUM

ISEH CONCUSSION MANAGEMENT AND RTP OPINIONS FROM LEADING AUTHORITIES AND GOVERNING BODIES

Chairs

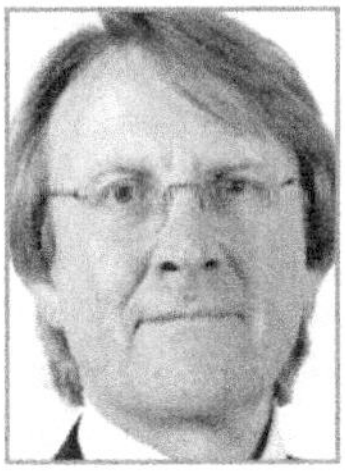

Peter Hamlyn
(London, United Kingdom)

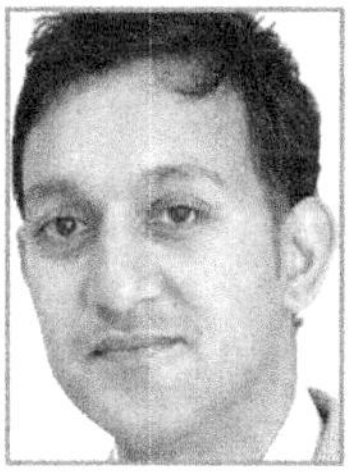

Akbar de' Medici
(London, United Kingdom)

13:00 Rugby World Cup 2015, what we learnt
Simon Kemp (Wimbledon, United Kingdom)

13:15 Challenges of creating a national guideline
Ian Beasley (United Kingdom)

13:30 TBD

13:45 Specialist management of sports related complex concussion, an MDT approach
Peter Hamlyn, Richard Sylvester (London, United Kingdom)

14:00 Discussion

14:30 End of the Workshop

Saturday 9th April (afternoon)
MOUNTBATTEN ROOM (sixth floor)

SYMPOSIUM

3D BIOMECHANICS IN RETURN TO PLAY DECISION MAKING AFTER ACL RECONSTRUCTION

Chairs

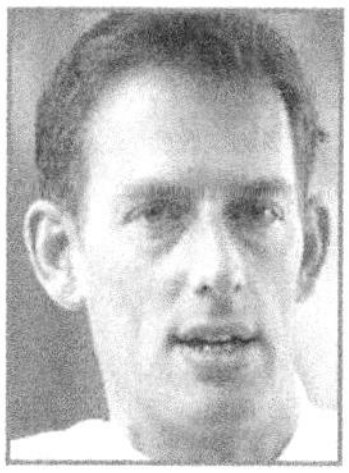

Andy Franklyn Miller
(Dublin, Ireland)

13:00	Return to play: whose decision is it anyway? **Andy Franklyn Miller (Dublin, Ireland)**
13:10	What is successful outcome after ACL reconstruction? **Enda King (Dublin, Ireland)**
13:20	3D biomechanical assessment after ACL reconstructions: What tests, what variables, what Analysis to run? **Chris Richter (Dublin, Ireland)**
13:40	What does a fully rehabilitated ACL look like and why? **Enda King (Dublin, Ireland)**
14:20	Discussion
14:30	End of the session

Saturday 9th April (afternoon)
DARWIN ROOM (sixth floor)

SYMPOSIUM

TURN DATA INTO INTELLIGENCE: HOW SOFTWARE CAN PLAY A ROLE IN SPORTS MEDICINE

Chairs

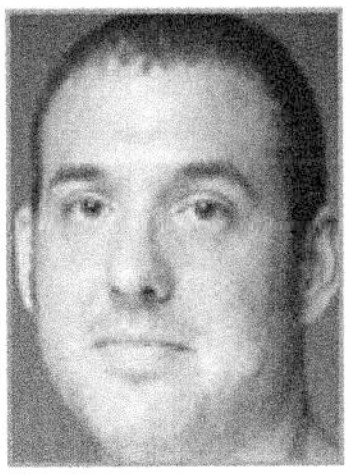

Gregori Ortanobas
(Barcelona, Spain)

13:00	Introducing MDM Systems
13:10	What is Soccer System Pro about?
13:40	Best practice: Qatar foundation
14:20	Discussion
14:30	End of the workshop

Saturday 9th April (afternoon)
PICKWICK SUITE (first floor)

SYMPOSIUM

WHOLE BODY CRYOTHERAPY IN ELITE SPORTS

Chairs

Liam Hennessy
(Dublin, Ireland)

11:30	Whole Body Cryotherapy in Elite Sports **Liam Hennessy (Dublin, Ireland)**
12:30	Discussion
13:00	End of the Workshop

Saturday 9th April (afternoon)
MOUNTBATTEN ROOM (sixth floor)

SYMPOSIUM

IAHA TAILOR TREATMENT FOR ATHLETES WITH DIFFERENT NEEDS

Chairs

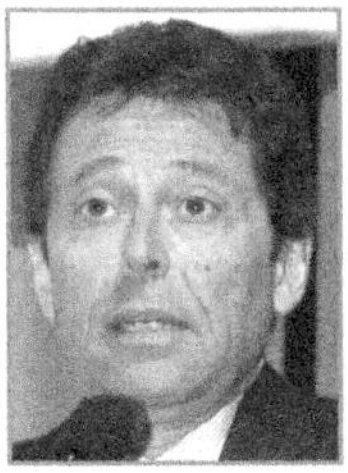

Francesco Benazzo
(Pavia, Italy)

14.30	Hymovis: From clinical to practical experience **Francesco Benazzo (Pavia, Italy)**
14.50	Hyaluronic Acid treatment of overuse disorders in athletes **Oliver Tobolski (Cologne, Germany)**
15.10	Hyaluronic Acid in elite basketball players **Marco Bigoni (Monza, Italy)**
15.30	Discussion
16:00	End of the workshop

1

HYMOVIS: FROM CLINICAL TO PRACTICAL EXPERIENCE...

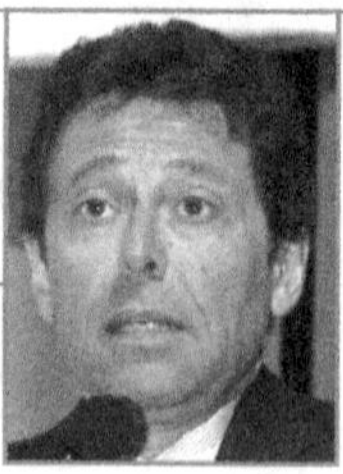

Benazzo F, Perticarini L

Fondazione IRCCS Policlinico San Matteo, Clinica Ortopedica e Traumatologica, Pavia, Italy

Hyaluronan (HA) is known to be the most used local therapy for the treatment and prevention of Osteoarthritis (OA). The mechanical features and the biological activity of this polysaccharide play a key role in the clinical efficacy of the treatments.

The HYADD 4 (Fidia Farmaceutici, Abano Terme, Italy) hydrogel is the result of a chemical modification of a native molecule of hyaluronan, and it is claimed to have enhanced rheological stability in response to mechanical stresses and to show a slower in vivo degradation resulting in a prolonged permanence in the joint, with no increase of the native molecular weight.

HYADD 4 has shown the efficacy in in vitro and in vivo studies.

In an multi-centre, open label investigation we have realized in a cohort of patients affected by knee OA, four intra-articular injections of HYADD 4 (2 at baseline, and 2 after 6 months) has brought a clear improvement in 93% of the patients at 26 weeks (no pain, or mild pain)as well as at 52 weeks (no pain in 56 % of the patients, mild pain in 44%). Moreover, the joint space width was assessed to evaluate the radiological progression of the knee OA (Rosenberg views) in this study over a 1-year period, was reduced of 0.2 mm (lower compared to other published literature).

These results, and those coming form similar investigations, have confirmed the hypothesis that this molecule is effective in relieving symptoms related to OA; being the efficacy prolonged in time, the mechanism of action could not only be due to the supposed mechanism of protection of cartilage against load (which could be also defined as overload relatively to the already damaged cartilage), but also to the lubricating and anti-inflammatory actions in form of biological activities. Based on this assumption, the use of HYADD 4 could be advocated in the prevention and treatment of the possible damages in the lower limb joints (hip, knee and ankle), in a younger, and active population, including athletes of different sports.

HYALURONIC ACID TREATMENT OF OVERUSE DISORDERS IN ATHLETES

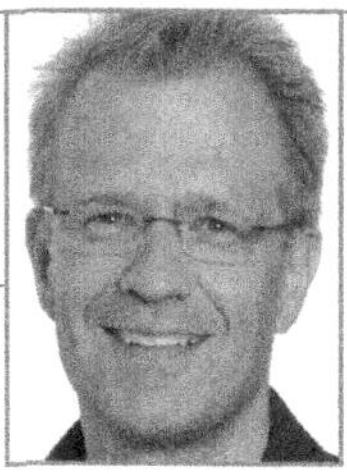

Tobolski O

Sporthomedic, Cologne, Germany

Within the framework of an observational study, the efficiency of hyaluronic acid in top athletes was put on trial.
In the past, degenerative cartilage defects caused by osteoarthritis up to Outerbridge stage III had commonly been treated with conventional hyaluronic acid which had led to measureable improvements of the Western Ontario and McMaster Universities Osteoarthritis Index (WOMAC) score and thus to a verifiable proof of the effects of the hyaluronic acid used.
Nevertheless, hyaluronic acid treatment of overuse syndroms (synovitic irritations/degenerative changes due to overuse), still showed unsatisfactory results, particularly in top athletes.
Thereupon such patients with overuse syndroms were treated with a next-generation hyaluronic acid (Hymovis), accompanied by case observations to monitor its effectiveness.
The evaluation of the results gathered showed a significant improvement of Magnetic Resonance Imaging-proven overuse syndroms (synovitis, hoffaitis, tendonitis, cartilage irritations, even bone bruise) in performance-oriented athletes who reported a substantial pain reduction subsequent to the treatment with Hymovis and, as a result, were able to resume their sport activities within a short period of time.

3

HYALURONIC ACID IN ELITE BASKETBALL PLAYERS

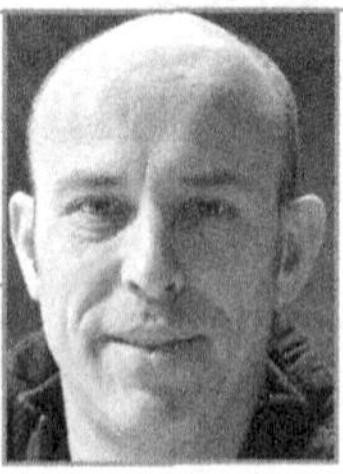

Bigoni M, Gaddi D, Piatti M, Giani E, Acquati M

Clinica Ortopedica Università Milano-Bicocca, Ospedale San Gerardo, Monza, Italy

Hyaluronic Acid (HA) has been widely used to improve knee function and pain relief. High performance professional athletes often complain with knee pain, and high percentage of day off is due to knee pain, especially in sports with repetitive jumps like basketball. This problem could also influence performance and tends to reduce muscle strength in a vicious cycle.
HA is a good choice in prevention and treatment of this clinical condition.
We present a case series of 10 professional basketball players with knee pain that underwent programmed injections with Hymovis (Fidia Farmaceutici, Abano Terme, Italy).
We report pain score (Visual Analogue Scale: VAS) and knee function at isokinetic test.
All sportsmen were investigated clinically and with Magnetic Resonance Imaging, after the first injection we performed the second about 2-3 weeks, and then one injection every month till the end of the season.
Initial mean pain, obtained from VAS evaluation, was 6.6/10 (range from 5 to 8), after two months reduction of pain was 42% in the group.
At the end of the season the mean reduction of pain was 58% and knee function was 30% higher.
We supposed that Hymovis was effective reducing knee pain and helped the basketball players in improving performance.

Saturday 9th April 2016 (afternoon)
DARWIN ROOM (sixth floor)

SYMPOSIUM

TENSOMYOGRAPHY AND RETURN TO PLAY

Chairs

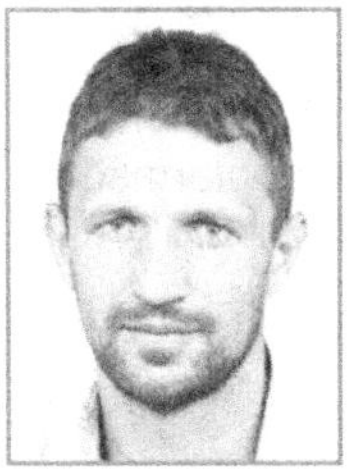

Boštjan Šimunič
(Ljubliana, Slovenia)

Andrej Žigon
(Ljubliana, Slovenia)

16:30	Introduction
16:45	Prediction monitoring, practical approach
17:00	Tensiomyography (TMG) as a tool for objective evaluation of functional muscle diagnostics. How TMG works?
17:15	TMG based return to play case study
17:30	Discussion
18:00	End of the workshop

1

MONITORING OF PRE- AND POST-OPERATIVE MUSCLE ADAPTATION OF ACL RECONSTRUCTION REHABILITATION PROCESS

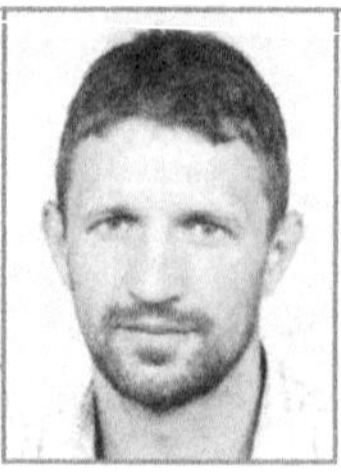

Šimunič B[1,2], Rozman S[1], Djordjevič S[1,2], Stok R[3], Pišot R[2]

[1]TMG-BMC Ltd, Ljubljana; [2]Institute for Kinesiology, Science and Research Centre of Koper, University of Primorska; [3]Orthopedic Clinic, Ljubljana, Slovenia

Introduction

For diagnosing Anterior Cruciate Ligament (ACL) tears there are many common used and reliable subjective methods, such are anterior drawer and Lachman tests and objective methods like stress arthrometry testing and Magnetic Resonance Imaging (MRI). But there are not many selective and objective tools available for testing muscle atrophy, as one of the most important accompanied effects. Any additional methods for fast, relevant diagnostic of functional skeletal muscle disorders can be useful for further understanding, prevention and return to play strategy in sport.
Tensiomyography (TMG) is non-invasive and selective method for measuring skeletal muscle mechanical contractile properties. In this study data gathered by measuring patients just before and after ACL reconstruction will be presented. The sensitivity of the TMG method monitoring muscle atrophy and hypertrophy during rehabilitation process and its ability to provide the information when muscle function is back to normal so subjects can resume maximal training intensity and return to play will be demonstrated.

Methods

Fifty-eight (43 male and 15 female) subjects (age 27.2±9.7 years) participated in the research. During the testing subjects were placed in standard measurement position (1) for measuring three heads of quadriceps muscle (Vastus Lateralis: VL; Vastus Medialis: VM; Rectus Femoris: RF) and one head of hamstring muscles (Biceps Femoris: BF). Each muscle was trans-cutaneous twitch stimulated via two bipolar electrodes placed on the skin surface above the muscle head. Supra-maximal muscle response was than recorded using TMG method and stored on Personal Computer (PC) for further analysis.
From each response the maximal amplitude (Displacement: Dm) was calculated and compared to healthy co-lateral side. The percentage of lateral symmetry coefficient of the each muscle was calculated, as division of Dm on the injured and healthy side (symmetry of 100% represents total symmetry). Four subjects were measured one day before the surgery and rest of them were grouped in weekly analysis. Some subjects were measured more frequently, as part of rehabilitation process. We also included six subjects that were measured one year after the surgery to stress the rehabilitation process results.

Results

Measurement results show that BF and VM had a huge asymmetry before the surgery and that VL and RF were very symmetrical. In first few weeks after the surgery the VL was the most affected muscle.
Huge drop in the symmetry was evident on VM and BF, from 141% to 83% and 196% to 84%, respectively.
The asymmetry reaches maximum simultaneously for all four observed muscles but with big difference in the absolute value. BF had by far the greatest asymmetry following VM, RF and VL. In about 24 weeks all of four muscles were fully recovered from the tone symmetry point of view.

Conclusions

The muscle tone of the skeletal muscle could be affected by atrophy and hypertrophy of muscle fibers. Atrophy is the process that takes time in about 7-10 days after the muscle inactivity. But before that a muscle inhibition takes place as a result of mechanical intervention during surgery, swallowing and tendon issues. Imbalance on BF and VM muscle of the injured side could be explained by the voluntary activation deficit alone and/or pain inhibition. From TMG response all three processes typical for ACL rehabilitation have been detected and timing for each separate muscle has been demonstrated. Consequently TMG monitoring of the muscle functional and structural atrophy and symmetry of knee extensors/flexors muscles after ACL surgery can significantly improve the rehabilitation process and help precisely determining return to play moment.

References

1. Dahmane R, Valen i V, Knez N, Er en I. Evaluation of the ability to make non-invasive estimation of muscle contractile properties on the basis of the muscle belly response. Med Biol Eng Comput 2001; 39: 51-55

Sunday 10th April (morning)
PICKWICK SUITE (first floor)

SYMPOSIUM

UTC IMAGING, NOVEL APPROACHES FOR THE MANAGEMENT OF TENDINOPATHY

Chairs

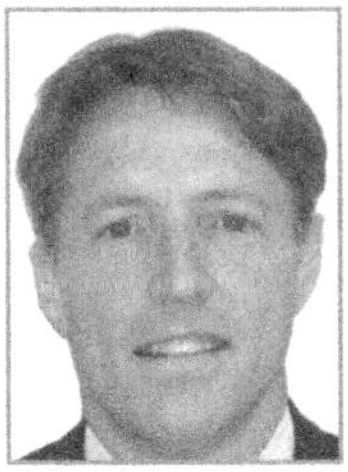

Hakan Alfredson
(Umea, Sweden)

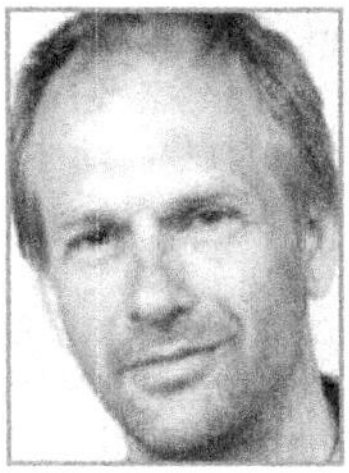

Erik Witvrouw
(Doha, Qatar)

8:00 Fundamentals of UTC imaging
Hans van Schie (Stein, The Netherlands)

8:12 UTC imaging for managing elite athletes
Jarrod Antflick (London, Unitd Kingdom)

8:24 UTC imaging for managing players at FC Barcelona
Gemma Hernandez, Gil Rodas (Barcelona, Spain)

8:36 UTC imaging in tendinopathy clinic; diagnosis and monitoring surgical cases **Lorenzo Masci (London, United Kingdom)**

8:48 Research into relationship between integrity and elasticity
Amy Fu (Hong Kong, China)

9:00 Discussion: UTC imaging, where does it fit in your prevention and management of tendinopathy

9:30 End of the workshop

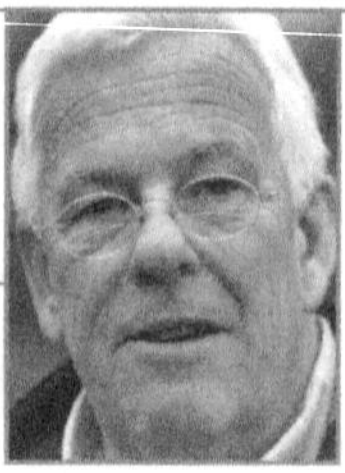

FUNDAMENTALS OF ULTRASOUND TISSUE CHARACTERIZATION (UTC)

Van Schie HTM

UTC Imaging, Stein, The Netherlands

Ultrasonography (US) can be used for the visualisation of tendons, although not standardized. The assessment of tendon integrity, however, is operator-dependent and subjective. For instance, scar tissue may generate US images with normal grey-levels too which indicates that US is not reliable to discriminate stages of integrity (2).

Main reason for the lack of discriminative power of US is that unique 3-D ultra-structure of tendons can not be visualized in single 2-D images. More so, 3-D structural integrity is reflected by real-time dynamism over contiguous 2-D images that are acquired while moving the US-transducer along the tendon. Due to the limits of spatial resolution, every US image is a mixture of structural reflections and interfering echoes, each with their characteristic dynamism in real-time US: relatively large structures, like secondary collagen bundles (fascicles), generate steady reflections, whereas smaller entities, like fibrils and cells, generate rapidly changing interfering echoes (2).

Ultrasound Tissue Characterisation (UTC) is based on standardized data-acquisition by means of a tracking device that moves the transducer automatically along the tendon while collecting transverse images at regular distances (600 over 12 cm). The compilation of these images creates a volume that can be used for (A) tomographic visualization and for (B) tissue characterization and quantification of integrity.

A. Tomographic visualization. The 3-D volume can be visualized in (1) transversal plane, (2) sagittal plane, (3) coronal plane, and (4) 3-D rendered coronal view. This inward view facilitates a reliable evaluation of 3-D ultra-structure that can be used e.g. for targeted and minimally invasive interventions.

B. Tissue characterization. Based on the quantification of dynamism of echo-patterns UTC-Algorithms can discriminate 4 different echo-types, with histo-morphology of tendon specimen as reference test:

Echo-type I, generated by intact and aligned fascicles, colored green in processed images;

Echo-type II, generated by waving, swollen and/or discontinuous fascicles, colored blue in processed images;

Echo-type III, generated by a mainly fibrillar matrix, colored red in processed images;

Echo-type IV, generated by a mainly amorphous matrix and fluid, colored black in processed images.

Fundamental research, by precisely matching UTC-processed images with exactly corresponding tendon specimen, revealed that ratios of these 4 echo-types are highly correlated with histo-morphological characteristics representing various stages of integrity (2).

Since 2005, UTC imaging is validated and implemented in sports medicine, till now mainly for Achilles and patellar tendons.

Some major observations are:

a. Inter- and intra- observer reliability of data-acquisition and analysis was tested at several research institutes. The intra-class correlation coefficient appeared to be 0.92-0.96, indicative for excellent reproducibility.

b. Normal tendons generate 65-85% echo-type I, 15-35% echo-type II and less than 5% echo-types III plus IV. Echo-types I and II may vary significantly, for instance with type of tendon (patellar tendons may generate more II compared to Achilles), localization in tendon (insertions generate more II compared to mid-portion), age (adolescents generate more II), and with physical activity (see the following point d.). This variation in echo-types I and II is physiological, in contrast to changes described in c.

c. Pathological changes are discriminated and quantified by means of significantly abnormal ratios of echo-types I-IV. Localized increase of echo-type II is indicative for fibrosis and localized or diffuse increase of echo-type III and/or IV is indicative for serious matrix disintegration (3).

d. Loading of tendons may lead to substantial increase of echo-type II, indicative for swollen fascicles (1). In case of overstraining besides II also echo-type III may increase, indicative for fascicular disintegration. These load-effects can still be reversible, if not this reactivity may lead to matrix degradation.

It is concluded that UTC imaging provides an inward view into ultra-structure and it quantifies tendon integrity with an excellent reliability. As such UTC imaging can be used for detection of load effects and early signs of matrix degradation, for staging of lesions, and for targeted therapy and guided rehabilitation, based on the stage of the lesion.

References

1. Rosengarten SD, Cook JL, Bryant AL, Cordy JT, Daffy J, Docking SI. Australian football players' Achilles tendons respond to game loads within 2 days: an ultrasound tissue characterisation (UTC) study. Br J Sports Med. 2015; 49: 183-187
2. Van Schie HT, Bakker EM, Jonker AM, van Weeren PR. Computerized ultrasonographic tissue characterization of equine superficial digital flexor tendons by means of stability quantification of echo patterns in contiguous transverse ultrasonographic images. Am J Vet Res 2003; 64: 366-375
3. Van Schie HT, de Vos RJ, de Jonge S, Bakker EM, Heijboer MP, Verhaar JA, Tol JL, Weinans H. Ultrasonographic tissue characterisation of human Achilles tendons: quantification of tendon structure through a novel non-invasive approach. Br J Sports Med 2010; 44: 1153-1159

ULTRASOUND TISSUE CHARACTERISATION (UTC) FOR MANAGING ELITE ATHLETES

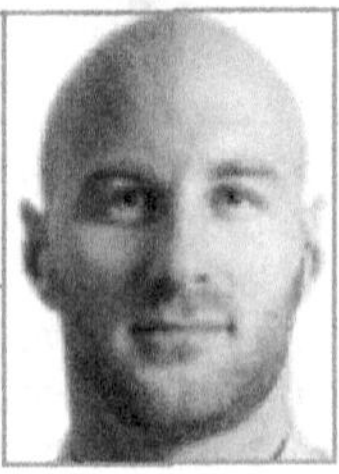

Antflick J

Tendon Performance, London, United Kingdom; Total Performance, New York, USA; Fortius Clinic, London, United Kingdom

A critical factor in the development of Achilles and patella tendinopathy is repeated high volume tendon load. Both cross-sectional and prospective studies on elite athletes from basketball, volleyball, ballet and Australian Rules football have demonstrated tendon pathology on imaging prior to the development of clinical symptoms (1). Risk factors in the development of Achilles tendinopathy include increasing pace and distance too quickly, high braking forces and reduced plantar flexor torques (2). Data from British Athletics suggests that the highest incidence rate is the period between March and July when athletes ready themselves to run quickly in preparation for the indoor season, increasing their elastic load requirements, and during high volume training at warm weather training camps. Early diagnostic and prevention strategies are therefore critical in keeping an athlete in training and competition.

The use of Ultrasound Tissue Characterisation (UTC) to monitor transient changes in tendon matrix structure is useful to minimise development of tendinopathy (3). It is a novel and exciting approach to risk mitigation by providing objective information on tendon quality. Structural change of the tendon matrix preceedes pain and athlete dysfunction. By preventing matrix disorganisation due to repeated high loads, an athlete can circumvet the onset of tendinopathy and reduce the abusive load stimulus.

It's use for monitoring transient intrinsic matrix changes of Achilles and patella tendons is being demonstrated in elite level National Basketball Association (NBA) to guide prophylactic loading and player exposures to repeated high tendon loads. An in press study looking at a cohort of elite level track and field athletes, aimed at recording the UTC profiles of male and female athletes. The study found a relationship between increasing age and history of tendinopathy. Increasing age was associated with an increase in type III & IV echo-types.

The use of UTC aids in the monitoring of interventions, including injection therapy and loading based strategies. A pilot study conducted at the Fortius clinic of seven males who failed conservative normal physiotherapy underwent an Ostenil injection followed by a high force loading program.

Follow-up at three months demonstrated an improvement in Visual Analogue Scale (VAS) (mean 5.1 to 1.6; P=0.007) and echo types Type I P=0.006, Type III P=0.019, Type IV P= 0.029. This improvement in structure correlated with a reduction in pain.

Sub classification of Achilles tendinopathy allows for differing loading and intervention strategies. UTC aids in the diagnosis of Achilles tendinopathy by visualising areas of tendon disintegration. Treatment for plantaris related mid-portion Achilles tendinopathy differs from intra-substance micro tears and para-tendinopathy. These discrete diagnoses can be made on normal ultrasound but with varying degrees of accuracy.

UTC visualises and quantifies the matrix disintegration or lesion site by providing a clear 3 dimensional and colour representation of these pathologies. A numerical output allows for on-going monitoring of intervention and load based strategies.

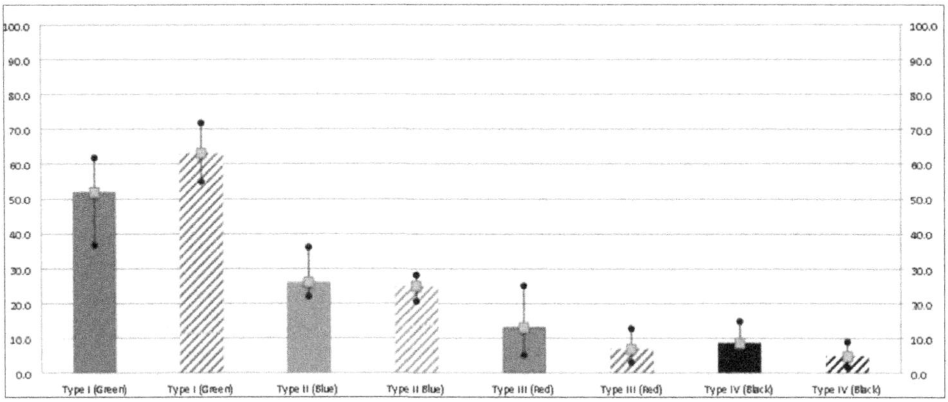

Figure 1. Comparison of Pre and Post Ostenil HVI injection in seven male subjects.

References

1. Cook JL, Khan KM, Kiss ZS, Coleman BD, Griffiths L. Asymptomatic hypoechoic regions on patellar tendon ultrasound: A 4-year clinical and ultrasound followup of 46 tendons. Scand J Med Sci Sports 2001; 11: 321-327
2. Lorimer AV, Hume PA. Achilles tendon injury risk factors associated with running. Sports Med 2014; 44: 1459-1472
3. Rosengarten SD, Cook JL, Bryant AL, Cordy JT, Daffy J, Docking SI. Australian football players' Achilles tendons respond to game loads within 2 days: an ultrasound tissue characterisation (UTC) study. Br J Sports Med 2015; 49: 183-187

ULTRASOUND TISSUE CHARACTERISATION (UTC) IN TENDINOPATHY CLINIC: DIAGNOSIS AND MONITORING OF SURGICAL CASES

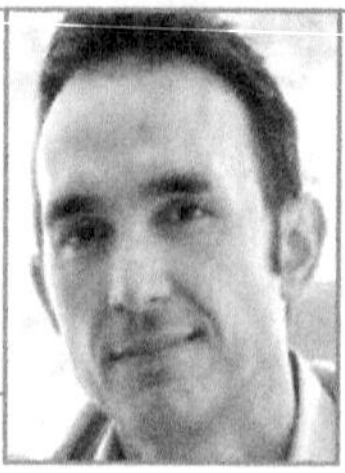

Masci L[1,2], Alfredson H[1]

[1]Pure Sports Medicine, London; Institute of Sport Exercise and Health (ISEH), London, United Kingdom

Visualising structure is an important adjunct to clinical presentation in managing tendon disease in a tendinopathy clinic. Ultrasound imaging demonstrates pathological changes of tendinopathy as heterogenicity and hypoechogenicity of tendon structure on B mode and increased tendon blood flow on colour-doppler. Despite importance in confirming a clinical diagnosis, ultrasound findings are subjective and lack reproducibility. This limits its applicability in the management of tendinopathy.

Ultrasound Tissue Characterisation (UTC) is a novel imaging modality that is able to visualise tendon structure and quantify tendon matrix integrity by assessing the stability of greyscale changes in contiguous images. By using a tracking machine, UTC is able to objectively quantify tendon matrix integrity in a reproducible manner. Therefore, in addition to providing diagnostic information, it can also monitor and objectify changes in tendon structure after intervention including rehabilitation and tendon surgery.

UTC has a practical utility in the management of specific clinical cases of tendinopathy, and can help in confirming diagnosis of difficult tendon presentations (i.e., a case of persistent medial Achilles pain where UTC confirmed a diagnosis of plantaris-associated midportion tendinopathy; a case of acute Achilles pain that was diagnosed as a partial tendon tear by using both B mode ultrasound and UTC).

UTC can also applied in monitoring tendon changes after surgical procedures to guide optimal loading and rehabilitation and can improve our ability to successfully manage return to play after tendon surgery (i.e., a case of patella tendinopathy that failed conservative treatment and required an arthroscopic surgical scraping procedure).

RESEARCH INTO RELATIONSHIP BETWEEN INTERGRITY AND ELASTICITY

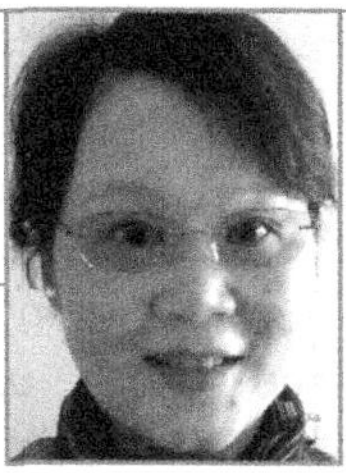

Fu A

Department of Rehabilitation Sciences, Hong Kong, China

Introduction

The relationship between tendon integrity and elasticity is currently unclear. Change in tendon elasticity observed in athletes with tendinopathy is partly contributed by changes in tendon integrity, such as micro-tears in the tendon fibrils (1). Investigation on tendon integrity and elasticity has been conducted in separate studies. This study conducted measurements on tendon integrity and elasticity on healthy and subjects with patellar tendinopathy to explore possible relationship between the two parameters.

Methods

This study was a cross-sectional observational study. 19 Healthy subjects (aged between 18 and 31 yrs; 10 male and 9 female) and 9 male athletes (aged between 21 and 33 yrs) with patellar tendinopathy participated in this study. Subject was asked to supine lying on the plinth with the knee positioned at 90 degrees knee flexion. The patellar tendon integrity was measured with a linear-array US transducer (SmartProbe 10L5,Terason 2000, Teratech, USA) mounted within a customized tracking device with motor drive and built-in acoustic standoff pad (UTC Tracker, UTC Imaging, The Netherlands) (1) and tendon elasticity with Supersonic Shear elastography (SSE, SuperSonic Imagine, Aix-en-Provence, France) at 0.5 cm and 1.5 cm from the proximal attachment of the patellar tendon. Four validated echo-types, related to tendon integrity, were discriminated from the Ultrasound Tissue Characterisation (UTC) echo-type I represents intact, continuous and aligned fibres and fasciculi, echo-type II represents less continuous and/or more wavy fibres and fasciculi, echo-type III represents a mainly fibrillar matrix and echo-type IV represents complete disintegration, with tendon tissue replaced by an amorphous matrix and fluid. These echo-types were quantified as relative percentages of the tendon in the region of interest. Tendon elasticity was quantified by a circular quantification box (Q-Box) centred at 0.5 cm and 1.5 cm from the inferior pole of the patellar. The diameter of the Q-Box was adjusted according to the thickness of the tendon (2). The mean shear elastic modulus was generated. Correlation tests were conducted between the percentage of echo type (1, II, III, IV) and the elastic modulus at the 2 sites.

Results

This study showed significant relationship between tendon integrity and elasticity in healthy patellar tendon. Shear modulus was positively related to percentage of echo type I (at 1.5 cm; rho =0.048; p<0.05) and negatively related to percentage of echo type II (at both 0.5 cm and 1.5cm; rho =-0.43 – -0.44; all p<0.05). A trend of positive correlation was detected between Shear modulus and echo type II (at 1.5 cm; rho= 0.59; p=0.074) in male athletes with patellar tendinopathy.

Conclusions

Patellar tendon integrity and elasticity are related in pain-free tendon and a trend of correlation in patellar tendon with patella tendinopathy. Greater percentage of echo type II is associated with less tendon stiffness in pain-free tendon but greater stiffness in tendinopathic tendon.

References

1. Van Schie HT, de Vos RJ, de Jonge S, Bakker EM, Heijboer MP, Verhaar JA, Tol JL, Weinans H. Ultraosographic tissue characterization of human Achillis tendons: quantification of tendon structure through a novel non-invasive approach. Br J Sports Med 2010; 44: 1153-1159
2. Zhang ZJ, Fu SN. Shear elastic modulus on patellar tendon captured from supersonic shear imaging: correlation with tangent traction modulus computed from material testing system and test–retest reliability. 2013; PLoS ONE 8: e68216.

Sunday 10th April (morning)
DARWIN ROOM (sixth floor)

SYMPOSIUM

SYMPOSIUM INDIBA ACTIV

Chairs

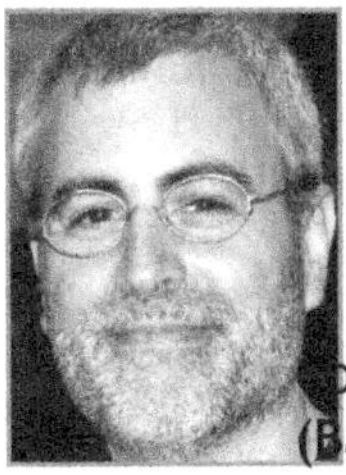

Corral-Baqués MI
(Barcelona, Spain)

9:30	Stem cell proliferation by 448 kHz frequency **Corral-Baqués MI (Barcelona, Spain)**
11:00	End of the workshop

STEM CELL PROLIFERATION BY 448 KHZ FREQUENCY

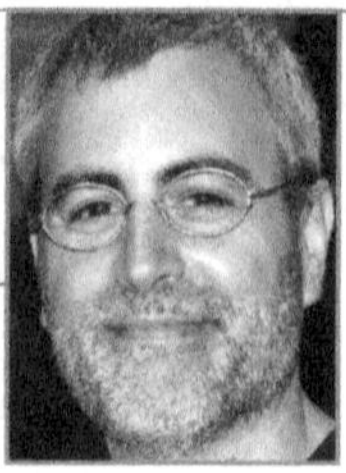

Corral-Baqués MI

Indiba, Barcelona, Spain

To know the physiological mechanism of action of any technique is the cornerstone to obtain optimal results. The latest findings regarding the INDIBA Activ 448 kHz electromagnetic field suggests that the bio-stimulating effect of these currents at sub-thermal doses influences the promotion of stem cells that regenerate tissues or injured organs (1).
Whilst other radiofrequencies only base their effects on the hyperthermal properties on tissues, the Bioelectromagnetic Research department from Ramon y Cajal University Hospital has proven that 448 kHz radiofrequency at a subthermal power stimulates stem cell proliferation, thus increasing their number and these new cells can perfectly differentiate between bone and cartilaginous tissues (1). These results explain the regenerative properties of INDIBA Activ in bone traumas and chondropathies.
This stimulatory action, that includes other effects apart from promoting the proliferation of stem cells, is described as the Proionic System and results in the promotion of cellular functionality, biostimulation and other biological phenomena that results in an increase of local blood circulation alongside an anti-inflammatory and draining effect that together promote wound healing (2).
Classic radiofrequencies cannot be used on acute conditions where heat is contraindicated, however the Proionic System by means of subthermal doses is an ideal proven solution to post-traumatic inflammation and oedema thus reducing the rehabilitation time during the recovery process (2).
The use of INDIBA in professional football injuries has proven to be of great help in a fast reduction of oedema and VAS pain scale, thus shortening the down time and allowing a quick return to professional competition.

References

1. Hernández-Bule ML, Paíno CL, Trillo MÁ, Úbeda A. Electric stimulation at 448 kHz promotes proliferation of human mesenchymal stem cells. Cell Physiol Biochem 2014; 34: 1741-1755
2. Naranjo P, López R, Pinto H. First assessment of the proioni effects resulting from non-themal application of 448 kHz monopolar radiofrequency for reduction of edema caused by fractional CO2 laser facial rejuvenation treatments. Journal of Surgery 2015; 3: 21-24

Sunday 10th April (afternoon)
FLEMING ROOM (third floor)

SYMPOSIUM

MUSCLETECH TECHNOLOGY AND RETURN TO PLAY

Chairs

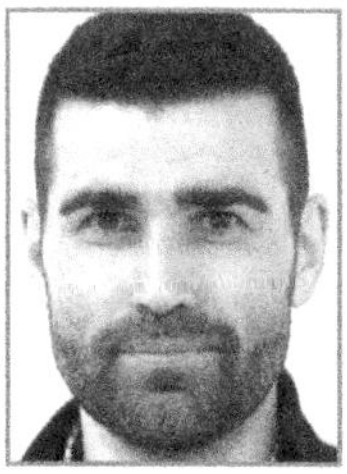

Raul Peláez
(Barcelona, Spain)

13:00	Current concepts of Tech in football **Steve Palmer**
13:15	Current concepts of Tech in sports medicine **Francisco Ayala (Alicante, Spain)**
13:30	Tech at Football Club Barcelona: GPS monitoring: why? **Eduard Pons (Barcelona, Spain)**
13:40	Tech at Football Club Barcelona: sports medicine monitoring tools **Daniel Medina (Barcelona, Spain)**
13:50	Tech for return to play in football **Ricard Pruna (Barcelona, Spain)**
14:00	Tech for return to play in other sports **Gil Rodas (Barcelona, Spain)**
14:10	Discussion
14:30	End of the workshop

Sunday 10th April (afternoon)
CHURCHILL AUDITORIUM (ground floor)

SYMPOSIUM

EVIDENCE BASED MEDICINE IN MUSCLES, LIGAMENTS AND TENDON DISORDERS: ISMULT GUIDELINES

Chairs

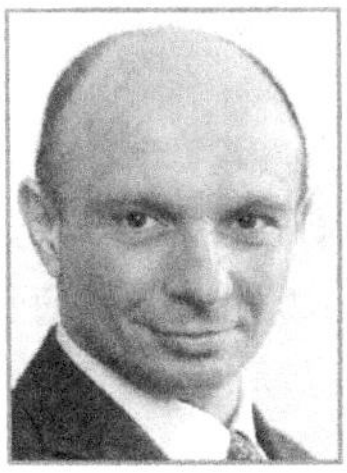

Nicola Maffulli
(Salerno, Italy)

13:00	Introduction
13:10	Management of rotator cuff tears: when conservative and when surgical **Francesco Oliva (Rome, Italy)**
13:25	Muscles injuries: from classification to treatment **Gianni Nanni (Bologna, Italy)**
13:40	What to do after first patellar dislocation : conservative and surgical evidences **Mario Vetrano (Rome, Italy)**
13:55	What about Hyaluronic Acid in Musculoskeletal applications: 2016 ISMuLT guidelines **Antonio Frizziero (Padova, Italy)**
14:10	Discussion
14:30	End of the workshop

1

ISMULT ROTATOR CUFF TEARS GUIDELINES

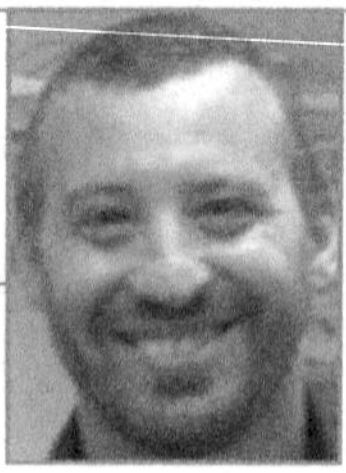

Oliva F

Department of Orthopaedics and Traumatology,
University of Rome Tor Vergata, Rome, Italy

Despite the high level achieved in the field of shoulder surgery, a global consensus on rotator cuff tears management in lacking. This work is divided into two main sessions: in the first, we set questions about hot topics involved in the rotator cuff tears, from the etio-pathogenesis to the surgical treatment. In the second, we answered these questions by mentioning Evidence Based Medicine that supports the questions.
The aim of the present work is to provide easily accessible guidelines: they could be considered as recommendations for a good clinical practice developed through a process of systematic review of the literature and expert opinion, in order to improve the quality of care and rationalize the use of resources.

2

ISMULT GUIDELINES FOR MUSCLE INJURIES

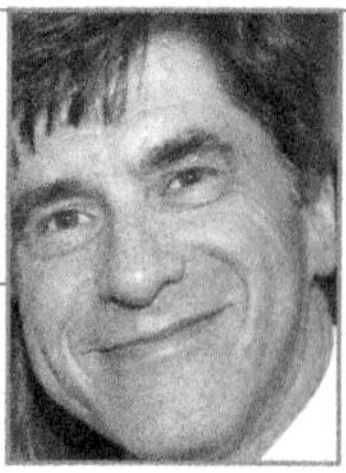

Nanni G

Isokinetic Medical Group, FIFA Medical Centre of Excellence, Bologna, Italy

No guidelines are available in the scientific literature. ISMuLT, the Italian Society of Muscles, Ligaments and Tendons, in line with its multidisciplinary mission, is proud to cover this gap.
Muscle injuries are frequent in high demand sports, accounting for 10 to 55% of all acute sports injuries. The muscles and muscle groups more frequently involved are the hamstrings, Rectus Femoris, and the medial head of the Gastrocnemius. Although the diagnosis is usually clinical, imaging tools are often advocated to better identify the extent and site of lesion, which can be relevant prognostic factors predictive of recovery time, return to pre-injury sport activity, and risk of recurrence.
A number of treatments is available for muscle injuries, including the PRICE (Protection, Rest, Ice, Compression, Elevation) and POLICE (Protection, Optimal Load, Ice, Compression, Elevation) protocols, passive and active stretching, physical therapies, functional rehabilitation and general athletic reconditioning.
The present guidance includes several treatments that have been used for the management of muscle injuries, and aims to reduce the uncertainty and variations in practice that remain in some areas of their diagnosis and management. Up to date recommendations are provided on:
- Classification of muscle injuries
- Diagnosis: clinical and at imaging
- The most effective method of management based on type of lesion

3

WHAT TO DO AFTER FIRST PATELLAR DISLOCATION: CONSERVATIVE AND SURGICAL EVIDENCES

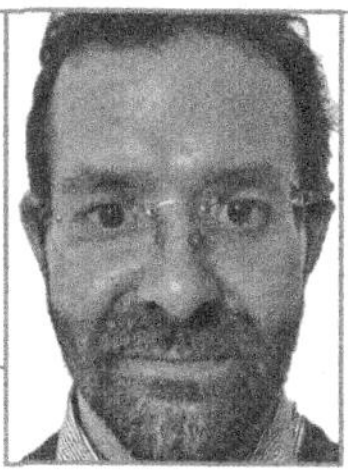

Vetrano M

Sant'Andrea Hospital, Sapienza University of Rome, Italy

Acute patellar dislocation is a common knee joint disorder in the practice of knee specialists, mainly affecting adolescents and active young adult populations.
In spite of the relatively high incidence of this pathologic condition, there remains a significant controversy regarding the ideal treatment protocol.
Treatment is essential to minimize sequelae, such as recurrent dislocation, painful subluxation and osteoarthritis. Management of first patellar dislocation has historically been conservative, with early operative treatment reserved for patients with associated osteochondral injuries or fractures.
Several Authors assert that surgical treatment after acute primary patellar dislocation significantly reduces the risk of re-dislocation and provides excellent results on Visual Analogue Scale (VAS) and other clinical scales. On the contrary, analysis of performance tests shows significantly better results after conservative treatment, which also provides significantly lower risk of minor complications. In many patients, however, both the surgical and conservative treatment for this injury does not restore patients to their pre-injury function.

4

ISMULT GUIDELINES FOR THE TREATMENT OF HYALURONIC ACID IN MUSCULOSKELETAL DISEASE

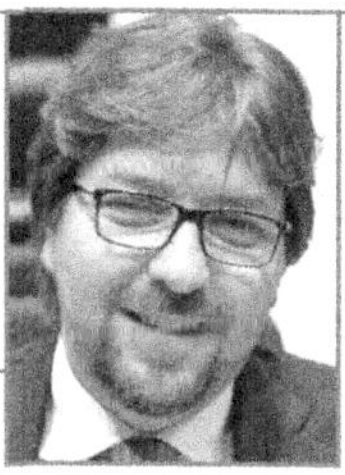

Frizziero A

Department of Physical and Rehabilitation Medicine, University of Padua, Italy

Hyaluronic Acid (HA) injections are commonly used for local treatment of Osteoarthritis (OA) and other musculoskeletal disease like tendinopathies, bursitis, considering its good tolerance.
In commerce there are a lot of products with different molecular weight and with a linear or reticulated structure.
Hyaluronic acid has demonstrated moderate but significant efficacy versus placebo in terms of pain and function, with a high rate of responders (60-70%) in knee osteoarthritis. It permits reduction of assumption of opioid analgesics and Non-Steroidal Anti-Inflammatory Drugs (NSAIDs).
Good clinical results have also been observed versus corticosteroids both in joints and in peri-tendon sites but the real efficacy of Hyaluronic acid and the modality of therapeutic administration are a matter of ingoing debate. Results have been disappointing in hip osteoarthritis but promising in ankle and shoulder OA (with and without rotator cuff tear). Our aim for this year it will be to offer easily accessible guidelines as recommendations for a good clinical practice developed through a process of systematic review of the literature and expert opinion.

Sunday 10th April (afternoon)
DARWIN ROOM (sixth floor)

SYMPOSIUM

MUSCLE ACTIVATION DATA (EMG) FROM WEARABLES IN INJURY PREVENTION AND REHABILITATION

Chairs

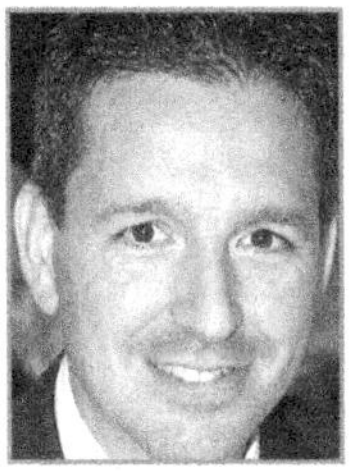

David Díaz Cueli
(Barcelona, Spain)

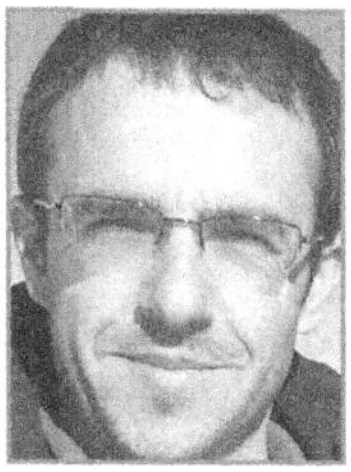

Xavier Gasol Santa
(Barcelona, Spain)

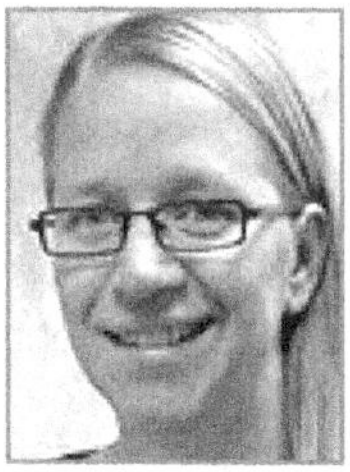

Merja Hoffrén-Mikkola
(Kuortane, Finland)

13:00	Introduction **Merja Hoffrén-Mikkola (Kuortane, Finland)**
13:10	Use of Mbody to detect muscle imbalances and muscle loading Merja **Hoffrén-Mikkola (Kuortane, Finland)**
13:25	Practical applications of Mbody shorts in Real Club Deportivo Espanyol of Barcelona **David Díaz Cueli (Barcelona, Spain)**
13:45	Practical demonstration of Mbody shorts **David Díaz Cueli, Xavier Gasol Santa (Barcelona, Spain)**
14:15	Discussion
14:30	End of the workshop

MUSCLE ACTIVATION DATA (EMG) FROM WEARABLES IN INJURY PREVENTION AND REHABILITATION

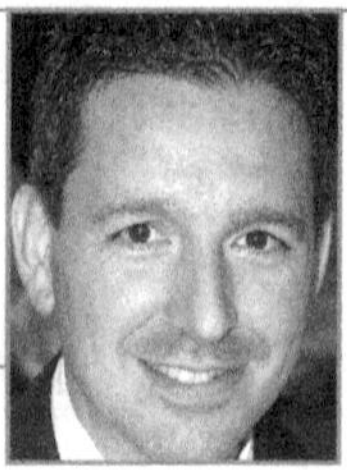

Díaz-Cueli D[1], Turmo-Garuz A[1,2,3], Gasol-Santa X[1], Cacciatori E[1], Hoffrén-Mikkola M[4]

[1]RCD Espanyol of Barcelona, Spain;
[2]High Performance Center of Sant Cugat, Consorci Sanitari de Terrassa, Spain;
[3]Professional Sports Medicine School, University of Barcelona, Spain;
[4]Kuortane Olympic Training Center, Finland

Introduction

Most soccer injuries occur in the lower extremities and result to significant loss of training hours and game participation. Training-related hamstring injury rates have increased substantially in European men football leagues since 2001 and currently 22% of players sustain at least one hamstring injury during a season (1). To decrease the number of injuries, monitor the rehabilitation process and avoid return to practice and play re-injuries, there is an increasing demand for objective monitoring of players physical performance, muscle loading and muscle function.

Methods

Myontec MBody (Myontec Ltd, Kuopio, Finland) offers a wearable device to monitor Electromyographic activity (EMG) on lower leg muscle groups (quadriceps, hamstrings, glutes). The washable textile electrodes permit the screening of muscle activities both in laboratory and field settings without any inconvenience to the players. The method has been validated against traditional surface EMG and has been shown to be a reliable tool to assess EMG both in static and dynamic exercises (2). Therefore it offers an objective assessment of muscle loading during training, games and throughout the rehabilitation programs. Balance between right and left leg can be monitored in order to quantify possible muscle imbalances as well as average EMGs (aEMG) during different trials recorded in order to estimate the level of force production in different exercises. EMG relations of lower leg muscle groups (quadriceps/hamstrings, glutes/hamstrings) give professionals information about the players technique and muscle activation profiles (activation/deactivation cycles) may reveal the potential problems related to current condition of nervous system.

Practical applications

Using Mbody Kalema et al. (3) reported that aEMG during soccer match decreased towards the end of the game the most probably due to muscle fatigue and proposed that those players with highest decrease in aEMG could be most potentially exposed to injuries. Therefore, wearable EMG may help to reduce the risk of injuries during match.
In addition Mbody shorts allow football club professionals the tool to analyze quadriceps and/or hamstrings EMG balance on acceleration sprints at different speeds on the field. It is suggested that since running is a complex task it can reveal some imbalances that are not present in more basic exercises, when the player is at the final phase of the rehabilitation process. Therefore the EMG data recorded in field conditions during fast high-intensity exercises may reveal vitally important information that may help professionals to decide whether it really is safe for the player to return to play and avoid further injuries.

References

1. Ekstrand J, Waldén M, Hägglund M. Hamstring injuries have increased by 4% annually in men's professional football, since 2001: a 13-year longitudinal analysis of the UEFA Elite Club injury study. Br J Sports Med 2016 Jan 8. pii: bjsports-2015-095359. doi: 10.1136/bjsports-2015-095359. [Epub ahead of print]
2. Finni T, Hu M, Kettunen P, Vilavuo T & Cheng S. Measurement of EMG activity with textile electrodes embedded into clothing. Physiol Meas 2007; 28: 1405-1419
3. Kalema R. Quadriceps and hamstring muscle EMG activity during a football match. Master's Thesis 2012; University of Jyväskylä. https://jyx.jyu.fi/dspace/handle/123456789/41027

Sunday 10th April (afternoon)
DARWIN ROOM (sixth floor)

SYMPOSIUM

BIOMECHANICS AND PODIATRY IN ELITE FOOTBALL

Chairs

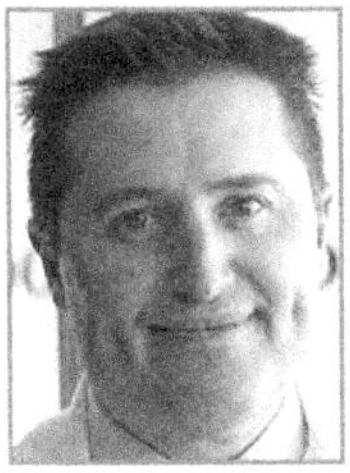

Javier Alfaro
(Madrid, Spain)

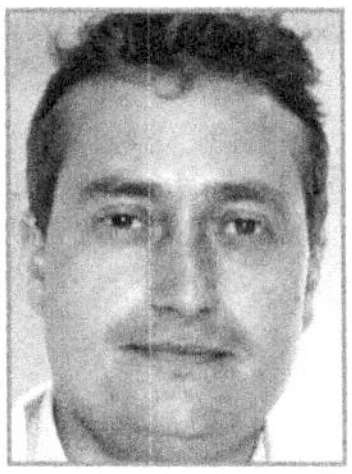

Víctor Alfaro
(Madrid, Spain)

14:30	Introduction
14:40	Podiatry assessment and treatment in elite football players **Javier Alfaro (Madrid, Spain)**
15:10	Biomechanical evaluation in top football players **Víctor Alfaro (Madrid, Spain)**
15:30	Customized Protection Technologies in elite football **Ismael Fernández-Cuevas (Madrid, Spain)**
15:45	Discussion
16:00	End of the workshop

Monday 11th April, 2016 (morning)
CURCHILL AUDITORIUM

INVITED SPEAKERS

4th Science and Football Summit

YOUTH ATHLETIC DEVELOPMENT

Chairs

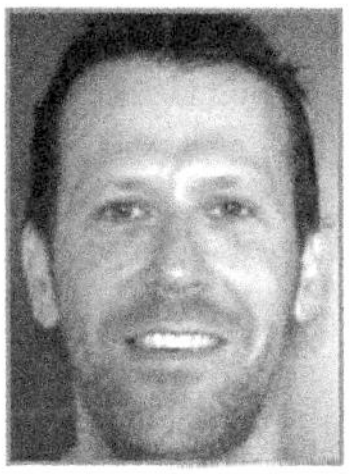

Warren Greson
(Liverpool,
United Kingdom)

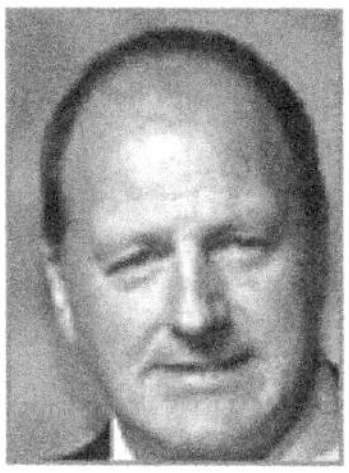

Ged Roddy
(Liverpool,
United kingdom)

9:15	Managing change in youth development **Greson Roddy (Liverpool, United Kingdom)**
9:30	The Belgium vision on youth development **Bob Browaeys (Brussels, Belgium)**
9:45	Managing and launching great talents: "cantera" of FC Barcelona **Daniel Medina (Barcelona, Spain)**
10:00	Tracking the player: 10 years injury histories and performance in French football academy **Alan McCall (Paris, France)**
10:15	Medical services in academies: the vision of Manchester City **Grant Downie (Manchester, United Kingdom)**
10:30	Youth athletic development in the USA: are we specializing too early? **Holly Silvers-Granelli (Santa Monica, USA)**
10:45	Discussion
11:00	End of the session

1

MANAGING CHANGE IN YOUTH DEVELOPMENT

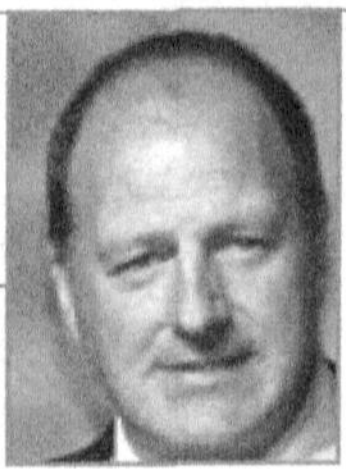

Roddy G

Premier League, United Kingdom

The Elite Player Performance Plan (EPPP) is a long term plan which promotes the development of a world leading Academy System across the Premier League and Football League. It aims to deliver an environment that promotes excellence, nurtures talent and systematically converts this talent into professional players capable of playing first team football at the club that develops them. The EPPP should promote technical excellence and ensure financial viability now and in the future.
To achieve this, the modernised Academy system will be regularly and independently audited, updated and improved.
The EPPP is inextricably linked to the development of a new Classification System for youth development and this new approach to the classification will be guided by the EPPP.
New Rules and Regulations and a new Compensation formula have been agreed to ensure the effective implementation of the new system.
Our mission is: to produce more and better home grown players
Our objectives are summarised in table 1.

STAFF	PLAYERS	ENVIRONMENT
-Develop the world's leading youth coaching fraternity. -Provide world class education via innovative and inspirational teaching. -Establish sports science and medicine as the trusted support service for all players.	-evelop technically excellent players who are tactically astute and independent decision makers, fully equipped for a successful career as a professional (Premier League) footballer. -Develop educationally rounded people through the delivery of a holistic approach to player care.	-Consistently measure and evaluate the academy system to provide benchmarked performance feedback to all Clubs. -Use these measures to refine understanding of the key characteristics of the elite environment. -Provide inspirational facilities capable of delivering an innovative Games Programme.

THE BELGIAN YOUTH DEVELOPMENT MODEL IN FOOTBALL

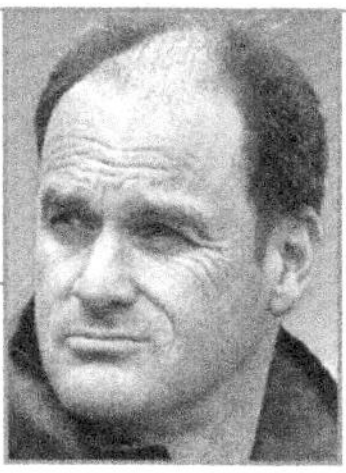

Browaeys B

Royal Belgian Football Association, Brussels, Belgium

Is the current 1st place on the FIFA-ranking of the Belgian A-team and the 3th place in the World Cup U17 2015 based on pure coincidence or is there a relationship between the worldclass Belgian football players and the Belgian Youth Development Model?
It's difficult to prove a scientific based link between performance of a sports team and a long term vision on youth development. However the purpose of the presentation is to describe the Belgian Vision on Youth Development and the different projects the Belgian Football Association (FA) launched since 2000 to produce world class football players.
The Belgian Vision on Youth Development is based on Vision 2000 which has been developed, taught and constantly adapted to new international football trends during the last 15 years.
The vision has initially been tested in practice at the Top Sport Schools and in the National Youth Teams. After a large consultation with feedback given by experts it has been spread towards all Belgian FA projects and Belgian clubs. Fun and Formation, game oriented learning, age appropriate learning objectives and player oriented approach still remain the keywords of this unique vision.
Small sides games (2v2, 5v5, 8v8) offer children from 5 to 12 year old a strong learning environment in which dribblings, passings, scoring opportunities and decision making processes occur more frequently than in 11v11 games. Different levels in youth competitions give all Belgian players the chance to play on the right level and to learn effectively as challenge and confidence are in balance.
The Belgian Talent Identification program is based on six competences (winner's mentality, emotional stability, personality, speed, insight in the game and ball and body control) and on specific characteristics within several player's profiles, not contaminated by the relative age effect and the biologic maturity of the player. The purpose is to identify as fast as possible high potentials for the future.
The aim of the National Youth Team System is to provide high quality development according to the Belgian FA vision during training sessions, training camps and international games where the best are playing with the best against the best and to prepare the most talented players per age group for a professional and international career and finally for the A-team.
In several Topsport Schools the Belgian FA offer the most talented boys and girls from 14 year to 18 year a supplementary quality education of four additional training sessions a week, which is complementary to their development in the club.
High quality Coach Education based on reality based learning, long life learning and self regulation must produce better Belgian youth players and better performances by senior teams.
The quality of the Club and Academy Management is since 2004 objectively and independently measured by the Foot PASS Instrument that classifies the clubs in different quality labels and gives recommendations to the youth academy directors about how to improve the quality of their educational programs.
Finally, club support managers from the Belgian FA are giving to the Youth Academy Directors continuously professional advice based on the Foot PASS reporting in accordance with the Belgian Vision on Youth Development.
World class football players can be produced by a small country as Belgium (11 million habitants) because of a Long Term Player Development based on a well defined vision and ignited by projects where high potential youth players are submerged by a quality educational programm in National Youth Teams, Top Sport School and Club Academies.

THE ROLE OF A MEDICAL DEPARTMENT IN THE ELITE ACADEMY SETTING. THE MANCHESTER CITY FC PHILOSOPHY

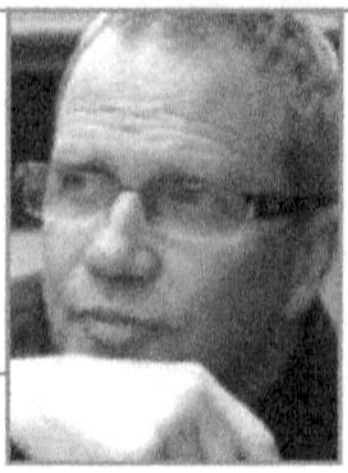

Downie G

Manchester City FC, The City Football Group, Manchester, United Kingdom

In five year time, we see city players globally that know how to win and look after their body, mind and soul, and we are all proud in the football brand.

Manchester City FC (MCFC) Performance Philosophy:

- Sky high standards
- Great people, who know how to deliver & can "connect"
- Development is everything
- No fear No failure
- Reflect & Learn
- Celebrate our practice (successes & failings)
- Team within a team

Added Value will make the difference. We go the extra mile and can learn from anyone.

As such MCFC Academy do not have a medical department, but a performance department who has "medics" who work for it.
We look on an injury as part of the football journey and as a great opportunity to get physically and mentally tougher. Therefore return a more robust player and person who knows a little more about his body and how to use it.
We will take scholars on a journey of guided discovery and empowerment, and get them to own their own journey. Every Second counts...

Conclusion

Athlete centered approach at developing the person so they have the skills and knowledge to deal with injuries throughout their football journey.

YOUTH ATHLETIC DEVELOPMENT IN THE USA: ARE WE SPECIALIZING TOO EARLY?

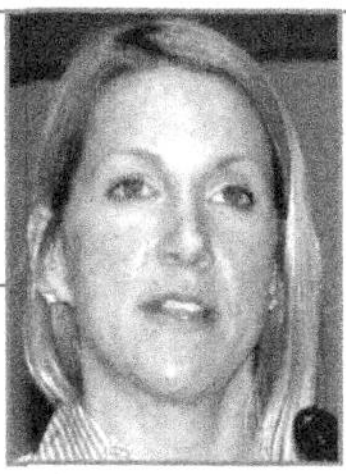

Silvers-Granelli H

University of Delaware, Newark, USA

In the United States of America, there are approximately 30 to 60 million athletes between the ages of 6 to 18 that participate in organized or recreational sport. There is a plethora of evidence that supports early specialization in skill acquisition. Ericsson et al. studied the effects of practice and training on learning acquisition and speculated that early specialization; "deliberate practice" (i.e. effortful practice that lacks inherent enjoyment done with the sole purpose of improving current levels of performance), was essential to the development of expertise (Ericsson KA, Krampe RT, Heizmann S. Can we create gifted people? Ciba Found Symp 1993; 178: 222-231).

Research examining the effects of prolonged practice and the rate of learning has indicated that performance increases directly according to a power function. This finding, better known as the log-log linear learning law, has been validated in various genres (Newell A, Rosenbloom PS. Mechanisms of skill acquisition and the law of practice. In J. R. Anderson (Ed.), Cognitive skills and their acquisition. Erlbaum, Hillsdale 1981: 1-55). However, at what cost does this occur? Why do we overemphasize the development and acquisition of skill over the child driven recreational aspect of play? How do we factor in the role of repetitive overuse injury, season ending injury, burn-out, attrition, social isolation, and myopic and limited overall motor skill acquisition? Diversified training that include similar, but not identical, performance element that are phase out with increasing chronological age can be consider a viable alternative to early specialization.

Youth athletes that specialize in a single sport account for 50% of overuse injuries in young athletes. Seventy percent of children participating in sport in the US and France drop out of sports by the age of 13-15 secondary to injury, stress and perceived pressure from coaches and parents (Delorme N, Boiche J, Raspaud M. Relative age and dropout in French male soccer. J Sports Sci 2010; 28: 717-722). Myer et. al found that children who specialized early in a single sport led to higher rates of adult physical inactivity. Those who commit to one sport at a young age are often the first to quit, and suffer a lifetime of negative sequelae (1). Jayanthi et. al found that early specialization of 1214 athletes in a single sport is one of the strongest predictors of injury. Athletes in the study who specialized were 70% to 93% more likely to be injured than children who played multiple sports. Children who specialize early are at a far greater risk for burnout due to stress, decreased motivation and lack of enjoyment (Jayanthi N, Pinkham C, Dugas L, Patrick B, Labella C. Sports specialization in young athletes: evidence-based recommendations. Sports Health 2013; 5: 251-257). Early sport specialization in female basketball, soccer and volleyball players is associated with increased risk of anterior knee pain disorders including PFP, Osgood Schlatter and Sinding Larsen-Johansson compared to multi-sport athletes, and may lead to higher rates of future ACL tears (Hall R, Barber Foss K, Hewett TE, Myer GD.

Sport specialization's association with an increased risk of developing anterior knee pain in adolescent female athletes. J Sport Rehabil 2015; 24: 31-35).

Research has shown that early participation in multiple sports leads to better overall motor and athletic development, longer playing careers, increased ability to transfer sports skills other sports and increased motivation, ownership of the sports experience, and confidence (Capranica L, Millard-Stafford ML. Youth sport specialization: how to manage competition and training? Int J Sports Physiol Perform 2011; 6: 572-579).

Multi-sport participation at younger ages has been shown to develop improved decision making and pattern recognition, as well as increased creativity (Baker J, Cote J, Abernethy B. Sport-specific practice and the development of expert decision-making in team ball sports. J Appl Sport Psychol 2003; 15: 12-25). A significant association between the number of sports participated in at the ages of 11, 13, and 15 and the standard of competition between 16 and 18 years was found. Individuals who competed in three sports were significantly more likely to compete at a national compared with club standard between the ages of 16 and 18 than those who participated in only one sport (Bridge MW, Toms MR. The specialising or sampling debate: a retrospective analysis of adolescent sports participation in the UK. J Sports Sci 2013; 31: 87-96). A study by DiFiori et al. found that 88% of college athletes surveyed participated in more than one sport as a youth athlete (DiFiori JP, Benjamin HJ, Brenner J, Gregory A, Jayanthi N, Landry GL, Luke A. Overuse injuries and burnout in youth sports: a position statement from the American Medical Society for Sports Medicine. Clin J Sport Med 2014; 24: 3-20).

A literature review regarding sport specific practice in The Sports Gene, David Epstein found that most elite competitors require far less than 10,000 hours of deliberate practice. Specifically, studies have shown that basketball (4000), field hockey (4000) and wrestling (6000) all require far less than the ubiquitous 10,000 hour rule (Baker J, Cobley S, Fraser-Thomas J. What do we know about early sport specialization? Not much! High Ability Studies 2009; 20: 77-89). A 2003 study on professional ice hockey players found that while most professionals had certainly allocated 10,000 hours or more involved in sports prior to age 20, only 3,000 of those hours were involved in hockey specific deliberate practice (and only 450 of those hours were prior to age 12) (Soberlak P, Cote J. The developmental activities of elite ice hockey players. J Appl Sport Psychol 2003; 15: 41-49). Clinicians, parents and coaches should provide opportunities for unstructured play outside of the sport of choice to enhance motor skill development. Young athletes should be encouraged to participate in a variety of different sports and dissuaded from participating solely in one sport in order to optimally develop diversified motor planning skills. For athletes who do specialize in a single sport at an early age, intense specialized training and sport specific activities should be closely monitored for psychological burnout, repetitive overuse injury, or decrease in overall performance and accuracy due to overtraining. There is compelling evidence to suggest that young athletes should practice strength and conditioning programs that encompass age appropriate neuromuscular training in order to help them prepare for the demands of competitive sport participation. Those athletes that individually choose to specialize in a single sport should plan periods of rest and time off during the course of the year, proprioceptive and neuromuscular training to enhance diverse motor skill development and reduce their inherent risk to injury (1, 2). Future research in this area should continue to assess the correlation of overuse and high-risk injury to specialized training while controlling for intensity and year-round training. Additionally, a comparison between multi-sport athletes and specialized athletes at various ages and stages of development would be prudent to analyze the impact of sport diversification versus specialization.

References

1. Myer GD, Jayanthi N, Difiori JP, Faigenbaum AD, Kiefer AW, Logerstedt D, Micheli LJ. Sport Specialization. Part I: does early sports specialization increase negative outcomes and reduce the opportunity for success in young athletes? Sports Health 2015; 7: 437-442
2. Myer GD, Jayanthi N, DiFiori JP, Faigenbaum AD, Kiefer AW, Logerstedt D, Micheli LJ. Sports Specialization, Part II: Alternative Solutions to Early Sport Specialization in Youth Athletes. Sports Health 2016; 8: 65-73

Monday 11th April, 2016 (morning)
CHURCHILL AUDITORIUM

KEYNOTE LECTURE

MANAGING YOUNG PLAYERS

Chairs

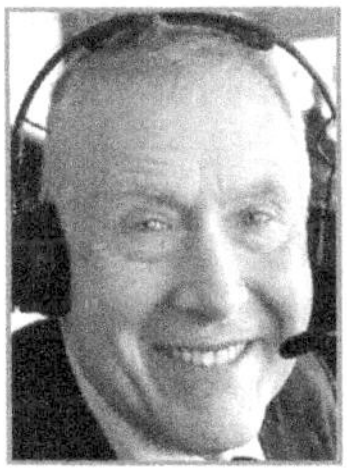

Martin Tyler
(Surrey, United Kingdom)

11:30	Managing youth players **TDB**
12:00	End of the session

Monday 11th April, 2016 (morning)
CURCHILL AUDITORIUM

INVITED SPEAKERS

4th Science and Football Summit

MANAGING LOAD ON YOUNG FOOTBALLERS

Chairs

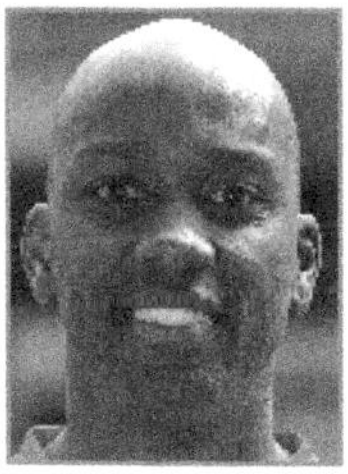
John Iga
(London, United Kingdom)

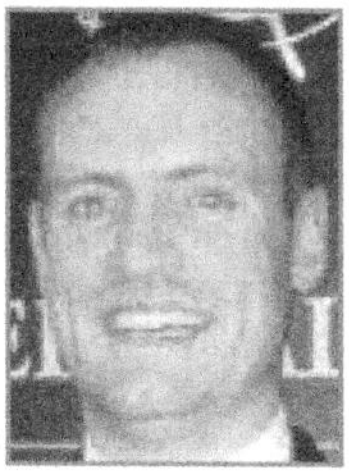
Andrew Massey
(Liverpool, United kingdom)

12:00	General principles of load management in academies **Barry Drust (Liverpool, United Kingdom)**
12:15	Optimising neuromuscular performance in young footballers **Alberto José Mendez-Villanueva (Doha, Qatar)**
12:30	Athletic development strategies for adolescent athletes **Bill Knowles (Philadelphia, USA)**
12:45	Monitoring training load in elite adolescent athletes **Will Abbott (Brighton, United Kingdom)**
13:00	Monitoring workloads in young footballers **Koen Lemmink (Groningen, The Nederlands)**
13:15	Discussion
13:30	End of the session

1

GENERAL PRINCIPLES OF LOAD MANAGEMENT IN ACADEMIES

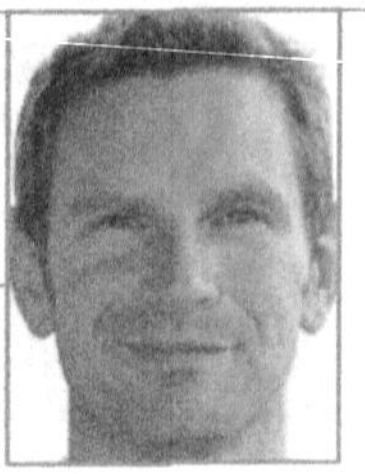

Drust B

Liverpool John Moores University and Liverpool Football Club, Liverpool, United Kingdom

Improving a talented individual to become an elite footballer is a complicated process.
Effective talent development in football requires players to improve their tactical and technical skills, psychological attributes and their physical capabilities.
Systematic training programmes represent effective ways to provide the stimulus necessary to improve these attributes.
The training load completed by players is an important determinant of the outcomes associated with any training programme from a physical perspective.
An effective training load can be highly variable and is dependent on an individual internal response (the internal training load) to a given exercise prescription (the external training load).
Understanding the external and internal training load requires the application of a monitoring strategy.
Monitoring key aspects of both the exercise completed, and the individual players response to this exercise, provides a basis for evaluating the extent to which a given training session may improve an individual fitness. It may also provide useful insights in the potential for that training to lead to negative adaptations that may ultimately lead to injury.

OPTIMISING NEUROMUSCULAR PERFORMANCE IN YOUNG FOOTBALLERS

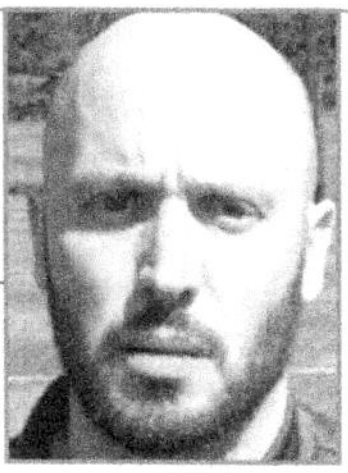

Mendez-Villanueva A

ASPIRE Academy, Football Performance & Science Department, Doha, Qatar

High-intensity actions such as sprints, turns, quick accelerations, sudden decelerations, jumps and 1vs1 situations with physical contact are often linked with many match-winning situations such as scoring a goal, outrunning an opponent or regaining ball possession. As such, the ability to perform high intensity actions is an important prerequisite for successful participation in football. These actions can also be associated with some of the most common injuries (e.g., ankle and knee sprains or hamstring muscles strains) occurring in football. Given the importance of high-intensity actions for both, on-field physical performance and protection against injury, training strategies that ensure their optimal development are continuously being searched for.

In addition to metabolic, morphological and other biological factors, neuromuscular aspects such as motor control, strength and power are key determinants of high-intensity actions in football. Thus, long-term player development programs should ensure that those neuromuscular factors are properly addressed across the developmental years, such that the player can optimize the gains in functional performance and minimize the risk of future injury. In this regard, it has been well established that the more specific a training exercise is to the competition environment the greater the transfer of the training effect to performance. Subsequently, for an aspiring, young football player is important to recognize the physical requirements of the game, the specific positional and tactical demands of the game model and the player physiological profile to determine the best training methods to employ.

Due to the multiple motor demands of soccer (e.g., running, sprinting, jumping, turning, changing direction, etc.) a combination of different training approaches appears to be needed to ensure enough specific overload of those neuromuscular factors. In this regard, in addition to the football-specific training exercises, high-intensity running, speed and agility drills, core stability, proprioceptive skills and various forms of resistance training are concurrently employed.

With training time at a premium, the search for training methods able to concurrently target different neuromuscular factors relevant to both on-field performance and injury prevention appears warranted.

MONITORING LOAD AND RECOVERY IN YOUNG FOOTBALLERS

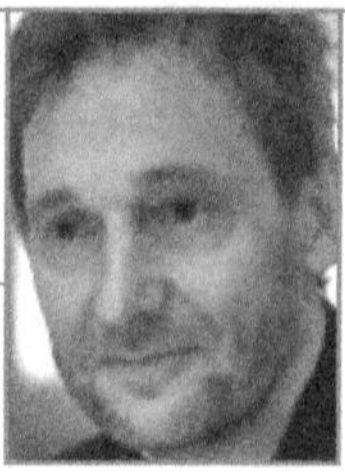

Lemmink K, Brink M

Center for Human Movement Sciences, University Medical Center, University of Groningen, Groningen, the Netherlands

Introduction

To reach the top in professional football, extensive training over an extended period of time is needed. On average, young elite football players train 4-6 times a week and play one match. The challenge is to balance load and recovery of training and matches in order to optimize performance development and prevent injuries, illnesses and overtraining. Recent insights indicate that, next to physical stress and recovery, psychosocial stress and recovery needs to be incorporated as well when monitoring young football players (2). An important step in developing a monitor system for young football players is to relate load and recovery parameters to performance development and the occurrence of injuries, illnesses and overtraining during the competitive season in young elite football players. So, the aim was to relate physical and psychosocial stress and recovery parameters to performance and health problems in young elite football players.

Methods

Three monitor studies were conducted to explore: 1) the relation between training load, recovery, and field test performance in 18 young elite football players during a full season; 2) the relation between load and recovery and injuries and illnesses in 53 young elite football players during two seasons, and 3) the relation between load and recovery and underperformance in 94 young elite football players during two competitive seasons (1). In these studies the perceived training load and recovery were determined by session Ratings of Perceived Exertion (duration x RPE) and Total Quality of Recovery (TQR). The Recovery Stress Questionnaire (RESTQ-Sport) was administered monthly to assess the psychosocial stress-recovery state of the players. Performance, i.e. interval endurance capacity, was measured with the Interval Shuttle Run Test on a monthly basis. Finally, Injury and illness data were collected using the standardised FIFA registration system.

Results

Main results showed that: 1) duration of training and matches as an indicator of training load was related to increases in field-test performance, 2) training load was related to both injury and illness and psychosocial stress and recovery were related to the occurrence of illness, and 3) an unfavourable recovery state appeared two months before underperformance compared to reference values at the start of the season with being in shape and fatigue as the most sensitive scales.

Conclusions

Outcomes highlight the importance of monitoring training load and recovery as well as psychosocial stress and recovery in order to optimize performance and prevent young players from illnesses, injuries and overtraining. Based on the findings, individualized warning systems can be built into these monitoring systems. Future studies should look for effective load and recovery interventions. Since compliance is key to successful monitoring, there is a need for simple and practical monitor tools. Technological innovations can help to collect important training and match information. Finally, it is of utmost importance that monitoring load and recovery parameters on a daily basis is fully integrated in the daily routines of a football academies and in the mind-set of the young elite football players.

References

1. Brink MS, Visscher C, Coutts AJ, Lemmink KAPM. Changes in perceived stress and recovery in overreached young elite soccer players. Scand J Med Sci Sports 2012; 22: 285-292
2. Kentta G, Hassmen P. Overtraining and recovery. A conceptual model. Sports Med 1998; 26: 1-16

Monday 11th April, 2016 (afternoon)
CHURCHILL AUDITORIUM

INVITED SPEAKERS

4th Science and Football Summit

HOW TO PREVENT AND TREAT THE MOST FREQUENT INJURIES

Chairs

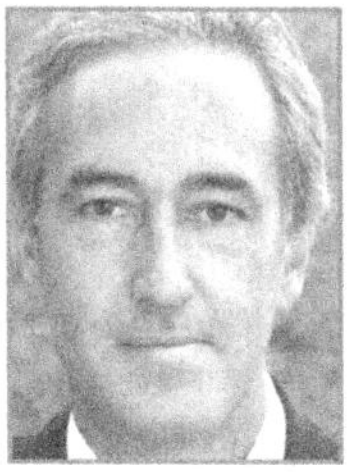

Angelo De Carli
(Rome, Italy)

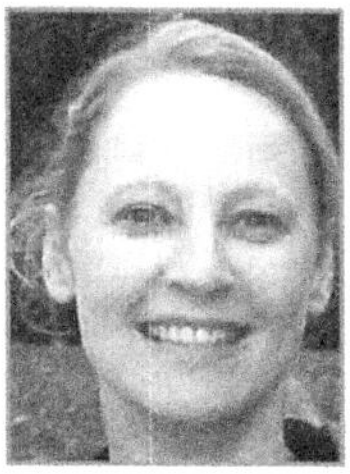

Elvire Servien
(Lyon, France)

14:30	Severe injuries in children football players: an epidemiological study **Jiří Chomiak (Prague, Czech Republic)**
14:45	Anterior cruciate ligament and meniscus injuries in adolescent players **Romain Seil (Luxembourg, Luxembourg)**
15:00	Low back pain in adolescent players **Michael Mayer (Münich, Germany)**
15:15	Medico legal and ethics implications in adolescent's return to play **Helen Millson (Ipswich, United Kingdom)**
15:30	Discussion
16:00	End of the session

SEVERE INJURIES IN CHILDREN FOOTBALL PLAYERS: AN EPIDEMIOLOGICAL STUDY

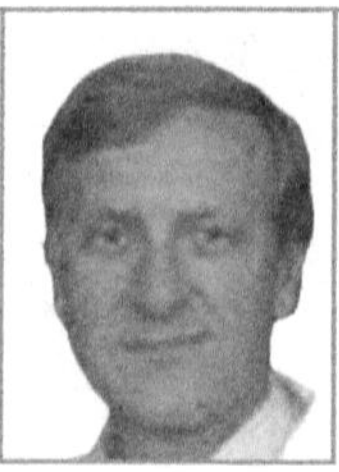

Chomiak J[1], Faude O[2], Rössler R[2], Němec K[1], Junge A[3]

[1]FIFA-MCOE Prague, Department of Orthopaedics,
1st Faculty of Medicine, Charles University and Hospital Na Bulovce, Prague, Czech Republic;
[2]Departement für Sport, Bewegung und Gesundheit Universität Basel, Switzerland;
[3]FIFA Medical Assessment and Research Centre, Zürich, Switzerland

Introduction

The aim of this study was to analyze the incidence and characteristic of severe football injuries in children age between 7 to 12 years according to international consensus statement on injury definitions and procedures for epidemiological studies

Methods

This study represents part of the epidemiological study on football injuries in children which was realized in Switzerland and Czech Republic in football seasons 2012-2013 and 2013-2014. The players (boys and girls) participating in regular training and playing in officially registered football clubs were included to the study. The children were subdivided to the three age categories, namely 7-8 years, 9-10 years and 11-12 years. The data were acquired according to above mentioned international consensus statement and include the injury severity, location, type and diagnosis as well as training and match exposure. Severe injuries were classified according to the duration of absence from games and training sessions for more than 4 weeks and any fractures and dislocations or serious damage to the visceral organs.

Results

Of 417 injuries incurred in all investigated players, 112 injuries (25%) were considered severe and all were documented in detail.
Concerning the incidences of severe injuries per 1,000 hours of exposure, the incidence in matches prevailed in all age groups, but it was significantly higher in the age group of 11-12 year old (1.13), followed by group of 9-10 years (0.82) and the lowest was in age group of 7-8 years (0.57).
In the training, similar distribution occurred, but the incidence was much-folds lower: 0.29 in group of 11-12 vs. 0.14 in group of 9-10 and 0.1 in group of 7-8.
Total incidence per exposure was highest in the group of 11-12 years (0.41), then in group 8-9 years (0.22) and lowest in age of 7-8 (0.15).

Injuries were sustained mainly in lower extremity (65%) and then in upper extremity (31%). There were only single injuries of head (brain concussion), thorax (rib fracture) as well as spine problem (spondylolisthesis).
The injuries were most prevalent in the foot (N =21; 19.8%) and hand and wrist (N=19; 17.7%), and were followed by the knee (N=17; 15.9%), ankle (N=15; 14.0%) and by hip/groin (N=7) and thigh (N=6) and shoulder, forearm and lower leg (N=5 each) and arm/elbow (N=3).
Regarding the type of injury, there were 42 traumatic fractures (39.6%) and 2 fatigue fractures (1.8%), 12 joint sprains and 12 specific growth problems (11.3% of each), followed by 10 muscle strains (9.43%) and 7 ligament ruptures/joint dislocations and 6 joint/tendon synovitis and (6.6% each) and 6 contusions (5.7%).
Regarding the mechanism of injuries there were 77 traumatic injuries (68.8%) and 29 overuse injuries (31.2%). 64 injuries (60.3%) occurred during training and 42 injuries (39.6%) during the match, but the real incidence of injuries per 1,000 hours of exposure prevailed in matches.
Injuries during training mostly occurred in situations similar to the games. The circumstances of traumatic injuries involved contact in 61 cases and non-contact in 16 cases. From the contact injuries, contact with opponents prevailed (31 cases; 51.6%), whereas contact with the pitch after the fall was observed in 18 cases (29.0%). 11 injuries (17.7%) sustained after the contact with ball and only one after the contact with pitch-equipment (1.6%). Only seven contact injuries were reported as caused by opposing foul play. No severe injury of player was reported as caused by a foul that he had committed.

Conclusions

Looking across the age groups, fractures prevailed in each age group.
There was a general tendency for an increase in relative proportion of muscle strains-ruptures and growth related pain and non-specific pain, and a decrease of joint sprains and contusions and joint or tendon synovitis with increasing age.
This study offers the baseline statistics for injury prevention program in youth football.

LOW BACK PAIN IN ADOLESCENT FOOTBALL PLAYERS

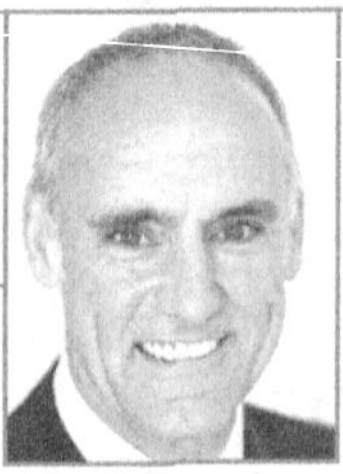

Mayer M, Schneider C, Haag T

Schön Klinik München Harlaching, FIFA Medical Centre of Excellence Munich, Germany and Paracescus Medical University Salzburg, Austria

In football players, low back pain account for more than 30 % of complaints unrelated to injuries. It is responsible for a premature end of the career in 22% of professionals.
The prevalence of low back pain in the normal adolescent population between 8-17 yrs of age ranges between 26 and 74%. There is only scarce scientific information about the prevalence of low back pain in young football players as well as about the effect of football on low back pain.
In the first part of our epidemiologic study on 1,110 players we found an increasing annual prevalence of low back pain of 30.4%, 43.9% and 46.2% in male players for U15, U17 and U19 respectively. The prevalence seemed to be higher in high-level players. Significant positive confounders were gender, age and years of training.

In a second study we compared U11-U14 players with children who did not do any sport and those who were only occasionally active. The annual prevalence in the football players was 33.2% as compared to 63.2% in the non-active group. There was an increasing prevalence with increasing Body Mass Index (BMI) as well as with age, training hours/week and club years. The lowest incidence of low back pain was found with 5-6 training hours/ week.
In a third study we looked at the youngest football player population (U8 - U10). The annual prevalence of low back pain was 28% and was thus higher as compared to all football injuries experienced during the same time span. There were two peaks of low back pain which could be observed at the end of the first and the start of the second growth spurt. Also in this group there was a strong correlation of low back pain with the BMI and the playing hours/week.

The conclusions from these studies are:
- Football might have a positive effect on low back pain.
- Back pain correlates with age, BMI and traing hours/week.
- Back pain cumulates during the growth spurts.
- A nomogram to determine the potential risk for low back pain was developed.

MEDICO-LEGAL AND ETHICAL IMPLICATION IN ADOLESCENTS' RETURN TO PLAY

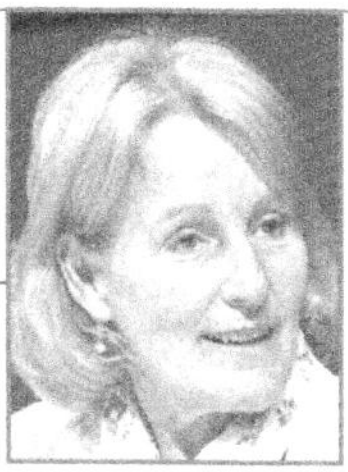

Millson H

Ipswich, United Kingdom

Sports people, particularly professional athletes, can place significant demands on clinicians to provide rapid injury resolution. The decision about Return To Play (RTP) at all levels of sports is just one of the many issues fraught with ethical dilemmas that a sports clinician must negotiate.

In professional sports, there are numerous stakeholders with potentially competing interests, along with huge financial risks and rewards for all concerned. Challenges may be due to internal and external pressures from coaching staff, management, sponsors and fans, with clinical decisions often made in this unique pressure cooker environment. Objectives of the team may conflict with the health and well being of the athlete, and clinicians may find themselves in complex situations. Even at the high school level there may be pressure from the school coaches and parents.

Management of the adolescent athlete requires an in-depth knowledge and awareness of the medico-legal ethical issues involved (1, 2). The interests must be for the athlete's long-term health and should not be influenced by any pressures which may affect the clinician's medical decision making. Whether it is letting a player compete with a "minor" injury or deciding on a quick return to sport versus better long-term outcomes, the outcome can be very serious for the athlete.

Thus sports clinicians may face moral and ethical issues relating to informed consent, third party involvement, advertising, confidentiality and even drug taking.

Thus the traditional Clinician-Patient relationship (which holds confidentiality and patient best interests as central concerns) may be compromised by the unique structure in sports medicine. There is often an untimely return of players to competitive duty following injury and compromises are often made concerning full recovery and return to competition.

There are limited studies of standardized objective criteria to accurately assess an athlete's ability to progress the end stages of rehabilitation and safe return to sport. A structured, quantified rehabilitation programme based on routine fitness and skills exercises and a graded subjective assessment of performance can provide an auditable record of a player's recovery from injury and a transparent exit point from rehabilitation.

Most importantly, all these factors apply to the skeletally immature athlete where the tissues most vulnerable to injury are the cartilaginous growth centers and must be taken into consideration when structuring a RTP strategy.

One of the areas of complexity regarding RTP is that of concussion, which is a minefield regarding RTP and particularly when dealing with the adolescent athlete (3). It has been recommended that a longer recovery of full cognitive function in younger athletes compared with college-aged or professional athletes should be the norm, even if they are asymptomatic.

Apart from the physical preparedness for RTP, the injured players cognitive appraisals and emotional and behavioural responses vary during different phases of the injury rehabilitation. The clinician needs to recognise the particular vulnerabilities and physiological and developmental characteristics of children in sport, and the short and long-term risks (physical and psychological) of training regimes, competition and RTP strategies on children.

Thus with the Young/Adolescent athlete and the RTP and Medico-Legal Ethical issues involved (1, 2), the clinician must take into consideration the following:

1. Make sure that the sports clinician is thoroughly educated on the Medico-Legal Ethical guidelines for clinicians dealing with the young adolescent athlete.
2. RTP should be individualised, with awareness of a physical, physiological and biological time progression in the young athlete.
3. The context of the specific sport and the level of expected RTP are key.
4. Return to previous non-injury markers, if available.
5. The objective of each phase of rehabilitation must be achieved and the clinician must have well documented, transparent rehabilitation and RTP notes. In a court of law this is paramount and the main plank of defence.
6. The clinician should be aware of the psychological and emotional aspects of the sport including: training, competition, sporting success/failure, which may have an impact on RTP.
7. Inform the athlete of the potential harm associated with RTP, including the likelihood and severity of further injury and the implications of injury on quality of life and future career. This advice may include the parent/guardian and should be recorded.
8. Advocate for the patient where the adolescent athlete is being pressured into taking high levels of risk. The young athlete is particularly vulnerable.
9. A sports clinician is under no obligation to assist an athlete to RTP following an injury, if the clinician considers the risk is unacceptable. External pressure must not be a contributory factor. The decision making process is made by contributions of the entire medical team, the athlete and possibly the coach. Depending on the age, the parent/guardian may have to be part of this decision making process.
10. The athlete should be enabled to give "informed consent" to participate, empowered with knowledge and then allowed to choose, placing current gain in the context of long-term risk. Depending on the age, parental/guardian consent may be mandatory.
11. If the adolescent athlete demands RTP in spite of medical advice to restrain him/her from RTP, a waiver should be signed accordingly. This should abide by the medico-legal age structure and depending on the age may have to be assessed to be Gillick Competent. The parent /guardian may have to be involved.
12. If the adolescent athlete is concussed, recent studies have fully advocated that this must be recognised and the young athlete removed. This is imperative from the legal and ethical perspective.
13. During the rehabilitation process, the athlete should be exposed to varied load so he/she is not apprehensive of the injury and understands the rehabilitation process. The adolescent athlete must feel that he/she has an input into the process of rehabilitation and RTP.

Conclusions

In the adolescent athlete there are different issues and legalities regarding consent and management and it is vital to take cognizance of these important implications in the young athlete when rehabilitating and structuring RTP criteria. Distinct ethical and medico-legal issues exist that include divided loyalties, athlete autonomy, informed consent, privacy and confidentiality, and the weighing of potential risks.

The organizational pressures involved in winning and success often compel team officials (and the athlete) to return to competition as quickly as possible. Health care professionals who work with adolescent athletes need to be prepared to deal with ethical issues as they arise. Given that these issues are ubiquitous and often part of routine clinical decision making, clinicians must be properly trained and knowledgeable in ethical decision making. It is vital to never be pressurized and to detail, with structured, transparent notes, all the rehabilitation and RTP strategies.

We highlight the importance of having Objective Criteria for Rehabilitation and RTP from the Medico-Legal and Ethical aspect, when dealing with the adolescent athlete. Most importantly, one should never compromise one's own ethics and the ethics of a medical practitioner in the sports medicine domain.

Monday 11th April, 2016 (afternoon)
CHURCHILL AUDITORIUM

INVITED SPEAKERS

4th Science and Football Summit

BUILDING A YOUTH PLAYER DEVELOPMENT CONSENSUS STATEMENT

Chairs

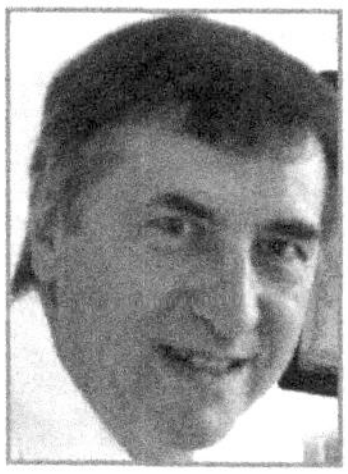

Neil Armstrong
(Exeter, United Kingdom)

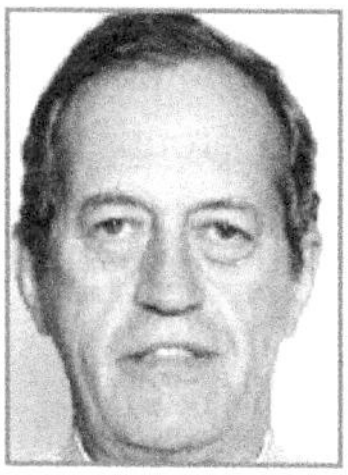

Peter Brukner
(Melbourne, Australia)

16:00	FIFA 11+kids **Mario Bizzini (Zürich, Switzerland)**
16:15	USA STOP Programme **Bruce Reider (Chicago, USA)**
16:30	OIC: Young Player Development **Neil Armstrong (Exeter, United Kingdom)**
16:45	Discussion
17:00	End of the session

FIFA 11+ KIDS

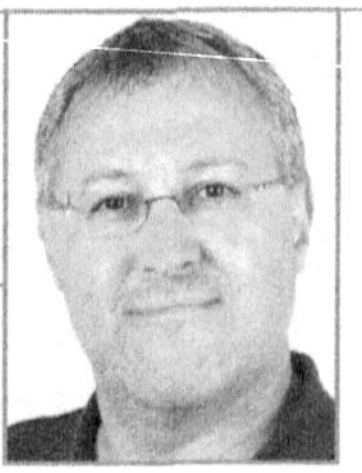

Bizzini M, Rössler R, Faude O, Dvorak J

FIFA Medical Assessment & Research Centre (F-MARC), Zürich, Switzerland

Introduction

In 2009 the Fédération Internationale de Football Association (FIFA) decided to promote and disseminate the FIFA 11+ injury prevention programme worldwide, developed and studied by its Medical Assessment and Research Centre (F-MARC). At that time, one randomised controlled study and one countrywide campaign in amateur football, both showing a significant impact in reducing injuries and health-care costs, were the strongest arguments behind this decision (Junge A, Lamprecht M, Stamm H, Hasler H, Bizzini M, Tschopp M, Reuter H, Wyss H, Chilvers C, Dvorak J. Countrywide campaign to prevent soccer injuries in Swiss amateur players. Am J Sports Med 2011; 39: 57-63).
In the following 6 years important publications have confirmed the preventive effects of FIFA 11+ (about 30-50% less non-contact injuries) and have evaluated its performance effects in both female and male amateur football. Furthermore, implementation strategies of this prevention programme have also been studied, and FIFA 11+ has been implemented at a large scale in the real world of amateur football players (Bizzini M, Dvorak J. FIFA 11+: an effective programme to prevent football injuries in various player groups worldwide-a narrative review. Br J Sports Med 2015 May; 49: 577-579; Bizzini M, Junge A, Dvorak J. Implementation of the FIFA 11+ football warm up program: how to approach and convince the Football associations to invest in prevention. Br J Sports Med 2013; 47: 803-806).
At December 18, 2015, a total of 27 peer-reviewed publications were available, with the most recent one presenting the FIFA 11+ KIDS, an adaptation of the injury prevention programme for children (Rössler R, Junge A, Chomiak J, Dvorak J, Faude O. Soccer Injuries in Players Aged 7 to 12 Years: A Descriptive Epidemiological Study Over 2 Seasons. Am J Sports Med. 2015 Dec 8. pii: 0363546515614816. [Epub ahead of print]; Soligard T, Myklebust G, Steffen K, Holme I, Silvers H, Bizzini M, Junge A, Dvorak J, Bahr R, Andersen TE. Comprehensive warm-up programme to prevent injuries in young female footballers: cluster randomised controlled trial. BMJ 2008 Dec 9; 337:a2469. doi: 10.1136/bmj.a2469; Steffen K, Meeuwisse WH, Romiti M, Kang J, McKay C, Bizzini M, Dvorak J, Finch C, Myklebust G, Emery CA. Evaluation of how different implementation strategies of an injury prevention programme (FIFA 11+) impact team adherence and injury risk in Canadian female youth football players: a cluster-randomised trial. Br J Sports Med 2013; 47: 480-487).

Methods

The FIFA 11+ KIDS program was developed, similarly than the original FIFA 11+, by F-MARC via international cooperation and following epidemiological studies in children in the age range 8-12 years old.
FIFA 11+ KIDS (a 15 minutes warm up format) consists of 7 different exercises: a running game, two jumping exercises, a balance/coordination task, two exercises targeting body stability, and an exercise to improve falling technique.
The intervention study was a large multicentre Randomised Controlled Trials (RCT) in four European countries, involving about 4,000 kids (age range 8-12 years old).

Results

The overall injury incidence rate (rate ratio 0.62, 95% CI 0.50-0.77) and the lower extremity injury incidence (rate ratio 0.58, 95% CI 0.46-074) were significantly ($P<0.001$) reduced in those teams practising the FIFA 11+ Kids as a warm up session before training (RCT results not yet published). Another RCT study (published) on motor performance effects of the programme showed that FIFA 11+ KIDS can significantly improve dynamic balance and agility skills in children.

Conclusion

The FIFA 11+ KIDS represents the adapted evidence-based version of the successful FIFA 11+ injury prevention programme, with also a similar impact in terms of injury reduction in children.

THE STOP PROGRAM: SPORTS TRAUMA AND OVERUSE PREVENTION

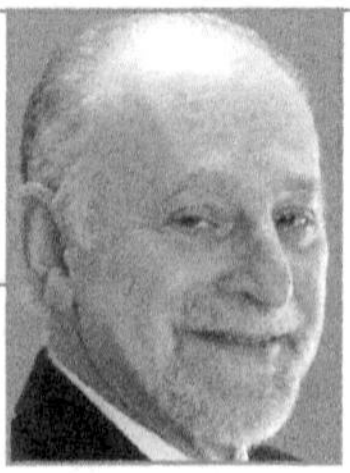

Reider B

University of Chicago; American Journal of Sports Medicine; Orthopaedic Journal of Sports Medicine; Chicago, USA

The Sports Trauma and Overuse Prevention (STOP) program is a public service initiative of the American Orthopaedic Society for Sports Medicine (AOSSM). It was initiated in 2010 in response to a perceived increase in youth sports related injuries in the United States. Although both traumatic and overuse injuries were included, there was a particular concern for overuse injuries. The president of the AOSSM at the time, James Andrews, was especially concerned about the number of youth baseball players he was seeing with overuse injuries.

In the US, 30 million children currently participate in organized sports, with 7.3 million in organized high school sports. According the Center for Disease Control (CDC) high school sports account for more than 2 million injuries annually, 500,000 doctor visits and 30,000 hospitalizations.

The goal of STOP is to serve as a reliable source of information of youth sports injuries and prevention in a form that can be easily understood by parents, coaches, older youth athletes themselves and other lay stakeholders. The strategy has been to build a network of support from AOSSM members and other health care professionals and organizations. Education is provided via printed and electronic materials focused on 25 different sports and 8 common injuries, as well as help organizing live educational sessions conducted by AOSSM members. These latter activities help members, who are orthopaedic surgeons, to be involved in injury prevention in their home communities.

At this time, 958 different organization have signed on as supporters of the program. These include 46 Professional Health Organizations, such as the American Academy of Orthopedic Surgeons, American Academy of Pediatrics, American Medical Society for Sports Medicine, National Athletic Trainers' Association and the National Strength and Conditioning Association; 95 medical institutions; 668 individual sports medicine practices; 42 child health and safety organizations and 107 sports organizations.

The program has proven very popular with the target audience. In 2015, STOP received over 1,500 media references in traditional news outlets. It has 12,115 Twitter followers and a reach of 285,026 Twitter followers. Its web site received 460,000 visits in 2015 alone. Although about ¾ of the visitors are from America, the rest are well-distributed among the remaining continents.

Page views of sport-specific "Sports Tips" have tended to follow the popularity of the covered sports among US youth. The top 10 include American Football, Soccer (Football), Volleyball, Baseball, Basketball, Softball, Gymnastics, Dance, Swimming and Ice Hockey.

Aside from Sports Tips, website features include links to sports injury research, tools to assist health care professional for planning a community educational events, issues of "In the Game" newsletter for the lay public and announcements about upcoming live or online events.

YOUNG PLAYER DEVELOPMENT: THE GROWTH, MATURATION AND TRAINABILITY OF SOCCER PLAYERS

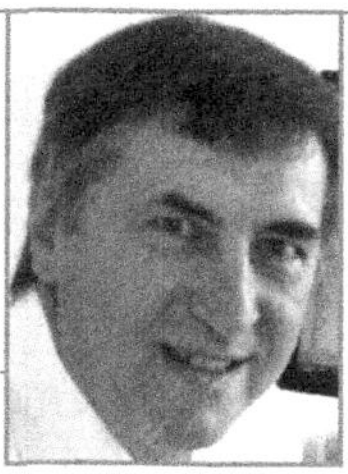

Armstrong N

University Of Exeter, Exeter, United Kingdom

Soccer performance during youth is founded on a range of sex - Chronological Age (CA) - and Biological Maturation (BM)-related physical and physiological variables. Investigations of body size, body shape, body composition, muscle structure, muscle strength, muscle metabolism, anaerobic performance/fitness and aerobic fitness include data derived from a variety of conventional and emerging technologies. The data on responses to exercise present a consistent but incomplete picture with sexual dimorphism and CA-related changes well-documented but independent BM-related effects on performance elusive to establish. Selection and retention in youth sports are often driven by BM and in soccer this is reflected by the relative age effect which is particularly prevalent in male CA-group teams (1-3).

The non-linear and asynchronous transition from pre-puberty through puberty to an adult physical and physiological profile has confounded the long-term prediction of performance.

Muscle strength increases in a near-linear manner with CA from early childhood until ~13-15 years of age when there is marked surge in boys' muscle strength followed by a slower increase into the early, mid, or even late twenties. Although substantial soccer-related benefits do not become apparent until late puberty earlier maturing boys enjoy significant advantages over similarly aged but later maturing peers. Girls do not experience a pubertal spurt and their muscle strength begins to plateau in late puberty.

Anaerobic performance/fitness and aerobic fitness are enhanced by both CA and BM but they increase with different magnitudes and rates and this impacts on the tempo of changes in soccer performance during youth. From 12-17 years, anaerobic performance/fitness (i.e. peak power output) increases by ~120% in boys and ~65% in girls. Increases in aerobic fitness (i.e. peak oxygen uptake) over the same age range are somewhat smaller at ~70% and ~25% for boys and girls respectively.

Running speed is an example of how a vital component of soccer performance is reliant on a complex amalgam of physical and physiological factors influenced by CA and BM. Pre-pubescent boys and girls show similar progression in sprint speed with CA, which probably reflects the development of the central nervous system, motor skills, and biomechanical coordination. From ~12 years of age running speed development in girls is diminished compared with boys with the disparity likely due to differential changes in muscle metabolism, muscle strength, muscle power, body shape, body size, and body composition in accord with BM (1-3).

There are no persuasive data to suggest that intensive exercise training influences stature, the length of body segments, or the timing or tempo of BM. Both pre-pubertal and pubertal soccer players benefit from appropriate exercise training. Children of 5–6 years of age have made noticeable improvements in muscle strength following exposure to appropriate resistance exercise. The trainability of muscle strength increases slightly with CA and BM but there is no discernible spurt in the ability to enhance muscle strength through training in puberty. There is a minor sex-associated effect on absolute and relative muscle strength gains following training among pre-pubertal children. However, in puberty sex-associated differences in trainability emerge with boys generally showing significantly greater training-induced muscle strength gains than girls. Aerobic fitness and anaerobic performance/fitness are augmented with appropriate training. Training-induced increases in aerobic and anaerobic fitness are independent of CA, BM and sex. There is no convincing evidence of a 'maturational threshold' or 'trigger point' below which appropriate training is ineffective. Physiological justifications for 'early soccer specialisation', 'specified hours of practice (e.g. 10,000 hours)' or 'windows of opportunity' as hypothesised in well-established long-term athlete development models remain to be proven (2,3).

A sound knowledge foundation of developmental exercise physiology has been established but the lack of rigorously designed youth- and soccer-specific laboratory and field testing environments has compromised physiological monitoring of young players and clouded the interpretation of data in real life situations. Critical analysis of extant knowledge and the translation of laboratory and field research into the optimisation of young player development are required.

References

1. Armstrong N, Barker AR, McManus AM. Muscle metabolism changes with age and maturation: How do they relate to youth sport performance? Br J Sports Med 2015; 49: 860-864
2. Armstrong N, McManus AM (eds). The Elite Young Athlete. Karger; Basel 2011, pp. 1-205.
3. Armstrong N, van Mechelen W (eds). Oxford Textbook of Children's Sport and Exercise Medicine. Oxford; Oxford University Press, 2016 (in press).

INDEX OF AUTHORS

INDEX OF SUBJECTS

Finito di stampare nel mese
di MARZO 2016
dalla Tipolitografia Sat - San Giustino (Pg, Italy)

Made in United States
North Haven, CT
10 November 2026

22100371R00280